Cardiovascular

• Palpate peripheral pulses for rate, rhythm, quality, and symmetry. (See *Pulses, peripheral.*)

Peripheral pulses

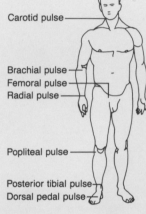

Carotid pulse

Brachial pulse
Femoral pulse
Radial pulse

Popliteal pulse

Posterior tibial pulse
Dorsal pedal pulse

• Inspect for jugular venous distention. (See *Jugular venous pressure.*)
• Inspect and palpate extremities for edema, mottling and cyanosis, and temperature change. (See *Edema, pitting; Skin mottling.*)
• Auscultate heart sounds for timing, intensity, pitch, and

Heart sounds

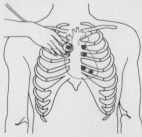

quality, noting murmurs, rubs, or extra sounds. (See *Heart exam: auscultation.*)

Gastrointestinal

• Inspect the abdomen for signs of trauma or distention. (See *Abdominal exam: inspection.*)
• Inspect any vomitus or stool for amount, color, presence of blood, and consistency.
• Auscultate the abdomen for bowel sounds before you pal-

Abdominal auscultation

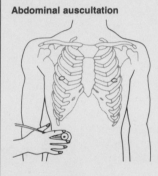

pate. (See *Abdominal exam: auscultation.*)
• Palpate the abdomen for pain, rebound tenderness, or

Rebound tenderness

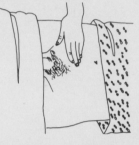

Percussing for ascites

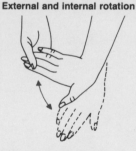

rigidity; percuss for ascites. (See *Abdominal exam: palpation; Abdominal rigidity.*)

Genitourinary

• Inspect the external genitalia for bleeding, ecchymoses, edema, or hematoma. Look for skin lesions and for a discharge. (See *STD: physical exam.*)
• Palpate the abdomen for suprapubic pain and the ex-

Bladder assessment

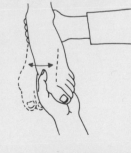

ternal genitalia for pain and tenderness. (See *Bladder assessment.*)
• Palpate and percuss for costovertebral angle tenderness. (See *Abdominal exam: percussion.*)

Musculoskeletal

• Inspect the body for trauma and deformities; the skin for ecchymoses, pigmentation, discoloration, and needle marks. Look at the patient's nailbeds for cyanosis and pallor. If your patient's dark-skinned, check his palms and soles, too. (See *Fracture assessment; Orthopedics: inspection.*)
• Palpate the cervical spine for tenderness and deformities; the pulses distal to any injury; and the area of suspected injury for tenderness, pain, and edema.
• Assess for motor and sensory responses and for nuchal rigidity. (See *Neurologic exam: assessment.*)
• For deep lacerations, also assess for peripheral nerve damage and tendon damage. (See *Nerve damage: peripheral; Lacerations: tendon damage.*)
• Observe the range of mo-

External and internal rotation

Eversion and inversion

tion of the injured body part. (See *Orthopedics: legs.*)

A B C D E F G H I J K L M N O P Q R S T U V W X Y Z

From the editors of *Nursing* magazine

Nurse's Quick Reference

An A-to-Z guide to 1,001 professional problems

Springhouse Corporation
Springhouse, Pennsylvania

Staff

Executive Director, Editorial
Stanley Loeb

Executive Director, Creative Services
Jean Robinson

Art Director
John Hubbard

Editor
Susan L. Jackson

Clinical Editor
Cynthia Weidman Haughey, RN, MSN

Copy Editors
Diane Armento, Jane V. Cray, Nancy Papsin, Doris Weinstock

Designers
Stephanie Peters (associate art director), Mary Stangl

Art Production
Robert Perry (manager), Anna Brindisi, Donald Knauss, Catherine Mace,
Robert Wieder

Typography
David Kosten (manager), Diane Paluba (assistant manager), Liz Bergman,
Joyce Rossi Biletz, Robin Rantz, Brent Rinedoller, Valerie Rosenberger

Manufacturing
Deborah Meiris (manager), T.A. Landis, Jennifer Suter

Production Coordination
Aline S. Miller (manager), Laurie J. Sander

Library of Congress Cataloging-in-Publication Data

Nurse's quick reference: an A-to-Z guide to 1,001 professional problems.
  p. cm.
Includes bibliographical references.
1. Nursing—Handbooks, manuals, etc.
I. Springhouse Corporation.
[DNLM: 1. Nursing—encyclopedias.
2. Nursing Care—encyclopedias. 3. Nursing Process—encyclopedias. 4. Nursing Services—encyclopedias. WY 13 N974]
RT51.N873 1990 610.73'—dc20
DNLM/DLC   89-21700
ISBN 0-87434-194-9   CIP

About this book

NURSE'S QUICK REFERENCE is an indispensable problem-solver for busy nurses—an A-to-Z guide to 1,001 professional problems at your fingertips. Its alphabetically arranged articles deal with nursing procedures, patient care, emergencies inside the hospital and out, legal matters, staff relations, career advancement, communication, patient teaching, and much, much more!

Yes, this book will help you solve all sorts of professional problems—counsel battered women, insert a contact lens, witness your dying patient's last words, connect a Holter monitor properly, plan a job change, detect melanoma, protect your patient from falls, remove a stubborn ring from a patient's finger, shampoo a bedridden patient, diagnose superficial thrombophlebitis, know when to withhold information from a patient, check for Queckenstedt's sign, and many other challenges.

We hope that every page will grab your attention. Look up *Sleep apnea*, for example, and you may find yourself reading about how to care for a snakebite!

Here's how to use this book: Look up your subject in alphabetical order as you would in an encyclopedia. You'll probably find it immediately. Or check in the back of the book, where an extensive index with cross-references can lead you to what you're looking for. For example, if you look up *contact lens insertion*, you'll find clear, step-by-step instructions on how to perform the procedure. And you'll see helpful illustrations that further clarify the instructions.

Turn to *Difficult doctors* and you'll find effective ways to head off problems before they start. Look up *MI: emergency intervention* and you'll be able to brush up on the latest technique and intervene immediately if a patient experiences a myocardial infarction.

Use this "how to" guide as a refresher on procedures you might not have performed in a while. Or use it to keep up-to-date on current nursing practices. Whether you're a student or a practicing nurse, and whether you work in a hospital or elsewhere, you'll find this book helpful because it encompasses such a wide range of topics. It doesn't cover every aspect of nursing, of course—no one book could. But it does deal with a host of common situations, and it invariably offers practical, sensible advice. Over 1,000 contributors from all over the country and Canada have shared their knowledge and expertise.

After you read the concise instructions, you'll no doubt feel more confident trying tasks you once hesitated to do before. If you still feel uncertain, check one of the Springhouse reference books listed in the back of this book or get help from someone with more experience in that particular area.

Sit back and enjoy the *Nurse's Quick Reference*. It'll supply you with a wealth of valuable information and hours of pleasure. It may prove to be the most useful book you've ever purchased!

The Editors

Contents and contributors

Abbreviations

a.m.	ante meridiem		EPA	Environmental Protection Agency
ABG	arterial blood gas		F.	Fahrenheit
AC	alternating current		FES	fat embolism syndrome
AIDS	acquired immunodeficiency syndrome		g	gram
AP	anteroposterior		GI	gastrointestinal
AST	aspartate aminotransferase		HCO_3	bicarbonate
ATN	acute tubular necrosis		HDCV	human diploid cell (rabies) vaccine
AV	arteriovenous		Hg	mercury
BSN	bachelor of science in nursing		HHNK	hyperglycemic hyperosmolar nonketotic coma
BUN	blood urea nitrogen		HIV	human immunodeficiency virus
C	cervical (vertebrae)		H_2O	water
C.	Celsius		hr	hour
CAPD	continuous ambulatory peritoneal dialysis		Hz	hertz
cc	cubic centimeter		IBD	inflammatory bowel disease
CCU	coronary care unit		ICP	intracranial pressure
CE	continuing education		ICS	intercostal space
CHF	congestive heart failure		ICU	intensive care unit
CIR	continent intestinal reservoir		ID	identification
cm	centimeter		IHSS	idiopathic hypertrophic subaortic stenosis
CMV	cytomegalovirus		I.M.	intramuscular
CO_2	carbon dioxide		IOP	intraocular pressure
COPD	chronic obstructive pulmonary disease		I.V.	intravenous
CPD	citrate-phosphate-dextrose		JVD	jugular venous distention
CPK	creatine phosphokinase		kg	kilogram
CPR	cardiopulmonary resuscitation		KS	Kaposi's sarcoma
CSF	cerebrospinal fluid		lb	pound
CT	computed tomography		LDG	lactic dehydrogenase
CVP	central venous pressure		LLQ	left lower quadrant
DPT	diphtheria-pertussis-tetanus (vaccine)		LSB	left sternal border
DT	diphtheria-tetanus (vaccine)		LUQ	left upper quadrant
DUS	Doppler ultrasound stethoscope		MAST	medical antishock trousers
DVT	deep vein thrombosis			
D_5W	dextrose (5%) in water			
ECG	electrocardiogram			
ED	emergency department			
EMS	emergency medical service			
EMT	emergency medical technician			

MCL	midclavicular line		**RLQ**	right lower quadrant
mEq	milliequivalent		**RN**	registered nurse
mg	milligram		**RR**	recovery room
mg/dl	milligrams per deciliter		**RSB**	right sternal border
MI	myocardial infarction		**RUQ**	right upper quadrant
ml	milliliter		**S.**	*Staphylococcus*
mm	millimeter		**SCI**	spinal cord injury
mOsm	milliosmole		**SGOT**	serum glutamic oxaloacetic transaminase
MRI	magnetic resonance imaging		**SGPT**	serum glutamic pyruvic transaminase
MS	multiple sclerosis		**SIDS**	sudden infant death syndrome
MSN	master of science in nursing		**SLE**	systemic lupus erythematosus
MUGA	multiple-gated acquisition (scanning)		**SN**	student nurse
NDE	near-death experience		**STD**	sexually transmitted disease
NG	nasogastric		**T**	thoracic (vertebrae)
NP	nurse practitioner		**T₃**	serum triiodothyronine
NPH	neutral protamine Hagedorn		**T₄**	serum thyroxine
NSS	normal saline solution		**TAC**	tetracaine, adrenaline, cocaine
OR	operating room		**TBSA**	total body surface area
oz	ounce		**Td**	tetanus-diphtheria (toxoid—adult)
PA	physicians' assistant		**TENS**	transcutaneous electrical nerve stimulation
PA	pulmonary artery		**TIG**	tetanus immune globulin
PaO₂	partial pressure of oxygen in arterial blood		**TPN**	total parenteral nutrition
PCA	patient-controlled analgesia		**TV**	television
PCO₂	partial pressure of carbon dioxide		**UTI**	urinary tract infection
PCWP	pulmonary capillary wedge pressure		**V₁**	chest lead 1
PD	peritoneal dialysis		**V₂**	chest lead 2
PEG	percutaneous endoscopic gastrostomy		**V₃**	chest lead 3
PERRLA	pupils equal, round, and reactive to light and accommodation		**V₄**	chest lead 4
pH	hydrogen ion concentration		**V₅**	chest lead 5
p.m.	post meridiem		**V₆**	chest lead 6
PMI	point of maximum impulse			
PO₂	partial pressure of oxygen			
PTCA	percutaneous transluminal coronary angioplasty			
PTT	partial thromboplastin time			
RBC	red blood cell			
RIG	rabies immune globulin			

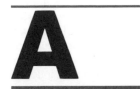

Abdominal exam: auscultation

Proper technique

Auscultation is done before percussion and palpation of the abdomen since it may alter the frequency of bowel sounds. Have the patient lie supine with his head on a pillow, arms at his sides, and knees slightly flexed. Drape him to expose the area from the sternum to the pubis.

Use the diaphragm of the stethoscope. Exerting only light pressure, listen for bowel sounds in all four quadrants and the epigastric area. Normally, air and fluid movement through the bowel create irregular bubbling or soft gurgling noises about every 5 to 15 seconds.

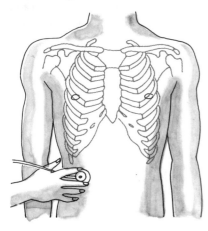

Auscultate for peristaltic sounds, noting their pitch, quality, and frequency. Extremely weak and infrequent bowel sounds or the complete absence of sounds for several minutes may indicate paralytic ileus and peritonitis. A loud, rushing, high-pitched tinkling sound frequently occurs in mechanical obstruction and is usually accompanied by a wave of pain. You may detect hypermotility in a patient who's hungry, who has functional hypermotility, or who has diarrhea.

Next, use the bell of your stethoscope to listen to vascular sounds. Place the bell lightly over the midline to check for bruits, blowing sounds that seem to elongate the pulsations normally heard over a vessel. Also check for bruits over the renal vessels. If you notice any in the abdominal aorta, assess arterial perfusion in the patient's legs. (See *Bruits: auscultation.*)

Abdominal exam: inspection

Conducting the exam properly

When a patient complains of abdominal pain, the first thing you must do is inspect his abdomen.

Position your patient so he's lying on his back, and stoop at his side to view his abdominal contour. A normal abdomen has a convex profile, even with the patient supine. A flat abdomen may be normal in an athlete or a muscular person. A hollow or scaphoid abdomen may indicate malnutrition. A distended or protuberant abdomen, usually having an everted umbilicus, could indicate excess air or fluid in the peritoneal cavity. Inspect the umbilicus for abnormalities besides eversion.

Next, stand at the foot of the bed and observe the patient's abdomen for symmetry of contour and for masses. An asymmetrical abdomen may result from previous abdominal trauma or surgery, an abnormal organ, or weak abdominal muscles.

Perform the rest of the examination from the patient's right side (if you're right-handed). Inspect the abdomen for movement from respiration, peristalsis, and arterial pulsations. Look for exaggerated abdominal movement during breathing that may indicate respiratory distress or severe anxiety. Normal peristaltic movement is rarely visible, even through a thin abdominal wall. If you can see strong contractions (peristaltic waves) crossing the patient's abdomen, report this finding to the doctor—it may indicate impending bowel or pyloric obstruction.

The only arterial pulsations you may see are those of the abdominal aorta, visible in the epigastric area. In a thin patient, you may see femoral arterial pulsations.

Inspect the abdominal skin thoroughly. Tense, glistening skin may indicate ascites or abdominal wall edema. Note any scars, lesions, ecchymoses, striae, rashes, or dilated veins. Also inspect for an abdominal hernia, which may become apparent when you ask the patient to cough. Draw a diagram of the abdomen's quadrants, and record the location—right upper quadrant (RUQ), left upper quadrant (LUQ),

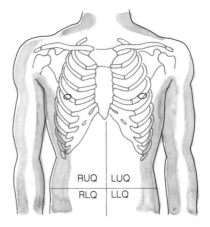

right lower quadrant (RLQ), or left lower quadrant (LLQ)—as well as the size and color of such abnormalities.

Abdominal exam: palpation

Recommended procedure

Before you begin palpation, determine if any areas are tender; palpate those areas last. (See also *Palpation.*)

Lightly palpate with fingertips of one hand all four quadrants for tenderness and masses. As you palpate, you'll recognize the aorta as a soft, pulsating mass in the upper abdomen left of midline. You may feel the sigmoid colon as a freely movable, slightly tender mass in the left lower quadrant. Estimate any muscle rigidity or tension in each quadrant. If the abdominal wall is rigid or tense, help the patient relax. You may detect reflex muscle spasm as a protective mechanism in an area where the peritoneal membrane is inflamed. Having the patient relax his muscles won't overcome this rigidity.

Performing light palpation

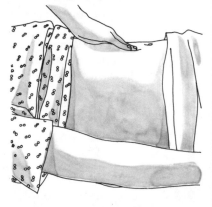

Now deeply palpate all four quadrants, using fingertips of one hand. Deep palpation allows you to identify abdominal organs and masses. You may have to use both hands for obese patients. Normally, you'll find some tenderness in the epigastric area. If so, determine the area of maximum intensity. (See *Abdominal exam: rebound tenderness.*)

Performing deep palpation

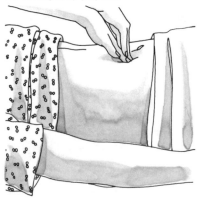

If you detect any mass, note the location, size, tenderness, contour and consistency, mobility, and pulsation.

The lower border of the liver is the only border that can be palpated. To identify that border, place your left hand posteriorly at the level of the eleventh and twelfth ribs and gently press your hand forward to move the liver more anteriorly. Start palpating at the upper level of the right lower quadrant at the midclavicular line. Using deep palpation, gently press your hand inward and upward. As the patient takes deep breaths, move your hand toward the costal margin until you feel the liver border.

Normally, the liver edge may be palpable just at the costal margin when the patient inhales deeply. In many cases, though, you can't feel the liver edge—only a sense of increased resistance. If you feel the liver below the costal margin, it might be enlarged—except if the patient has a barrel chest. In such a case, the patient's diaphragm may be flattened, forcing the liver downward. If you can palpate the liver, note any tenderness and whether its surface is smooth or nodular. (See also *Liver assessment: percussion.*)

When you're palpating kidneys, palpate them by placing one hand below the kidney and the other hand above and rotate your hands to check for each kidney's contour and size. Also, check for lumps and masses. (See *Splenomegaly* for spleen palpation.)

Abdominal exam: percussion

Types and technique

Percussion is the third step of the abdominal exam, done after inspection and auscultation. (See *Abdominal exam: auscultation; Abdominal exam: inspection.*) Percussion is used mainly to check the size of abdominal organs and to de-

tect excessive amounts of fluid or air in the abdomen. Percussion notes in each abdominal quadrant depend on its underlying structure. Keeping the positions of these underlying organs in mind, follow a clockwise pattern when you percuss. Abdominal percussion normally elicits tones ranging from dull or flat (over solids) to tympanic (over air). A sigmoid colon filled with stool produces dullness in the left lower quadrant. You'll usually hear high-pitched tympanic notes over a section of bowel filled with air (the degree of tympany reflects gaseous bowel distention). When ascites are present, you'll also detect dullness when you percuss the patient's flanks. (See *Ascites.*)

Over organs, such as the liver, spleen, or a full bladder, you'll detect dullness. Percussion (blunt) can also be used to detect tenderness. Percuss tender areas last in exam.

The three types of percussion are described here.

Mediate percussion is most frequently used to percuss the thorax and abdomen. You strike the middle

Mediate percussion

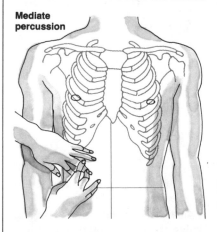

finger of one hand with the middle or index of the other hand. The finger that does the striking is called the *plexor*; the finger that is struck is called the *pleximeter*. To perform mediate percussion, place the distal phalanx of the pleximeter (not the entire finger) against the patient's body. (Keep the palm and other fingers of this hand raised off the skin.)

Then strike the base of the pleximeter's distal interphalangeal joint with the tip (not the fat pad) of the plexor.

To perform *immediate* percussion—an older technique used mainly to percuss an infant's thorax or adult sinuses—simply strike the patient's body with one hand. (The other hand is not involved.)

To perform *fist* percussion, place one hand flat against your patient's body, then strike the back of this

Fist percussion

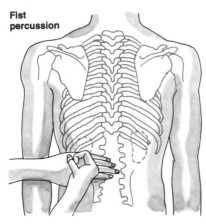

hand with your other hand, which is clenched in a fist. This form of percussion helps determine the presence of pain or tenderness.

Abdominal exam: rebound tenderness

Eliciting it

To elicit rebound tenderness, place the patient in a supine position, and push your fingers deeply and steadily into his abdomen. Then quickly release the pressure. If pain results from the rebound (rebound tenderness), suspect peritoneal inflammation or peritonitis.

You can also elicit this symptom on a miniature scale by percussing the patient's abdomen lightly and indirectly. (See *Abdominal exam: percussion.*) Better still, simply ask him to cough. This will allow you to elicit rebound tenderness without having to touch his abdomen and may also

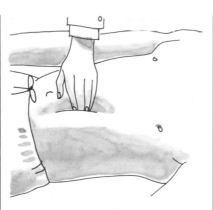

increase his cooperation, since he won't associate the exacerbation of his pain with your action.

Abdominal rigidity

Getting an accurate nursing assessment

Distinguishing voluntary and involuntary abdominal rigidity is essential for accurate nursing assessment.

Voluntary abdominal rigidity is characterized by:
• symmetry
• more rigidity on inspiration (expiration causes muscle relaxation)
• ease from relaxation techniques, such as positioning the patient comfortably and talking to him calmly and soothingly
• less pain when the patient sits up using his abdominal muscles alone.

Involuntary abdominal rigidity is characterized by:
• symmetry
• equal rigidity on inspiration and expiration
• little relief from relaxation techniques
• pain when the patient sits up using his abdominal muscles alone.

Acidosis, metabolic

Recognition and intervention

Serum potassium levels characteristically rise with acidosis. You can

expect high serum potassium level in a patient who has suffered extensive burns or crushed tissue as the dying cells release their potassium into the extracellular fluid. Similarly, you can expect it in a patient with metabolic acidosis because his kidneys cannot excrete potassium properly.

The patient's arterial blood gas (ABG) readings will show a low pH and a low bicarbonate level. In metabolic disorders, these values shift in the same direction.

Nursing interventions

Keep an eye on the status of any patient with metabolic acidosis. He may be dehydrated from diarrhea or vomiting, and this means you'll have to keep careful track of his intake and output. Assess his electrolyte balance frequently, too, paying special attention to neuromuscular signs of hyperkalemia—weakness, dysrhythmias, or even cardiac arrest.

Check also for a change in his level of consciousness. Remember, acidosis dulls the central nervous system. Never leave a disoriented patient alone with the side rails of his bed down. Frequently monitor his vital signs since changes can occur rapidly. And monitor his ABG levels as he begins to compensate or as treatment begins to correct his metabolic disorder. Acid-base status can be a constantly changing affair.

Acidosis, respiratory

Signs and symptoms

Early clinical signs and symptoms of respiratory acidosis result primarily from depression of the central nervous system. Arterial blood gas (ABG) readings will show a low pH and a high Pco_2.

The patient may be lethargic, very weak, drowsy or confused, and slow to respond to questions. He may experience nausea and vomiting, or have a headache from the vasodilation brought on by the high PCO_2 (hypercapnia). As his acidotic state worsens, his level of consciousness will decrease. Left untreated, his respiratory acidosis may result in coma.

Blood gas values

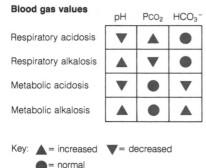

	pH	PCO_2	HCO_3^-
Respiratory acidosis	▼	▲	●
Respiratory alkalosis	▲	▼	●
Metabolic acidosis	▼	●	▼
Metabolic alkalosis	▲	●	▲

Key: ▲ = increased ▼ = decreased
● = normal

Nursing interventions
The most important thing you can do for the patient is monitor his clinical status while you try to improve his respiratory function.

A patent airway is essential. Nasopharyngeal or tracheal suctioning or chest physical therapy may be required if he can't clear his secretions. Avoid sedation unless the hypoventilation is caused by pain or he must be prepared for possible endotracheal intubation.

Hypoventilation, bringing a rising PCO_2, will inevitably bring hypoxemia to anyone breathing only room air. Yet this hypoxemia combined with acidosis produced by the PCO_2 may result in fatal dysrhythmias. Monitor his cardiac function closely.

Watch the patient's PO_2 in his ABG studies. Supplemental oxygen will surely be required. But remember to use caution in giving oxygen to patients with chronic obstructive pulmonary disease. They have come to tolerate such high CO_2 levels that their hypoxic drive may be their only remaining stimulus to breathe.

Note your patient's fluid and electrolyte balance and check his ABG levels frequently. The health care team's efforts at correction will probably be augmented by the patient's kidneys. The kidneys will attempt to compensate for the respiratory acidosis by excreting nonvolatile acids and conserving bicarbonate.

Adrenal crisis

Discharge teaching

Adrenocortical insufficiency can cause adrenal crisis with these signs and symptoms: hypotension, tachycardia and thready pulse, oliguria, cool and clammy skin, flaccid extremities, lethargy, confusion, restlessness, decreasing level of consciousness, and hyperpyrexia. To prevent this emergency and avoid additional hospitalization costs, review the following points with the patient before discharge:
• the pathology, signs, and symptoms of chronic adrenocortical insufficiency and the constant risk of adrenal crisis
• proper steroid self-administration, actions and doses of his prescribed medications, and signs and symptoms of excessive or insufficient drug use
• the need to avoid stopping the prescribed steroid or altering the dosage without first consulting the doctor (See also *Steroids.*)
• the need to avoid long fasts
• the importance of maintaining a high-carbohydrate, high-protein diet, with a daily sodium intake of up to 8 g (more during diaphoresis)
• the need to call his doctor to have his glucocorticoid dosage increased during stressful situations or to have his mineralocorticoid dosage increased if he sweats profusely for any reason
• the use of relaxation techniques to reduce stress (See *Relaxation techniques.*)
• the need to intersperse planned activities with rest periods (muscle weakness and decreased hepatic glycogen stores lead to fatigue).

Adrenalectomy

Preparing the patient for surgery

To help the patient withstand surgery and improve postoperative wound healing, administer parenteral cortisol (usually hydrocortisone) as ordered. This protects the patient from developing acute adrenal insufficiency during surgery. Provide a diet high in protein and vitamins to promote rebuilding of wasted tissue. To correct any electrolyte imbalances, make sure the patient receives appropriate supplements. For example, a patient with adrenocortical hyperfunction should receive potassium supplements as well as potassium-rich foods because he has a low serum potassium level.

If your patient had a bilateral adrenalectomy, he'll need adrenocortical hormones and adrenal medullary catecholamines. To prevent adrenal crisis, monitor him carefully and give fluids, electrolytes, and corticosteroids, as ordered.

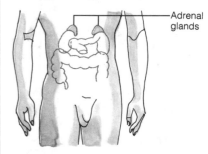

Adrenal glands

Postoperative blood pressure and fluid electrolyte levels may fluctuate widely, especially in the first 48 hours. You'll need to monitor the patient's ECG and arterial, central venous, and (if indicated) pulmonary capillary wedge pressures to evaluate his hemodynamic status.

Expect to give I.V. replacement glucocorticoids until the patient can tolerate oral form. The doctor may order fluid replacement with dextrose 5% in water and normal saline solution, as well as vasopressors to prevent hypovolemic shock.

Immediately after surgery, withhold foods and fluids. Introduce oral intake gradually, according to the patient's tolerance. Because his condition may rule out prolonged fasting, he'll probably require I.V. caloric supplements. After he begins eating, make sure he doesn't miss any meals, and offer him between-meal snacks. Stay alert for signs and symptoms of hypoglycemia. To reduce anxiety, anticipate stressful situations and try to prevent them. Provide for sufficient rest periods and comfort measures.

Resistance to infection is low because of a decrease in adrenal hormone. Infections also become more difficult to treat. To promote wound healing, scrupulously monitor the patient's temperature and wound drainage, and use strict aseptic technique when changing his dressings. To reduce pressure on the wound, make sure he splints it during coughing or turning. Watch closely for wound dehiscence and evisceration. (See *Wound assessment; Wound care dressings: changes.*)

Before his discharge, discuss the importance of taking cortisol supplements regularly to treat adrenocortical insufficiency and to prevent acute adrenal insufficiency. (See *Adrenal crisis.*)

Agitation

Assessment guidelines

Determine the severity of the patient's agitation by assessing the number and quality of agitation-induced behaviors, such as emotional lability, confusion, memory loss, hyperactivity, and hostility. If possible, obtain a history from the patient or a family member, including diet and known allergies. Ask if the patient is currently being treated for any illnesses. Has he had any recent infections, trauma, stress, or changes in sleep patterns? Ask about the use and dosage of any prescribed or over-the-counter drugs. Check for signs of drug abuse, such as needle tracks or dilated pupils. Ask about the patient's usual alcohol intake and the time of his last drink.

To obtain baseline data for future comparison, check and record his vital signs and neurologic status.

AIDS: home care

General safety precautions

By observing the following precautions in your care and teaching them to your patient, you can help protect him from infection and safeguard others from exposure.

Respiratory safeguards

First, advise keeping all rooms well ventilated to decrease the risk of airborne disease. If the patient catches a cold, make sure he always covers his mouth and nose with a tissue when coughing or sneezing.

Should those around the patient wear masks? Only if he has a productive cough, and if they'll be performing care that involves being in close contact with him. (Remember, a strong cough may spread droplets as far as 6′ [1.8 m] away.)

Secretions

The patient's razor, toothbrush, and other personal hygiene items that may come into contact with his body secretions must be his *alone*. The same is true for washcloths and towels between machine washings.

Good hand-washing technique is a necessity for everyone—the patient, his caregivers, and his family. (Here's where your example can speak volumes.)

Repeated hand washing, of course, may dry the skin, causing minute breaks and entry for infection. So recommend the use of moisturizing lotions. The caregiver should check her hands and if she has any cuts, wear gloves.

Naturally, the patient should flush body wastes down the toilet. But as his disease progresses, other people may be exposed to diarrheal or bloody secretions. If so, they should wear gloves. If they accidentally touch or get splashed by these secretions, they should wash the exposed skin with hydrogen peroxide or soap and water. They may want to wear a gown for practical as well as infection-control purposes. (See *AIDS: housekeeping precautions*.)

AIDS: housekeeping precautions

Cleaning the patient's home

Housekeeping techniques can protect the immunocompromised patient from infection while safeguarding others from exposure to AIDS. They're not much different than the techniques normally used in most homes.

Common household bleach effectively deactivates the human immunodeficiency virus found in AIDS patients. Spills (such as body secretions or bathwater) should be cleaned up with soap and water, and the area wiped with a solution of bleach and water: 1 part bleach to 10 parts water. This 1:10 solution is adequate for cleaning the bathroom; full-strength bleach is best for disinfecting the toilet bowl.

Dirty water from cleaning the bathroom (or spilled body secretions) should be flushed down the toilet. Mops and sponges used to clean up should be soaked for 5 minutes in the 1:10 solution; they should only be used for cleaning the bathroom, not for general household cleaning. Another set should be kept aside for cleaning spilled body secretions in other parts of the house. (See *AIDS: home care.*)

AIDS: kitchen precautions

Tips for cleaning your patient's kitchen

Tell family members who prepare the AIDS patient's food to first scour the kitchen counters, then rinse them to remove any potentially dangerous microbes. (Reserve one sponge for this purpose.) As in any home, food preparers must wash their hands before handling food—but not in the kitchen sink, where food may be rinsed.

A

Because the patient with AIDS is immunocompromised, he must watch what he eats and how it's prepared. For example, he shouldn't eat unpasteurized milk products (to avoid salmonella infections) or fruits and vegetables fertilized with manure (unless they're peeled or cooked). Meats must be thoroughly cooked.

Separating the AIDS patient's utensils from everyone else's isn't necessary; the family's utensils and dishes can be washed together in *hot,* soapy water and air-dried. Or they can be run through the dishwasher on the HOT setting.

Normal kitchen cleaning guards against infection. Keeping the refrigerator clean, for example, will prevent mold from forming. Washing the floor once a week (cleaning all spills immediately) can help prevent bacteria from growing.

AIDS: laundry precautions

Techniques for home care

Household detergents can easily deactivate the AIDS virus. Allow the detergent to circulate fully, and don't overload the washer.

Detergent and bleach (1 cup per load) added to hot water will work well for cottons and colorfast materials. Detergent and a phenolic disinfectant (such as Lysol) in warm water won't fade noncolorfast materials. A second wash and rinse without the phenolic disinfectant will remove any remaining chemicals.

Laundry can be machine-dried— but on a HIGH setting.

AIDS: neurologic assessment

What to look for

Life-threatening neurologic infections, HIV-related encephalopathy,

depression, fatigue, anxiety, pain, and adverse drug effects—any or all of these AIDS-related problems can cause your patient's mental status to deteriorate. So you'll need to assess his mental status and motor coordination frequently throughout his hospitalization. (See *Neurologic exam: coordination; Neurologic exam: mental status.*)

Assess his short-term memory first. Give him a short series of numbers and colors to remember (for example, "five, eight, and three," and "yellow, red, and green"). At the end of your examination, ask him to recall them.

When you assess his orientation, try testing his knowledge of current events. For example, you could ask him to name the mayor or invite him to talk about some recent news story. From his replies, you may find out more about his mental status than you'd ever learn simply by asking him the usual questions about person, place, and time.

To test your patient's ability to reason and think abstractly, ask him to explain a proverb, such as "a stitch in time saves nine." To test fine motor coordination, ask him to draw a simple connecting line figure, such as a star.

Throughout the examination, assess his ability to concentrate and his mood. For example, does he seem anxious, angry, or distracted? Document your observations with your other findings.

Here are some neurologic warning signs to watch for:
• Impairments in short-term memory, reasoning, or ability to perform sequential tasks (for example, telephone dialing or dressing) may indicate HIV, encephalopathy, toxoplasmosis, or some less common neurologic infection.
• Photophobia suggests cryptococcal meningitis, which can also cause mood swings, headaches, disorientation, and hallucinations. Cryptococcal infection of the optic nerve can lead to blindness.
• Dementia similar to Alzheimer's disease is typical of HIV-related en-

cephalopathy. A patient with this complication needs a lot of supervision and may need restraints.

AIDS: night sweats

Keeping the patient comfortable

To make your patient more comfortable, prepare a 1:10 concentration of isopropyl alcohol in tepid water. Put on sterile gloves and towel down the patient with the prepared solution. It will leave him feeling fresh and clean. Just keep the alcohol solution away from his eyes.

After you towel down the patient and help him into dry pajamas, change the bed. If your hospital stocks old flannel pads, use a few when you remake the bed—they're comfortable and absorbent, and could save you from having to change the whole bed if the patient has night sweats again. But don't use plastic-backed pads—they'll make him sweat even more.

AIDS: patient history

Asking the right questions

For a patient with AIDS, recent health changes can be especially revealing, so you should question him about:
• *his general health over the past few months.* Recent unexplained weight loss, fevers, night sweats, and diarrhea are signs and symptoms of AIDS-related complex, often a precursor of AIDS.
• *problems with cognition or memory.* Brain infections and HIV-related encephalopathy can cause intellectual and personality changes.
• *sexual changes.* Loss of sexual desire or testicular atrophy are common.
• *pain.* Headaches, abdominal pain, and rectal pain can all be symptoms of AIDS-related opportunistic diseases.

A

You also want to learn more about the patient's home life. For example, does he live with someone who can help him at home? Does he have any pets in the house? (Some opportunistic organisms can be transmitted in animal feces.)

AIDS: physical assessment

Performing a head to toe assessment

Here's the best way to examine your AIDS patient.

Head and neck

Look for lesions on the patient's head and neck, and examine his mouth for Kaposi's sarcoma (KS), which may appear on the hard palate and adjacent gums. Other mouth lesions may be caused by:

• *candidiasis (thrush),* which causes white plaques on the tongue and hard palate.

• *hairy leukoplakia,* which is similar in appearance to candidiasis but can appear and disappear rapidly—sometimes within the same day.

Examine the lymph nodes beneath the patient's jaw and on the back of his neck, and document their size. Assess his conjunctivas for signs of hypoxemia or anemia.

Also check your patient's vision and hearing (and reassess it regularly). When you check his vision, ask if he's noticed any recent changes in his field of vision, flashing lights, or cloudy spots. Examine his retinas with an ophthalmoscope, looking for hemorrhages (which suggest cytomegaloviral [CMV] infection) or "cotton wool" spots (which could indicate *Pneumocystis carinii* infection).

When you test his hearing ask if he's noticed any recent changes. Hearing loss may indicate cryptococcal infection of the otic nerve.

Chest

Next, auscultate and percuss his chest for signs of pulmonary problems. Keep in mind that *P. carinii*

doesn't necessarily cause the adventitious breath sounds typical of other pneumonias. But, like anyone else, a patient with AIDS could have an asthma attack or develop a conventional pneumonia. So document any wheezes, gurgles, crackles, or egophony.

Cardiovascular system

An AIDS patient's blood pressure and pulses may be abnormal for several reasons—malnutrition, hemorrhage, drug therapy, or dehydration from persistent diarrhea, for example. So document the patient's baseline findings, and monitor them for abnormal heart sounds. Kaposi's sarcoma can invade the heart wall, causing valvular dysfunctions and cardiac tamponade.

Abdomen, perineum, and rectum

When you examine the patient's abdomen, you may find an enlarged spleen; some patients develop AIDS-related thrombocytopenia. An enlarged liver may indicate an AIDS-related hepatic problem, such as *Mycobacterium avium-intracellulare* infection.

Check his rectum for:

• condyloma (venereal warts), which may appear as red or pink pinhead papules or cauliflower-like masses; they're usually painless.

• herpes simplex virus, which causes painful vesicles on an erythematous base.

Also note any excoriation and inflammation from chronic diarrhea. If you have to perform a digital rectal examination, do so gently. Check feces for occult blood.

Genitalia

Check your patient's genitalia for condyloma and herpes simplex virus as well as other abnormalities.

Assessing herpes lesions

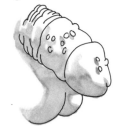

A swollen scrotum, for example, could be a sign that KS has invaded the inguinal area. Note testicular atrophy, a common complication of AIDS that's probably related to adrenal-testicular dysfunction caused by CMV or HIV infection. (See *Lymphadenopathy; Rectal exam; STD: physical exam.*)

AIDS: precautions around pets

Minimizing infection risks

Pets are a mixed blessing for an AIDS patient. They can provide emotional support, but their care requires infection precautions. For example, toxoplasmosis is spread by cat feces and can attack the immunocompromised patient's neurologic system; so he should wear gloves and a mask when cleaning the litter box. Bird droppings can spread psittacosis, possibly leading to pneumonia. So, advise the patient to wear gloves and a mask when he cleans the birdcage.

Mycobacterium, found in fish tanks, can cause devastating respiratory pathology, as well as damage the liver and spleen. The patient should *never* clean the tank; someone else should do it for him.

AIDS: self-protection

Safety precautions for nurses in the hospital

Follow these guidelines when caring for any patients who have AIDS and AIDS-related complex or who are known to be HIV-positive.

The blood and body fluid precautions are the same as you would follow for patients with hepatitis B, unless the patient has another infection that calls for additional safeguards.

1. *Rooms.* A private room isn't necessary unless a patient has special problems, such as severe diar-

A

rhea, bowel incontinence, or behavior changes from a central nervous system infection. AIDS patients shouldn't share rooms with patients who have other easily transmitted diseases, so use caution even when putting two AIDS patients together.

2. *Hand washing.* Wash your hands before and after caring for an AIDS patient, even if you've worn gloves. If your hands become contaminated with any of his body fluids, wash them immediately.

3. *Isolation clothing.* Wear latex gloves if you expect to touch the patient's blood or other body fluids; for example, starting I.V.s and emptying urine drainage bags. Also, wear a gown if body fluids might soil your clothes, and a mask or protective eyewear if blood or body fluids might splash your face. Wear gloves to handle a newborn until amniotic fluid has been removed from his skin.

4. *Resuscitation equipment.* Keep artificial airways and Ambu bags handy; avoid mouth-to-mouth resuscitation. Instead, use mouth-to-mask devices.

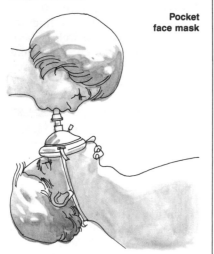

Pocket face mask

5. *Pregnancy risks.* Pregnant nurses aren't thought to be at greater risk for contracting AIDS. But many AIDS patients have cytomegalovirus, which causes fetal abnormalities and stillbirths, so pregnant nurses should follow blood and body fluid precautions meticulously.

6. *Sharp items.* Consider all sharp items potentially infective and handle them with care. Use disposable needles and syringes, and discard them in rigid, puncture-proof containers. Never recap, bend, or break a needle or remove it from the syringe. (See also *I.V. therapy: needle safety.*)

7. *Labeling.* Clearly label blood and other specimens with a sign such as "Blood/body fluid precautions," not "AIDS precautions." If the outside of the specimen container becomes contaminated with blood, clean it with a solution of 1 part household bleach in 10 parts water. Double-bag all blood specimens before transfer.

8. *Blood spills.* Clean up all spills immediately with bleach solution.

9. *Linens.* Bag, label, and process soiled linens as you would any other isolation linens.

10. *Eating utensils.* Special precautions (such as disposable dishes) aren't necessary.

11. *Disposable and nondisposable articles.* Incinerate or discard disposable items, following hospital policies for disposal of infectious waste. Bag and label nondisposable articles contaminated with blood or body fluids before sending them for decontamination and reprocessing.

12. *Sterilization.* Sterilize equipment following hepatitis B precautions. Decontaminate surgical instruments by machine or by hand after use; don't just rinse them in water.

13. *Transporting AIDS patients.* Follow blood and body fluid precautions. Be sure that workers in areas where AIDS patients will be transported know what precautions to take.

14. *Outpatients with AIDS.* Outpatients can use the same waiting rooms and bathrooms as other patients unless they have other infections requiring special precautions. (See also *Infection control.*)

AIDS: skin assessment

Examination guidelines

Use a systematic approach, as with any patient, paying special attention to the signs and symptoms pointed out below. Put on gloves, and you're ready to start.

Examine and palpate the patient's axillary and inguinal lymph nodes for swelling. (See *Lymphadenopathy.*) Also check his nail beds for signs of hypoxemia and anemia.

Look for lesions, especially in places that the patient can't easily see himself—for example, the back of his head and neck, behind his ears, his buttocks, and back, the axillary and dorsal surfaces of his upper arms, the backs of his legs, and the soles of his feet. (With a female patient, remember to examine the skin under her breasts.)

Assess for dermatitis, open wounds, and other lesions. If you see only a few lesions, note the location, size, color, and character of each. Look for:
• *Kaposi's sarcoma,* a vascular cancer that causes purplish macular or papular lesions that may first appear on the arms and legs. In some patients it grows slowly; in others, it spreads rapidly. Either kind can invade internal organs.
• *cutaneous T-cell lymphoma (mycosis fungoides),* which can cause scaling or nonscaling superficial plaques that thicken as the disease progresses.
• *Burkitt's lymphoma,* which can cause irregularly shaped, lumpy tumors deep beneath the skin on the upper chest and elsewhere.
• *herpes simplex virus,* causing painful vesicles and pustules on the lips, genital areas, and elsewhere.
• *herpes zoster (shingles),* which causes painful vesicles and pustules on an erythematous base distributed along nerve pathways.

Air embolism: prevention

Recognizing the patient at risk

Air embolism results when air enters a systemic vein and travels to the right ventricle through the vena cava.

Exactly how much air is lethal isn't known, but at least 10 to 20 cc are needed to produce the condition just described. And, if injected rapidly enough, this can be fatal.

The average lethal dose, however, is between 70 to 150 cc per second. A larger amount of air may be tolerated if it enters the venous system over a long period (as with a leaking catheter).

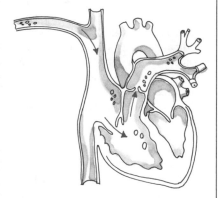

Various circumstances can cause air embolism. Air may be pulled into the circulation if the catheter is leaking or open or if the tubing is accidentally disconnected from the catheter. Also, air embolism can occur during catheter insertion or during the time between catheter removal and healing of the site.

Any patient with a central line risks air embolism. The danger increases if the patient has a line for central venous pressure monitoring, or if he is likely to disconnect the tubing or dislodge the catheter.

To determine if he is suffering from air embolism look for confusion, pallor, light-headedness, tachypnea, tachycardia, hypotension, anxiety, and unresponsiveness.

If you note any of these signs or symptoms, turn the patient on his left side in Trendelenburg's position. In this position, the pulmonary artery is below the right ventricle; the air rises to the wall of the right ventricle and blood flow from the ventricle improves.

Unless it's contraindicated, give him oxygen by mask, to achieve a higher blood concentration. Monitor his vital signs every 15 minutes. Throughout the emergency, reassure him and explain what you're doing. His lack of oxygen may make him very frightened.

To prevent air embolism, take the following precautions: During catheter insertion, place the patient in Trendelenburg's position. To increase intrathoracic pressure, have him perform Valsalva's maneuver. (He should also do this during tubing changes.)

Be sure all Luer-Lok connections are tight; use tape to anchor the tubing. Never use an implantable port without being sure the junction between the needle and tubing is securely connected. During catheter removal, again have the patient perform Valsalva's maneuver, and apply sterile occlusive gauze.

Teach the patient to look for warning signals. Make sure he understands that a leak or hole in the catheter is an emergency that should be evaluated as soon as possible. Also, tell him that if the catheter is accidentally cut or severed, he should call the nurse. (See also *Air embolism: treatment.*)

Air embolism: treatment

What to do in an emergency

Act quickly to prevent lethal complications if you suspect an air embolism in your patient's bloodstream. Unless your patient's had a cardiac arrest, follow these steps:

1. Immediately position the patient in the left lateral decubitus position with his head down, to increase intrathoracic pressure and to help prevent more air from flowing into the catheterized vein during inspiration. This position also helps air bubbles float toward the right atrium and away from the pulmonary artery, preventing obstruction of the outflow tract and allowing blood to enter the lungs.

2. While you're reassuring your patient, have someone notify the doctor, who may attempt to aspirate air from the catheter, particularly if the embolus is within the patient's right atrium or ventricle.

3. Administer 100% oxygen by mask unless contraindicated (such as for a patient with chronic obstructive pulmonary disease). Gas contained in an air embolus, which is 80% nitrogen, becomes trapped in the pulmonary vessels and can readily diffuse into the alveoli. By decreasing nitrogen levels in the alveoli, oxygen helps decrease the size of the embolus and supports the blood-deprived lung. (See *Air embolism: prevention.*)

Airway, esophageal gastric tube

Using one properly

The esophageal gastric tube airway consists of an esophageal tube, face mask, and a gastric tube (to remove stomach contents). To use it you'll

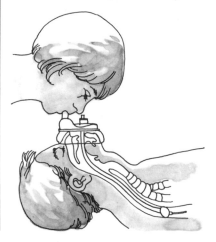

A

also need a 35-cc syringe for inflating the cuff and mask, a stethoscope, and a bag-valve mask.

• Connect the proximal end of the esophageal tube to the mask's lower port and lock it into place. Inflate and deflate the cuff to see that it's working properly.

• Place the patient's head in a neutral or slightly flexed position. Insert your thumb deeply into his mouth behind the base of his tongue, grasp the bony ridge of his lower jaw with your index and middle fingers, and lift straight up.

• With your other hand, advance the tube gently, following the natural curve of his throat. Don't force the tube. If it doesn't advance easily, either redirect it or withdraw it and start over. Advancing the tube into the right side of the mouth is usually easier, since the esophagus lies slightly to the right of and behind the trachea.

• Advance the tube until the mask is sealed tightly over the patient's nose and mouth. If the mask isn't sealed adequately, connect the syringe to the small valve on the mask and inject more air.

• Inflate the cuff by injecting 30 to 35 cc of air, and blow into the mask's ventilation port to see if the tube is in the esophagus. With the esophagus blocked, the air enters the trachea and lungs. You should see chest movement as another nurse listens for air moving in and out of the lungs. If you don't, the tube might be in the trachea. If so, immediately deflate the cuff, remove the tube, and reinsert it.

• Perform mouth-to-tube ventilation by breathing through the mask's ventilation port until you can connect a manual resuscitation bag.

Airway, oropharyngeal

Easy insertion

During an emergency, you may have to insert an artificial oropharyngeal airway to keep an unconscious patient's tongue from falling back and occluding his airway.

To insert this artificial airway, you can use the crossed-finger or tongue-depressor technique. For the crossed-finger technique, place your thumb on the patient's upper teeth and your index finger on his lower teeth, and gently push his mouth open. Then slide the tip of the curved airway upside down back over his tongue. (Attempting to insert the airway in its "normal" position may push his tongue back.) Or point the tip toward his cheek, push gently, then rotate the airway until it's pointing down.

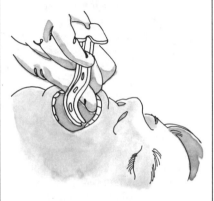

For the tongue-depressor technique, open the victim's mouth and depress his tongue with a tongue depressor. Guide the airway in the normal position over the back of his tongue until it's in place.

Airway obstruction: adults

Using the Heimlich maneuver

First, determine if the choking victim can speak by asking, "Are you choking?" If he can speak, cough, or breathe, stand by but don't intervene.

If he can't speak, cough, or breathe, call for help and then perform abdominal thrusts: Stand behind him, wrap your arms around his waist, and place the thumb side of one fist against his abdomen at midline (slightly above the navel, well below the xiphoid tip). Grasp the fist with your other hand and make quick upward thrusts. Repeat until you're successful or the victim loses consciousness.

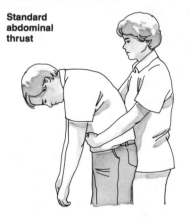

Standard abdominal thrust

If he becomes unconscious, position him supine and call for help again (or activate the emergency medical services system). Open his mouth with a tongue-jaw lift and sweep deeply into his mouth with your finger (finger sweep).

Open his airway with the head-tilt/chin-lift maneuver, and attempt to ventilate. (See also *CPR: technique.*)

If you don't succeed, straddle the victim's thighs and position the heel of one hand against his abdomen at the midline point. Place your other hand on top of it and deliver 6 to 10 abdominal thrusts. Use chest thrusts for obese victims and women in the late stages of pregnancy.

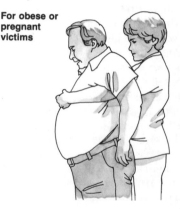

For obese or pregnant victims

Open the victim's mouth and perform a finger sweep. Then open his airway with the head-tilt/chin-lift maneuver, and attempt to ventilate. If unsuccessful, repeat the procedure as necessary. (See *Airway obstruction: unconscious victim.*)

Airway obstruction: infants

Emergency procedures

If a conscious infant appears to be choking, assess his condition by looking, listening, and feeling for breathing. Observe for blue lips. If the child can't cry, cough, or breathe, call for help and then begin the procedure.

To clear an obstruction, support his head and neck by holding his jaw with one hand. Position him over your arm with his head lower than his trunk. Use your thigh to support your forearm.

Deliver four forceful back blows between the shoulder blades with the heel of your hand.

Back blows

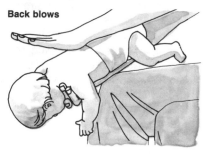

Next, sandwich the infant between your hands, and turn him on his back, head lower than trunk. Continue to support his head.

Chest thrusts

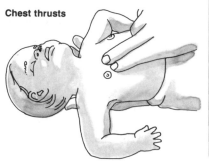

Deliver four chest thrusts in the midsternal region. Use the same technique you'd use to deliver chest compressions, but deliver at a slower rate. Repeat back blows and chest thrusts until you dislodge the foreign object or the infant becomes unconscious.

If he does, call for help and activate the emergency medical services system. Then open the airway with a tongue-jaw lift and look for the foreign body. Attempt to remove it only if you can see it. Open the infant's airway with a head-tilt/chin-lift maneuver and attempt to ventilate.

Ventilation

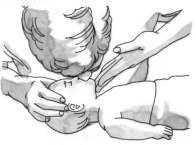

If you can't ventilate the infant, position him head-down, and deliver four back blows. Then, turn the infant and deliver four chest thrusts. Repeat the sequence until effective.

Airway obstruction: unconscious victim

Emergency procedures

If you find a victim who's unconscious for unknown reasons, follow these steps:
• Determine unresponsiveness by tapping or shaking his shoulder and shouting, "Are you OK?" Then call for help.
• Position him supine and open his airway with the head-tilt/chin-lift maneuver. (See also *CPR: technique.*)
• Look, listen, and feel for breathing for 3 to 5 seconds.

• If he's not breathing, attempt to ventilate. If you can't, reposition his head and try again.
• If you're still unsuccessful, activate the emergency medical services system.
• Straddle the victim and perform 6 to 10 abdominal thrusts.

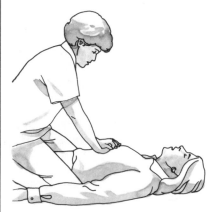

• Use the jaw-lift/chin-lift manuever to open his mouth. (See *Jaw-thrust maneuver.*) Perform a deep finger sweep to remove a foreign body, if present.
• Open his airway and attempt to ventilate. If you're unsuccessful, repeat this until help arrives.

Alcoholic nurse

Reporting an alcoholic colleague

Your professional obligation arises from paragraph 3.1 of the American Nurses' Association's Code (1976): "The nurse's primary commitment is to the client's care and safety. Hence, in the role of a client advocate, the nurse must be alert to and take appropriate action regarding any instances of incompetent, unethical, or illegal practices by any member of the health care team or system."

Your *legal* obligation is equally clear. To be aware of a colleague's possible drug or alcohol abuse and not report it to the appropriate authority may constitute negligence.

Can you be sued for slander (oral defamation) or libel (written defa-

A

mation) if you report a nurse for alcohol or drug abuse? You have two main defenses to a slander or libel charge: truth and privilege.

If you're right that the nurse is abusing alcohol or drugs, you will be absolutely immunized from liability because truth is an absolute defense.

If you're wrong, you'll still be immunized from liability if your charge meets these tests:
• If you have a professional reason or duty to report the information.
• If you report the information in good faith.
• If you report the information to a person who has a legitimate right to it.

Alcoholic patients

Caring for them effectively

Alcoholism is a pervasive problem in our society, so you're probably going to come across a patient who has this disease. If so:
• Determine if he is intoxicated by ordering a blood alcohol content test.
• Remember that getting a rational response from an intoxicated patient is nearly impossible.
• Deal with your own feelings about the alcoholic patient. Even if he can't follow what you're saying, he may still feel your resentment or concern at his noncompliance.
• Document changes in his orientation, speech, coordination, behavior, skin color, and breath. These observations support your nursing assessment of intoxication.
• Share your concerns with the patient's doctor in working out the best treatment for the patient. For example, should he be admitted to a substance abuse clinic?
• Try to screen visits from family members and friends, at least until you're sure they understand the necessity to withhold all alcohol from the patient. Also, determine if they'll back treatment for the patient and

consider a support program, such as Al-Anon, for themselves.

Most of all, when caring for the alcoholic patient, remember the need to show compassion. He's suffering, not merely weak.

Alkalosis, metabolic

Developing a care plan

Structure your care plan around cautious I.V. therapy, keen observation, and strict monitoring of the patient's status.
• Dilute potassium when giving it intravenously. Monitor the infusion rate to prevent damage to blood vessels; watch for signs of phlebitis. When administering 0.9% ammonium chloride, limit the infusion rate to 1 liter in 4 hours; faster administration may cause hemolysis of red blood cells. Avoid overdosage, since it may cause overcorrection to metabolic acidosis. Don't give ammonium chloride if patient has signs of hepatic or renal disease.
• Watch closely for signs of muscle weakness, tetany, or decreased activity. Monitor vital signs frequently, and record intake and output to evaluate respiratory, fluid, and electrolyte status. Remember, respiratory rate usually decreases in an effort to compensate for alkalosis. Hypotension and tachycardia may indicate electrolyte imbalance, especially hypokalemia.
• Observe seizure precautions. (See *Seizures: precautions.*)
• To prevent metabolic alkalosis, warn patients against overdosing with alkaline agents, such as sodium bicarbonate. Irrigate nasogastric tubes with normal saline solution instead of plain water to prevent excessive loss of gastric electrolytes. Monitor I.V. fluid concentrations of bicarbonate or lactate. Teach patients with ulcers to recognize signs of milk-alkali syndrome: anorexia, weakness, lethargy, and a distaste for milk. (See *Alkalosis detection, metabolic.*)

Alkalosis, respiratory

Recognition and intervention

Acidosis depresses the central nervous system, but alkalosis stimulates it, so the leading sign of hyperventilation is rapid (but not Kussmaul's) respirations. This in turn produces dizziness, sweating, tingling in the fingers and nose, muscle weakness, and muscle spasm (particularly carpopedal spasm because calcium does not ionize normally in an alkaline medium). The arterial blood gas (ABG) readings show a high pH with a low PCO_2.

Nursing interventions
Treatment of any acid-base imbalance is geared to reversing the underlying problem. Because this imbalance may cause muscle spasms (see *Trousseau's sign*) and possible tetany, prevent the alkalotic patient from hurting himself: Keep the side rails of his bed up, and have an airway at hand. (See also *Tetany.*) Monitor his cardiac status; dysrhythmias are common in alkalotic states.

If the alkalosis is caused by anxiety, your role is to calm and reassure the patient. Tell him why he needs to breathe more slowly. Have him breathe with you, with you starting at his rate and gradually breathing slower and slower. If he still can't follow your lead, let him breathe a minute or two into his cupped hands or a small paper bag. This may be sufficient to restore PCO_2 levels to normal and relieve his symptoms temporarily.

Alkalosis detection, metabolic

Detection and special precautions

With predictable effect, alkalosis renders the central nervous system overexcitable, leading to irritabiiity and belligerence. Disorientation may follow and—if the alkalosis is untreated—even tetany and convulsions.

Look for shallow, slow respirations as a compensatory attempt by the lungs. Because of abnormal loss of potassium from the extracellular fluid (in exchange for hydrogen ions), the patient may have muscle twitching or dysrhythmias. His arterial blood gas values will show a high pH and a high bicarbonate concentration. In fact, in metabolic acid-base imbalances, the pH and bicarbonate go hand in hand; they're both down or both up.

Nursing interventions
The doctor will treat the underlying cause of alkalosis, and the patient who's been vomiting or having gastric suctioning will need replacement fluid. When you irrigate the patient's gastric tube, use isotonic solutions, and offer isotonic fluids for vomiting.

Because he might have spasms and convulsions, always protect the patient by padding the side rails of his bed and leave them up whenever he's left alone.

Since excess antacids cause metabolic alkalosis, one extremely important follow-up for the patient who's been medicating himself with antacids is to teach him about their effects. (See *Alkalosis, metabolic.*)

Allen's test

Assessing collateral arterial blood supply

First, have your patient extend his forearm over a rolled towel with his

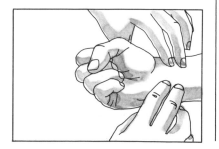

palm up. Tell him to close his hand while you occlude his radial and ulnar arteries for 5 to 10 seconds.

Next, have him open his hand. You should see blanching of the palm because of the impaired blood flow.

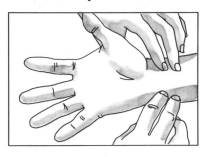

Then, release pressure on the ulnar artery. Color should return to the patient's hand in 15 seconds indicating adequate collateral circulation. You can then proceed with radial ar-

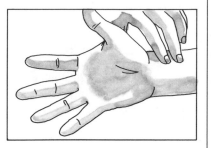

terial puncture. If the color doesn't return, repeat test on other arm. (See *Arterial puncture.*)

Alzheimer's disease

Teaching the patient's family

Because most patients with Alzheimer's disease become totally dependent on their families, much of your nursing care will be devoted to family teaching. Your primary goal: to help maintain the patient's mental and physical functions for as long as possible.

Tell family members to stick to a regular routine and keep furniture and appliances where the patient's used to seeing them. Suggest repeatedly reminding the patient of the day and date. To provide sen-

sory stimulation, they can show him family albums or read the newspaper out loud.

Even the simplest task must be broken down into steps. Something as mundane as brushing his teeth, for example, will prove too difficult for him unless he's shown each separate activity involved—taking the toothbrush in hand, removing the toothpaste cap, wetting the brush, squeezing the toothpaste onto the brush, and so forth.

When the family members go out, they should write down where they're going and leave notes reminding the patient to turn off the oven, to close the refrigerator, or to take the names and numbers of telephone callers. These steps would apply only during the early stages of Alzheimer's disease; the patient will eventually need constant supervision because of his forgetfulness and tendency to wander. Because he has a short attention span, relatives should keep their conversations with him brief and their instructions simple. To keep him physically active, a family member might take him for daily walks through the neighborhood, using the same route every time to minimize confusion. Short, brisk walks are essential to maintaining his mobility, muscle strength, joint movement, cardiac output, and sleep patterns.

The patient's diet needs close attention because he'll use up a lot of energy from constant pacing. And, as mentioned earlier, his eating habits may change drastically.

To counter growing disorientation, the family will need to take special precautions to ensure his safety. They must consider all sorts of hidden hazards since the patient will lose the ability to recognize potential danger—to discern sharp from dull, for example, or hot from cold. So, they should remove furniture that has sharp edges and lock up things like forks, knives, and medications. And they should always check the temperature of the patient's food and bathwater.

A

If the patient insists on driving, the family may have to hide the keys or distributor cap to his car. He'll be prone to wander from the house, so all doors and windows must be kept locked. Advise the family to put a locked gate at the top of the stairs. (Some families put a fence around the house.)

Recognizing the family's needs
Family members will feel they're "on call" 24 hours a day. They get very little sleep, have no time to relax, and eat sporadically.

They'll need some time to themselves, so arrange for someone—maybe a home health aide or a neighbor—to stay with the patient part-time. And then help find a facility where health care professionals can care for the patient during the day. (Reluctant at first, adult day-care centers are now opening their doors to Alzheimer's patients.) (See *Day care for adults*.)

Set up an appointment with a social services agency, which will help the family assess its financial status and handle legal matters, such as power of attorney. Refer family to support groups; they may find solace in knowing that others are going through the same devastating experience. To locate support groups in your area, contact your local Alzheimer's Disease and Related Disorders Association (ADRDA). And finally, listen to the family members—letting them express their feelings of stress and despair. (See also *Elderly patients: emotions.*)

Amputated finger

Emergency intervention

Just imagine you see one of your neighbors cut his hand with a chain saw—severing his thumb and two fingers. What can you do?

First, tell the victim to lie down, and quickly assess his airway, breathing, and circulation. Apply direct pressure to his wound with any material you can find: a clean rag, his shirt, or your slip. Look in your handbag and pockets; use a sanitary pad, gloves, or a scarf.

Elevate his arm above the level of his heart. If his wound is gaping, pack it and wrap his hand to control the bleeding. When the packing becomes soaked, don't remove it; just add more packing.

If direct pressure doesn't control the bleeding, go to the appropriate pressure point—in this case, the brachial artery. (See *Pulses, peripheral.*) Place your fingers flat over the artery, with your thumb on the outside of his arm.

Don't use your fingertips to apply pressure because they may slip off the artery if it rolls. Also, if you're not sure where the artery is, you're more likely to occlude it by placing your fingers flat over it, simply because you'll cover more area. And you'll be less likely to injure a nerve. Keep in mind, though, that when you occlude the artery, you're cutting off circulation to the arm.

If applying direct pressure, elevating the arm, and occluding the brachial artery still don't control the bleeding, apply a tourniquet. Do this only as a last resort—a tourniquet could cause tissue and nerve damage, and possibly loss of the hand from ischemia.

Apply a 1″ or 2″ (3 or 5 cm) wide tourniquet as close to the wound as possible, tight enough to occlude arterial flow but not so tight as to cut into tissue. Keep the tourniquet uncovered and write a large "T" on the victim's forearm so emergency personnel will know a tourniquet is in place. Release it slowly every 10 to 15 minutes, keep it released for a few seconds to allow some blood flow to the arm, then retighten it. If you must use a tourniquet, get the victim to a hospital immediately. (See also *Tourniquets.*)

Once the bleeding is controlled, locate the amputated fingers. (See *Amputated limb* for care of amputated fingers.) If someone has arrived to help, tell him to call an ambulance.

As you're doing all this, keep your eye on the victim's general appear-

ance. Also monitor his vital signs and level of consciousness. Continue to reassure him; if he panics, you may not be able to control the bleeding.

Don't try to wash the injured hand or replace any protruding bones. Once bleeding is controlled, get the victim to a hospital as soon as possible. If you must leave him to get help, have him continue to apply pressure to the wound.

When emergency personnel take over the victim's care, tell them what happened and what you did. If you applied a tourniquet, be sure to let them know how long it's been in place. Make certain the amputated fingers are kept with the victim.

Amputated limb

Caring for the amputated part

If a patient arrives in the ED with a traumatic amputation, you may be asked to preserve the amputated part for possible replantation. Here's a four-step procedure to follow:

1. Put on sterile gloves; then flush the amputated part with normal saline or Ringer's lactated solution. *Never use any other solution,* and don't try to scrub or debride the part.

2. Gently pat the part dry with sterile gauze. Then wrap it in saline-soaked sterile gauze. Wrap the gauze with a sterile towel. Then put the whole thing in a watertight container or bag and seal it.

3. Fill another plastic bag with ice water and place the part, still in its watertight container, inside the bag. Seal the bag. (Always protect the part from direct contact with ice—and *never* use dry ice—to prevent irreversible tissue damage; this would make the part unsuitable for replantation.) Keep this bag ice-cold

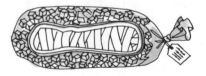

until the doctor's ready to do the replantation surgery.

4. Label the bag with your patient's name, identification of the amputated part, the hospital identification number, and the date and time when the part was put on ice.

Amputation, leg

Stump care

A properly applied bandage is crucial in stump care: It supports the soft tissue, controls edema, minimizes pain, and shrinks and molds the stump into a cone-shaped form so the prosthesis will fit snugly.

After the wound heals, encourage the patient to wrap the stump himself, if possible—it will foster his sense of independence. For an above-the-knee amputation, one 4-inch (10-cm) and two 3-inch (7.5-cm) elastic bandages are commonly used. The 4-inch bandage is used to secure the stump bandages and prevent slippage.

Tell the patient to be sure to extend the bandage well up into his groin to prevent an adductor roll or bulge from forming. Such a bulge could cause problems in fitting the prosthesis later. A prosthesis that

Above knee stump wrapping

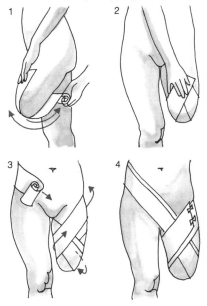

doesn't fit the stump snugly could cause the patient to "vault"—that is, move forward and slide out of his prosthesis with each step.

Suggest that the patient wrap his stump before getting out of bed in the morning. To support himself, he can lie on his back or side. Show him how to apply the bandages with even, moderate pressure, guarding against any tourniquetlike action. If the bandages become loose, they should be reapplied (See also *Bandage, roller.*)

Frequently, stump shrinkers—elastic stockings that fit over the stump and lower trunk area—are used instead of elastic bandages. These custom-fitted devices are simply pulled on—the same way as a trouser leg. Suggest that the patient have two shrinkers, so that one can be washed while the other is being worn.

Amputees

Teaching them exercises

Remind your patient that every day is "moving day" when stump conditioning is the goal. If the patient must spend most of his time lying down because of a medical condition, encourage him to turn from side to side and to assume an alternate position—usually on his stomach—for 20 to 30 minutes at least twice a day. Changing position will stretch his hip flexor muscles and prevent contractures.

Keeping his legs in a neutral position will prevent adduction deformity. Tell the patient never to prop up his stump, even though he may be tempted to do so.

Because moving can be painful for a new amputee, he may need pain medication about a half hour before his exercises. When the medication takes effect, he'll be able to move more easily, which should make him more willing to follow a regular exercise routine.

Also, schedule his walking periods throughout the day—at least

every 2 hours—to prevent contractures. Be sure he understands that if contractures do occur, fitting his stump to a prosthesis may become impossible. In other words, walking now, although difficult, will make walking easier for him later.

Some patients will never be considered candidates for a prosthesis—perhaps because of senility or a severe stroke affecting the side opposite the amputation. Even so, try to get such a patient to stand or walk if at all possible. Walking not only prevents contractures but strengthens hip and knee muscles and promotes wound healing as well. Also, try to gradually increase the distance the amputee walks every day.

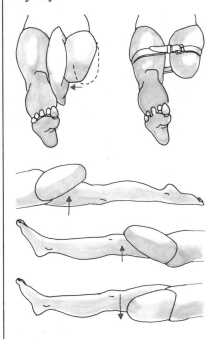

To further strengthen stump muscles before a prosthesis is fitted, the doctor may prescribe specific stump-conditioning exercises for the amputee. Since these exercises are usually carried out by a physical therapist, follow the therapist's lead in explaining and supervising them. Schedule these exercises around meal times to help the patient to remember to do them. Gradually, the patient should increase the exercises to 30 times, two or three times a day. Explain that these exercises will help him gain the muscle strength he needs to use crutches, a walker, or a prosthesis.

Analgesia, epidural

Nursing considerations

Epidural analgesia has been most commonly used with pregnant women. But now it's being used for many other postsurgical patients. Here's what you need to know.

As its name suggests, a catheter is inserted into the epidural space surrounding the spinal cord. Usually, the anesthesiologist inserts a flexible polyethylene catheter into the L3 and L5 interspace (the spinal cord ends at L1 and L2). Once he's sure of the placement, he advances the catheter and removes the needle. To make subsequent drug administration easier, he attaches a port or heparin lock adapter to the tubing's distal end. He then tapes the tubing onto the patient's back.

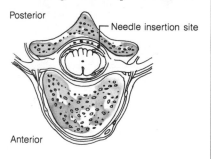

Posterior
— Needle insertion site
Anterior

Orders for all pain or sleeping medications should come from the anesthesiologist; check with him before administering any narcotics to the patient through other routes.

Be sure to assess the patient's pain before and after you administer an epidural analgesic to determine its effectiveness—and the need for a repeat injection. As in caring for any postoperative patient, use a pain scale to balance the information you get from the patient with your observations of pain-related behaviors (grimacing, restlessness, irritability, and so on).

Put your greatest emphasis, however, on the patient's judgment of the pain's intensity.

Keep in mind the onset, duration, and dosage of the narcotic the patient is receiving. Carefully assess him and intervene if he develops any of the most common adverse reactions: respiratory depression, urine retention, pruritus, and nausea and vomiting. (See *Pain detection; pain, postoperative.*)

Analgesia, patient-controlled

Setting up the unit

The patient-controlled analgesia (PCA) unit delivers small amounts of a narcotic at short intervals. This stabilizes serum narcotic concentrations, providing constant therapeutic blood levels.

The PCA unit has two other advantages. First, the narcotic is delivered I.V., not I.M., so absorption is faster and more predictable. Second, the patient doesn't have to depend on you to administer pain medication. When he feels the need for analgesia, he simply pushes the PCA control button.

Give the patient a complete explanation and a demonstration of how the unit works. Be sure to explain what the *ready* and *lockout interval* messages mean. Tell him that he should feel relief soon after pushing the button. If two consecutive doses don't relieve his pain, he should call you.

Here are some key features of the PCA unit: driver-release mechanism, display panel, touch key controls, and thumb-wheel controls.

Here's how to set up the unit:

1. Gather the following equipment: a PCA unit; PCA tubing with Y connector and slide clamp; primary I.V. tubing with clamp; an injector and a 30-ml vial of morphine or Demerol, as ordered; I.V. maintenance solution (such as D_5W); an

I.V. start kit; an I.V. catheter; and an I.V. pole.

2. Unlock the security door on the front of the PCA unit. This allows you to loosen the I.V. pole clamp on the back of the unit. (When the door is locked, you can only tighten the clamp.) Secure the unit to the I.V. pole.

3. Plug the unit into an electric outlet. To make sure the battery is charged, check the display panel. It should light up briefly. (If it isn't charged, you won't be able to set the touch key control in Step 9.)

4. Connect the vial of morphine or Demerol to the injector.

Connecting vial to injector

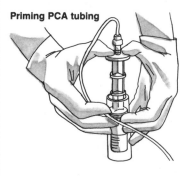

5. Attach the PCA tubing to the injector.

6. Invert the vial and gently push down on the injector to prime the PCA tubing. (The vial is overfilled by 2.5 ml for this purpose.) Clamp the PCA tubing above the Y connector.

Priming PCA tubing

7. Squeeze the driver-release mechanism and push it up as far as it'll go. Now insert the vial.

8. Squeeze the driver-release mechanism and slide it down until the vial locks in place. Make sure the PCA tubing isn't kinked below the vial.

9. After calculating the appropriate dosage and lockout interval, you're ready to set the controls. Push in the 4-hour limit touch key until the display panel shows the number of milliliters prescribed for 4 hours. Now use the thumb-wheel controls to set the dose volume in milliliters and the lockout interval in minutes.

10. After connecting the D_5W bag to the primary I.V. line and hanging the bag, attach the primary line to the Y connector on the PCA tubing.

11. Make sure the PCA tubing is clamped above the Y connector, then unclamp the primary I.V. line. This allows you to flush the PCA tubing below the Y connector with the D_5W (or other maintenance fluid).

12. Using the I.V. start kit, prepare the I.V. site. After inserting the catheter, attach the PCA tubing to it and unclamp the tubing. Cover the site with the transparent dressing included in the I.V. start kit.

13. Close the door on the unit; the display panel will briefly show all messages.

PCA unit

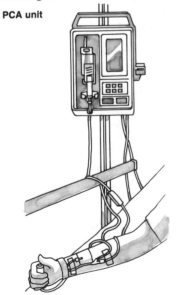

14. Give the pendant to the patient and tell him to push the button when he wants pain medication. To keep the pendant from sliding off the bed, you can pin it to the sheets or wrap it around the side rail.

Analgesia administration

Precautions

Assess the source of the pain before giving the analgesic. For example, the patient may actually be having chest pain when you assume he's having incisional pain.

• Individualize the drug, dosage, and interval between doses, if ordered this way.

• For later comparison, establish the patient's baseline vital signs and level of consciousness before giving the drug.

• Note that when giving rectal suppositories, the rectum should be empty to facilitate absorption.

• Before giving a parenteral analgesic, check for special administration procedures.

• During prolonged I.M. therapy, alternate sites and use large muscle groups for the injections. Check the sites for hardness and bruising.

• Observe the patient's response to the drug. Note degree and duration of pain relief and adverse effects.

• Try to prevent the pain rather than wait to relieve it. Tell your patient to let you know as soon as pain begins.

• Because narcotics and nonnarcotics relieve pain by different mechanisms, use a combination.

• Use noninvasive pain-relief techniques: distraction, relaxation exercises, and cutaneous stimulation.

• Explain the pain-relief plan to the patient. Document that you've done so on the nursing care plan. (See *Orders, sliding scale; Pain relief: distraction.*)

Anaphylaxis: emergency care

Intervening quickly

A patient who suddenly and unexpectedly exhibits the early signs and symptoms of anaphylaxis needs emergency attention with split-second timing.

Your first step is to identify the antigen and stop his exposure to it. Determine which possible antigen he's been exposed to—for example, a drug, food, contrast dye, or insect venom. Also ask him if he remembers having had an allergic reaction before. (Don't rule out anaphylaxis, however, even if he says no.)

Try to identify the antigen, but don't waste time doing so. In this emergency, your top priority is performing an emergency assessment and taking any action necessary to stabilize your patient's airway, breathing, and circulation. So unless another cause of the patient's signs and symptoms seems likely (for example, myocardial infarction, pulmonary embolism, or a vasovagal episode), take these steps:

1. Maintain the patient's airway. Keep in mind that the biggest threat is asphyxiation secondary to massive upper airway edema. Be prepared to assist with endotracheal intubation or, if laryngeal edema closes the patient's airway so intubation's impossible, with an emergency tracheotomy or cricothyrotomy. Remember that an oral airway won't keep the patient's airway open if he develops laryngeal edema. (See *Endotracheal tubes: insertion.*)

2. Administer oxygen and support his respirations. If he's not in severe distress, ask if his chest feels tight; auscultate for wheezes, crackles, and lack of air movement; note whether he's using accessory muscles for breathing. (See *Breath sounds, adventitious; Respiratory: auscultation.*) Unless contraindicated, help him into a sitting position so he can breathe more easily.

3. Administer epinephrine (Adrenalin) as ordered. Although epinephrine is the drug of choice for treating anaphylactic shock, be aware that a delicate balance exists between its therapeutic value and its adverse effects. If you're administering epinephrine I.V., even a slight overdose or a too-rapid infusion can cause

A

cardiac dysrhythmias and a sudden rise in blood pressure—even cerebral hemorrhage. When administering it subcutaneously, such adverse effects are of much less concern because it wouldn't be administered directly into the bloodstream.

If your patient's normotensive and not in severe distress, give 0.3 to 0.5 ml 1:1,000 subcutaneously, as ordered. Massage the injection site to speed absorption. Tell the patient he'll feel a faster, stronger heartbeat.

If he's in severe distress, give the same dose I.V. If an I.V. site isn't available, inject the drug in the vascular plexus at the base of the patient's tongue. Endotracheal tube administration is a last-resort method for administering epinephrine to a patient in severe shock—the medication is quickly absorbed into the bloodstream through lung tissue. (See *Medication, endotracheal.*)

The first epinephrine dose may immediately reverse the patient's signs and symptoms, especially if you administer it as soon as they appear. If signs and symptoms persist, however, repeat the dose in 5 to 10 minutes, as ordered.

Check your patient's vital signs frequently and monitor him for cardiac dysrhythmias.

4. Support his circulation. Because anaphylaxis depletes the intravascular fluid compartment by encouraging third-space fluid shifting and vasodilation, restore his circulating volume by administering one-half normal saline solution, normal saline solution, or plasma, as ordered. Infuse fluids through large-bore needles.

During fluid replacement therapy, monitor his blood pressure closely to assess his fluid requirements. Watch carefully for signs of fluid overload—particularly if he's elderly or has a pre-existing cardiac condition. Assess for jugular venous distention, S_3 gallop, and inspiratory crackles. If possible, monitor central venous pressure. Insert an indwelling Foley catheter, as ordered, and keep meticulous fluid intake and output measurements.

Don't let edema fool you: It indicates third-space fluid shifting, not fluid overload.

If fluid replacement fails to maintain your patient's blood pressure, the doctor may order a vasopressor—norepinephrine (Levophed) or dopamine (Intropin)—to improve cardiac contractility and to counteract vasodilation. This treatment can be dangerous, however, because vasoconstriction further compromises tissue perfusion. If possible, administer the vasopressor through a central venous line. This is because doing so prevents local tissue necrosis resulting from infiltration around a peripheral I.V. site. If you must give the medication through a peripheral line, keep phentolamine (Regitine) nearby to treat infiltration if it occurs. Assess the patient frequently for tachycardia, dysrhythmias, and signs of infiltration.

5. Give the patient continuous emotional support to keep him as calm as possible. Few experiences are as frightening as anaphylaxis. Your patient knows he's in danger—and his fear can increase his heart rate and oxygen needs.

Anaphylaxis: emergency kit

A kit for patients allergic to insect stings

If your patient's at risk for a severe anaphylactic reaction, advise him to carry an emergency kit with him at all times.

For a patient allergic to insect stings, for example, you might recommend any of the following:
• Ana-Kit (Hollister-Stier Laboratories), which includes epinephrine 1:1,000 (two 0.3-mg doses) in 1 ml; one disposable sterile syringe; chlorpheniramine maleate, 2 mg (four chewable tablets); sterile alcohol sponges (two each); tourniquet (one each).
• EpiPen Auto-Injector (Center Labs), which delivers a 0.3-mg I.M. dose of epinephrine 1:1,000 in 2-ml disposable injectors.

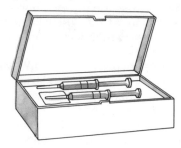

• EpiPen Jr. Auto-Injector (Center Labs), which delivers a 0.15-mg I.M. dose of epinephrine from epinephrine injection 1:2,000 in 2-ml disposable injectors.

Also advise the patient to wear a medical identification tag (such as a Medic Alert tag) to inform health care workers of his allergy. (See also *Anaphylaxis: emergency care.*)

Anesthesia, general

Rousing the patient after surgery

Here's the usual sequence that the patient's recovery process follows: unconsciousness, response to stimuli, drowsiness, awake but not oriented, and alert and oriented. As your patient awakens, voices may sound quite loud to him and his own thoughts may seem fuzzy and unclear. Next, he'll notice that his arms and legs feel heavy, like lead. In the drowsiness stage, voices seem even louder. He'll wonder where he is and he'll feel things in his mouth. When he opens his eyes, his vision will be blurred. Before he's fully awake, he'll become aware of sounds and tubes. Even at this stage he's likely to still feel drowsy and be disoriented to time and place. And he'll first realize that he hurts. All this adds up to a frightening experience for even a patient who's been told *before* his operation what to expect.

To arouse him, call him by name. Continually reorient him, assuring him that his surgery is completed. Otherwise he may think he's waking up during the operation. Address him in a normal tone, though; don't yell. And watch what you say when you're near him. He may seem to be only semiconscious, but hearing is the first sense to return. With his impaired judgment, he may grasp careless conversation and become frightened. Before doing anything to him, even when he appears unconscious, tell him what it is you'll be doing.

Be especially careful rousing a patient who's received ketamine. This injectable anesthetic may cause hallucinations, particularly in patients between 15 and 65 years old. To reduce this likelihood, don't overstimulate your patient.

You have four main areas of concern in recovery: adequate respiratory function, adequate cardiovascular function, proper fluid and electrolyte levels, and a safe environment with physical and emotional comfort. (See *Postanesthesia recovery.*)

Anger

Maintaining your professionalism

How you handle your anger can make or break how others judge your professionalism. Blowing up at every mistake or seething in silence won't help you resolve your anger. And neither approach is conducive to building a strong relationship with your staff. Instead, separate petty anger from serious anger. Then you can resolve the petty and express the serious in a controlled manner. Here's how:

First, make a list of the things that make you angry. If you feel angry at your supervisor, the administrator, or the hospital in general, jot that down. Next to each complaint, list reasons why they're to blame. In another column, write down your part in the problem. Seeing why you're angry and who's at fault will make changing your behavior or speaking to the person at fault much easier.

Second, when someone lashes out in anger at you, ask yourself why. If you can recognize that she's just having a bad day, you won't get angry in return.

Third, determine your own anger threshold. When you're hot, hungry, in a noisy environment, disturbed, or overworked, your anger threshold is lowered. Try counting to 100 before getting angry when you're under these pressures.

Fourth, stop saying "should." You only make yourself mad by telling yourself, "My staff should be working harder," or "My team leader should be more pleasant." Don't become obsessed with other people's failures to live up to your standards.

Fifth, laugh a little. Humor makes anger tolerable because you can't laugh and frown at the same time. (See *Humor.*)

Sixth, never be rude. Rudeness encourages anger by giving the other person a reason for getting angry, too. Force yourself to remain courteous. Your anger may dissipate, and you'll have a better chance to solve your problem.

Angina: psychological reactions

Helping your patient face his problems

Patients who suffer from unstable angina are especially prone to psychosocial problems. Fear of dying probably lies at the root of most of these problems. And from that can grow loss of self-esteem, loss of identity as a family member, and loss of confidence. (See *Angina, unstable.*)

First, encourage your patient to express his feelings so he can deal with them. Some patients won't have any problem with this; the feelings will come gushing out. Others will keep the feelings bottled up, creating an internal turmoil that eats away at their self-image. Be especially leery of the patient who tells you he can handle what's happened to him by himself. Chances are, he can't.

Besides expressing his feelings, your patient needs to know that he's the same person he was before the unstable angina attack, with the same qualities and abilities. Telling him this yourself will help, but he really needs to hear it from his family, friends, and even his co-workers. Most likely they're as uncertain about him as he is about himself, so besides encouraging them to help, you'll also have to support them in their efforts.

Finally, assure your patient and his family that every effort's been made to diagnose his condition accurately, and he's been given the appropriate medication. Assure him that if he follows the preventive and rehabilitative measures he has been taught, he'll ward off future attacks.

Angina, unstable

Usual management methods

Get the patient into bed, raise his head, and notify the doctor. Begin

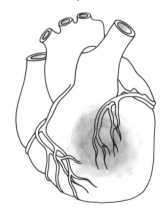

administering oxygen—preferably by nasal cannula, since a mask can make the patient feel smothered—plus any drugs that may be prescribed. Even though the patient will already be attached to a monitor or

A

telemetry, you'll want to get an ECG stat. (See *ECG, single channel.*)

Monitor his vital signs frequently (keep the blood pressure cuff in place), and carefully observe his color, respirations, skin condition, and level of consciousness. Listen to his heart, particularly for an S_3 sound, which indicates the left ventricle is compromised by ischemia. He's likely to be terrified and will need your constant reassurance.

Angina drugs

Adverse reactions

If your patient's receiving a beta-blocker, watch for indications of cardiac failure (for example, wheezing, shortness of breath, and GI upset). Notify the doctor immediately when these occur. If he orders the beta-blocker stopped, do it gradually, not abruptly, or your patient could suffer a myocardial infarction.

Calcium channel blockers offer another drug therapy for unstable angina. These drugs block the flow of calcium into the smooth muscle cells. Because calcium is necessary for muscle contraction, the reduced calcium flow produces a less forceful contraction. For the heart, a diminished contraction means reduced oxygen demand—the primary goal in treating unstable angina. (See also *Angina, unstable.*)

Angry co-workers

Dealing with them effectively

Angry people are hurting psychologically, and—despite their claims of objectivity and logic—emotions are ruling their lives. You can ease their pain, however. Some tips:

1. Soothe the bruise. Remember why the person is angry. She feels weak, devalued, out of control; she's using anger to give herself the illusion of control. So your first step is to send "valuing" statements to

her. These will show her that—despite what she has said or done—she's still important. For example, "I'm sorry you're upset, Karen. Our relationship is important to me, and I want to keep it."

2. Lance the boil. Next, tell her—and show her—that she has your undivided attention, and let her talk. This meets her need to drain the emotion that has built up inside her.

Listening won't be easy. (See *Listening to co-workers.*) Fight your own need to defend yourself when you hear your behavior interpreted in a way you never intended. But your defensive arguments at this point will only prompt more anger. Instead, hold your tongue. Let the person's anger drain out.

3. Find something you agree with. If you've listened to the other person with an open mind, you'll probably find at least one thing you agree with. Say so. Instead of retaliating with, "You're wrong," start by saying, "You have a point there." This will create a whole new environment, because it shifts the focus of the conversation away from the anger, toward agreement, and the start of finding a solution.

4. Identify exaggerations and bring the discussion closer to reality. Do this by pointing out the "always" and "never" statements angry people may make. Questions like these can usually help the other person realize what she's been saying: "Do I always make you wait?" ("Well, maybe not always.")

You can also ask for clarification: "Karen, you say I'm always on your back. Can you give me some examples so I know what we're talking about?" If you avoid sarcasm and treat the other person with respect and concern, she'll soon relax and be ready to talk more rationally.

Angry patients

Coping strategies

Approach the angry patient as you would any nursing problem: Assess

the situation and plan your actions. Within your limited time with the patient, you can't make him over, but you can use nursing interventions to make his hospital stay more tolerable for him, for you, and for the rest of the staff. Here are some suggestions.

Begin by acknowledging the situation. Your simple statement that "I know you're upset" could strike a patient as condescending or simplistic. And the word "angry" is too threatening for many patients. If you are genuinely concerned, your body language will reflect this. Knowing you're concerned with his feelings may sometimes give the patient enough relief to enable him to move from the irrational stage of anger toward thought and resolution.

Listening to your angry patient becomes a major nursing intervention when you listen actively rather than passively. To make your listening more active, experiment with techniques such as door-openers and perception checks. (See *Listening to patients.*)

A door-opener is a brief invitation to the patient to say more; "Go on," "Tell me more," and "Uh huh" may be all you need to say.

Perception checks help you make sure you've understood the patient correctly. For example, you could say to the patient: "You look frustrated with the doctor's latest orders. Are you?"

Encourage the patient's physical activity; this is one of the best-known ways to alleviate anger. If your patient's ambulatory, ask the occupational therapist to design an activity program adapted to the patient's particular physical capacity. Exercise in bed is helpful for non-ambulatory patients.

Allow the patient to participate in solving the problem. As in the classic problem-solving process, start by defining the problem. Help him clarify the situation by asking a question, such as "What would you like us to do?" Once you're both sure you have the same problem in mind, you can move on to discuss all the possible solutions with the patient, even those that seem far-fetched or absurd.

Set limits on the patient's angry behavior. If a patient continues to shout and act out his anger, make the limits clear at once. You might say, "The screaming and shouting upset me. When we've both calmed down, we can talk about what's troubling you." If a situation seems beyond your control, you may have to involve another person. Then you should say to your patient: "I think I need help in dealing with this problem. I'll call my supervisor. Maybe she can help us work something out." If you're facing a patient so angry you think he could do you physical harm, set limits immediately. Without seeming to threaten the patient, tell him: "I'd like you to try to calm down so I don't have to call for help."

Anticoagulants

What to teach your patient

Stress the importance of preventing bleeding. Teach the patient to:
• take his medication at the same time every day
• avoid excessively rough sports that could lead to injury and subsequent bleeding
• use a soft toothbrush
• use an electric razor instead of a razor blade
• eat a balanced diet, including a consistent amount of vitamin K–enriched foods (e.g., leafy green vegetables, tomatoes, cheese, egg yolk, fish, and liver)
• check with his doctor about how much alcohol he may drink because alcohol can affect how some anticoagulants work
• check with his doctor before taking any drugs (prescription and over-the-counter) for these may also affect how some anticoagulants work

• report any of these signs of excess bleeding: nosebleed, heavy menstrual flow, unexplained bruising on his skin, bleeding from his gums, melena, tarry stools, hematuria, and hematemesis.
• carry an identification card or wear a Medic Alert bracelet stating that he takes anticoagulants
• keep all appointments for prothrombin time testing.

Antiembolism stockings

Applying them properly

After covering the foot, gather the loose part of the stocking up to the toes and carry only this portion up to the heel. Then, gather the loose part of the stocking at the ankle and

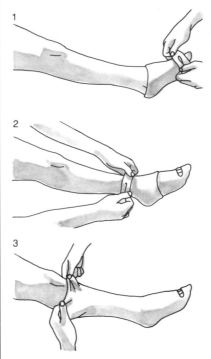

bring it over the heel with short, alternating front and back pulls. Next, using both hands, insert your index and middle fingers into the gathered part of the stocking at the ankle and carry the stocking to the top by rocking it slightly up and down.

Antineoplastic drugs: handling

Recommendations for safe use

The mutagenic, teratogenic, carcinogenic, and local irritative properties of many cytotoxic agents are well established and pose a possible hazard to the health of occupationally exposed individuals. These potential hazards require special procedures for the handling, preparation, and administration of these drugs and the proper disposal of residues and wastes.

Preparation for administration
1. Wash hands thoroughly before putting on gloves and after gloves are removed.
2. Take care to avoid puncturing of gloves and possible self-inoculation.
3. Use syringes and I.V. sets with Luer-Lok fittings whenever possible to avoid spills from disconnection.
4. To minimize aerosolization, vent vials containing cytotoxic agents with a hydrophobic filter to equalize internal pressure, or use negative pressure technique.
5. Before opening ampules, take care to ensure that no liquid remains in the tip of the ampule. Wrap a sterile disposable alcohol sponge

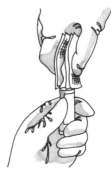

around the neck of the ampule to reduce aerosolization. Break ampules in a direction away from your body.
6. For sealed vials, perform final drug measurement before removing

A

the needle from the stopper of the vial and after the pressure has been equalized.

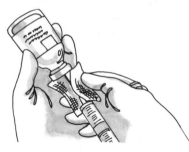

7. Make sure a closed collection vessel is available in the biological safety cabinet. Or use the original vessel to hold discarded excess drug solutions.

8. Make sure cytotoxic agents are labeled to identify the need for caution in handling (for example, "Chemotherapy: Dispose of Properly").

9. Be certain the final prepared dosage is protected from leakage or breakage by being sealed in a transparent plastic container labeled "Do Not Open if Contents Appear to be Broken."

Precautions for administration

1. Wear disposable surgical latex gloves during administration of cytotoxic agents. Wash hands thoroughly before putting on gloves and after gloves are removed.

2. Wear protective barrier garments. Such garments should have a closed front, long sleeves, and closed cuffs (either elastic or knit).

3. Use syringes and I.V. sets with Luer-Lok fittings whenever possible.

4. Take special care in priming I.V. sets. The distal tip or needle cover must be removed before priming. Priming can be performed into a sterile, alcohol-dampened gauze pad. Other acceptable methods of priming include closed receptacles (such as evacuated containers) or back-filling of I.V. sets. Do not prime sets or syringes into the sink or any open receptacle.

Disposal procedures

1. Place contaminated materials in a lead-lined, puncture-proof container appropriately marked as hazardous chemical waste. These

containers should be suitable to collect bottles, vials, gloves, disposable gowns, and other materials used in the preparation and administration of cytotoxic agents.

2. Dispose of contaminated needles, syringes, sets, and tubing intact. To prevent aerosolization, do not clip needles and syringes.

3. Make sure cytotoxic drug waste is transported according to your institution's procedures for hazardous material.

4. Presently, no preferred method is recommended for disposal of cytotoxic drug waste. One acceptable method for disposal of hazardous waste is by incineration in an Environmental Protection Agency (EPA) permitted hazardous waste incinerator. Another acceptable method of disposal is by burial at an EPA permitted hazardous waste site. A licensed hazardous waste disposal company may be consulted for information concerning available methods of disposal in the local area.

Anuria

Important steps to take

If you detect anuria, notify the doctor and prepare to catheterize the patient to relieve any lower urinary tract obstruction and to check for residual urine. You may find that an obstruction hinders catheter insertion and that urine return is cloudy and foul-smelling. If you collect more than 75 ml of urine, suspect lower urinary tract obstruction; if less than 75 ml, renal dysfunction or an obstruction higher in the urinary tract.

Next, take the patient's vital signs and obtain a complete history. Also ask about drug use.

Inspect and palpate the patient's abdomen for asymmetry, distention, or bulging. Inspect the flank area for edema or erythema, and percuss and palpate the bladder. Palpate the kidneys both anteriorly and posteriorly, and percuss them

at the costovertebral angle (See *Abdominal exam: palpation.*) Auscultate over the renal arteries, listening for bruits. (See *Bruits: auscultation.*)

Anxiety: assessment

Correct procedure

If the patient displays acute, severe anxiety, quickly take his vital signs and determine his chief complaint. Because anxiety is a notoriously nonspecific symptom, you'll need this information to guide your subsequent assessment and interventions. For example, if the patient's severe anxiety were accompanied by chest pain and shortness of breath, you might suspect myocardial infarction and act accordingly. (See *MI: emergency intervention.*)

During your assessment, try to calm the patient as much as possible. Suggest relaxation techniques, and talk to him in a reassuring, soothing voice. (See *Relaxation techniques.*) Remember that uncontrolled anxiety can alter vital signs and often exacerbate the causative disorder.

If the patient displays mild or moderate anxiety, ask about its duration. Is his anxiety constant or sporadic? Did he notice any precipitating factors? Find out if his anxiety is exacerbated by stress, lack of sleep, or excessive caffeine intake, and alleviated by rest, tranquilizers, or exercise.

Obtain a complete medical history, especially noting drug use. Then perform a physical examination, focusing on any complaints that may trigger or be aggravated by anxiety.

If the patient's anxiety isn't accompanied by significant physical signs, suspect a psychological cause. Assess the patient's level of consciousness and observe his behavior. If appropriate, refer him for psychiatric evaluation. (See also *Panic attacks.*)

Anxiety: counseling

Providing good support

Before you can help a patient cope with fear, determine why he reacts the way he does by answering as many of the following questions as possible:
• Does he seem to have only one or two coping mechanisms?
• Is he an introvert or an extrovert?
• How does he usually handle stress?
• Does he talk warmly about his family and friends, or does he criticize them?
• Does he have someone to confide in?
• Who makes the decisions in his family?
• Has he ever had a serious illness before?
• Have any of his family or friends been seriously ill? What was the outcome of the illness?
• Does he think a sick person should be the center of attention?
• Does he think illness is a sign of weakness?
• Does he think chronic illness makes a person less deserving of love?
• Does he expect his present illness to leave him an invalid?
• Does he expect to be completely cured?
• Does he expect others to take care of *all* his needs, even those he should be able to meet himself?
• Does he believe the doctor is the only caregiver who can share medical information or help with a problem?
    Obtaining answers to these questions will help you help him. (See also *Anxiety: detection.*)

Anxiety: detection

Understanding patients' fears

Here's a two-part therapeutic interview technique that works won-

ders. It requires more than simply being a good listener—you must set specific goals for yourself and your patient and consciously direct each interview. Follow these steps.
    First, you need to uncover the problem. Try to help your patient verbalize his fears. Then determine if they're rational or not and validate the ones that are. Since most people are fearful *before* they're even admitted to the hospital, the earlier you schedule this meeting, the better. Ask the patient's spouse or a close family member or friend to be present.
    Explain that your interview will last about 15 minutes. Then gradually introduce the subject of fear, using open-ended statements such as: "I'd like to discuss any worries or concerns you might have" or "Many patients have worries. Can you tell me if anything's bothering you?" A few of your patients may admit right away that something's worrying them.
    But if your patient's reluctant to talk or if he hasn't had time to clarify his fears in his own mind yet, he may need gentle encouragement. Name some common fears, such as fear of pain, disfigurement, disability, and death. Then ask if he's feeling them. Many patients also have secondary fears—of suffering indignities while hospitalized, facing restrictions in their life-styles, or becoming a burden to their families after discharge, for example.
    After you find out what your patient's fears are, you can then decide whether they're rational or not.
    Rational fear is a *normal* response to a legitimate threat. A woman who's had one breast removed and worries about developing breast cancer in the other breast is experiencing a rational fear. But a woman with no family history of breast cancer who's convinced she'll develop it is exhibiting an irrational fear.
    If you decide that your patient's fear is rational, validate it: Convey that such a reaction is completely understandable and normal.

Conclude the first interview by briefly summarizing your discussion. Then schedule a second interview—on the same day, if possible—to discuss how the patient can cope with his fears.
    Now you're ready to offer solutions. Help your patient learn how to cope with his fears by teaching him techniques such as deep breathing or visualization and imagery.
    Suggest biofeedback to control body responses to fear. But simply giving more information about his condition may be the only intervention necessary. (See *Anxiety: counseling.*)

Aortic dissection

Crisis intervention

Stay with the patient and call for another nurse. Ask someone to contact his doctor. Although you're trying to stabilize him, his condition may rapidly deteriorate. Cardiac tamponade is one of the most devastating secondary effects of aortic dissection, so ask for a crash cart and pericardiocentesis tray. And watch for signs of cardiac tamponade—decreasing blood pressure and pulsus paradoxus. (See also *Cardiac tamponade.*)
    While delegating nursing activities, watch the patient for changes that indicate the dissection is progressing, such as confusion, ab-

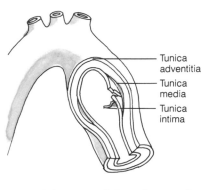

Tunica adventitia
Tunica media
Tunica intima

normal heart and breath sounds, significantly different blood pressure readings between the arms, decreased peripheral pulses, and increased pain.

Direct your co-workers to administer oxygen by nasal cannula at 4 liters/minute. Obtain a 12-lead ECG. Continue to monitor the patient's heart rhythm with a cardiac monitor, and hook him up to an automatic blood pressure machine (See *Blood pressure monitoring.*) Call for a stat chest X-ray. Insert two large-bore I.V. cannulas. Make sure a multiple-speed infusion pump is available. Draw blood for stat electrolyte, blood urea nitrogen, and creatinine tests; a complete blood count; cardiac enzyme analysis; and typing and cross matching. Insert an indwelling urinary catheter and obtain a specimen for urinalysis.

The rapidity and extent of an aortic dissection depend on the force of the patient's blood pressure. If your patient's blood pressure is high, his doctor will probably order antihypertensive drugs to bring his systolic pressure down to about 100 to 120 mm Hg. The drop in blood pressure will also help to ease the patient's pain, but the doctor may want to give morphine to control both pain and anxiety.

The doctor may also order nitroprusside (Nipride) or trimethaphan camsylate (Arfonad). Both drugs will decrease preload and afterload. Nipride is a short-acting antihypertensive that begins to work instantly, but it also increases heart rate. Propranolol (Inderal) may also be added to counteract the reflex tachycardia induced by the Nipride.

You may give these medications in D_5W. Start the infusion of Nipride at 0.5 to 10 mcg/kg/minute. Your patient's blood pressure should start to drop within 5 minutes. Administer 1 to 3 mg of Inderal not to exceed 1 mg/minute. If you're using Arfonad, start the infusion at 1 to 2 mg/minute. The patient's blood pressure should drop within 5 to 10 minutes. To enhance Arfonad's hypotensive effects, place 4" to 6" (10 to 15 cm) blocks under the head of the patient's bed. Remember, before you administer any of these medi-

cations or titrate the doses, check his blood pressure and heart rate.

What to do later

After you start the patient's blood therapy, transfer him to the ICU or take him immediately to the angiography department for an aortogram. Make sure the operating room is on standby. Talk with the patient's family about what has happened and what's likely to occur in the next few hours.

Apnea

Emergency actions

Your first priority is to establish and maintain a patent airway. Position the patient supine and open his airway using the head-tilt/chin-lift technique. If he has an obvious or suspected head or neck injury, use the jaw-thrust technique to avoid hyperextending his neck. (See *Jaw-thrust maneuver.*)

Next, quickly look, listen, and feel for spontaneous respirations. If they're absent, begin artificial ventilation until spontaneous respirations resume or until mechanical ventilation can be started.

Because apnea may result from cardiac arrest (or may cause it), assess the patient's carotid pulse immediately after you've established a patent airway. (See *Carotid artery: palpation.*) If the patient is an infant or small child, assess the brachial pulse. If you can't palpate a pulse, begin cardiopulmonary resuscitation.

Once you're satisfied that the patient's respirations and cardiac status are stable, begin to investigate what caused the apnea. The most common causes include trauma, cardiac arrest, neurologic disease, aspiration of foreign objects, bronchospasm, and drug overdose.

Ask the patient (or, if he can't answer, anyone who witnessed the episode) about the onset of apnea and the events immediately preceding it. Next, take a history, noting especially any reports of headache,

chest pain, muscle weakness, sore throat, or dyspnea. Ask about any history of respiratory, cardiac, or neurologic disease and about allergies and drug use.

Inspect the patient's head, face, neck, and trunk for soft tissue injury, hemorrhage, or skeletal deformity. Don't overlook obvious clues. Oral and nasal secretions, for example, indicate fluid-filled airways and alveoli. Facial soot and singed nasal hair suggest thermal injury to the tracheobronchial tree.

Auscultate over all lung fields for adventitious breath sounds, particularly crackles and gurgles, and percuss the lung fields for increased dullness or hyperresonance. Move on to the heart, auscultating for murmurs, pericardial friction rub, and dysrhythmias. Check for cyanosis, pallor, jugular venous distention, and edema.

If appropriate, perform a neurologic assessment. Evaluate the patient's level of consciousness and orientation. Test cranial nerve function and motor function, sensation, and reflexes in all extremities. (See *Neurologic exam: assessment.*)

Appendicitis

Assessment and intervention

Your patient will need surgery once the diagnosis of appendicitis has been confirmed. If his temperature's elevated, expect to administer antipyretics to reduce it. Place him in the Fowler's position to reduce his pain and make him as comfortable as possible. Avoid giving him large doses of pain medications because these may mask symptoms of perforation. Continue I.V. fluids to keep him hydrated. Make sure you *don't* apply heat to his lower right quadrant, and *don't* give him enemas or cathartics. *These may cause the appendix to rupture.* Give him nothing by mouth. While you're preparing him for surgery, explain the procedure to him and his family.

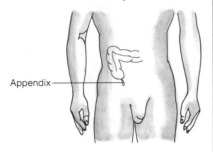

Appendix

If the patient's appendix ruptures before surgery and he has signs and symptoms of peritonitis, you'll also need to monitor his fluid and electrolytes carefully and to give replacements I.V. Administer antibiotics, as ordered.

Appraisals: management

Getting feedback on your performance

If you want to know how you're doing—as team leader, head nurse, or supervisor—turn the tables on your staff nurses.

Ask them to fill out a review form, rating your performance as a manager, but not signing their name. Here are some questions you might include:
• Does your supervisor show interest in you as an individual?
• Is she a good listener who tries to understand your point of view?
• Does she give you understanding and support when you're having a bad day?
• Does she make sure you get the training you need for new procedures?
• Does she assign work clearly and fairly?
• Does she set a good example with her appearance, attendance, punctuality, and commitment?
• Does she encourage questions and complaints about the way the unit's run?
• Is she receptive to suggestions?

• Does she give criticism in a fair, considerate manner?
• Does she admit her mistakes?
• Does she discuss your performance and how it'll be measured before review time?
• Does she give your review on schedule?

Appraisals: records

Keeping notes

When you have to evaluate other staff members, make your task easier by keeping a written log of incidents related to their performance. Then, when it's time to write a formal evaluation, you'll have all the concrete information you need.
Here are some hints:
• Write your notes regularly—for example, twice a week.
• List enough specific information about the incident so you can remember it clearly a few months later. This is particularly important when you're doing an employee's annual evaluation.
• Document both good and poor performances equally. Notes that reflect only all positives or all negatives can be unfair.
• Don't write a note immediately after an incident—especially if it's negative. Wait until the next day, when you're more detached.

Appraisals: technique

Giving your reviews constructively

To be fair when giving employee evaluations, avoid these 10 common errors:
1. Clustering everyone in the middle—keeping employees close to the middle point on a rating scale. (This may result from the fear of rating too high or too low.)
2. Latest behavior myopia—focusing only on recent events and

overlooking past problems or accomplishments. (This error usually occurs when employees are rated every 6 or 12 months.)
3. Spillover effect—allowing past evaluations to boost or diminish a current rating, even though the employee's performance has changed.
4. Leniency—awarding high ratings to avoid conflict.
5. Strictness—being overly critical.
6. Stereotyping or clinging to first impressions—giving more weight to conscious or unconscious stereotypes or prejudices than to the employee's actual performance.
7. Halo effect—rating all aspects of an employee's performance based on a single positive trait. (Example: giving a staff nurse high ratings across the board because she has good communication skills.)
8. Horn effect—letting one poor rating influence other ratings, leading to a lower overall evaluation.
9. Projection—giving higher ratings to people who are like you and lower ratings to those who aren't. (Example: "She reminds me of myself when I first started out, a real go-getter.")
10. Comparative judgment—basing an employee's evaluation on a comparison with others. (This wouldn't be fair if another employee's ratings were inflated because of favorable circumstances, not actual performance.)

Arterial puncture

Recommended techniques for blood gas analysis

To perform an arterial puncture for blood gas analysis, you'll need the following equipment: a 10-ml glass Luer-Lok syringe with a cork or capping device; 1 ml of aqueous heparin (1:1,000); one ½" needle (22- or 23-gauge); povidone-iodine (Betadine) and alcohol sponges; a 4" × 4" gauze pad; 1-inch adhesive dressing or tape; and an iced specimen bag with label. (Kits contain-

A

ing all the necessary equipment are available.)

Heparinizing the needle and syringe

Before entering the patient's room, heparinize the syringe and needle to help prevent the specimen from clotting on its way to the laboratory. Here's how: After washing your hands, attach a 22- or 23-gauge needle to the syringe. Draw 1 ml of heparin into the syringe while simultaneously pulling the plunger back past the 7-ml mark and rotating the barrel. Then, holding the syringe upright and tilting it slightly to prevent heparin from running down the side of the needle, force the heparin toward the syringe hub and expel all but 0.1 ml. Finally, push the plunger all the way up to eject the remaining heparin.

Choosing a site

The radial artery is the best artery to use when drawing arterial blood specimens for blood gas analysis. It's a superficial artery that's easily accessible, and isn't located directly over a vein. (Arterial blood specimens may also be drawn from the brachial or femoral arteries—in most cases by a doctor.)

Another advantage of using the radial artery is the presence of the ulnar artery. This artery allows for collateral circulation in case of injury to the radial artery— the greatest hazard of drawing arterial blood. Because an injury to the radial artery could occlude circulation to the surrounding tissue, you must always use the Allen's test to assess ulnar artery circulation before performing a radial puncture. (See *Allen's test.*)

Performing the puncture

After explaining the procedure to the patient, choosing the site, and performing the Allen's test, you're ready to obtain the specimen. Before you start, get into a comfortable position, sitting or kneeling, so you don't have to lean over or turn awkwardly to reach the site. Then, perform the following steps:

• Hyperextend the patient's wrist over a rolled towel for support.

• After washing your hands thoroughly, palpate the site with your first two fingers held slightly apart. Take your time to get a "feel" for the location of the sides and center of the artery, noting the strength of the pulsations. Then, prepare the site with Betadine and alcohol, according to your hospital's policy.

• Palpate again with one finger, holding the needle at a 45-degree angle over the radial artery. Then with the bevel up to avoid arterial trauma, carefully puncture the skin. (You may find it easier to anchor the artery by holding your fingers on each side of the vessel. Then, enter the artery between your finger tips with the needle at a 45-degree angle.) If the arterial puncture is successful, blood will automatically fill the syringe.

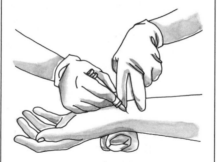

• You might see a momentary flow of blood into the hub of the needle that stops before the syringe fills. This may indicate that you've penetrated the artery or rested the needle against the arterial wall. If this happens, pull the needle back gently and slowly. To avoid arterial damage or getting a venous sample, don't draw back on the barrel of the syringe. If you note swelling of the area while moving the needle, withdraw the syringe and apply pressure. If the patient's blood pressure is low, you may have to draw back on the plunger to obtain the specimen.

• After you've drawn 3 to 5 ml of blood, withdraw the needle. (If you can't get more than a 2-ml specimen, ask the laboratory to run a microsample.) Then, apply pressure to the site for at least 5 minutes or for 15 minutes or more if the

patient's receiving anticoagulant therapy or has a prolonged clotting time. Apply a pressure bandage over the puncture site when the bleeding has stopped.

• An air bubble in the specimen can alter PaO_2 and $PaCO_2$ measurements. To eject an air bubble, tap the syringe lightly with your finger. If the bubble remains, hold the syringe upright and force some of the blood out of the syringe after piercing a $2'' \times 2''$ gauze pad with the needle to catch the blood.

• Insert the needle into the rubber stopper, or remove the needle and place the rubber cap on the needle hub, to prevent the specimen from leaking and to keep air out of the syringe.

• Put the labeled specimen in the ice-filled bag. Attach a request slip and send the specimen to the laboratory immediately.

Arthritis aids

Making crocheting and writing painless

For an elderly patient who has arthritis, holding a crochet hook can become painful and difficult. Rather than let her abandon her favorite pastime, make grips for the hooks with small Styrofoam balls. Simply poke a hook through a ball, and let the patient slide the ball to a position on the hook where she can grip it comfortably and move if efficiently.

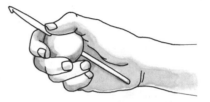

This idea can be adapted for pens and pencils, too. Experiment with different-sized Styrofoam balls until you find one that gives your patient the most comfortable grip. (See also *Shampooing: arthritic patient.*)

Ascites

Distinguishing it from other causes of distention

To differentiate ascites from other causes of distention, check for shifting dullness, fluid wave, or puddle sign, as described here.

Shifting dullness

1. With the patient supine, percuss from the umbilicus outward to the flank. Draw a line on the patient's skin to mark the change from tympany to dullness (See *Abdominal exam: percussion.*)

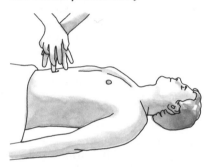

2. Turn him onto his side, which causes any ascitic fluid to shift. Percuss again and mark the change from tympany to dullness. Any difference between these lines can indicate ascites.

Fluid wave

Have another nurse press deeply into the patient's midline to prevent

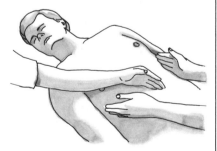

vibration from traveling along the abdominal wall. Place one of your palms on one of the patient's flanks. Strike the opposite flank with your other hand. If you feel the blow in the opposite palm, ascitic fluid is present.

Puddle sign

Position the patient on his elbows and knees, which will cause any

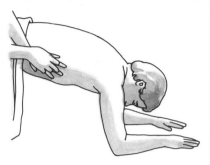

ascitic fluid to pool in the most dependent part of the abdomen. Percuss the abdomen from the flank to the midline. The percussion note becomes louder at the edge of the puddle, or ascitic pool.

Assertive behavior

Using nonverbal language to get what you want

If you find yourself agreeing to do things you don't want to do, you're not alone. Many nurses have a hard time saying no—to doctors, managers, co-workers, patients, and family members. But not standing up in the face of pressure from others can lead to burnout, fatigue, overwork, and a poor self-image. Here's how to stand up for yourself:

First, learn to speak in a normal voice. Some people know what they want, but they have so little confidence about expressing their wishes that they whisper. Others get so nervous—or so angry at the thought that they might not get their wishes—they *shout* their message. A moderate volume is most effective.

Second, plan what you're going to say so you won't stammer or stutter—and thus make other people think you don't really believe you deserve what you're asking for.

Third, look at the person you're talking to and make sure your posture and facial expression give the same message as your words. If you're angry, look the other person

in the eye. Don't look at your feet or at the other person's chin. If you're serious, don't smile.

And whatever your feelings, stand up straight and keep your arms relaxed at your side, not closed across your chest or in your pockets. The more relaxed and in control you look, the more relaxed and in control you'll feel.

Fourth, stand close enough to the person you're talking to so he knows he's the one you're addressing.

Fifth, fit your behavior to the situation. Let's say you've always provided coffee for one of the doctors when he asked for it. In the past, you've been afraid to say no. Today, you decide you're not going to be the "gofer" anymore. But don't launch into a speech about your proper responsibilities in front of the entire medical staff—a situation sure to embarrass and anger the doctor. Instead, wait till you and the doctor are alone to discuss your proper responsibilities. (See *Assertiveness.*)

Assertiveness

Standing up for yourself

Learning to be assertive is easier when you break the process down into manageable steps. Assess your current style. Get a notebook and jot down any situations that leave you feeling used or uncomfortable during the week. Describe what you did and how you felt as objectively as possible.

Analyze your nonverbal and verbal behavior. For example, how did you speak to the other person? How loudly? Did you look the person in the eye? Did you agree to do what the person asked or did you refuse?

Start looking for patterns. Do you frequently avoid looking people in the eye? Do you make excuses about why you can't do something—instead of saying you don't *want* to?

Write down what you wish you'd done—and why you didn't.

A

Think of someone you respect who asserts herself, and observe the way she handles herself. This will help you imagine yourself as an assertive person. When you see how others respond to your role model, you'll gain courage. You'll see that people don't ignore her, get mad at her, call her names behind her back, or do any of the other things you may fear. Most people respect her for her honesty. And they'll feel the same way about you.

Think of a situation where you'd like to be assertive. The less important the situation, the better. Now, imagine your usual reaction to that situation. If you're nonassertive, you probably say nothing. If you're aggressive, you probably raise your voice. Map out the ways you could respond to the situation more assertively.

Imagine yourself choosing an assertive response. Think about the nonverbal behavior you'd use. Then, practice your assertive response out loud until you're comfortable saying the actual words. The more you practice, the better you'll look—and sound.

Practice your assertive response with a friend, too. She can see nonassertive behavior you might not see in yourself. She can also respond in various ways to your assertiveness so you get a feel for what may happen in public.

Try it out. Once you've chosen an assertive response and practiced, you have to take the big step and try it out. Of course, you can't go looking for someone to jump in front of you at the bank. But similar situations crop up often, so you shouldn't have trouble practicing. (See *Assertive behavior.*)

Asthma

Preventing acute attacks

The key to managing asthma is preventing airway irritation. Review these preventive measures with your asthmatic patient:

"Seek treatment if you notice signs or symptoms of bacterial or viral infection. Get a flu inoculation every year and a pneumococcal inoculation every 5 years.

"Keep your home as dust-free as possible.

Cross sections of bronchioles

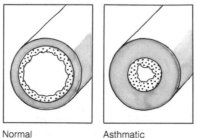

Normal   Asthmatic

"Don't let yourself become dehydrated as this would make your airways more susceptible to irritation. But limit your intake of coffee, tea, and alcohol because all of these can have a diuretic effect.

"Avoid excesses of aspirin, tartrazine (yellow dye #5), and exercise. They can trigger an attack.

"Know the signs and symptoms of infection (increased coughing with sputum, fever, and malaise) and bronchial irritation (increased coughing without sputum or with decreased sputum, increased shortness of breath, and wheezing). If any of these signs and symptoms occur, you should retrace your steps for the previous 24 hours to try identifying the offending substance. Also, perform bronchial hygiene techniques. If these signs and symptoms persist for 24 hours, notify your doctor."

Autonomic dysreflexia

Helping the quadriplegic patient

Some quadriplegic patients can develop severe hypertension caused by autonomic dysreflexia. If that happens, the patient could develop an intracerebral hemorrhage and die. If you can locate the noxious stimulus (usually caused by bladder or bowel distention or skin irritation), you can bring the patient's blood pressure back to normal.

Symptoms you might find are a bright red face and neck, heavy perspiration, pale and cool skin, irregular pulse, and high blood pressure. You must quickly locate and remove the stimulus that's causing this reaction.

First, elevate the head of his bed. Because his spinal cord is injured, he'll probably have an exaggerated orthostatic hypotensive response. Take his blood pressure and leave the cuff on his arm so you can check it every 3 to 5 minutes. Summon help, and tell the nurse who responds to page a doctor. Ask her to get a urinary catheter kit, nonsterile gloves, a lubricant, and an anesthetic cream or ointment. Stay with him and reassure him that you know what's wrong and that you're taking steps to correct the problem.

Now, begin a systematic search for the cause of the response. Be sure to have someone monitor his blood pressure to determine the effect of your interventions. Bladder irritation or distention is the most common stimulus, so start by examining his catheter for kinks. Irrigate the catheter with normal saline solution to determine patency. If it's clogged and irrigation doesn't help, remove the catheter and do a straight catheterization at once.

If the patient has no catheter in place, do a straight catheterization. Don't perform Credé's maneuver, which would increase stimulation. (See *Credé's maneuver.*)

If you rule out a bladder problem, digitally examine the rectum for fecal impaction. (See *Rectal exam.*) A word of caution: To prevent the digital exam from causing further stimulation, first apply an anesthetic around the anus and in the rectum. If you find an impaction, gently remove it.

If your assessment of the bladder and bowel reveals no problems, examine his skin, especially over pressure points. Look for reddened areas, rashes, and ulcerations. If you think his position is causing pain or pressure, reposition him.

Recheck his blood pressure. If it remains elevated, you must administer a rapidly acting antihypertensive. Get an order for diazoxide (Hyperstat), hydralazine (Apresoline), or a similar drug used for hypertensive emergencies.

After giving the drug, continue to monitor his blood pressure. Make sure a vasopressor has also been ordered; if you find and remove the stimulus after administering the antihypertensive, his blood pressure may drop significantly.

Later, monitor his pulse and blood pressure every 1 to 2 hours for the next 8 hours, more frequently if you administered an antihypertensive. Explain to him what happened; he's probably very frightened. Reassure him that the problem can be prevented.

Document the incident, including your assessment, interventions, and the patient's response to each intervention. Be sure to discuss what happened with all health care professionals caring for him. Patients who've already experienced autonomic dysreflexia are more likely to do so again.

Autotransfusion problems

Preventing them

Despite its advantages, autotransfusion can cause complications. To avoid them, follow these guidelines.
Embolism prevention
• Check the entire system for air leaks before reinfusing blood.
• Use extra in-line micropore filters.
• Administer corticosteroids, as or-

dered, when performing massive autotransfusion.
Hemolysis prevention
• Keep the suction device tip below the blood's surface (preferably at the bottom of the blood pool) to decrease blood-air contact.
• Limit suction pressure to 15 mm Hg.
• Try to prevent acidosis, dehydration, and shock.
Sepsis prevention
• Don't reinfuse shed blood that's been stored for more than 4 hours.
• Never add autotransfusion blood to the donor pool (autotransfusion blood can't be stored).
• Use in-line micropore filters to trap contaminants.
• Don't perform autotransfusion if you know or suspect that your patient has a systemic or cardiopulmonary infection, a cancerous lesion in the hemorrhage area, or a thoracoabdominal injury with possible intestinal contamination, or if he has any signs or symptoms of GI tract disruption.
• If you suspect your patient may be developing an infection, give broad-spectrum systemic antibiotics, as ordered.
• Never use the same autotransfusion device for two patients. Discard the entire device when your patient no longer needs it.
Coagulopathy prevention
• Add an anticoagulant, such as citrate phosphate dextrose, as ordered.
• Try to avoid transfusing more than 4,000 ml of blood. If you must transfuse more, supplement it with fresh-frozen plasma and platelets, as ordered.
Equipment malfunction prevention
• Don't let furniture, bed linens, or other items block the autotransfusion device's atmospheric vent.
• When using the Receptal ATS, check for drainage overflow into the Receptaseal canister to prevent valve malfunction. (See *Autotransfusion system.*)

Autotransfusion system

Setting one up properly

Autotransfusion—the collection, filtration, and infusion of a patient's own blood—is being performed in more and more emergency departments and trauma centers today, most commonly for hemothorax. The reasons are basic: It's fast and it's safe. Here's how to set up the Receptal ATS Trauma System, one of the most widely used autotransfusion systems:

1. Gather the following equipment: suction apparatus; 1,900-ml rigid plastic canister that attaches to a standard I.V. pole; chest tube with suction tubing; sterile collection and infusion liner; microemboli blood filter tubing; 500-ml bottle of anticoagulant citrate phosphate dextrose (CPD) solution; and burette I.V. tubing.

2. The sterile liner used for collecting and infusing blood, which also has a 1,900-ml volume capacity, fits into the plastic canister. A smaller reservoir bag is located inside the larger one—this filters the blood as it is collected.

3. Place the liner inside the plastic canister, snapping the lid on tightly so air can't leak out.

4. Connect the tubing on the liner lid to the suction apparatus, using the sterile spacer joined to the canister tee. (If a wall unit isn't available, use any suction source.)

5. Attach the chest drainage tubing to the port on top of the liner lid. Later, you'll connect the capped end of the tubing to the chest tube.

6. Open the bottle of CPD solution, remove its diaphragm, and attach the I.V. burette, using sterile technique. Then hang the bottle and burette on the I.V. pole. Remove the yellow cap from the anticoagulant connector on the distal end of the chest drainage tubing.

B

7. Attach the flushed line from the bottle of CPD solution and burette to the anticoagulant connector. Prime the burette with 100 ml of I.V. solution; set the drip rate so 25 to 60 ml of CPD solution mixes with every 500 ml of blood collected.

8. The autotransfusion system is now assembled and ready to use, once the doctor inserts the chest tube. When the tube is inserted, turn on the suction to 10 to 30 mm Hg—gentle suction won't damage red blood cells.

Blood collection

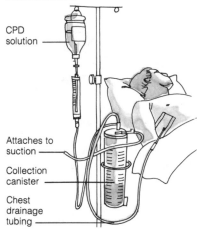

CPD solution

Attaches to suction

Collection canister

Chest drainage tubing

9. Monitor the patient as blood aspirated from his chest collects in the sterile liner. When between 500 and 1,000 ml of blood are collected, you're ready to begin infusing.

10. After clamping the chest tube to prevent pneumothorax, disconnect the chest drainage tubing attached to the anticoagulant connector from the port on top of the liner lid.

11. Remove and discard the sterile spacer.

12. Remove the liner from the canister, squeezing out the air. Clamp the liner lid tubing, and cap the port on the lid with the tubing connector.

13. To begin the infusion, remove the white cap at the bottom of the liner, then insert a 40-micron blood filter tubing into the liner, and prime the tubing. (You can use any standard I.V. blood tubing to filter clots

and debris from the blood as it's infused.)

14. The patient's blood is infused by gravity through a peripheral I.V. line. A central I.V. line may also be used. The rate of infusion depends on the patient's clinical condition and doctor's orders. (See *Autotransfusion problems; Blood transfusion technique.*)

Bandage, roller

Wrapping one

Follow this procedure when wrapping a roller bandage:
• Don't wrap the bandage too tight; excessive pressure can interfere with circulation and nerve function.
• Don't cover the patient's fingers and toes; you won't be able to perform a neurovascular assessment.
• Use the proper size bandage.
• Wrap from the distal to the proximal part of the arm or leg to promote venous return.

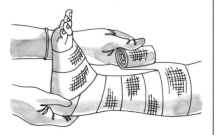

• Keep the unrolled part of the bandage close to the arm or leg to give you more control and to maintain even pressure as you wrap.
• Use spiral turns, covering one-third to one-half of each previous wrap.
• Check distal pulses and capillary refill.
• Remind the patient to elevate and rest the bandaged arm or leg.

Bathing

Teaching immobilized patients

For a patient who has one arm or one hand immobilized, using a washcloth is difficult. A sponge will be easier for him to handle. It'll fit into his hand, can be wrung out easily, and won't require folding as a washcloth does.

A sponge is also effective for arthritic patients, since the squeezing action helps loosen up stiff joints.

Battered women

Understanding their dilemma

When you suspect battering, immediately take the victim someplace where you can speak privately. If she has come to the hospital with her partner, you might hear some objections but they'll probably come from him, not her. Most battered women welcome an opportunity to talk. If he asks to stay, tell him matter-of-factly, "I need to talk to your wife (or girlfriend), to check her. We'll come back when we're finished."

When you're alone, ask her compassionately what happened. If she's reluctant to speak, gently point out how the bruise on her neck, for instance, doesn't fit in with her tripping on the sidewalk. Or ask her why she didn't seek treatment for these injuries earlier.

And don't be afraid to use such words as "battered," "abused," or "hit." You might say, for example, "A lot of women are ashamed to say their husband hit them. If that's what happened, don't be ashamed to share it with me."

Tell her that many women are battered. If she says anything about being at fault, assure her that she didn't deserve to be beaten because of it. Criticize the beating but not the man who did it.

• Encourage her to talk about her family life and job. Stir up her self-confidence by pointing out her strengths.

• Help her understand the effects that violence can have on her children.

• Help her explore her options. Ask her where she plans to go after leaving the hospital. If she doesn't want to go home but says she's too ashamed to stay with a relative or friend, try to help her ease these feelings. If she still resists taking your advice, give her the names of a women's shelter, YWCA, and other social agencies that can offer help.

Be sure to give her this information as well as any pamphlets you have on local resources, even if she denies she's been abused.

Now, what of the woman who wants to go home? Try—almost like one friend to another—to find out if she thinks she'll really be safe. Just thinking about it may help change her mind. But if she still wants to go home, arguing with her won't stop her; it's just another thing that will convince her you don't understand.

Instead, help her plan for a fast escape if the man tries to batter her again. Discuss whom she should call and where she should go. And encourage her to pack an emergency bag with such things as extra money, clothes, a spare set of car keys, and important papers. Now besides knowing what to do, she's prepared, and your advice may give her the courage to take action. (See *Battering.*)

Battering

Recognizing the signs

Battering is so common that you should assume it in any woman with trauma until you get evidence to the contrary. Be suspicious if you note any of these signs in the history or physical examination:

• The patient's injuries don't match her story. Would she, you should ask

yourself, be likely to suffer these fractures and lacerations in a fall down the stairs? In fact, multiple injuries should *always* be suspected.

• Her injuries are at multiple stages of healing, indicating she's been injured previously.

• The present injuries are several hours or even days old. Battered women often wait for the right opportunity—perhaps when their husband or boyfriend goes to work—to seek medical help.

• She has abdominal injuries and is either pregnant or has spontaneously aborted. Many women feel that their husbands or boyfriends deliberately beat them to make them abort. To many of these men, a new child only means new problems and new stresses.

• If she comes in with her husband or boyfriend and seems especially uneasy with him. Perhaps she glances at him in a frightened way or flinches when he moves.

• She has a history of somatic or emotional complaints. These may be related to the stresses of being battered or perhaps to her turning to drugs or alcohol as an escape.

• She was abused as a child.

• She refers to her partner as jealous, a drinker, or a drug user.

• She says her injuries are too insignificant to have warranted medical attention. Although she hasn't come right out and said she's been abused, this may be her cry for help. (See *Battered women.*)

Bed positioning

Helping weak patients sit up in bed

What if one of your home care patients is a big man who's too debilitated to pull himself up in bed? Twist a flat bed sheet into a rope and place it across the bed, under the patient's shoulders. Bring the

ends of the sheet under his armpits, over his shoulders, and over the head of the bed. Then grip each end,

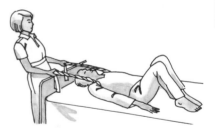

with the patient pushing with his feet, and pull him up in bed. (See *Bedridden patients.*)

Bedridden patients

Helping them with head elevation

A bedridden patient sometimes needs the head of his bed raised for comfort. Unless he's in a hospital bed, suggest the following:

• Wedge a bean-bag chair between the mattress and box spring. The chair will raise the head of the bed about 30 degrees.

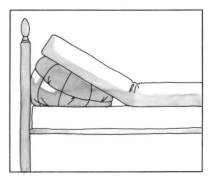

• Put a few boards or books under the legs at the head of the bed.

• Slant a wide board (or a few boards) from the middle of the bed to the top of the headboard. Then secure the boards to the headboard and bed to keep them in place, and pad the boards with sheets, blankets, and pillows.

Whatever method the patient chooses, he'll have the comfort of a hospital bed without the expense. (See also *Bed positioning.*)

Bed-wetting

Helping a child have dry nights

No single treatment for bed-wetting is always effective, but these recommendations for parents can help their child achieve bladder control.
• Restrict the child's fluid intake—especially of cola drinks—after supper.
• Make sure he urinates before bedtime. Wake him once during the night to go to the bathroom.
• Reward him after each dry night with praise and encouragement.
• Keep a progress chart, marking each dry night with a sticker. Reward a certain number of consecutive dry nights with a book, small toy, or special activity.
• Always give him emotional support. Never punish him if he wets the bed, but reassure him that he will learn to achieve bladder control. Remember that most children simply "outgrow" bed-wetting. However, periods of wet and dry nights will occur before he develops a constant pattern of dryness.

Bite, dog

Emergency intervention

Control bleeding, as needed. Support and splint the injured areas. For a laceration, assist with wound care—including thorough cleaning, debridement, and copious irrigation, usually with normal saline solution. The doctor may or may not suture the wound, although he'll probably suture a facial wound.

For a puncture wound, assist with cleaning and excising devitalized tissue; irrigation is not performed. (Alternatively, the entire wound may be excised and closed.)

If the dog is a stray, contact the local public health department to determine the need for rabies prophylaxis. Administer tetanus and rabies prophylaxis, as ordered.

Bite, human

What to do

Explore the wound to determine the depth and severity of the injury. Clean and irrigate it. Then, culture the wound site, and start antibiotic therapy, as ordered (usually with cephalosporins). Administer tetanus prophylaxis, as ordered. Assist with debridement of the infected wound or devitalized tissue, if ordered. The doctor probably won't close the wound unless it's on the patient's face.

Bite, tick

Nursing care

Remove the tick by covering it with a tissue or gauze pad saturated with alcohol or mineral oil, which blocks the tick's breathing pores and causes it to withdraw from the skin.

Wood tick	Deer tick

Approximate size 4mm	Approximate size 1mm

If the tick still doesn't withdraw after using alcohol or mineral oil, remove the tick with tweezers (make sure you get the entire tick).

Wash the area with soap and water, and apply an anesthetic. If the patient develops respiratory failure, assist with mechanical ventilation, as ordered.

Bladder assessment

Inspection, palpation, and percussion

You should assess the bladder only when it's full. Begin by inspecting the suprapubic area. Observe the contour of the patient's lower abdomen for bladder distention.

Now, palpate the bladder, starting at the umbilicus and moving toward

Bladder palpation

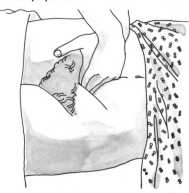

the symphysis pubis. You may palpate (and percuss) a full bladder as far up as the umbilicus. If the patient's bladder is greatly distended from urine retention, you may be able to palpate it above the umbilicus. In a patient with chronic urine retention, the bladder walls will feel flabby. (See *Palpation.*)

As you palpate, note any masses, which may indicate bladder lesions or calculi. If the patient feels pain during palpation, proceed carefully. Suprapubic pain or tenderness is often associated with cystitis.

Percussing the bladder can help you determine the degree of urine retention. Start percussing at the symphysis pubis, and move up toward the umbilicus. The farther up

Bladder percussion

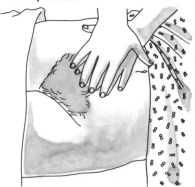

you continue hearing a dull percussion sound, the fuller the bladder. (See *Bladder distention.*)

Bladder distention

History taking and assessment

If the patient has *severe distention,* insert an indwelling urethral catheter, as ordered, to help relieve discomfort and prevent bladder rupture.

If distention isn't severe, begin your assessment by reviewing the patient's voiding patterns. Find out the time and amount of his last voiding and the amount of fluid consumed since then. Ask if he has difficulty initiating urination. Does he ever use Valsalva's or Credé's maneuver to initiate it? (See *Credé's maneuver; Valsalva's maneuver.*) Also ask if urination occurs with urgency or without warning and if it causes pain or irritation. Remember to ask about the force and continuity of his urine stream and if he feels that his bladder is empty after voiding.

Ask your patient if he has had a history of urinary tract obstruction or infections; sexually transmitted diseases; neurologic, intestinal, or pelvic surgery; lower abdominal or urinary tract trauma; and systemic or neurologic disorders. Note his drug history as well, including use of over-the-counter preparations.

Take his vital signs, and percuss and palpate his bladder. Remember that an empty bladder can't be palpated through the abdominal wall. (See *Bladder assessment.*) Inspect the urinary meatus and measure its diameter. Describe the appearance and amount of any discharge. Test for perineal sensation and anal sphincter tone, and in the male patient examine the prostate. Document your findings.

Bladder rupture

Quick intervention

Your trauma patient with a pelvic fracture has signs and symptoms pointing to either a ruptured bladder or a lacerated urethra. What should you do?

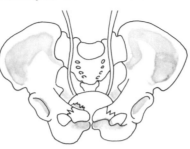

Don't insert a urinary catheter. If you do, a partial tear could become a complete one, introducing the risk of hemorrhage. Tell the doctor what you've discovered and wait for a urologist. He'll insert the catheter when he does a retrograde urethrogram or cystogram. Hematuria doesn't reflect the severity of an injury, so these studies will clarify if the patient has a ruptured bladder or a urethral tear.

Gently palpate her abdomen to identify any suprapubic mass or firmness and to assess her pain. (See *Abdominal exam: palpation.*) Examine her for vaginal bleeding; the bony spicule could also have lacerated her vagina. Check her bowel sounds frequently—if they're diminished or if the patient starts feeling nauseated and vomits, you can assume that the tear has led to intraperitoneal extravasation of urine. Insert a nasogastric tube and connect it to low intermittent suction to empty her stomach and prevent aspiration.

Draw blood for a complete blood count with differential, electrolyte profile, and blood urea nitrogen and creatinine levels. Closely monitor her vital signs for hypovolemic shock. (See *Shock: recognition.*) Remember, if she has a pelvic fracture, it can cause hemorrhaging. You may need to insert another large-bore (#14 or #16 French) catheter to start an I.V. infusion of lactated Ringer's or normal saline solution.

To check for occult blood, perform a dipstick test on any urine specimen you've obtained. Send it to the laboratory for culture and sensitivity testing. Antibiotics may be ordered as prophylaxis for her traumatic injuries.

If the cystogram reveals a ruptured bladder, the doctor will order surgery to repair the bladder, stabilize the fracture, and examine the vagina.

Bleeding disorders: assessment

Checking for thrombi and hemorrhage

If your patient has an acquired or congenital bleeding disorder, you need to:
• Measure intake and output hourly. Notify the doctor if urine output falls below 30 ml/hour. This could mean that acute tubular necrosis has developed secondary to thrombi, hemorrhage, or hypovolemia. Look for increased blood urea nitrogen and creatinine levels. Also look for hematuria.
• Assess every 1 to 2 hours for crackles, wheezes, stridor, dyspnea, tachypnea, cyanosis, and hemoptysis—these simple measures can help you detect early signs of respiratory failure caused by thrombi or hemorrhage. Help him cough and deep-breathe every 2 hours.
• Assess for changes in mental status every 3 to 4 hours. Look for confusion, lethargy, obtundation, coma, or seizures, all of which may be caused by cerebral hemorrhage or emboli.
• Assess for petechiae, purpura, and ecchymoses.
• Check frequently for changes in pulse, blood pressure, and peripheral perfusion. Note the color and temperature of his arms and legs and the presence of peripheral pulses. Inspect his skin for acrocyanosis. Monitor hematocrit and hemoglobin levels and any other coagulation studies.

Also assess every 4 hours for neck-vein distention, extra heart

B

sounds (S_3, S_4), and murmurs. Every 3 hours assess for thrombosis in the leg by checking for pain with dorsiflexion of the foot—Homans' sign. (See *Homans' sign*.) Also, look for bleeding from any body orifice or I.V. site. Test all stools, nasogastric drainage, vomitus, and urine for blood.

Help your patient with range of motion and position changes every 1 to 2 hours. Immobility predisposes him to thrombi formation, particularly if he has coagulopathy.

Check for shock caused by the rampant depositing of fibrin in the microcirculation. This will decrease venous return and consequently lower cardiac output. Clotting in the lungs can increase central venous pressure and produce signs of pulmonary edema.

Bleeding precautions

Teaching the high-risk patient

Explain to your patient that he's predisposed to bleeding because his blood lacks a clotting factor. Then teach him to:
• wear shoes at all times
• use a soft toothbrush
• use an electric shaver
• avoid cuts and puncture wounds
• advise his dentist and other health care practitioners of his bleeding disorder. (He will need cryoprecipitate prophylactically before certain dental and medical procedures.)

Teach him to recognize and report early signs of bleeding, such as bruising. Make sure he understands that he's not to take aspirin and he should always read the labels on medications to be sure they don't contain aspirin (a surprising number do).

How can he stop bleeding? Local measures include applying gentle pressure for at least 5 minutes, and possibly cold packs, also. If this doesn't work, he should call the doctor immediately.

Blind patients

Teaching them self-medication

If a blind patient is taking various medications in tablet form, and wants to take them himself, use this system: Using letters cut from sandpaper, label seven envelopes with the days of the week. Place the tablets in small Ziploc plastic bags labeled with sandpaper numbers, according to the time the tablets are to be taken. Then, place the bags inside the envelopes, and file the envelopes in a shoe box within his reach.

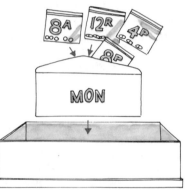

Each morning, he simply pulls the first envelope from the box, "reads" the numbers on the plastic bags with his fingers, and takes his tablets at the designated hours. He should have a braille clock or a radio to listen for the time.

This system not only gives him independence, but it also gives you an accurate way to tell whether he's taken all of his tablets.

Blood gases

Ensuring accurate test results

Even if your hospital policy doesn't allow you to draw arterial blood specimens (see *Arterial puncture*) for blood gas analysis, you're still responsible for ensuring an accurate report. Follow these guidelines:

• Take the patient's temperature and note it on the laboratory request slip as well as on the patient's chart. Temperature extremes will alter oxygen and carbon dioxide readings (especially if a patient's temperature is below 95° F. [35° C.] or above 102° F. [39° C.]). Knowing the patient's temperature will allow the laboratory to adjust for hypothermia or hyperthermia.
• If the patient's receiving oxygen, note and document the fraction of inspired oxygen. He must receive his prescribed oxygen concentration for at least 15 minutes before the blood's drawn. If no oxygen's in use, document that on the chart and laboratory request slip. Don't turn off a patient's oxygen to get a blood sample unless the doctor orders it.

A patient receiving positive end-expiratory pressure should be on the ventilator for at least 30 minutes before blood is drawn for analysis. Note any recent setting changes made on the ventilator.
• If possible, avoid suctioning the patient for at least 20 minutes before blood is drawn.
• Note and document activity and its effect on his respirations. Even such activity as morning care may cause labored breathing in a patient with chronic obstructive pulmonary disease, altering his arterial blood gas results.
• Because anxiety and accompanying hyperventilation can alter his $PaCO_2$ results, be calm and reassuring. Prepare the needle and ice outside the patient's room.
• Note if he's receiving (or has recently received) anticoagulant therapy. If so, you'll need to apply pressure to the puncture site for 15 minutes or longer.

Blood loss assessment

Taking serial extremity measurements

Use calipers instead of a tape measure so the patient won't have to lift the extremity you're measuring.

Let's say you're monitoring your patient's left arm.

• Using an indelible marker, put a dot on the arm's medial aspect, several inches above the injury site.

• Mark a second dot at a parallel site on the arm's lateral aspect. Continuing to move up from the injury site, mark pairs of dots—each pair 1 inch above the other—until your marks extend all the way up the arm.

• Now open the calipers and close the jaw's tips lightly on the pair of dots closest to the injury site.

• Read the measurement on the calipers' outer scale, document it, then repeat for each pair of dots.

• Repeat the measurement every 15 to 30 minutes or as ordered. Notify the doctor if you detect any increase in the arm's diameter. (See also *Blood loss measurement.*)

Blood loss measurement

Checking abdominal girth

Using a string (or tape measure), measure the distance across the patient's abdomen from one side of the hip to the other. If you're using a

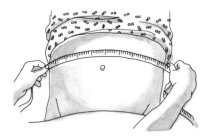

string, cut it, then remeasure every 15 minutes to determine if his abdominal girth has expanded. Or, pass a tape measure behind the patient's back and completely around his abdomen to measure its full circumference. (Don't use this method if moving the patient is contraindicated—for example, if he has a suspected spinal cord injury.)

For either method, use an indelible marker and measure the abdomen in the same place each time,

using the same reference points. Try marking your measurements on both sides of the tape to ensure accurate placement. (See *Blood loss assessment.*)

Blood pressure, orthostatic

Assessing for hypovolemia

Orthostatic vital signs may help you assess a patient with volume depletion or with a side effect of a medication.

Take your patient's blood pressure and pulse when he's supine, sitting, and standing. (Wait at least 1 minute between each position change.) Consider a systolic blood pressure decrease of 10 mm Hg or more between positions or a pulse rate increase of 10 beats/minute or more a sign of possible volume depletion or a side effect of a medication. (See *Blood pressure measurement.*)

Blood pressure measurement

Ensuring accuracy

When taking your patient's blood pressure, begin by applying the cuff properly. Then be alert for these common pitfalls:

• *Wrong size cuff.* Select the appropriate size cuff for your patient. For example, if the cuff bladder is too narrow, the reading will be falsely high. If the arm circumference is less than 13″ (33 cm), select a regular-sized cuff; if between 13″ and

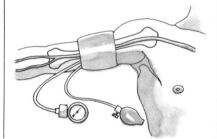

16½″ (41 cm), a large-sized cuff; if more than 16½″, a thigh cuff. Pediatric cuffs are also available.

• *Slow cuff deflation, causing venous congestion in the arm.* Don't deflate the cuff more slowly than 2 mm Hg/heartbeat or you'll get a spuriously high reading.

• *Cuff wrapped too loosely, reducing its effective width.* Tighten the cuff to avoid a falsely elevated reading.

• *Mercury column not read at eye level.* If the column is below eye level, you may record a falsely low reading; if it's above eye level, a falsely high reading.

• *Tilted mercury column.* Keep the mercury column vertical to avoid a spuriously high reading.

• *Poorly timed measurement.* Don't take blood pressure if the patient appears anxious or has just eaten or been walking; you'll get a falsely high reading.

• *Cuff overinflation, causing venospasm or pain.* You'll get a falsely high reading.

• *Inaudibility of feeble sounds.* Before reinflating the cuff, have the patient raise his arm to reduce venous pressure and to amplify low-volume sounds. After inflating the cuff, lower his arm. Then deflate the cuff and listen. Or, with his arm positioned at heart level, inflate the cuff and have him make a fist. Have him rapidly open and close his hand 10 times before you begin to deflate the cuff. Then listen. Be sure to document that the blood pressure reading was augmented. (See *Blood pressure monitoring.*)

Blood pressure monitoring

Using an automatic monitor

There are two commonly used blood pressure monitors—the continuous automatic blood pressure monitor and the ambulatory continuous automatic monitor. You're more likely to use the first one.

Its features include:
• mean arterial pressure (MAP) readout
• heart rate and minutes elapsed since the last cuff inflation
• systolic arterial pressure readout
• diastolic arterial pressure readout
• switches for setting the time interval between cuff inflations
• a switch for an immediate blood pressure readout
• a switch for setting high and low MAP alarm limits.

To use this monitor, apply the blood pressure cuff as you would for a manual reading. Then, turn on the machine and set the MAP limits and the time interval between cuff inflations (1 to 160 minutes).

When the preset time interval has elapsed, air passes through the hoses and automatically inflates the cuff to 160 mm Hg. The next cuff inflation will reach a pressure 35 mm Hg higher than the previous systolic reading.

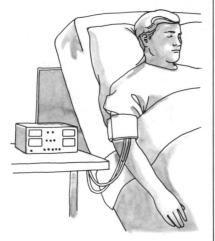

This highly sensitive system can detect blood pressures 2 to 6 mm Hg higher than you can palpate or auscultate. However, sometimes this sensitivity can cause problems. For example, if your patient flexes his arm while the cuff's deflating, you'll see an inaccurately high reading. To guard against this, make sure you take a baseline pressure reading when you first set up the monitor.

A patient's positional change can also cause a blood pressure rise

with the next readout. So, try to keep the patient in the same position he was in when you obtained baseline pressure. If you get a suspiciously high reading, always check the patient's position.

Keep these other important points in mind when using a continuous monitor:
• Check cuff position periodically. Use a proper size cuff. A cuff that slips from the proper position will cause an inaccurately low reading; a cuff that's too small, an inaccurately high reading.
• When you take manual blood pressure measurements to double-check monitor accuracy, always use the same arm to which the monitor was attached.
• If your patient's attached to an ECG machine that shows a higher pulse rate than the monitor, check the patient for cardiac dysfunction. The monitor detects only peripheral pulsations; it won't detect dysrhythmias such as premature ventricular contractions.
• Remember that although the machine's sensitive and reliable, it's no substitute for your expert nursing skills. Assess your patient frequently and intervene as necessary. (See *Blood pressure measurement.*)

Blood specimen: elderly patients

Tailoring your technique

Don't use a tourniquet to dilate an elderly patient's veins before performing a venipuncture. His veins may look healthy but may actually be quite fragile; a tourniquet could cause a hematoma when the needle pierces the vein.

Instead, have the patient hang his arm at his side for a few minutes while he opens and closes his fist. Then lightly tap the area around the vein to dilate it.

If you must use a tourniquet, use only light pressure.

Blood specimen: infants

Getting blood easily

If you have to get enough blood from an infant for a specimen, hold his feet in warm water for 5 to 10 minutes. (Better still, let his parent do the soak.) Then, with just one stick, you should be able to obtain an adequate specimen.

Blood transfusion, massive

Recognizing the hazards

Stored blood transfusions can save your patient's life when he's suffered serious GI bleeding. However, massive transfusions pose their own risks. Citrate-phosphate-dextrose, used to preserve whole blood, reduces blood's oxygen-carrying capacity. Also, storage causes various changes that may lead to complications (blood may be stored up to 35 days before transfusion).

If your patient's receiving massive transfusions, give him supplemental oxygen, as ordered, and monitor him carefully for the following complications:
• hyperkalemia (stored blood has a high potassium content from red blood cell aging)
• hypocalcemia (stored blood lacks ionized calcium)
• acid-base imbalance (stored blood acidifies gradually)
• ammonia intoxication (stored blood has an increased ammonia level)
• citrate intoxication (stored blood contains citrate, which binds to serum calcium)
• coagulation disturbances (stored blood may have low levels of platelets and other clotting factors)

• bacterial and viral infections (stored blood may come from infected donors)
• circulatory overload (from excessive volume replacement)
• hypothermia (from rapid infusion of cold blood). (See *Blood transfusion preparation; Blood transfusion reaction; Blood transfusion technique.*)

Blood transfusion preparation

Warming blood

Before you administer any blood to your patient, you might want to run it through a blood warmer. This is especially important if you're giving blood through a central line or if your patient's at high risk for hypothermia—for example, if he's very young, elderly, or suffering from multi-system disease or trauma.

Warming blood will:
• help prevent ventricular fibrillation from hypothermia
• help prevent a hypothermia-related decrease in metabolism of acid and potassium, which could lead to acidosis
• help minimize the patient's expenditure of energy to maintain normal body termperature. (Otherwise, his shock state will deepen as he struggles to get enough oxygen to counteract hypoxia from hypothermia.)

Adding a blood warmer to the equipment used to infuse blood or I.V. fluids may reduce the flow, but this is offset when the warmed fluid dilates the veins and decreases their resistance.

Never infuse *overheated* blood or fluids, which could overheat your patient's veins or cause hemolysis. Be sure the blood warmer you use has a built-in thermostat with an upper limit of 106.8° F. (41.6° C.). Never place blood components in a microwave oven for warming. (See also *Blood transfusion technique.*)

Blood transfusion reaction

Emergency care

A patient receiving blood calls out that he doesn't feel right—he has chills and a pain in his back. You stop the transfusion and quickly take his vital signs. His temperature is 102° F. (39° C.); his blood pressure, 96/62; his pulse, 128; and his respiratory rate, 32. He is experiencing a blood transfusion reaction.

Check to see if you've given the wrong blood by comparing the name and identification number on his wristband against the same information on the blood component identification tag. Hemolytic transfusion reactions almost always result from mismatched blood. The patient's chills and back pain are classic symptoms of an acute hemolytic reaction, as are fever, hypotension, tachycardia, tachypnea, and dyspnea. The earlier a reaction occurs during a transfusion, the more severe it's likely to be.

Let's say you discover that the blood is mismatched. First, disconnect the transfusion administration set from the I.V. device's hub. Begin administering normal saline solution to maintain the line's patency. Then call for the doctor and notify the blood bank of the patient's reaction. Briefly tell the patient what's happened and help him into an upright position to make breathing easier.

Next, working carefully, to avoid mechanical hemolysis, draw two tubes of blood from the arm that wasn't receiving the transfusion. (Or have a lab technician draw blood.) Send one sample to the blood bank along with a transfusion reaction slip, the bag containing the blood, and the blood administration set. Send the other sample to the laboratory so it can be tested for free hemoglobin in the plasma. Then obtain a urine specimen to be tested for hemoglobinuria. Be sure

to document his condition and your interventions.

Then, monitor him for signs and symptoms of shock; if they appear, place him in a supine position, call for an ECG technician to hook up the cardiac monitor, and begin administering oxygen. Insert an indwelling Foley catheter so you can monitor his urine output. Reassure him that more help is coming.

When the doctor arrives, tell him the patient's status. If urine output has dropped, he may order osmotic and diuretic drugs, such as mannitol and furosemide. He may also order dopamine to improve perfusion to vital organs. Infuse I.V. fluids and administer oxygen as ordered.

Later, continue to assess the patient's vital signs and general condition; monitor his intake and urine output hourly. His output should be at least 100 ml/hour for 24 hours to prevent renal tubular damage. If diuresis occurs, maintain his fluid volume with I.V. infusions. If diuresis fails to occur, he may need dialysis.

After the crisis, determine how the wrong blood was given and how this error could have been prevented. (See *Blood transfusion technique.*)

By following these guidelines, you can prevent most blood transfusion reactions. You may want to suggest that your hospital sponsor a staff-development program on the latest protocols for transfusions. (See also *Blood transfusion preparation; Blood transfusion, massive.*)

Blood transfusion technique

Doing it correctly

When you administer blood, always follow hospital policy and procedure. But keep these important guidelines in mind as well:
• Carefully compare patient and donor unit identification. Most hemolytic transfusion reactions associ-

B

ated with ABO mismatching stem from identification errors.
• Always administer blood through a filter that removes cellular debris (preferably a microaggregate filter).
• Always use normal saline solution to prime the tubing. Never mix a drug or another solution with blood. Once you begin the transfusion, monitor the patient for signs and symptoms of immediate transfusion reaction: fever, chills, hypotension, chest and lumbar pain, nausea, vomiting, wheal formation, eyelid edema, bronchospasm, hives, and itching.

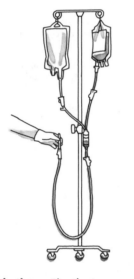

• Check the patient's temperature and vital signs before you start the transfusion. Notify the doctor of any temperature elevation and note any increase from baseline temperature, which may indicate transfusion reaction. Document baseline hemodynamic parameters, breath sounds, and urine output.
• Always warm banked blood to body temperature (98.6° F. [37° C.]) before administration for massive transfusions (replacement of 50% or more of the patient's blood volume at one time or replacement of the patient's total blood volume within 24 hours). Exchange transfusions and potent cold agglutinins also require warming. Banked blood—stored at 33° to 43° F. (1° to 6° C.)—may cause hypothermia if administered without warming.

Use an electric blood warmer, if available—this automatically heats blood to body temperature. Never warm blood above body temperature or above 107° F. (42° C.) because excessive warming causes hemolysis.
• Provide psychological support. The patient and his family may react to the prospect of a blood transfusion with both relief (because it's a lifesaving measure) and fear (because they perceive it as a last-ditch effort). They may also worry about becoming infected with AIDS or hepatitis. (See *Blood transfusion preparation; Blood transfusion reaction; Blood transfusion, massive.*)

Body mechanics

Protecting your back

Using proper body mechanics when moving patients can prevent back injuries. But a device is also available that reduces the risk even more. It's called the *Patented Smooth Mover Patient Mover.* Besides protecting your back, it makes the transfer easier on the patient.

The device is nothing more than a smooth polyethylene board, measuring 22″ × 72″ (55 × 180 cm), with handholds along its edges. Unlike some of the complicated transfer devices available, this works on the basic principle of decreasing friction. You simply slip it under the patient, then slide the patient across the bed to the stretcher.

Similar devices are available, but this seems to be the easiest to use.

One-person transfer from bed to stretcher
Explain to the patient what you're about to do. Then lock all the wheels on the bed and raise the far side rail. Raise the bed to your working level. Position the patient on his side with his back to you, as close to the far edge of the bed as possible. Lift up the drawsheet and slide the transfer device under him.

Have the patient roll back onto the device, and center his body on

it. Then place the stretcher next to the bed and lock all its wheels. Raise or lower the bed so it's even with the stretcher. Tuck the drawsheet close to the patient's side.

Then, ask him to rest his arms across his body. Holding his legs with one hand, grasp the handhold on the lower half of the transfer device with your other hand. Pull the lower half of the transfer device across to the stretcher; the upper half should follow part of the way.

One-person transfer

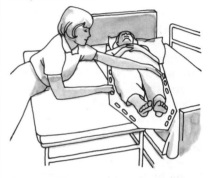

Next, place your arm across the patient's chest. Then, positioning yourself at the center of the stretcher to keep him from rolling off, grasp the upper handhold and pull the upper half of the transfer device toward you.

Lastly, center the transfer device on the stretcher. Raise the side rails, unlock the wheels, and you're ready to transport him.

Two-person transfer from bed to stretcher
First, place the stretcher next to the bed and lock the wheels on both. Raise or lower the bed so it's even with the stretcher. Then have your assistant use the drawsheet to roll the patient onto his side. Place the transfer device as far under him as possible.

Roll him back so he's lying on the transfer device. Ask him to rest his arms across his body, then tuck the drawsheet close to his side. Have your assistant get into position. Then grasp the handholds, having your assistant do the same. On the count of three, together slide (not lift) the transfer device across the bed to the stretcher.

Two-person transfer

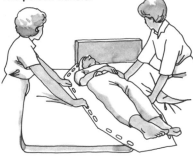

Then, have your assistant push and guide the device as you pull and guide it. Stop when the patient and device are centered on the stretcher.

Use the drawsheet to roll him toward you, allowing your assistant to remove the transfer device. Then roll the patient onto his back, raise the stretcher's side rails, unlock the wheels, and transport him. You may leave the transfer device under the patient during transport, so you can easily move him when you arrive at your destination. It can also be left in place during an X-ray.

Bowel disease, inflammatory

Helping your patient cope

Your patients with Crohn's disease and ulcerative colitis need your expert nursing care. Keep a bedpan and wipes within easy reach, and put a deodorizer in the room. Try to empty the bedpan as soon as possible after it's used. Administer antidiarrheals, as ordered. And document the number of stools and their appearance. Are they fatty? Or bloody?

Routinely check for perianal fissures, fistulas, or abscesses, which often result from prolonged diarrhea. Also give (or teach the patient to perform) meticulous perianal skin care, using clear water on lesions and mild soap on surrounding areas. Then, dry the skin and apply a lotion or cream. A cream containing a topical anesthetic (such as Nupercainal) will provide temporary relief from the pain, itching, and burning that follow frequent bowel movements.

Give the patient some tips on controlling diarrhea at home, too. Tell him to fast during an attack. Or he may eat small, frequent meals and reduce the amount of roughage in his diet. Explain that a combination of diet restrictions and antidiarrheals can ameliorate his long-term diarrhea.

Helping the patient maintain good nutrition poses a real problem because certain foods may exacerbate the disease. In some cases, I.V. therapy or total parenteral nutrition may be necessary.

To monitor the patient's nutritional status, record his weight and his intake and output daily. Also, observe him for signs of nutritional deficiencies. If the patient is a child, look for growth retardation.

When the patient is able to eat, ask the dietician which foods are likely to be tolerated. If the patient can tolerate only a few foods at first, he may need nutritional supplements. (See *Nutritional supplement.*)

One of the best things you can do, of course, is to help ease the patient's pain. Try positioning him with his knees flexed. Applying heat to his abdomen may also provide welcome relief.

Most likely, the patient's doctor will order antispasmodics and analgesics, which should help. But be sure to encourage the patient to report his pain. Some patients may try to tolerate the pain rather than ask for analgesics.

Understandably, inflammatory bowel disease (IBD) puts a considerable strain on social relationships. A child with IBD, for example, may be teased because of the extra time he spends in the rest room or because of the odor from diarrhea. His parents may become overprotective, putting too much emphasis on the child's limitations. Adults with IBD can have difficulty maintaining relationships, too. Some sufferers, convinced that others can't understand their predicament, simply shut people out of their lives.

This is where you come in. Probably the most important thing you can do for a hospitalized IBD patient is to establish a trusting relationship. Encourage the patient to discuss his feelings and fears. And let him know that you recognize how difficult it is to carry on a normal life.

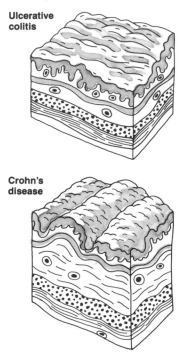

Ulcerative colitis

Crohn's disease

Keep in mind that the exhaustion brought on by the disease will tend to magnify the patient's problems. When you plan your care, be sure to allow him plenty of time to rest.

Also, discuss changes he can make in his life to make it easier for him to cope with IBD. He may want to consider adding a second bathroom to his home or buying special equipment, such as commodes or bedpans. And he should join a local support group for people with IBD.

Talk to the patient about the importance of using his time constructively, working within the limitations imposed by his disease. Suggest that he try doing some normal tasks even when he has an at-

B

B

tack. For instance, he might keep some clothes that need mending in the bathroom. By noting the patterns of their signs and symptoms, most IBD patients can estimate how much uninterrupted time will be available for an activity.

Bowel retraining

How to institute a program

You can help your patient control his bowel by instituting a bowel retraining program. Here's how:
• First, establish a specific time for defecation. A typical schedule: once a day or once every other day after a meal, usually breakfast. However, be flexible when establishing this schedule, and consider the patient's normal habits and preferences.
• If necessary, help ensure regularity by administering a suppository, either glycerin or bisacodyl, about 30 minutes before the time scheduled for defecation. Avoid the routine use of enemas or laxatives, as they can cause dependence.
• Provide privacy and a relaxed environment to encourage regularity. If "accidents" occur, assure the patient that they're to be expected and don't represent a failure of the retraining program.
• Adjust the patient's diet to provide adequate bulk and fiber; encourage him to eat more raw fruits and vegetables and whole grains. Ensure a fluid intake of at least 1,000 ml/day.
• If appropriate, encourage him to exercise regularly to help stimulate peristalsis.
• Be sure to keep accurate intake and elimination records.

Bradycardia

Managing a severe case

Bradycardia can signal a life-threatening disorder when accompanied by pain, shortness of breath, and other symptoms; by a prolonged exposure to cold; or by head or neck

trauma. In such a case, quickly take vital signs and have another nurse immediately notify the doctor. Connect the patient to a cardiac monitor, and insert an I.V. line. Depending on the cause, you'll need to administer fluids, atropine, steroids, or thyroid medication, as ordered. If indicated, insert an indwelling (Foley) catheter. Assist with intubation and mechanical ventilation if the patient's respiratory rate falls (See *Endotracheal tubes: insertion.*)

If appropriate, perform a focused assessment to help pinpoint the cause of bradycardia. Ask, for example, about pain. Viselike, crushing, or burning chest pain that radiates to the arms, back, or jaw may indicate acute myocardial infarction (MI); a severe headache may signal increased intracranial pressure. Also ask about nausea, vomiting, or shortness of breath—symptoms associated with acute MI and cardiomyopathy. Look for thyroidectomy scar because severe bradycardia may result from hypothyroidism caused by failure to take thyroid hormone replacements.

Breast biopsy

Assisting with one-needle biopsy

Prepare the patient by explaining the procedure and describing the equipment. If she's undergoing a superficial-tissue biopsy, tell her she'll feel discomfort similar to what she'd feel during venipuncture. (If she's undergoing a deep-tissue biopsy, she'll receive a local anesthetic.)
• Document baseline vital signs and make sure she has signed a consent form, if required.
• Position her comfortably. Ask her to remain still during the procedure, but tell her to signal with her hand if she needs to cough or say something.
• Remain with her and help her relax during the procedure.

• Apply pressure to the site afterward, using a sterile gauze pad.
• Tell her to report swelling, bleeding, or signs of infection.

Breast exam: guidelines

When your patient has a lump

If your patient reports a lump, ask her the following questions: How and when did she discover it? Does the size and tenderness of the lump vary with her menstrual cycle? Has the lump changed since she first noticed it? Is she aware of any other breast signs, such as discharge or nipple changes? Find out if she's noticed a change in breast shape, size, or contour. Is she lactating? Does she have fever, chills, fatigue, or other flu-like symptoms? Ask her to describe any pain or tenderness associated with the lump. Is the pain in one breast only? Has she sustained recent trauma to the breast?

Explore her medical and family history for these special risks of breast cancer: a high-fat diet; a mother or sister with breast cancer; or history of cancers, especially cancer in the other breast; multiparity; a first pregnancy after age 30; and early menarche or late menopause.

Next, perform a thorough breast examination. Pay special attention to the upper outer quadrant of each breast, where half the ductal tissue is located. This is the most common site of breast cancers.

Carefully palpate any suspected breast nodule, noting its location, shape, size, consistency, mobility, and delineation. Does the nodule feel soft, rubbery, and elastic, or hard? Is it mobile, slipping away from your fingers as you palpate it, or is it firmly fixed to adjacent tissue? Does it seem to limit the mobility of the entire breast? Note the delineation of the nodule. Are its borders clearly defined or indefinite? Or does the area feel more like a hardness or diffuse induration than a nodule with definite borders?

Do you feel one nodule or several small ones? Is the shape round, oval, lobular, or irregular? Inspect and palpate the skin over the nodule for warmth, redness, and edema. Palpate the lymph nodes of the breast and axilla for enlargement (See *Lymphadenopathy*.)

Observe the contour of your patient's breasts, looking for asymmetry and irregularities. Be alert for signs of retraction, such as skin dimpling and nipple deviation, retraction, or flattening. (To exaggerate dimpling, have your patient raise her arms over her head or press her hands against her hips.)

Gently pull the breast skin toward the clavicle. Is dimpling evident? Mold the breast skin and again observe for dimpling.

Be alert for nipple discharge that's spontaneous, unilateral, and non-milky (serous, bloody, or purulent). Be careful not to confuse it with the grayish discharge that can often be elicited from the nipples of a woman who has recently been pregnant. (See also *Breast exam: patient teaching*.)

Breast exam: patient teaching

Guidelines to give your patient

Tell your patient that examining her breasts at least once a month will help detect any abnormalities early. Tell her to perform this examination on the 4th to 7th day after her menstrual period ends, when her breasts are least congested. If she's past menopause, tell her to choose the same date each month. Then instruct her to follow these steps, and call her doctor if she notices any abnormalities.

"Undress to the waist, then stand in front of a mirror with your arms at your sides. Carefully look for the following: changes in breast shape, size, or symmetry; skin puckering or dimpling; ulceration; lumps; nipple secretions; or retraction of the skin, nipple, or areola. Repeat the inspection with your arms over your head, and with your hands on your hips and elbows out to the sides.

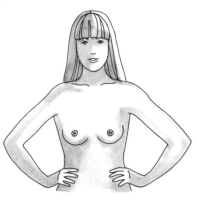

"Now, examine your left breast with your right hand. Using the pads of your fingers, move clockwise around your breast to feel for lumps; don't be afraid to press firmly. Start at the outer area of your breast and work inward toward the nipple. You may feel a ridge of firm tissue along the lower part of your breast; this is normal. Repeat the procedure, examining your right breast with your left hand. You may prefer to examine your breasts while standing in the shower, with one hand placed behind your head.

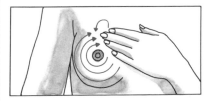

"Also using the pads of your fingers, feel the opposite armpit. Repeat the examination on the other armpit. Don't be alarmed if you feel a small lump that moves freely; this area contains the lymph glands. But check the size of the lump daily. If it doesn't go away or if it gets larger, notify your doctor.

"Next, check your nipples for secretions by gently squeezing the nipple between your thumb and forefinger. Notify your doctor if you see any secretions, and describe the color and amount.

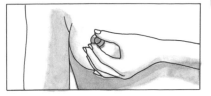

"Now, lie down with a rolled-up towel or a small pillow under your right shoulder and your arm behind your head. Using your left hand, examine your right breast and armpit as you did while standing. Repeat the procedure with your left breast.

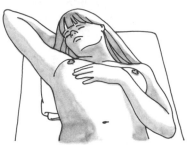

"If you do feel a lump while examining your breasts, note if you can easily lift the skin covering it, if the lump moves under the skin, and if it's soft or hard. Be sure to give your doctor this information when you call him." (See *Breast exam: guidelines*.)

Breast-feeding

Making it less painful

A new mother who wants to breast-feed her baby but whose nipples are sore might appreciate this advice.

Just before breast-feeding, tell her to wrap some ice chips in a cloth and apply it to the nipple. In a minute, the nipple will be numb; the baby can start sucking; and the mother won't feel the soreness that usually accompanies the first moments of breast-feeding. (The cold will also make the nipple more erect, and easier to grasp.)

B

Breathing devices

Using a bag-valve mask

With the oropharyngeal airway in place (see *Airway, oropharyngeal*), position yourself at the head of the patient's bed so you can use the bag-valve mask properly. If the headboard can be removed, take it off the bed. Keep the patient's neck hyperextended and his lower jaw elevated. Then cover his mouth and nose with the mask, as shown.

• Place the third, fourth, and fifth fingers of one hand on the patient's lower jaw, as shown, to keep it elevated.

• Then place your thumb and index finger on either side of the mask's valve connection. This helps create a tight seal against the patient's face. To maintain the seal, lightly squeeze the mask.

• Make sure the patient's head is properly tilted back, then squeeze the bag with your other hand. Observe his chest to see whether it rises as you squeeze the bag and falls as you release it. Ask another nurse to auscultate the chest for signs of lung expansion. Someone should also be setting up suctioning equipment and supplemental oxygen.

Bag-valve mask

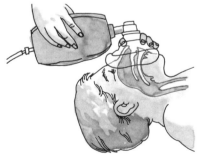

As soon as possible, the supplemental oxygen source should be attached to the oxygen inlet valve. Adjust the flow rate for 10 to 12 liters/minute. This setting will provide a 40% to 90% oxygen concentration, depending on how fully the patient's airway is open, how tight the mask-face seal is, how hard you can squeeze the bag, and how much supplemental oxygen is delivered.

Provide one full lung inflation every 5 seconds—ventilating the patient's lungs 12 times/minute as you'd do in mouth-to-mouth ventilation. Closely observe the mask so you'll see immediately if the patient vomits. If he does, remove the mask, turn him onto his side, and suction his airway. (See also *Airway, esophageal gastric tube*.)

Breath sounds, adventitious

Recognition guidelines

The four adventitious breath sounds are crackles, gurgles, wheezes, and rubs. Usually, when you hear one of these, your patient has some form of pulmonary disease.

Crackles (formerly called rales) result from air moving through airways that contain fluid. Typically heard on inspiration, crackles are discrete sounds that vary in pitch and intensity. They are classified as fine, medium, or coarse.

Fine crackles are high-pitched sounds heard near the end of inspiration. To produce a similar sound, hold several strands of hair close to your ear and roll them between your fingers. Fine crackles can result from fluid in small airways or small atelectatic areas that expand when the patient breathes deeply. You may hear these adventitious sounds in a patient who has congestive heart failure or pneumonia. Usually, fine crackles are first detected in the lung bases. They usually don't clear with coughing.

Medium crackles are produced by fluid in slightly larger airways—the bronchioles, for instance. They're lower pitched and coarser than fine crackles. You'll hear them during the middle or latter part of inspiration. Medium crackles won't clear when the patient breathes deeply and coughs.

Coarse crackles are loud, bubbling, gurgling sounds, resulting from a large amount of fluid or exudate in the larger upper airways, including the mainstem bronchi and the large bronchi. You'll hear these sounds on both inspiration and expiration. Usually, coarse crackles can't be cleared by breathing deeply and coughing. They indicate increasing pulmonary congestion.

Gurgles (formerly called rhonchi) develop when thick secretions partially obstruct air flow through large upper airways. Loud, coarse, and low-pitched, they sound a lot like snoring. You'll hear gurgles mostly on expiration and sometimes on inspiration, too. A patient may be able to clear gurgles by coughing up secretions. Gurgles may indicate chronic obstructive pulmonary disease, tumors, or acute bronchitis.

Like gurgles, *wheezes* occur on expiration and sometimes on inspiration. Wheezes are continuous, high-pitched, musical squeaks. You'll hear them when air moves rapidly through airways narrowed by asthma or partially obstructed by a tumor or foreign body. In a patient with mild asthma, you'll probably hear bilateral wheezes on expiration. But if his condition worsens, you'd hear wheezes on both expiration and inspiration. Unilateral, isolated wheezes usually indicate an obstruction.

A pleural friction rub has a distinctive grating sound. It may remind you of the sound made by rubbing leather. As the name indicates, these breath sounds are caused by inflamed visceral and parietal pleurae rubbing together. (See *Breath sounds, normal; Respiratory exam: auscultation*.)

Breath sounds, normal

Where to find them

Normal breath sounds are caused by air moving through the respiratory tract. Depending on their characteristic sound and their location, normal breath sounds are classified as bronchial, bronchovesicular, or vesicular. To distinguish among the three, listen closely to the duration, pitch, and intensity of the sound you hear.

Posterior chest

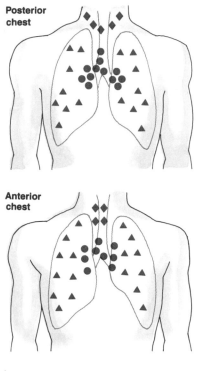

Anterior chest

◆ = Bronchial
● = Bronchovesicular
▲ = Vesicular

You'll auscultate bronchial breath sounds over the largest airway, the trachea. On the posterior chest, this will be on both sides of the spinal column from the C7 to T4 vertebrae. On the anterior chest, the trachea extends to about the level of the sternal angle.

Bronchial breath sounds are loud and high pitched. They may remind you of wind blowing through a tunnel. You'll hear the inspiratory phase for just a short time, but the expiratory phase will sound long and loud.

If you hear bronchial breath sounds in any other area besides over the trachea, suspect consoli-

dation. For example, if there is consolidation in the lower right lung lobe, you'll hear bronchial breath sounds instead of normal vesicular sounds over that area.

Bronchovesicular breath sounds are heard over the mainstem bronchi. So listen between the scapulae from the T4 to T7 vertebrae on the posterior chest and from the sternal angle to the fourth ribs on the anterior chest. These sounds have a medium pitch and intensity. With bronchovesicular breath sounds, the inspiratory and expiratory phases will last the same amount of time.

You'll hear *vesicular* breath sounds over most of the peripheral lung fields where air moves through small airways. So expect these soft, breezy, low-pitched sounds when you're auscultating away from the trachea and mainstem bronchi. With vesicular sounds, inspiration will sound longer than expiration.

Remember that solid tissue transmits sound better than air or fluid does. So over an area of consolidation, breath sounds (as well as spoken or whispered sounds) will be louder than they should be. But if there's pus, fluid, or air in the pleural space, breath sounds will be quieter than normal. If a foreign body or secretions are obstructing a bronchus, breath sounds will be diminished or absent over distal lung tissue. (See *Breath sounds, adventitious; Respiratory exam: auscultation.*)

Breath sounds: ventilator patient

Auscultation method

You should auscultate your ventilator patient's breath sounds every hour to verify adequate ventilation and to detect secretions or atelectasis. Normally, you'll be able to hear breath sounds easily in ventilator patients. Document diminished breath sounds, and report

them at once. They may indicate inadequate ventilation, possibly from fluid accumulation and atelectasis. The absence of breath sounds, of course, is an ominous finding. Usually, it's a sign of pneumothorax, a potential (and common) complication of mechanical ventilation, or improper intubation.

Remember to auscultate breath sounds immediately after repositioning the patient or manipulating his endotracheal tube. This will confirm that the tube is still properly positioned. You'll notice numbers on the side of the tube. Document the position of the tube on the Kardex by recording the number that's closest to the patient's lips.

A dislodged endotracheal tube may wind up in the right mainstem bronchus, which is straighter and wider at the tracheal bifurcation than the left bronchus. The result will be diminished breath sounds over the left lung.

If you hear breath sounds equally diminished on both sides, with harsh or noisy breath sounds coming from the patient's mouth, the tube may have been pulled out or the cuff may be deflated or broken. (See *Breath sounds, normal; Respiratory exam: auscultation.*)

Brudzinski's sign

When you suspect meningeal irritation

Here's how to test for Brudzinski's sign: With the patient in a supine position, place your hands behind his

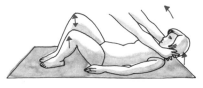

neck and lift his head toward his chest. If he has meningeal irritation, he'll flex his hips and knees in response to the passive neck flexion.

Bruits: assessment

What they mean

Bruits are most significant when heard over the patient's abdominal aorta; the renal, carotid, femoral, popliteal, and subclavian arteries; and the thyroid gland. They're also significant when heard consistently despite changes in patient position and when heard during diastole.

If you detect bruits over the abdominal aorta, check for Cullen's sign. (See *Cullen's sign.*) Either sign—or severe, tearing pain in the abdomen, flank, or lower back—may signal life-threatening dissection of an aortic aneurysm. If you suspect this, notify the doctor immediately; emergency surgery may be necessary.

If you detect bruits over the thyroid gland, ask the patient if he has a history of hyperthyroidism. Notify the doctor promptly if you discover any signs and symptoms of life-threatening thyroid storm, such as tremor, restlessness, diarrhea, abdominal pain, and hepatomegaly.

If you detect bruits over the carotid artery, be alert for signs and symptoms of a transient ischemic attack, such as dizziness, diplopia, slurred speech, and syncope, which may indicate an impending cerebrovascular accident. (See *Carotid artery: auscultation.*)

If you detect bruits over the patient's femoral, popliteal, or subclavian arteries, watch for signs of decreased or absent peripheral circulation—edema, weakness, and paresthesias. Frequently check the patient's distal pulses and skin color and temperature. Immediately report to the doctor sudden absence of pulse, pallor, or coolness, which may indicate a threat to the affected limb.

If you detect a bruit over any vessel, be sure to check for further vascular damage. (See also *Bruits: auscultation.*)

Bruits: auscultation

Using the stethoscope correctly

Typically, bruits result from arterial luminal narrowing or arterial dilation. But bruits can also result from excessive pressure applied to the stethoscope's bell during auscultation. This compresses the artery, creating turbulent blood flow and a false bruit.

Normal blood flow, no bruit

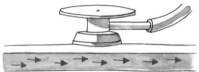

Bruit (aneurysm)

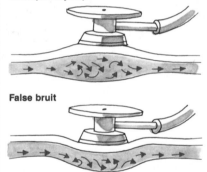

False bruit

To prevent this, place the bell lightly on the patient's skin. Also, if you're auscultating for a popliteal bruit, you'll need to position the patient supine, place your hand behind his ankle, and lift his leg slightly before placing the bell behind his knee. (See *Bruits: assessment; Stethoscope, acoustic.*)

Burnout

Warning signs

Pay attention to these important signs that indicate you're burned out:

• *Feeling overwhelmed.* Unrelieved stress can soon make you feel as if you'll never get things back under control. Do you wonder what to do first when you've got so much to do? Do you feel that you'll never make a dent in your work no matter how hard you try?

• *Fatigue, angry outbursts, and depression.* As you continue to feel overwhelmed, you may start using ineffective coping methods—such as repression. Do you feel tired all the time? The effort of holding in your feelings might be draining your energy.

Of course, you can't repress your feelings forever. When they begin to overflow, you may become irritable or angry, flying off the handle at things that wouldn't have bothered you several months ago. Or you may turn your anger inward, becoming depressed, quiet, and withdrawn.

• *Forgetfulness and disorganization.* With mounting stress, you can't seem to think clearly. Your once-comfortable routine becomes haphazard and you begin to make mistakes. Do you notice yourself filling out more incident reports for simple mistakes you always avoided in the past? Do you forget to do routine jobs?

• *Guilt and self-sacrifice.* The forgetfulness and disorganization that accompany unrelieved stress frequently lead to this inappropriate coping device: working even harder to catch up. Do you feel indispensable, unable to stay home when you're ill? Do you find yourself skipping lunch breaks and working overtime more than your colleagues?

• *Feeling disillusioned.* Feelings of powerlessness and fatigue slowly drain your enthusiasm, leaving you feeling disillusioned and cheated. Do you find yourself thinking, "This isn't what I expected from nursing"?

• *Passivity.* Exhausted, you may try to cope by giving in. Do you find yourself tolerating rudeness and unreasonable behavior or accepting unrealistic assignments because it's easier than arguing?

• *Distancing.* As your emotional resources drain, you may be unable to offer emotional support to others. You cope ineffectively with this problem by increasing the psychological distance between yourself and your patients—by concentrating only on the technical aspects of nursing. Do you find yourself referring to the patients as diseases—"the coronary in 207"? Or do you become irritated when patients' questions "interrupt" your efforts to give an injection or perform other technical tasks?

• *Letting yourself go.* When you feel powerless to change anything, you may simply stop trying. Besides showing up in your work, stress shows up in your appearance. Have you stopped keeping your uniform spotless and pressed? Have you lost or gained several pounds in the past few weeks?

• *Substance abuse.* As depression, fatigue, and anxiety increase, you may try disguising or escaping them inappropriately. Are you drinking more coffee and smoking more cigarettes than you used to? Are you taking tranquilizers or sedatives inappropriately or using alcohol to help you escape?

• *Physical illness.* Stress can lead to increased illness and physical discomfort. You may notice you've had more colds, headaches, or gastrointestinal problems than you used to. (See *Burnout victims.*)

Burnout victims

Helping others

Some nurses recover from burnout only because someone else helps them. Here's how:

• Develop a supportive relationship, but listen and accept what the person has to say without passing judgment. Let an optimistic attitude do the talking.

• Listen actively. Let her know you want to understand what she's feeling. Research shows that burned out people feel no one understands. (See *Listening to co-workers.*)

• Ask questions. Start off with simple requests for information such as "How did the meeting go?" Later, ask about feelings with questions such as "What feelings do you have when you go to work in the morning?"

• Level with people. When questions don't work, state your feelings about the situation that's troubling the victim. Doing so can help her see the situation from another perspective and may encourage her to share her views.

Listening, questioning, and leveling have one aim in common: To help the person verbalize her frustrations. (See *Burnout.*)

Burns: bedside debridement

Performing the procedure

If this is your patient's first bedside debridement, explain the procedure to him to encourage his cooperation. Limit the number of people in his room to prevent bacterial contamination of the exposed wound. Then do the following:

• Administer an analgesic 20 minutes before starting debridement, as ordered.

• Wash your hands and put on a sterile cap, mask, gown or apron, and gloves.

• Remove any existing burn dressings, then gently clean the wound with povidone-iodine (Betadine) or another appropriate cleaning agent.

• Shave all hair 2″ (5 cm) from the wound site.

• Change to a fresh sterile gown or apron and gloves.

• Pick up loosened edges of the eschar with sterile forceps. Then, with the blunt edge of sterile scissors or another forceps, probe the eschar and cut the dead tissue away from the wound with the scissors. Leave a ¼″ (.5 cm) edge of remaining eschar, to avoid cutting into viable tissue. *Don't* debride closed blisters.

• Because debridement removes only dead tissue, bleeding should be minimal. If significant bleeding occurs, apply gentle pressure on the wound with dry, sterile 4″ × 4″ gauze pads or apply a hemostatic agent, such as a silver nitrate stick. If the bleeding persists, notify the doctor and maintain pressure on the wound until he can control the bleeding with sutures or electrocauterization.

• Rinse the wound surface with saline-soaked gauze sponges, then place a sterile burn pad under the cleaned body part. Obtain wound cultures, as ordered.

• Remove the contaminated gown and put on another pair of sterile gloves.

• Replace dressing or antimicrobial ointment, as ordered.

• To prevent chilling and fluid loss from evaporation, keep your patient warm and avoid exposing large areas of his body. Don't debride more than a 4-inch-square (10-cm²) area per procedure.

• As you know, debridement can be extremely painful. Try to complete the procedure quickly to spare your patient unnecessary pain. If possible, ask another nurse to assist you, and limit the entire procedure to 20 minutes. (See also *Burns: tub debridement.*)

Burns: chemical

Emergency steps for eye contamination

First, find out what's in the patient's eye. If it's a caustic solution, his eye will need *immediate* attention to prevent a severe chemical burn and blindness.

Ask someone to call an ambulance or to get a car so you can take the patient to the hospital. Then check quickly to see if he's wearing contact lenses. If he is, no matter how urgent the emergency, you must remove them first. (See *Contact lens removal.*) Then, lead the patient to the nearest sink to flush his eyes with water.

Adjust the tap water to a tepid temperature and moderate pressure. Then place his head sideways under the faucet, with the affected

B

eye downward. (This keeps the caustic solution from splashing into his other eye.) Tell the patient to keep his eyes open and to roll them so the water can wash out as much of the solution as possible. Make sure he doesn't rub his eyes with his hands. Restraining him might be necessary. Remember, he may panic again at any time.

While you flush the patient's eyes, ask someone to fill a large container with fresh water and to find a cup. You'll need the extra water and cup to flush the patient's eyes on the way to the hospital. Also have someone carefully pour a little of the caustic solution into a bottle. The ED will use this to identify what's burning the patient's eye. (See also *Eye irrigation.*)

Burns: depth measurement

Classification procedure

First-and second-degree burns are partial-thickness burns, and third-degree burns are full-thickness burns. But determining burn depth can be difficult because most burns aren't solely partial-thickness or full-thickness; they're mixtures of both. Also, skin thickness varies according to age and body area.

Burn depth is also difficult to assess right away. With electric burns, for example, the patient may show only minimal external tissue damage, but he may have considerable internal damage along nerve and vascular pathways. The electric current makes an entrance and an exit wound just like a gunshot. At first you may see only two small burns on the palm of the hand. But 10 days later, the patient's whole arm may be necrotic.

In fact, final determination of burn depth usually can't be made until several days after a severe burn, but that shouldn't delay a decision to transfer a patient to a burn center. In both the young child and

elderly person, many burns that at first appear to be partial-thickness are full-thickness.

First-degree burns

As you know, a first-degree burn is the most superficial, involving only the epidermis. Common causes are

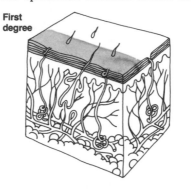

First degree

sun exposure or very brief contact with intense heat following flash explosions. The main characteristic is erythema. Pain occurs because nerve endings are injured and exposed. Because the deeper layers of the dermis aren't destroyed, regeneration takes place without scarring.

Healing occurs within a week by a scaling process. During this time, the patient experiences dryness and itching because of increased vascularization, destroyed sebaceous glands, and increased perspiration.

Second-degree burns

A second-degree burn involves the entire thickness of epidermis and part of the dermis. Commonly caused

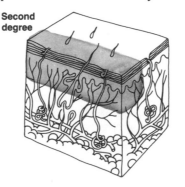

Second degree

by hot liquid or by a flash from an explosion, it forms large, thick-walled blisters. (Blisters also occur in full-thickness burns from steam trapped in the epidermis.) The skin is usually mottled red or pink, moist and sensi-

tive to touch. Reddened areas blanch when touched. Healing takes 10 to 14 days.

Third-degree burns

A third-degree burn involves the epidermis, dermis, and subcutaneous tissue. The most common cause is flame injury.

Elasticity of the dermis is destroyed, and the wound appears dry, hard, and leathery. It's waxy, white, cherry red, brown, or black, with extensive subcutaneous edema. If red, the burn remains red with no blanching when touched. Thrombosed blood vessels are characteristic. Scarring occurs because deeper layers are affected. Since the nerve endings are destroyed, the wound is usually insensitive to touch.

Healing doesn't occur because all layers of the skin are involved. The

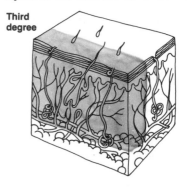

Third degree

destroyed tissue, called eschar, is removed, and skin is grafted to the injured site from another area. (See *Burns: skin grafts.*)

Burns: dressings

Applying a Sulfamylon sandwich

This dressing is used in burn care because it helps promote graft viablity, reduce pain, and prevent infection. Here's how to apply it:

1. Apply a layer of fine-mesh gauze soaked with normal saline solution over the graft site. (Use warm solution for patient comfort.)

2. Wrap a single layer of normal saline-solution-soaked Kling wrap around the gauze.

3. Next, fill up a normal saline-solution-soaked Intersorb pad with Sulfamylon, then place it over the Kling wrap. Center the pad in the graft area; don't place it over healed skin.

Sulfamylon sandwich layers

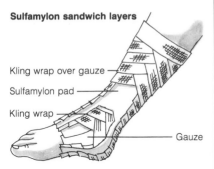

Kling wrap over gauze
Sulfamylon pad
Kling wrap
Gauze

4. Apply another Intersorb pad, also soaked in normal saline solution, over the Sulfamylon layer. Secure the entire dressing with Kling wrap and soak it in normal saline solution. (See *Burns: skin grafts.*)

Burns: emergency care

Emergency department care

Many burn patients have been in automobile accidents or explosion, so they also have traumatic injuries. These injuries should be treated before the burns, experts say. Remember, burns probably won't kill during the first few hours, but traumatic injuries might.

Start by assessing the patient's ABCs—his airway, breathing, and circulation. Administer humidified oxygen, if needed, and have a trach tray handy for an emergency.

As you check his respirations, determine whether he suffered any inhalation burn injury. He may have an inhalation burn but show no signs of body surface burns. Are the hairs inside his nose singed? Smell his breath as he exhales—does it smell like smoke or charcoal? Does he have burns on his face or neck? Consider also how the accident happened: Was there an explosion? Did the patient run and fan the flames?

Or was he in an enclosed space? All these may indicate an inhalation injury. If so, he may have to be intubated.

Now, check his heart rate, blood pressure, peripheral pulses, and temperature. If he's suffered an electric burn, the electric current may have caused cardiac fibrillation or asystole. If his blood pressure is normal, elevate his head and upper torso slightly to reduce edema and to help him breathe easier.

As you check him for other injuries, such as head contusions, blunt trauma fractures, or lacerations, ask him questions to determine his level of consciousness. Also, reassure him about what's happening.

As you're doing this assessment, collect as much information as you can about the accident, the patient's past medical history (including allergies), and his present physical condition. The time you take to record this information will help the burn center or your hospital's critical care unit (CCU) determine the best treatment.

If the emergency medical team has already started one I.V. line, you may have to assist while the doctor inserts a central venous line for I.V. therapy. Any time you do a venipuncture, draw a blood sample for the necessary diagnostic tests, which include complete blood count, type and cross match, creatinine, blood urea nitrogen, total serum protein, albumin, globulin, and electrolytes. Also, draw an arterial blood sample for blood gas measurements. (See *Arterial puncture.*)

And for any patient with burns over more than 15% of his body, insert an indwelling Foley catheter. It's the only reliable means of determining his output, which is measured hourly during the first 48 hours. Get a urine sample for urinalysis, too.

Then, when the patient's condition has stabilized, make sure he has a chest X-ray and an electrocardiogram. Administer tetanus

toxoid prophylactically after checking to make sure he's not allergic to it.

Whether he's transferred to a burn center or merely to your CCU, use sterile gauze and a mild antiseptic solution to remove any gross debris from his burns. He'll get a more thorough wound cleansing later. If you apply a topical bactericidal agent like silver sulfadiazine (Silvadene), apply only a thin layer.

To prevent wound contamination and possible pain caused by circulating air, cover your patient with a sterile sheet or blanket. Or you can use a space blanket, readily available from sporting goods stores, to keep him warm during the transfer. (See *Burns: depth measurement; Burns: extent measurement.*)

Burns: emotional support

Helping your patient cope

After discharge, the patient with a major burn will have to adjust to the following:
• temporary or permanent functional loss
• cosmetic disfigurement
• other people's reactions.

His ability to make these adjustments depends on how he coped before his burn, the severity and the site of his burn, and others' reactions.

Remember, too, that the stress of disfigurement may alter the patient's behavior after discharge. He may benefit from a social worker's help.

Burns: exercise

Home care planning

A major goal in home care planning is to prevent excessive scar formation by exercising, splinting, applying pressure, applying dressings, and, if necessary, undergoing corrective surgery. If the patient is recovering from a major burn, he may need 12 to 18 months to achieve this goal. He'll need to work with a physical therapist, an occupational therapist, a home care nurse, and a social worker.

Before he's discharged, help him work out a plan for exercise, splinting, and wearing pressure garments at home. (See *Burns: scar maturation.*) He may need to go to daily therapy sessions for several weeks or months; this can cause problems if he can't get to and from the sessions alone. You can help by offering solutions—for example, a transport service or home therapy with a physical therapist.

Burns: extent measurement

Calculation method

The "Rule of Nines" is the simplest and most widely used method for assessing the extent of total body surface area (TBSA) burned. According to this method, the head

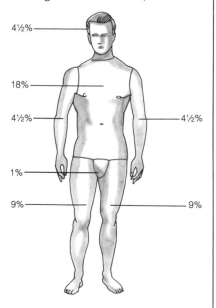

(including the neck) and arms each represent 9% of the TBSA (total, 27%); the chest, back, and each leg separately represent 18% (total,

72%); and the perineal area represents 1%. The larger the TBSA involved, the greater the threat to the patient.

Because the Rule of Nines gives a quick estimate of the extent of a patient's burns, it's useful in triage of burn patients. But used hastily during a life-threatening burn emergency, it may produce an inaccurate estimate that hinders later medical effort.

The Berkow method provides a more accurate and comprehensive method of determining the extent of burn injury. It assigns percentage values for each body area, as the Rule of Nines does. But these values vary across six different age brackets, allowing more precise assessment of children.

Here's how to use it:
• First shade the body diagrams to match the burned areas on your patient's body.
• Next, using the patient's age as a guide, record the numbers appearing in those shaded areas in the appropriate columns, depending on whether the burns are second- or third-degree. Is only a fraction of an area burned? Multiply that fraction by the number, and record the answer.
• Remember, as a child grows, his body proportions change—mostly in his head, thighs, and legs. So the percentages for these areas vary according to age.
• Now, add all the numbers you've recorded to get the percentage of second- and third-degree burns. Then, add these subtotals to get the final percentage of total body surface area burned.
• As a check, perform the same calculation on the unburned area. The two percentages should add up to 100. If they don't, you've made an error and should check your calculations.

So, you can use the Rule of Nines to get a general impression of how extensively your patient's burned. But for a more exact assessment, use the Berkow method.

To determine the percentage of body surface burned, use the Rule of Nines. (The same percentages apply to the backs of the body parts shown here, except for the genital area.)

Burns: follow-up care

What to tell your patient

Two important aspects of planning home care for the patient with major burns are community resources and vocational counseling. The establishment of regional burn care centers means that he may receive his initial treatment several hundred miles from home. When he's discharged, he not only loses the burn team's support, but he might not know who to turn to at home. His family doctor—or perhaps a doctor he's never seen before—may be the only professional aware of his return.

Your planning can make his return easier. Ask his burn team doctor to contact the patient's family doctor to plan a medical follow-up. Other members of the burn team (physical therapist, social worker, and occupational therapist) may also contact their counterparts in the community to plan follow-up care. He may need additional support from a psychologist, psychiatrist, or a community mental health agency before discharge.

Finally, consider vocational counseling. If the burn injury caused loss of joint function or some other physical limitation that will prevent him from doing his former job, he will need job retraining. Contact the local office of the state labor and industry board to help the patient find out what's available. Even if retraining can't begin for several months, the contact with vocational counselors and the anticipation of retraining may help him look beyond his immediate problems and think of the future.

How you plan his home care will influence his adjustment when he's discharged. The effort you put into this planning will stay with him long after he's left your care. (See *Burns: home care.*)

Burns: home care

Planning

Early home care planning for the patient with major burns accomplishes two goals. First, it helps resolve problems before they develop. For example, if his house was burned and needs to be repaired, the family may need to relocate. This could be done before he's discharged, thus preventing the added stress of moving after the discharge.

Second, early home care planning emphasizes the future. If you consistently discuss plans for home care, he and his family will realize that he will indeed get well and will return home.

Start with a patient interview. Ask about his home environment, his ability to adapt that environment to meet his needs, and any family problems that may affect his cooperation with the treatment—either in the hospital or at home.

He should understand each of the five major areas of home care—wound management, pain relief, exercise therapy, scar maturation, and emotional support. He should be given verbal as well as written instructions (perhaps in the form of a booklet). (See *Burns: emotional support; Burns: exercise; Burns: follow-up care; Burns: pain; Burns: scar maturation; Burns: wound care.*)

Burns: infection

Nursing considerations

Sepsis is the leading cause of death from burns, particularly with burns on more than 25% of the body. The normal barrier to outside infection has been destroyed; dead tissue (eschar) provides an excellent me-

dium for bacteria; and the immunologic system has been severely depressed.

Topical agents such as mafenide acetate (Sulfamylon) and silver sulfadiazine (Silvadene) retard but don't eliminate bacterial growth. Sulfamylon may cause kidney and lung problems in some patients; Silvadene is less powerful and less penetrating. Don't use prophylactic antibiotics until a specific bacteria has been identified. You'll only encourage development of resistant strains. (The sole exception: an open scald wound that might be exposed to a streptococcal infection. This is particularly devastating to younger burn patients.)

How sterile should the patient's environment be to inhibit the growth of infectious microorganisms? Nobody knows for sure. Some burn centers use the barrier isolation technique (including laminar flow units for individual patients). Other centers rely on the aseptic technique. All of these centers report similarly low rates of infection for burn patients.

To reduce the risk of infecting your patient, wear a mask, gown, cap, and surgical gloves when treating him in his room. And to prevent cross-contamination of burn wounds, replace your gloves frequently during dressing changes.

Burns: management

Replacing fluids and electrolytes

Major complications for a burn patient during the first 5 days of hospitalization usually stem from fluid and electrolyte changes. In the first 48 to 72 hours after a burn, fluid suddenly shifts from vascular to interstitial spaces. With small burns, this is a local process. But with burns of 25% or more of total body surface area (TBSA), it happens throughout the body and can cause burn shock, a form of hypovolemic shock.

Fluid therapy will restore cardiac output by putting fluid back into the blood vessels. The volume must be calculated from the TBSA burned and the patient's weight. (See *Burns: extent measurement.*) Ideally, it should begin within an hour after a severe burn. A central venous line inserted into a vein permits rapid administration of fluid and electrolytes. A patient with 40% to 70% TBSA burns, for example, requires 3 to 5 liters per day for replacement.

Several different fluid resuscitation formulas exist: crystalloid, Evans, Moore's burn budget, hypertonic, Brooke, or a modification of any of these. The crystalloid resuscitation formula is approved for the Emergency Department by the Committee on Trauma of the American College of Surgeons and is the formula most commonly used. But remember that any formula the doctor chooses serves only as a guideline: The patient's response must still be closely monitored.

During the first 48 hours, urine output rate is the most reliable measure for determining that response. Output should be measured every hour. Usually, a urine flow of 30 to 50 ml/hour is sufficient for an adult; at least 15 ml/hour for infants, and 25 ml/hour for older children. If output rises above or falls below these figures, fluid therapy must be adjusted accordingly. Lack of urine output may indicate insufficient fluids or acute tubular necrosis.

After the first 48 to 72 hours, urine output is no longer a reliable guide to the patient's fluid needs. Water deprivation may occur even when the urine output for an adult is 1,000 ml/day or more. So, his needs are better determined by measuring serum electrolyte levels.

Burns: pain

Relief for the severely burned

Patients with partial-thickness burns usually have much pain be-

B

cause nerve endings are exposed. Even the slightest air current across sensitive tissue causes extreme discomfort. Patients with full-thickness burns, however, may have little pain because their nerve endings are destroyed (See *Burns: depth measurement.*) And many patients in "burn shock" don't complain about pain.

To assess your patient's pain as accurately as possible, follow this simple rule: Pain is what he says it is, not what you *think* it is. By encouraging him to tell you about his pain, you do more than just get assessment data. You also acknowledge his pain as a personal experience, in which he alone is the final authority.

Not all burn patients need analgesics or narcotics for pain relief, of course. Diversion techniques help many patients, especially children. And tender care from you and the other nurses during dressing changes can certainly help comfort patients.

But if your patient requires pain medication, don't let your fear of overmedication or addiction hamper your efforts. Burn pain defies stereotyped notions of "proper" dosage. Give your patient the least amount of medication that will free him from pain or make his pain tolerable—not some preconceived limit. (See *Orders, sliding scale.*)

The *only* time you should limit your patient's medication is during the *early* stages of a severe burn. Most burn centers avoid sedating the patient during that time because of the dangers of respiratory depression and overdose. Fluid shifts in the first 72 hours after a severe burn cause blood pressure fluctuation. If you give pain medication intramuscularly when your patient's blood pressure is low, it may not be absorbed immediately. When the patient's pressure rises again, another injection may cause a dangerous overdose.

Burns: scar maturation

Patient teaching

Pressure garments and masks help decrease the formation of thick, disfiguring scars. But the patient's acceptance of these aids will probably be a problem. These garments are uncomfortable and make the patient warm, especially during hot weather. They must be tight enough to produce the 24 mm Hg of pressure required to exceed capillary pressure, reducing edema and scar formation. And he must wear the garments 24 hours a day for 6 to 12 months. The masks will probably be even more unappealing to him, although the new clearer plastic face masks are a slight improvement.

Teach him as much as possible about scar formation and the therapy needed to prevent it. Make sure he understands the normal course of scar maturation and what can be realistically accomplished through plastic and reconstructive surgery.

Scar maturation is often difficult for the patient to understand. If he has survived a burn over 50% of his body, he'll be disheartened to hear that his scars are going to get worse before they get better. Learning that his scars may take 6 months to 2 years to mature completely is even more discouraging.

This information may depress him, but it's better than allowing him to go home and realize several weeks or months later that his wounds look worse, not better. If he knows from the beginning that this will happen, but that eventually the scars will fade and soften, he'll be able to cope better.

Discussing reconstructive surgery is another aspect of home care planning for the patient with a major burn. Although planning specific reconstructive procedures may be impossible at discharge time, you should give him some realistic expectations of what the surgery can and can't do. If follow-up and reconstructive surgery will be performed by a doctor who hasn't yet been involved in his care, arrange for him to meet that doctor as soon after discharge as possible.

Burns: skin grafts

Caring for temporary grafts

A patient with deep partial-thickness or full-thickness burns will need skin grafts to prevent infection and to promote healing of the wounds. Grafts may be applied as soon as eschar is removed. Extremely serious burns may require temporary grafts to provide early wound closure until autografting (permanent grafting of skin taken from the patient's own body) can be done. Grafts, also called biological dressings, prevent the loss of large amounts of fluid and protein, and protect the wounds from infection. They also protect exposed structures such as nerves, blood vessels, and tendons.

Whatever type of temporary graft your burned patient receives, he'll need constant care to ensure that his burns heal properly and are protected from infection. So be sure to follow these guidelines when caring for a patient with a temporary graft:
• Keep the graft exposed to air, or dress it as ordered, and protect it from pressure.
• Inspect the burn site frequently. The temporary graft "takes" by adhering tightly to the wound. If separation or sloughing occurs, notify the doctor. He may have to replace the graft.
• Assist the doctor in changing the temporary graft if rejection occurs.
• Watch for signs and symptoms of systemic infection and infection at the graft site. Infection may necessitate removal of the graft; if this occurs, expect to treat the burn site

with antimicrobial ointment and the patient with systemic antibiotics.
• You may use a synthetic material, such as Op-Site, to temporarily cover superficial partial-thickness burns. (See *Burns: infection.*)

Burns: tub debridement

Proper procedure

Here's what to do:
• To prevent cross contamination, make sure the tub, all equipment, and the tub room are thoroughly cleaned and disinfected before beginning hydrotherapy. You may line the tub with a sterile plastic liner for extra protection against infection.
• Fill the tub with water heated to 98° to 100° F. (36.7° to 37.7° C.), turn on the agitator (if appropriate), and add electrolyte solutions and germicidal solutions as ordered. Make sure the air temperature is 80° to 85° F. (26.7° to 29.4° C.) or that heat lamps are in place, so your patient won't be chilled when he enters or exits the tub.
• If this is the patient's first tub debridement, explain the procedure to him.

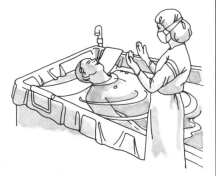

• Administer an analgesic 20 minutes before beginning the procedure, as ordered.
• Wash your hands and put on a sterile gown, shoe covers, mask, surgical cap, and arm-length sterile gloves.
• Place your patient on the plinth, then lower him into the tank so the headrest supports his head. Allow him to soak for 3 to 5 minutes.
• Clean all unburned areas (encourage your patient to do this himself if he can). Wash the unburned skin (shave the hair near the wound), shampoo his scalp, and give mouth care. Provide perineal care (often done before tubbing, too), and clean inside your patient's nose and the folds of his ears and eyes with cotton-tipped applicators.
• Change into a fresh sterile gown and gloves, and gently wash burned areas with gauze pads or sponges to remove topical agents, exudate, necrotic tissue, and other debris.
• Turn off the agitator and use sterile forceps and scissors to debride, as needed.
• When the debridement is complete, spray-rinse the patient's entire body to remove all debris.
• Transfer the patient to a stretcher covered with a sterile sheet and bath blanket; then cover him with a warm, sterile sheet (a blanket may be added for warmth), and pat unburned areas dry.
• Replace dressings or antimicrobial ointment, as ordered, before returning the patient to his room.

Here are some special considerations to keep in mind while performing debridement:
• Remain with the patient at all times during the procedure, to prevent him from injuring himself in the tub.
• Limit hydrotherapy to 30 minutes, to avoid electrolyte loss.
• During the procedure, watch your patient for signs of chilling or fatigue, for altered vital signs, and for unusual pain. Inspect the burn site and surrounding tissues carefully for signs of infection.
• Hydrotherapy is contraindicated if your patient has an electrolyte or fluid imbalance; a body temperature above 103° F. (39.4° C.); or a sudden increase or decrease in respiration, pulse, or blood pressure. It's also contraindicated for a patient who has a mending fracture, an endotracheal tube, a tracheostomy, or has respiratory assistance.

• In some centers, hydrotherapy has been discontinued in favor of suspending the patient over a tank and spray-rinsing him. This is done to prevent cross contamination and sepsis. (See *Burns: bedside debridement.*)

Burns: wound care

Teaching your patient

Make sure you give the patient written instructions, including the name and phone number of a doctor or nurse he can contact if he has questions or problems concerning his care. Tailor the instructions to his needs, considering the nature of his wound and his home environment.

Tell him how to do every step of the wound care procedure. Don't assume, for instance, he'll know how to use a sterile tongue depressor to apply ointment. Again, reinforce your verbal instructions with written ones.

Your instructions should also include how to care for healed grafted and nongrafted areas, and areas that may blister and break down after discharge.

Bypass, arteriofemoral

What your patient needs to know

When your patient starts walking—usually by the second postop day—instruct him not to do any unnecessary sitting. Why? Because sitting involves bending the knees and feet and putting pressure on the popliteal area, leading to possible swelling and pooling of blood in the legs. Explain that he'll be allowed to use the toilet and to sit for meals—but for no more than 10 to 15 minutes at a time. Tell him to avoid crossing his legs while sitting because that constricts the veins behind the crossed knee.

Discharge instructions

Before discharge, instruct your patient as follows:

"Avoid prolonged sitting, change your position frequently, and alternate between walking and reclining. Use a reclining chair to elevate your feet.

"Develop a good balance between rest and exercise, but gradually increase your activities. Exercise and walk short distances daily.

"It's important to recognize signs and symptoms that might indicate circulatory problems—pain, pallor, loss of pulses, numbness, coldness, or ulceration.

"Always dress warmly in cool or cold weather (this will help maintain blood flow to your legs and feet) and avoid tight clothing." (Tell female patients to avoid girdles, garters, and knee-high stockings.)

"Avoid temperature extremes—for example, putting ice or heat on your legs.

"Take medications correctly. Observe your dosage schedule and be aware of possible adverse reactions.

"Obesity puts an extra load on the circulatory system, so avoid excess weight gain. Avoiding foods high in saturated fats can also help reduce your risk of atherosclerosis—which probably contributed to your need for bypass surgery.

"Nicotine in cigarettes constricts blood vessels, interfering with circulation.

"Resume your sexual activity, as your doctor advises."

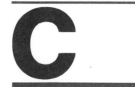

Cancer, oral

Assessment guidelines

To evaluate your patient's risk, first ask whether he smokes, and if he uses or has ever used snuff or chewing tobacco. Then ask about his work history, dental hygiene measures, diet, and alcohol use.

Ask if he's noticed a sore throat, difficulty in swallowing, changes in salivation, or discomfort when eating. Has he discovered sores or white, thickened patches in his mouth that won't heal? These patches, called oral leukoplakia, are significant because many become cancerous. Most common among smokeless tobacco users, they appear on the mucous membranes of the lips, cheeks, gums, or tongue. They can't be scraped off and many must be surgically removed, although they may disappear when a patient stops using smokeless tobacco.

Continue your assessment by noting the quality of the patient's voice; advanced oral cancer can paralyze the vocal cords. Note also his breath odor, since some cancerous lesions produce a foul smell.

Next, observe his face and neck for symmetry and any swelling, masses, or lesions. Palpate facial bones, especially the jaw, for tenderness and deformity. Assess also for neurologic impairment, such as paresthesia, facial weakness, or impaired cranial nerve function (see *Cranial nerve assessment.*)

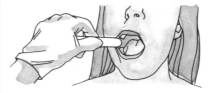

Finally, inspect his mouth for leukoplakia, ulcers, areas of drainage, and tongue immobility. If you find anything suspicious, report it immediately.

Cancer care

Nursing interventions

The patient needs time and space to adjust to a diagnosis of cancer. He will probably be preoccupied with thoughts and questions about his life, interpersonal relationships, and death. He may feel angry, isolated, and confused by the information. He may have both misconceptions and realistic fears.

Give the patient only the information he needs. Answer specific questions, but don't bombard him with unessential information. You may need to repeat things. Ask the patient for verbal feedback so you can assess his understanding. Suggest he use a pocket calendar to record appointment times, locations, diagnostic tests, test preparations, and questions. Other patients familiar with the treatment regimen might reinforce the information you give. Encourage the patient to share his thoughts and feelings.

Assess the patient's fears by asking him and his family about their knowledge and experience with other people who have cancer. Determine what the doctor has told the patient about his illness and treatment and what conclusions the patient has reached. Set up an effective communication system with the patient's doctor (try to be present when he talks to the patient). Work with the doctor to correct the patient's or family's misconceptions. (See also *Cancer recurrence; Cancer treatment.*)

Cancer recurrence

Reassuring the patient

If cancer recurs, the patient and his family must face a dismal future. Give them privacy and time to share feelings. Encourage them to resolve their conflicts and concerns. Help, as needed. Remember, sometimes a patient is more prepared than his family to face the reality of his death. If so, encourage him to support his family members. Listen to him and encourage him to highlight and reinforce past accomplishments. Discuss hospice care. (See *Hospice philosophy.*)

Encourage him to maintain his sense of control as long as possible. For instance, you might say, "I know you'd like to do it, but would you mind if I do it?" Keep the patient comfortable and free from pain. Don't feel rejected if your attempts to set up a relationship with the patient are unsuccessful. Perhaps the only psychosocial support he needs is a person sitting quietly by his bedside.

Cancer treatment

Helping your patient cope

Your patient's treatment is aimed at a cure. Treatment will end when the patient and family learn the results of its effectiveness.

During the treatment phase, the patient and family members are coping with the adverse reactions to the treatment and changes in lifestyle: frequent disruptions in activities of daily living, altered work schedule, role changes, and so forth. They may feel ambivalent as they await test results to determine the treatment's effectiveness. This can create feelings of helplessness, so help the patient and family maintain control by giving them information about the treatment and its purpose, its adverse reactions and how to minimize them, and signs and symptoms to report to the doctor or to you.

Encourage the patient and family to express their feelings. Work with the doctor to explain test results and other information. Explore the patient's and family's understanding about any further treatment; plan follow-up visits. Maintain channels of communication between doctor and patient to reinforce information and correct any misconceptions. (See also *Cancer care; Cancer recurrence.*)

Canes

Keeping them within easy reach

Here's a tip for any patient who uses a cane. Instruct him to attach a small piece of Velcro to the handle of his cane and attach matching pieces to his belt, workbench, filing cabinet, kitchen counter, and wherever else he usually props his cane.

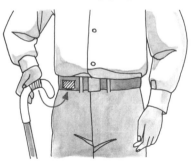

Then whenever he has to use both hands, he can hang his cane on the Velcro, and it will stay upright until he needs it again.

Cardiac output

When it's altered

Cardiac alteration causes changes in thought processes and reduces activity tolerance. With this diagnosis, your goal is to maintain hemodynamic stability. Hemodynamic monitoring—measurement of pulmonary artery end-diastolic pressure, mean pulmonary capillary wedge pressure (PCWP), and cardiac output—is a useful tool for assessing the patient's response to treatment and maintaining hemodynamic stability. PCWP is probably the most accurate indicator of impending heart failure, but measurement of cardiac output is also useful. Congestive heart failure always reduces cardiac output, causing hypoperfusion. (See *Congestive heart failure: complications.*)

In acute failure, if nitroprusside and a positive inotropic agent have failed to restore hemodynamic stability, the doctor may insert an intra-aortic balloon pump (IABP) until the patient's condition stabilizes or until valve replacement. (See *Congestive heart failure, acute.*)

What should you do?

1. *Position the patient properly.* Correct positioning helps maintain hemodynamic stability. Unless an IABP has been inserted, place the patient in a semirecumbent position in bed or in an armchair to decrease venous return. If the patient's in bed, elevate the head of the bed on 8″ to 12″ (20 to 30 cm) blocks. Support his arms with pillows. If the patient is orthopneic, have him sit on the side of the bed, supporting his head and arms on an overbed table. Place a pillow behind his lumbosacral spine, and support his feet.

2. *Promote rest.* Provide supportive care to reduce cardiac work load. Provide a bedside commode to prevent overexertion. Make sure the patient's room is quiet, cool, and well ventilated. Also, limit the number of visitors, eliminate unnecessary physical exams, and allow the patient to rest between care procedures, before and after meals, and several times during the day.

To promote sound sleep, administer oxygen, as ordered, to decrease respiratory effort and increase comfort. (See *ICU noise.*) Provide a night-light to help prevent disorientation for the patient who awakens at night. If the dyspneic patient insists on leaving his bed at night, position him comfortably in an armchair. Avoid using restraints. Instead, administer a mild sedative, as ordered—but do so carefully to prevent respiratory depression. Also, realize that because of poor hepatic and renal function, drugs will clear more slowly.

Cardiac tamponade

Responding quickly

When a patient's had coronary artery bypass surgery, he runs the risk of experiencing acute cardiac tamponade. Fluid starts escaping from the left ventricle into the pericardium, increasing pericardial pressure and impeding left ventricular return. As a result, blood pressure and cardiac output start failing rapidly despite a rising central venous

C

pressure. The patient has difficulty breathing and becomes restless and agitated. His urine output drops.

Call a code—you have no time for a confirming chest X-ray, ECG, or echocardiogram. If the patient is not already receiving supplemental oxygen, start it.

Administer plasma volume expanders, such as dextran, whole blood, and albumin. These will temporarily increase preload or volume, thus improving cardiac output. Also, isoproterenol (isoprenaline, Isuprel) will increase myocardial contractility and decrease peripheral vascular resistance.

Monitor the patient's vital signs, particularly his blood pressure, respiratory rate and rhythm, and central venous and pulmonary artery pressures.

Then set up for pericardiocentesis, making sure emergency equipment is at hand—including a defibrillator and pacemaker. To begin, place the patient in semi-Fowler's position. Attach him to a continuous ECG monitor. (See *Pericardiocentesis.*)

Once the procedure is over, obtain a chest X-ray. You can compare it with the one done before the coronary artery bypass surgery. Note the heart's size and position. This X-ray also may disclose complications from the pericardiocentesis—for example, pneumothorax.

What to do later
Closely monitor hemodynamic, respiratory, and renal functions.

Because the patient's blood pressure may not improve immediately, you may need to administer plasma volume expanders and vasopressors (for example, dopamine). To be sure cardiac compression isn't recurring, frequently assess intracardiac filling pressures, systemic vascular resistance, and cardiac output and index. Also, check for muffled heart sounds, pericardial friction rub, and jugular vein distention. (See *Heart sounds: abnormalities; Jugular venous pressure.*)

Be on the alert for dysrhythmias; promptly report any changes in heart rate or rhythm. Obtain a 12-lead ECG—fluctuations in QRS complexes indicate myocardial penetration.

In monitoring the patient's respiratory status, check arterial blood gases to be sure tissue perfusion is adequate. If acidosis occurs, administer oxygen. (Keep in mind, though, that mechanical ventilation might impede cardiac output by increasing intrathoracic pressure.)

Every hour, check urine output. Also, monitor blood urea nitrogen and creatinine levels to assess renal function.

And don't forget emotional support: Reassure the patient and his family, explaining why you're monitoring him so closely. Encourage them to express their concerns and ask questions.

Cardiogenic shock care

When you suspect it

If you think your patient's going into cardiogenic shock, you'll probably follow this protocol:
• Place him in low-Fowler's position. If he's unconscious or semiconscious or his blood pressure's low, assist maximum blood flow to the brain.
• Notify the doctor and emergency support staff.
• Administer oxygen to promote adequate tissue oxygenation.
• Start an I.V. or check the patency of the existing I.V. line, and start another line.
• Connect a cardiac monitor and obtain a 12-lead ECG to help determine the extent of myocardial damage.
• Draw blood for arterial blood gas measurements (see *Arterial puncture*) and for cardiac isoenzyme studies, as ordered.
• Insert a Foley catheter, and measure urine output hourly.
• Provide emotional support for him and his family. Explain all procedures and what to expect after his transfer to the coronary care unit (CCU). By giving him emotional support, you'll reduce his stress and help to decrease the compensatory sympathetic response.
• Prepare him for transfer to the CCU. There, he'll receive continuous cardiac and arterial blood pressure monitoring, intracardiac pressure monitoring with a pulmonary artery catheter, and (if necessary) mechanical ventilation.

Possible treatments to improve cardiac output and to maintain pump efficiency will be initiated after invasive cardiac monitoring: plasma volume expanders to increase stroke volume, vasopressors or vasodilators to alter peripheral resistance, inotropic drugs and drugs that correct acidosis and hypoxemia to improve contractility, antiarrhythmics and beta-blockers to control heart rate and rhythm, and an intra-aortic balloon pump is used to assist cardiac function in extreme cases of cardiogenic shock. (See *Cardiogenic shock detection.*)

Cardiogenic shock detection

Pointers for recognition

Any patient with impaired cardiac function can suddenly slip into cardiogenic shock. But the prime candidate is the patient who's recently suffered a myocardial infarction with more than 40% percent of his left ventricle damaged.

One sign of cardiogenic shock is hypoperfusion; you'll note cool, clammy, mottled skin and decreased or absent peripheral pulses. You'll also hear crackles in the lungs and abnormal heart sounds—usually an S_3 or a ventricular gallop.

Hypotension—a systolic blood pressure reading less than 80 mm Hg (or if the patient's hypertensive, 30 mm Hg below his norm)—also may signal cardiogenic shock. But remember that these indicators are valid only if obtained via arterial cannulation. If you're using a cuff, look for a systolic reading of 90 mm Hg or less.

Watch for these other signs and symptoms of poor tissue perfusion: depressed sensorium, altered level of consciousness, hypoxemia, lactic acidosis, and—most important—a urine output of less than 20 ml/hour. And remember that your patient may not experience all of them simultaneously or continuously.

What's the best way to spot cardiogenic shock early? Keep looking for trends: Don't rely on any single reading. And keep comparing these trends with baseline values. This way, you may uncover subtle clues that warrant early intervention.

Don't forget that by the time your patient exhibits definite signs and symptoms of cardiogenic shock, he'll already be in acute danger—and even immediate supportive measures may not save him. (See *Cardiogenic shock care.*)

Cardiovascular assessment

Techniques to use with children

When assessing a child's cardiovascular system, tailor your assessment to his size and anatomic traits. Consider these points:

Inspection
An infant or a young child breathes with his diaphragm. Assess his breathing pattern by observing his abdomen. Cardiac bulging can mean left ventricular hypertrophy, associated with certain heart defects. Observe for cyanosis.

Palpation
In a child under age 7, feel for the point of maximal impulse (PMI) at the third or fourth intercostal space, and to the left of the midclavicular lines. In an older child, you'll find the PMI at the fifth intercostal space. Femoral pulses should also be pal-

pated; their absence may indicate coarctation of the aorta. (See also *Heart exam: palpation.*)

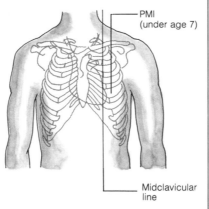

PMI
(under age 7)

Midclavicular line

Percussion
Use light percussion to identify the child's heart size and location. Heart borders should be triangular.

Auscultation
Heart sounds are louder in a child than in an adult because of the child's thinner chest wall. Expect sinus arrhythmia, which speeds the heart rate during inspiration and slows it during expiration, in an infant or young child. Ask the child to hold his breath as you auscultate; the sinus arrhythmia should temporarily disappear.

When listening, you may hear S_3 and systolic murmurs—normal in some children and young adults. *Still's murmur,* common in children 3 to 8 years old, sounds like a vibrating groan or croak. This murmur may arise from occasional vibration of pulmonic leaflets. (See *Heart sounds: abnormalities; Heart sounds: diagnosis.*)

Blood pressure reading
When measuring a child's blood pressure, you may have trouble hearing the diastolic sound. In a patient under age 1, you may not hear the systolic sounds either. In this case, use the flush technique to measure blood pressure: Elevate the infant's arm or thigh. After the skin blanches, apply the proper size pressure cuff and inflate it to about 75 mm Hg. Lower the limb and begin deflating the cuff. The pressure reading that appears when the en-

tire limb flushes with color shows the infant's mean blood pressure.

Expect a pulse pressure of 20 to 50 mm Hg in children. If it's less than 20 mm Hg and you've used the proper size pressure cuff, suspect patent ductus arteriosus or aortic regurgitation. (See also *Blood pressure measurement.*)

C

Career advancement: new responsibilities

Making time for more responsibility

When you're promoted to a managerial position, you may worry about stretching your time and expertise to cover your expanded responsibilities. These ideas should help:

1. *Cultivate an ally.* An ally is someone you can use as a resource for information about people, policies, and politics—the kind of information that can make or break you as a new leader. Your best resource might be your manager, an experienced team leader, or a staff nurse. But don't ignore possible allies a few rungs below you—staff members who've been around for a while know the ropes.

2. *Identify staff members' strengths.* Interview them during the first 6 weeks to begin sorting out their strengths and weaknesses. Move beyond surface judgments by varying each staff member's assignments, and noting how well she handles them.

3. *Make daily rounds.* During your first weeks as head nurse, some days will be so demanding and hectic you'll look for ways to cut corners like skipping rounds.

You can probably rely on staff members to keep you informed. But you're wrong if you think no one will miss you when you skip rounds. Everyone will miss you: You matter—you're the boss. When the sky seems to be falling, you're the pillar that holds it up.

C

4. *Write objectives.* You need a written game plan to help guide you when you want to change things and to support you when times get rough. For each objective, list:
• what you want to accomplish
• what percentage of your time, energy, and attention you plan to give this objective in comparison with others
• individual tasks that give you a step-by-step strategy for accomplishing the objective
• tests that'll indicate whether you're on the right track
• milestone date and completion checklist for each task. (See *Leadership skills; Leadership strategies; Time management.*)

Career advancement: promotions

When you move ahead

If you've just been promoted over your co-workers, you'll need to convert their friendship to respect. How can you do this?
• Don't accept favors from them.
• Don't do special favors just to be liked.
• Don't try to make popular decisions—try to make the right ones.
• Don't be soft about enforcing discipline.
• Don't socialize with them.
The going might be rough for a while. But soon, your subordinates will see that you're fair, and appreciate it. (See *Career advancement: new responsibilities.*)

Career strategies

Ensuring your success

Before trying to move up the career ladder, evaluate your power base. For example, if you're interested in a new job where you already work, ask yourself, "Has my supervisor formally recognized my clinical and management skills? Do I have good working relationships with subordinates and with personnel in other departments?" Having a strong power base will help you reach your goal.

Next, consider the following questions:

1. *What credentials does the job require?* An advanced degree increases your credibility. Investigate the degree programs offered at schools in your area, and enroll in one that meets your needs. Then, if an interviewer asks your plans for further education, you'll have your answer ready. Earning certification while working toward your degree may also increase your chances for the job. The American Nurses' Association has certification programs in many specialty areas.

2. *How has your experience prepared you for the job?* Look for your strengths and weaknesses.

3. *What's your management style?* If you usually ask others for their opinion about decisions that will affect them, you might be a participatory manager. If you like to keep the decision-making power to yourself, you're more of an authoritarian. Most good managers combine both of these styles. Whatever your style, make sure it fits the job you're seeking.

4. *Have you presented yourself in the best possible light?* If you're applying for a job at another hospital, your resumé may determine whether or not you're called for an interview. Make sure that it accurately reflects your achievements in your current and previous positions.

Take extra copies of your resumé and any other materials that help highlight your accomplishments to the interview. (See *Resumés.*)

Care plans

Writing better ones

Care plans provide critical documentation in the event of a lawsuit. Also, they're necessary for reimbursement agencies that believe "if it wasn't documented, it wasn't done."

Care plans provide a central source of information about the patient's problems, needs, and goals; your necessary actions; and documentation of progress in solving his problems.

They include assessment of his medical condition, the nursing diagnosis, insights into his personality and his family, and knowledge of your facility's resources.

They serve as a communication tool for everyone involved in patient care—nonprofessionals and professionals (temporary staff nurses, for

Sample care plan

Name: BETH JACKSON Age: 70 Admitted: 12/1/87 Room: 440

Height: 5 FEET 4 INCHES Weight: 105 POUNDS Suggested weight range: 110 – 130 POUNDS

Medical diagnosis: CEREBROVASCULAR ACCIDENT WITH RESIDUAL LEFT HEMIPLEGIA. HYPERTENSION, ANOREXIA, PRESSURE SORE ON LEFT BUTTOCK

Nursing diagnosis: ALTERATION IN NUTRITION, IMPAIRMENT OF SKIN INTEGRITY

Problems	Desired outcomes	Interventions	Evaluation
WEIGHT LOSS TO 105 POUNDS DUE TO ANOREXIA. IDEAL BODY WEIGHT = 110 TO 130 POUNDS. PATIENT'S NORMAL WEIGHT IS 115 POUNDS.	WITHIN IDEAL BODY WEIGHT BY 2/6/88.	1. MODIFY DIET FOR FOOD PREFERENCES (DIETARY). 2. SUPPLEMENTAL FEEDINGS (NURSING). 3. WEIGH EVERY 3RD DAY (NURSING). 4. RECORD INTAKE BY FOOD GROUP EACH MEAL (DIETARY). 5. EVALUATE FOR POSSIBLE PSYCHIATRIC REFERRAL DUE TO ANOREXIA (NURSING).	1. ADD BREAD, FRUIT TO EACH MEAL 12/5/87. 2. 10 A.M. AND BEDTIME SNACK. 3. SEE GRAPHIC SHEET. 4. SEE DIET INTAKE FORM. 5. REFERRED 12/7/87.

example) whose contact with one another is limited.

Once you've assessed the patient, you'll focus on two things:
• comprehensive information about the patient. This includes identifying data, medical and nursing diagnoses, and details about the patient's ability to care for himself.
• the patient's problems and needs. These may be physical, emotional, medical, social, or spiritual. They may also be immediate, chronic, or potential.

Concentrate on two types of goals—long-term and short-term. Long-term goals are broad, meaningful, and derived from problems you and other health care workers identify. Short-term goals derive from these problems or long-term goals. They're measurable, realistic, and time-limited so you can objectively evaluate progress toward a goal and how the plan is being used.

Interventions should be individualized and based on the patient's condition and preferences. Note the specific date you deliver care. To comply with Medicaid and Medicare standards in long-term care facilities, also identify the person or department responsible for implementing and evaluating each short-term goal or objective. Interventions should show coordination among the caregivers responsible for the plan.

Finally, all nursing progress notes should address the problems, goals, and interventions on the plan. Make sure each paragraph addresses a single problem, not several. Think of them as a quick reference to help decide whether the care plan should be continued or changed. (See *Documentation.*)

Carotid artery: auscultation

Proper procedure

Bruits are best heard with a stethoscope bell. They sound similar to murmurs. However, they're caused by vascular, not cardiac, blood turbulence.

To approximate the sound of a bruit, press gently on a normal carotid artery. Be careful—too much pressure will occlude blood flow. Now, auscultate the artery above the point where you're pressing. What you hear will sound like bruit.

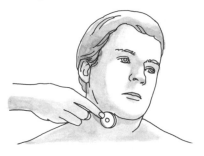

To auscultate a carotid artery, begin at the base of the neck and move gradually toward the jaw. Ask the patient to hold his breath for a moment so breath sounds don't obscure the sound of blood rushing through the carotid artery. If you detect a bruit, note its pitch, intensity, location, and timing in the cardiac cycle. Bruits may be the first indication of extracranial carotid disease, which can be an early warning sign of a cerebrovascular accident. If bruits become more intense as you move the stethoscope toward the jaw, their source is probably in the cranium. Bruits that are more intense near the base of the neck probably originate in the great vessels of the heart. (See also *Carotid artery: inspection; Carotid artery: palpation.*)

Carotid artery: inspection

Good technique

A good time to assess carotid arterial pulsations is just before or after you assess the jugular veins. For the assessment, the patient should lie supine, with the head of the bed elevated about 15 to 30 degrees. To inspect the right common carotid artery, turn the patient's head slightly to the left. Now, focusing on the medial border of the sternocleidomastoid muscle, inspect the carotid artery for forceful pulsations. You can inspect the left common carotid in the same way, with the patient's head turned slightly to the right.

An *absent* or *diminished* carotid pulse usually indicates arterial occlusion or stenosis. A *bounding pulse* may result from hypertension, aortic regurgitation, or thyrotoxicosis. If the patient has a carotid aneurysm, the artery will dilate with each heartbeat. (See *Carotid artery: auscultation; Carotid artery: palpation.*)

Carotid artery: laceration

Emergency action

What do you do when you find a patient bleeding from a self-inflicted lacerated carotid artery? If you don't stop the bleeding immediately, he could exsanguinate and die, so you need to get him to surgery at once so they can repair his wound. In the meantime, you need to control the bleeding. Here's how:

First, apply direct pressure on the artery, using your fingers and a bath towel if you're able to reach one. At

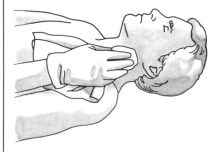

the same time, call for help and turn on the emergency call light. When someone arrives, tell her to get the crash cart (see *Crash cart*) and have the unit secretary call a surgeon or the trauma team. Tell her also to

C

have the secretary call the blood bank to send a unit of type O–negative blood.

When the crash cart arrives, have someone else apply pressure on the artery while you insert at least two large-gauge I.V. catheters. Draw blood samples to be typed, cross matched, and tested for hemoglobin and hematocrit levels; send them to the laboratory. If the doctor's ordered it, begin a rapid infusion of lactated Ringer's solution at one I.V. site and begin transfusing the O–negative blood at the other. Replace this blood with typed and cross matched blood as soon as it arrives.

Have someone help you move the patient and put him in bed. Be sure to maintain pressure on the artery while he's being moved. Begin administering oxygen, and be prepared to assist with endotracheal intubation or a tracheotomy if necessary. (See *Endotracheal tubes: insertion.*)

Observe the patient for cyanosis, stridor, and hemoptysis—all signs of respiratory distress and possible tracheal injury. The trachea may also be deviated by hematomas, thereby increasing respiratory distress. If he appears to have a tracheal injury, also look for signs of pharyngeal and esophageal injury, such as dysphagia and hematemesis. If the vagus nerve has been injured, he may not be able to speak or cough, and he may lose his gag and swallowing reflexes. Remember that all of these conditions threaten the airway, either by obstruction or aspiration.

Keep the patient supine and still, with his neck in a neutral position to avoid putting pressure on the uninjured side.

He will need prompt surgical repair of his carotid artery to prevent cerebral ischemia, which can lead to neurologic deficits and death. Until he's transferred to the operating room, continue to monitor his vital signs and cardiac status. Reassure him that the situation is under con-

trol, and have someone notify his family. Stay with him until he's taken to surgery.

Carotid artery: palpation

Using the proper procedure

To palpate the common carotid arteries, first ask the patient to turn his head slightly to the side you'll be palpating. That will relax the sternocleidomastoid muscle. Then, with the tips of your index and middle fingers, palpate one carotid artery at a time—*not* both at once as you might with other peripheral pulses. (See *Pulses, peripheral.*) You don't want to impair blood flow in both carotid arteries at the same time because diminished flow to the brain could produce syncope. Also,

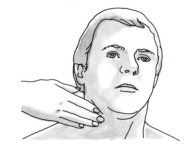

be sure to use light palpation. If you use too much pressure, you might occlude a carotid artery, especially if the patient has atherosclerosis.

Remember that the carotid pulse and the first heart sound (S_1) occur almost simultaneously. So if you have trouble locating the carotid artery, try palpating while you auscultate for S_1. (See *Heart exam: auscultation.*)

Cast, leg

Positioning your patient's leg

Tell him to use one of his crutches to prop up his casted leg.

After the patient sits down, he should adjust the crutch to the shortest position, then place it between his chair and thigh, with the hand grip pointing away from him. He can place his casted leg over the crutch so his ankle is supported by the hand grip and his foot rests below the grip.

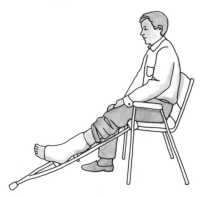

Because the crutch goes wherever the patient goes, he'll always be able to keep his leg elevated and still while sitting. (See also *Casts.*)

Casts

Management tips

Casts require special care, especially synthetic ones. Depending on the material, the cast sets in 3 to 15 minutes and can bear weight in 30 minutes. You'll need to perform a neurovascular assessment every 30 minutes for several hours after it's applied, and every 4 hours the first day or two. Check skin color and temperature, pulse, swelling, and sensation in fingers or toes of the casted arm or leg. Remember possible complications with the five "Ps": Pain, Pulselessness, Pallor, Paresthesia, and Paralysis.

Also, note any drainage or unusual odor from the cast. Although the patient isn't as restricted as he would be with a plaster cast, caution him to avoid activity that could affect alignment of the fracture.

If the patient is allowed to get the cast wet, tell him to use a mild soap and apply only a small amount near the cast. If he has a leg cast, stress that good footing is important when getting in or out of the tub or shower—a wet cast can be slippery (see *Cast, leg*). After swimming, bathing, or showering, he should flush the cast with water and dry it thoroughly to prevent skin irritation and maceration.

To dry it, the patient should first remove excess water by blotting it with a towel. Then he should use a blow dryer (set on a cool or warm setting) in a sweeping motion over the entire cast until it's completely dry. This whole procedure takes about an hour. If it isn't thoroughly dry, he may feel a cold, clammy sensation, similar to that produced by a wet bathing suit.

If he isn't willing to follow this procedure every time, he should avoid getting his cast wet.

Also, tell him to keep dirt, sand, and other foreign particles away from the cast. If they do get under it, he should rinse them out and dry the cast thoroughly.

Some additional tips

If you're caring for an infant who has his legs in casts, here's a way to keep the top of the casts clean and odor-free. Put a terry cloth wristband on each of the infant's legs above the cast. (Make sure, of course, that the band isn't too tight.) The band will absorb any urine or moisture and can be removed regularly for cleaning.

For a patient in a body cast, even the simplest tasks are difficult. Here are some ways you could advise him to make life easier for himself:

• Since he can't get regular trousers over his cast, tell him to make some "custom-fit" pants by hemming a large piece of material at two opposite edges, putting a drawstring through each hem, and sewing some Velcro on the two remaining edges.

To put pants on, he just brings the material between his legs so one hem is in front, one in back. Then he ties the drawstrings together at both sides of his waist and attaches

the Velcro to itself around each leg. (A female patient can simply wear a wraparound skirt.)

• To keep the cast from scraping paint off the toilet seat or gouging it, tell him to cut a piece of heavy vinyl into an oval-shape the same shape as the toilet seat. Tell him to sew Velcro tabs to the sides of the vinyl oval. Before he sits on the toilet seat, he can place the vinyl on the seat, lift the seat, and attach the Velcro to itself underneath each side of the seat.

Tell him to take the seat cover along when he visits friends so he won't have to worry about damaging someone else's toilet seat.

• Because he can't carry anything while he's in a body cast and on crutches, suggest that he wear a carpenter's apron with lots of pockets. That way, he can carry almost anything he needs.

Cataract surgery

Preop and postop care

For the first 24 to 48 hours, your patient will probably be wearing an eye patch. Depending on the type of surgery and the doctor's preference, he may continue to wear it for up to a week. Or he may wear cycloplegic-style dark glasses during the day and an eye shield at night to protect the eye from injury. Show the patient what the eye shield looks like and how it will be secured.

Also, prepare him for the temporary vision loss he'll experience while his eye is patched. Familiarize him with his surroundings to reduce the risk of postoperative disorientation. Explain that for his own safety, the side rails of his bed will be raised for at least 24 hours. Tell him you'll place the call light within his reach, and ask him not to leave his bed without calling for help. (See *Visually-impaired patients.*)

Explain that vision will be blurred after the patch is removed, but that cataract eyeglasses or a contact lens will eventually correct this. If your

patient received an intraocular lens during surgery, he'll probably be able to see clearly at once.

Preoperative care

Before surgery, trim the patient's eyelashes to a length of about 3 mm, if this is a nursing responsibility in your hospital. Ask him to keep his eyes closed while you work. (You can prevent clippings from dropping into his eye by applying a dab of petrolatum to the scissors.) Remember to explain why trimming lashes is necessary, and reassure him that they'll grow back quickly.

Take conjunctival specimens for culture, if ordered, with a sterile cotton-tipped applicator.

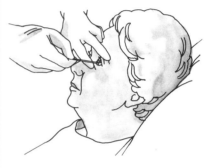

Instill topical antibiotic drops and apply ointment to the eye scheduled for surgery (or both eyes), as ordered. (See *Eye ointments.*)

The evening and morning before surgery, have the patient thoroughly wash his face with a cleansing solution, such as pHisoDerm. Caution him to keep the solution out of his eyes, since it will irritate them.

Shortly before surgery, instill any ordered mydriatic and cycloplegic drops. Administer preanesthetic medications as ordered.

Postoperative care

After your patient returns from surgery, follow these guidelines:

• Position the head of his bed at a 30-degree angle, as ordered. Lying flat may strain the suture line.

• Closely monitor vital signs, and watch for sudden, sharp, or excessive bloody or purulent drainage, temperature elevation, and other signs and symptoms of postoperative complications.

C

• Try to prevent any activity that may increase intraocular tension, such as bending at the waist, vomiting, sneezing, coughing, straining during elimination, and lifting more than 5 lbs (2.3 kg).
• Ask him not to squeeze, scratch, or manipulate his eyelid or to lie on his affected side.
• If he seems disoriented after surgery, consider having a family member stay to prevent him from touching his eye. Take steps to reorient him. Obtain an order for arm restraints only as a last resort.
• Be prepared to help with even the simplest activities and tasks. Remember, when one eye's patched, depth perception is lost. And if the other eye has a well-developed cataract, or is aphakic (without a lens) from prior cataract surgery, he may have little vision. If he wears glasses, help him put them on.
• Arrange personal belongings within easy reach on his unaffected side. Also, always approach him from his unaffected side.
• Instill eyedrops, as ordered. For instance, if he received an intraocular lens implant, the doctor may order miotic eyedrops after surgery to constrict the pupil and reduce the risk of lens displacement.
• Teach him to instill the ordered eyedrops, since he'll need them after discharge. (See *Eyedrops: patient teaching.*) Also, show how to tape an eye shield in place before

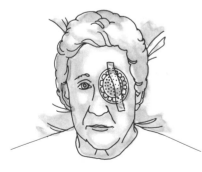

going to sleep. If he lives with family or friends, teach them, so they can also help. Determine whether he'll need help from the local visiting

nurses' association, and make the necessary arrangements.
• Teach him about activity restrictions after discharge, while healing continues. Also, if he's to receive cataract eyeglasses or a hard contact lens, explain that he'll need several weeks to fully adjust to them. The adjustment period for a soft lens is shorter.

If the patient is to receive a soft contact lens, you may need to know how to insert and remove it. (See *Contact lens insertion; Contact lens removal.*)

Catheterization: patient teaching

Guidelines for spinal-cord-injured women

A spinal-cord-injured woman who lacks fine motor movement in her fingers often has difficulty performing self-catheterization. A surgical retractor will help. It will enable her to

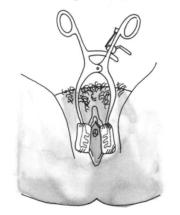

spread the labia and keep it spread, preventing contamination of the urethra and the catheter.

You can teach the patient to use a blunt-tipped Weitlaner retractor. It requires only minimal hand strength to open and is self-retained, so both hands are free for self-catheterization. The patient should pad the tips of the retractor with 2" × 2" gauze pads for use during catheterization. Afterward, she should release the bar to close

the retractor, then sterilize the retractor in boiling water. (See also *Catheterization: technique.*)

Catheterization: technique

Special procedure for paraplegics

Catheterizing a paraplegic woman can be embarrassing to her, and awkward for you to perform if you don't have someone to help you.

Here's a suggestion. Place the patient on her side with an abductor pillow between her lower legs. Insert the catheter posteriorly, as you would for a patient with a fractured hip.

Or you could place her in a frog-like position (knees out, soles together). To keep her feet from sliding, buttress them with rolled blankets or pillows at the foot of the bed. Then insert the catheter.

You could also use a wheelchair and transfer her to an examining table. Place her legs in stirrups and insert the catheter.

Another option would be to place a bedpan or fracture pan upside down on the bed with a pad over it. Then position the patient's buttocks on the pan. You'll be able to see the area better, and catheter insertion will be easier. (See also *Catheterization: patient teaching.*)

Central line: blood specimen

Obtaining one from a triple-lumen catheter

Gather the following equipment: a 10-ml syringe with needle; a needle and syringe for withdrawing the blood specimen (size depends on size of specimen ordered); 5 ml of bacteriostatic saline solution in a syringe with needle; 1.5 ml of 10 units/ml heparin flush in a 3-ml syringe with needle; blood specimen tubes; alcohol sponge; and non-sterile gloves.

If fluids are being infused through one or two lumen ports, turn off the infusions 5 minutes before drawing a blood specimen. Put on the gloves. Then follow these steps:

1. Clean the Luer-Lok cap with the alcohol sponge. Apply pressure to create friction.

2. To check the lumen for patency, use the 10-ml syringe and needle to withdraw 5 ml of blood. Discard the needle, syringe, and blood. (Each catheter lumen contains between 0.4 cc and 0.5 cc of dead space, depending on the lumen gauge.)

If the lumen isn't patent, follow the procedure for removing the clot as described in *Central line: clots.*

3. Next, using the needle and syringe you have ready for the blood specimen, withdraw the amount of blood needed. Inject the blood into the specimen tubes and discard the needle and syringe.

4. To maintain catheter patency, first flush the lumen port with 5 ml of bacteriostatic saline solution, then with 1.5 ml of 10 units/ml heparin flush solution.

Take these steps every time you use the port to withdraw blood.

Central line: care

Pointers for using a Groshong catheter

The Groshong catheter is made of silicone. Its soft and flexible nature makes it less irritating. And its small diameter makes it good to use for very thin veins.

When working with this catheter, keep these points in mind:
• Don't use acetone on or near the catheter. It will cause the catheter to deteriorate.
• Keep sharp objects, such as scissors, away from it.
• Use needles measuring 5/8″ to 1″— no longer.
• Pull back *slowly* on the syringe's

plunger when you're aspirating blood. If you pull back too quickly, the catheter will collapse.
• Don't use excessive force when you're flushing the catheter. But be sure you flush it briskly to clean it thoroughly. Remember to withdraw the needle while injecting the last 0.5 ml of saline solution. This is important so you won't create a vacuum in the syringe and blood won't flow back into the catheter.
• For continuous infusion, use a direct Luer-Lok connection to decrease the strain on the catheter.

When a Groshong central venous catheter is not used for continuous infusion, irrigate it every 7 days with 5 ml of bacteriostatic sodium chloride.

Central line: clots

Clearing them from a triple-lumen catheter

If the catheter lumen contains a clot that you can't aspirate through a needle, prepare to tackle the problem by gathering the following equipment: a Luer-Lok cap; 5 ml of bacteriostatic saline solution in a syringe with needle; 3 ml of 10 units/ml heparin flush solution in a syringe with needle; and an empty 5-ml syringe.

Flush the air from the Luer-Lok cap with 2 ml of heparin flush solution. Then follow these steps:

1. Clamp the occluded lumen and remove the cap. Place the empty 5-

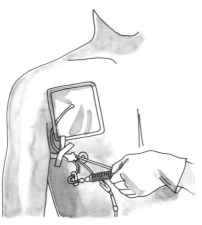

ml syringe on the port. Then, unclamp the lumen and aspirate the clot. If you can't aspirate the clot, clamp the lumen and notify the doctor. *Never* attempt to flush an occluded lumen.

After reclamping the lumen, remove and discard the blood-filled syringe and replace it with the new Luer-Lok cap.

2. Unclamp the lumen and flush it, first with 5 ml of saline solution, then with the remaining heparin flush solution.

Central line: damage

Repairing a double-lumen catheter

Here's how to repair a double-lumen catheter damaged between the Y junction and a point more than 6″ (15 cm) from the chest wall. Four hours after the repair, you can use the lumen again. However, the catheter won't be back to full mechanical strength for 48 hours—so handle it carefully.

1. Assemble these sterile supplies: a towel, two pairs of gloves, povidone-iodine sponges, alcohol sponges, a smooth-edged clamp, scissors, two 22-gauge needles and two 1-ml syringes with heparinized saline solution, a needle and 10-ml syringe with normal saline solution, a 1″ (3 cm) piece of vinyl tubing split lengthwise, and a repair kit. For a Raff 2.2 double-lumen catheter, the repair kit contains a new section of double-lumen catheter with a sleeve to cover the repair junction, two catheter caps, a tube of adhesive, and a blunt needle with a 1-ml syringe.

2. Put on a pair of sterile gloves, then place the sterile towel under the catheter. Clean the catheter with povidone-iodine sponges and alcohol sponges. Allow it to dry.

3. If necessary, remove the first pair of gloves and put on the second pair. Then remove the plunger from the syringe that comes with the repair kit. Now squeeze some adhe-

C

sive into the barrel and reinsert the plunger.

4. Clamp the catheter between the chest wall and the damaged area. Using scissors, cut off the damaged section of the catheter.

5. Place the two new catheter caps on the two lumens of the new section of catheter. Now prime both lumens with heparinized saline solution.

6. Using the syringe of normal saline solution, wet the two ends you'll be joining together—the one on the catheter and the one on the new section of catheter. This will make it easier to slide the sleeve over the repair junction. Next, insert the adapter on the new section into the end of the catheter. Push until both tubings touch the ridge of the adapter. Then, pull the sleeve over the junction.

7. With the sleeve in place, inject adhesive under it until all voids are filled.

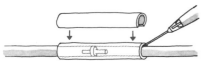

8. Place the piece of vinyl tubing over the sleeve. This tubing keeps adhesive off the patient and helps support the repaired section.

Unclamp the catheter and try to gently aspirate, then try to flush with heparinized saline solution. If you feel resistance, stop. Forcing the solution can damage the repair. If you can't flush it, the catheter may be clotted. You'll have to wait 4 hours until the adhesive sets before you can use a fibrinolytic agent, such as urokinase. Manipulate the catheter and instill the fibrinolytic agent gently; otherwise, the repaired section may separate.

Unfortunately, catheter damage within 6″ of the chest wall cannot be repaired. In this case, a new catheter must be inserted. (See also *Central line: defects; Central line: repair.*)

Central line: defects

Dealing with small holes or tears in the lumen

Gather the following sterile equipment: a towel, two pairs of gloves, povidone-iodine sponges, alcohol sponges, silicone Type A adhesive, and two 1″ (3 cm) pieces of vinyl tubing split lengthwise. You can use vinyl I.V. or nasogastric tubing.

1. Put on a pair of sterile gloves, then place the sterile towel under the catheter.

2. Prep the area you'll be repairing, using povidone-iodine sponges and alcohol sponges. Let it dry.

3. If necessary, remove the first pair of gloves and put on the second pair. Apply the adhesive to the damaged area of the catheter.

4. Take one piece of vinyl tubing and open it lengthwise. Then apply the adhesive along the inside of the tubing. Place the tubing over the damaged area of the catheter.

5. Open the other piece of tubing lengthwise and place it over the first piece of tubing, covering the split. This will seal and reinforce the re-

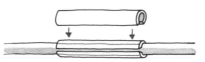

paired area while the adhesive is drying. (See also *Central line: damage; Central line: repair.*)

Central line: displacement

Correcting a dislodged line

Any catheter can become displaced, of course, and for any number of reasons. The most common cause of displacement of a central line is severe coughing or vomiting. As with all central line complications, displacement may occur just after insertion or not until weeks or even months later.

Watch for these indications of catheter displacement in a patient with a central line:
• no blood return from the catheter
• swelling in the chest wall during infusion
• leaking at the catheter site
• pain or discomfort with infusion.

Always check a central line for blood return. If you can't get a blood return, recommend chest X-ray or contrast flow studies to determine placement, particularly before chemotherapy.

Teach the patient that if flushing creates discomfort, he should notify the nurse or doctor, and any leak or swelling must be evaluated.

Central line: dressings

Changing dressings and I.V. equipment

First, gather the following equipment: I.V. fluid (as ordered), I.V. tubing, I.V. extension tubing, surgical mask, two povidone-iodine sponges, two alcohol sponges, culture swab, skin preparation, tincture of benzoin and gauze sponges (to use if the patient is diaphoretic), clear occlusive dressing, clear plastic tape, pair of sterile gloves, pair of nonsterile gloves, and bed protector pad.

After washing your hands, attach the extension tubing to the I.V. tubing, spike the container of I.V. fluid, and hang it on the patient's I.V. pole. Prime the tubing and cap it. Then, follow these steps:

1. Explain the procedure to the patient and position the bed protector pad under his shoulder. Then put on the mask.

2. Put on the nonsterile gloves and remove the dressing. Then discard the dressing and examine the site. If you see drainage, inflammation, or other signs of infection, obtain a specimen with the culture swab.

3. Remove and discard the gloves. Using aseptic technique, open the sterile equipment (let the packaging serve as a sterile field for each piece of equipment), and put on the sterile gloves.

4. Using an alcohol sponge, begin cleansing at the catheter insertion site and work outward in a circular motion. As you work, apply pressure to create friction. Discard the sponge and repeat the process with the second alcohol sponge.

5. Following the same procedure, cleanse the same area with both povidone-iodine sponges. Allow the area to dry naturally for 2 minutes.

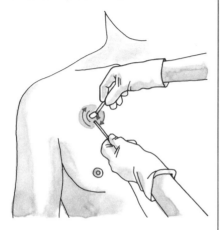

6. Apply the skin preparation to the outer edges of the cleansed area. (If the patient is diaphoretic, use tincture of benzoin so the dressing will adhere better.)

7. Cover the site with the clear occlusive dressing.

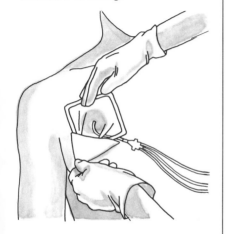

Now, prepare to change the I.V. equipment by clamping the catheter lumen tubing with the slide clamp. Remove the cap from the I.V. tubing that you primed earlier.

8. Disconnect the old I.V. tubing from the lumen port and insert the new tubing.

9. Unclamp the lumen and regulate the flow rate as ordered. Remove your gloves and label the dressing with the date, time, and your initials.

10. To secure the catheter and dressing, cut a strip of tape, slide it under the catheter sticky side up, and criss-cross the tape over the catheter.

11. Place a second strip of tape over the first. Then, label the I.V. tubing and document the procedure.

Central line: infection control

Prevention guidelines

Several things can lead to infection in a patient with a central line. The normal flora emanating from him or hospital personnel—for example, *S. aureus, S. epidermidis,* and *Candida albicans*—can cause a localized infection. The catheter may also become colonized with microbial growth during a systemic infection (usually bacteremia) and serve as a secondary site of infection. Infection can occur both within the catheter lumen and around the insertion site.

Immunosuppressed patients undergoing chemotherapy or radiation are at greater risk for catheter-related sepsis. So are those receiving total parenteral nutrition (TPN) or antibiotic or steroid therapy.

Other contributory factors include prolonged hospitalization, malnutrition, contamination from surgery or dressing changes, an occluded catheter, or a fibrin sheath at the catheter tip.

Common signs and symptoms of infection are fever and chills; red-ness, drainage, or swelling at the insertion site; tachypnea, diaphoresis, or confusion; elevated leukocyte count (in some cases); and hypotension and shock (in severe cases).

To prevent infections, make sure you use aseptic technique when you irrigate or flush the line. When you change dressings or use an implantable port, follow strict sterile technique. (See *Central line: dressings.*) If a long-term atrial catheter (such as a Hickman or Broviac catheter) has been inserted and the wound at the insertion site has healed adequately (2 to 4 weeks), and if hospital policy permits, you can use clean technique.

Remember, the less manipulation, the less chance for infection from breaks in an aseptic technique. Try to change tubing at the same time you change the bottle. The Centers for Disease Control recommends changing all I.V. tubing, except for TPN tubing, every 48 hours. (Many hospitals, however, require a change in central line tubing every 24 hours.)

At most hospitals you would insert a 0.22-micron filter to prevent contaminants or debris from reaching the patient. Change the needle each time you administer an antibiotic, even if you don't change the tubing.

Many central lines are inserted for outpatients, so thorough patient and family teaching is critical. Follow your hospital's teaching protocol. If it doesn't have one, make sure the patient and his family at least understand aseptic technique before the patient is discharged. Also, teach them the signs and symptoms of infection. At home, the patient or a family member may be the first to notice redness at the site or a low-grade fever. In particular, emphasize that sepsis, whatever its cause, is an emergency for the already immunocompromised cancer patient. (See also *Hickman catheter:*

patient teaching; Venous access device: continuous infusions.)

Central line: insertion

Assisting with the procedure

Explain the insertion procedure to the patient and teach him how to perform Valsalva's maneuver. Then place him in Trendelenburg's position to dilate his neck and shoulder blood vessels, which will make insertion easier. Turn his head away from the insertion site and cover his nose and mouth with a mask, if required.

After draping the area with sterile towels, the doctor will clean the site with a povidone-iodine sponge. The doctor will inject lidocaine (lignocaine, Xylocaine) to anesthetize the site. He'll then insert the needle and check for blood return to make sure he's punctured the subclavian vein, not the artery. Next, he'll remove the syringe and insert the catheter through the needle and into the vein. Tell the patient to perform Valsalva's maneuver. If he's unconscious or intubated, you can produce Valsalva's maneuver for him using a manual resuscitation bag. Maintain the inspiratory phase for 3 to 4 seconds while the catheter's being inserted.

Once the catheter's in place, the doctor will remove the needle and place a hub connection with a catheter guard into the end of the catheter. Then you can set up an I.V. bag containing an isotonic solution. Set the I.V. to flow at a keep-vein-open rate.

The doctor will suture the catheter in place and apply a sterile dressing. Once the dressing's in place, loop the I.V. tubing so it won't catch on the patient's bedclothes. Then have an X-ray done of the patient's chest to verify that the catheter's been placed in the superior vena cava proximal to the right atrium, where it won't cause atrial or ventricular irritation.

Central line: patency

Preventing clots in subclavian catheters

To prevent blood clots from obstructing subclavian catheters, try this: Flush the catheter with 1.5 to 2.0 ml of 1,000 units/ml of heparin. Just before you've finished injecting this heparin, clamp the catheter to prevent any blood backflow.

If a clot develops despite this preventive measure, try to open the catheter by gently infusing a solution containing 3 ml of 1,000 units/ml of heparin. The gentle force of the infusion and the anticoagulant action of the heparin should unclot the catheter.

If the heparin solution doesn't work, get a doctor's order for streptokinase or, in some special circumstances, urokinase. These two agents dissolve clots by converting plasminogen to plasmin—the substance that breaks down fibrin, the protein matrix of clots. Inject a streptokinase solution of 100,000 to 250,000 units/3 ml and clamp the catheter for 3 hours. Be sure to have diphenhydramine (Benadryl) on hand in case the patient develops an allergic reaction, and have epinephrine and fluids in case he develops an anaphylactic reaction. With a patient who has a known allergy to streptokinase or a high streptokinase antibody titer, inject 2.5 ml of 2,500 units/ml of urokinase and clamp the catheter for 3 hours.

If one injection of streptokinase or urokinase doesn't work, try a second injection. When the clot does dissolve, flush the catheter with 3 ml of 1,000 units/ml of heparin. Remember to clamp the catheter before you stop injecting the heparin.

If the clot doesn't dissolve after the heparin flush and two injections of streptokinase or urokinase, you may need to have the doctor replace the catheter.

Central line: preparation

Care before and after insertion

The procedure for inserting a quad-lumen I.V. catheter is similar to that of any central venous catheter. (See *Central line: insertion.*) First, explain to the patient what's going to happen and answer his questions. Then prime each lumen with heparin flush or I.V. solution. The doctor will insert the catheter, usually into the patient's jugular or subclavian vein. He may also order X-rays to verify its position.

Assessing your patient and the catheter frequently will help you identify and prevent complications. Suppose, for example, you administer only two I.V. solutions. What happens to the remaining lumens? You can preserve them by covering each unused port with heparin lock caps and by flushing each lumen with 100 units of heparin every 6 hours. Also flush the lumen after every use.

Follow your hospital's policy when changing the tubing, heparin caps, or dressings. (See *Central line: dressings.*) After the catheter has been inserted, apply povidone-iodine ointment over the insertion site and cover it with a sterile dressing.

Besides the usual precautions you'd take to secure a standard catheter, take these for the bulkier quad-lumen catheter: Tape the four

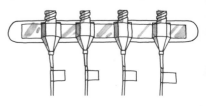

lumens to a tongue depressor, for example, to prevent tangles and keep the lumens close together for easy access; for comfort, pad the tongue depressor; and label each lumen to show what's being infused through it.

Central line: repair

When the hub cracks

You'll need these sterile supplies: a towel, two pairs of gloves, povidone-iodine sponges, alcohol sponges, a smooth-edged clamp, a new hub, a new injection cap, two 22-gauge needles, and two 5-ml syringes filled with heparinized saline solution. Use a smooth-edged clamp to avoid damaging the catheter.

1. After putting on the sterile gloves, lay the sterile towel under the catheter. Clean the catheter first with povidone-iodine, then with alcohol.

2. If necessary, remove the first pair of gloves and put on the second pair. Clamp the catheter below the damaged hub.

3. Attach the new injection cap to the new hub. Then prime the hub with heparinized saline solution.

4. To remove the damaged hub and the old injection cap, hold the catheter firmly while gently twisting and pulling the hub.

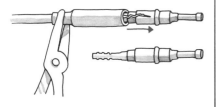

5. Now twist the new hub and injection cap into the distal end of the catheter.

6. After unclamping the catheter, flush it with heparinized saline solution. Check carefully for leaks. (See also *Central line: damage; Central line: defects.*)

Central line: thrombosis

Managing complications

Thrombosis can occur in many forms, ranging from a thin fibrin sheath over the catheter tip to a full-size thrombus. If a fibrin sheath forms over the catheter tip, you could still flush the line and infuse medication, but you wouldn't be able to withdraw blood. With a full thrombus, you can't flush the line, infuse medication, or withdraw blood.

Watch for these indications of thrombosis in a patient with a central line:
• edema of the arm closest to the catheter insertion site (or the arm in which the catheter is inserted) because of inadequate circulation
• mild to moderate neck pain, which usually radiates down the arm or to the back
• jugular venous distention.

In assessing the patient's catheter—which you'll do continually—look for resistance during flushing or lack of a blood return. Promptly report these warning signals to the doctor. Thrombosis can lead to emergencies such as impaired circulation to the arm, superior vena cava syndrome, and, in rare cases, pulmonary embolism.

Even if the patient shows no signs or symptoms of thrombosis, the doctor may order the thrombolytic agent urokinase if the drip rate through the central line slows or stops, or if you're unable to flush or withdraw blood. Only nurses or others with the proper education and experience, however, should attempt to declot a catheter by administering urokinase or aspirating the clot. (See *Central line: patency.*)

In more severe cases of thrombosis, the doctor may begin heparin or Coumadin therapy. This would require you to monitor the patient's coagulation studies closely.

Also, caution the patient and his family to watch for problems in flushing the catheter, neck vein distention, or any swelling of the arm; tell them to report these signs at once to you or to the doctor.

Cerebrospinal fluid

Testing your patient for drainage

If your patient can sit up, have him bend forward and watch for drainage from his nose.

If you see drainage, use this simple test to determine whether it's cerebrospinal fluid (CSF): Test for glucose with Dextrostix or Tes-Tape. CSF tests positive for glucose.

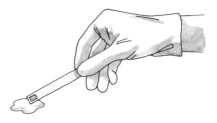

Also, check his pillowcase and sheets for stains indicating CSF leakage. If you see stains, look for the *halo* or *double-ring* sign, which indicates bloody CSF. On cloth, blood aggregates at the center of the stain and a halo of clear CSF surrounds it.

Change

Effective strategies for decreasing stress

To decrease the stress that can accompany change, follow these steps:

1. *Get information.* Learn all you can about the proposed change. Ask your supervisor to tell you:
• why the change is necessary
• when it will occur
• exactly how it'll affect your daily routine.

C

2. *Stay flexible.* If you can look at change as just another way of doing something, you'll quickly recognize that you've successfully adjusted to many such changes—for example, from the team care model to the primary care model.

Keep in mind, too, that institutions must also be flexible enough to cope with the need for change. So administrative changes that seem threatening may actually mean that your hospital's healthy and growing.

3. *Initiate change yourself.* Don't always expect change to start at some level above you and just filter down. Sometimes, you should be the one to initiate change on your unit or in administrative policy. Staff nurses are in a key position to identify both patient care problems and administrative problems.

Assessment and problem identification are initial steps in the nursing process, and applying the same two skills to formulate a change in policy or procedure will help solve problems on the unit.

You could also be the first to identify a need for change in administrative policy. Here again, collecting information could be the key.

Chemotherapy, intraperitoneal

Performing it safely

Intraperitoneal chemotherapy (IPC) is used in the treatment of ovarian cancer patients with peritoneal metastasis. Set up like a peritoneal dialysis system, IPC is performed using a Tenckhoff catheter that's been surgically implanted into the patient's abdomen. (See *Peritoneal dialysis: patient preparation.*)
Warm the solution first
Because the chemotherapy solution must be at body temperature, first immerse the bottle of solution in a basin filled with hot water. Check the water temperature with a thermometer. It should be 98.6° F. (37° C.).

Then set up the chemotherapy administration system and the drainage system with a peritoneal dialysis drainage bag. Close all three roller clamps and connect the drainage bag to the tubing with the drainage arm. Secure this connection with adhesive tape.

Next, while wearing gloves and a face mask, remove the bottle of chemotherapy solution from the water. After drying it, use sterile technique to attach it to the tubing with the drip chamber. Then hang it from an I.V. pole. Be careful not to contaminate the tubing.

Now, tear off the top of a foil alcohol-wipe packet. Gently press the sides of the packet together to form a pouch. Remove the cap from the patient end of the peritoneal tubing without touching the tip. Unclamp the bottle of chemotherapy solution and the patient's I.V. lines. To clear air from the tubing, prime it with the solution and let it run into the kidney basin.

Close the clamps to both the bottle and the patient lines. Place the tip of the tubing that connects to the Tenckhoff catheter into the open alcohol-wipe packet. Put on a pair of sterile gloves to remove the old dressing. Inspect the site for erythema and drainage, then discard the gloves.
Cleaning the catheter and catheter tip
Use sterile technique to pour povidone-iodine into the solution container of a peritoneal dialysis catheter tray. Wearing sterile gloves, place a sterile fenestrated towel under the Tenckhoff catheter. Soak several 4″ × 4″ gauze pads in povidone-iodine solution; leave two pads dry.

Sandwich the catheter tip between two povidone-iodine-soaked gauze pads held in each hand. Scrub the catheter from its tip to the end of the connector for 3 minutes. While holding the catheter inside one of the povidone-iodine-soaked pads, discard the other pad.

With a dry gauze pad, pull back the catheter cap until you see the first rung of the catheter. Again, sandwich the tip between two povidone-iodine-soaked pads and repeat the 3-minute scrub. Discard the gauze from one hand and grasp the catheter. Remove the catheter cap, using a dry, sterile gauze pad.

Shake off the alcohol-wipe packet in which you placed the tubing tip. Attach the tubing to the Tenckhoff catheter. Then, starting close to the patient end, wipe down the catheter with a povidone-iodine-soaked 4″ × 4″ gauze pad. Wash the exit site of the Tenckhoff catheter with povidone-iodine and apply a sterile dressing. Reinforce the catheter tubing connection with sterile adhesive tape. Loop the tubing and tape it to the patient.
Instilling the solution
You'll instill 2 liters of the chemotherapy solution. The second liter of solution is warming while the first is being infused. Depending on the doctor's orders, the solution remains in the abdominal cavity about 1 to 4 hours. After that time, you'll open the roller clamps to let the solution drain from the patient into the peritoneal drainage bag.

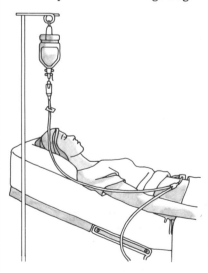

Sometimes 2 additional liters of solution will be ordered. Warm these solutions just as you did the previous ones. After putting on a mask and sterile gloves, remove the protective cap from the new bottle and remove the spike from the empty bottle. Insert the spike into the solution to be infused. (See also *Peritoneal dialysis: exchange.*)

Discontinuing the procedure

When it's time to stop IPC, first remove the dressing and inspect the site. Then, using sterile technique, open up another peritoneal dialysis catheter tray. Pour povidone-iodine into the solution container, open the catheter cap, and place it on a sterile field.

Remove the tape from the Tenckhoff catheter and disconnect the chemotherapy solution tubing. While wearing sterile gloves, place the Tenckhoff catheter on a sterile towel.

Just as you did earlier, soak several 4″ × 4″ gauze pads in povidone-iodine; scrub the catheter and catheter tip for a total of 6 minutes, changing gauze pads after 3 minutes. Using a dry gauze pad, separate the catheter from the tubing. Put a sterile cap on the catheter up to the second ridge.

Wash the exit site of the Tenckhoff catheter with povidone-iodine. Apply a sterile, precut gauze pad to the patient's abdomen, around the catheter. Wipe off the catheter's red cap with alcohol and flush it with heparin. To prevent skin irritation, curl the catheter on top of a gauze pad. Cover the catheter and exit site with a plain, sterile dressing. Tape the dressing, but don't cover it completely.

Chest drainage bottles

Managing them properly

To empty an Emerson bottle, you and another nurse will need a sterile towel, sterile graduated cylinder, and sterile normal saline solution. Here's how:

Take the chest tube—or tubes— and *double clamp* it (or them)

in opposite directions as close to the patient's body as possible. Wait a few moments after clamping to see how the patient tolerates having the tubes clamped. Then turn off the Emerson pump. Undo the bottle lid, lift the pipette out of the bottle—maintaining its sterility—and wrap it in a sterile towel.

Double clamping

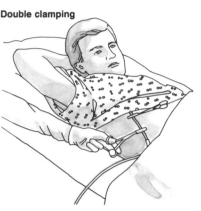

Then pour and measure the drainage in the graduated cylinder and replace 1,500 ml of normal saline solution in the drainage bottle. Last, return the pipette to the bottle, making sure the ends are immersed in at least 2″ (5 cm) of saline solution and the lid is securely placed on the bottle. Always keep the drainage bottle below the level of the patient's chest even though

Emptying bottle

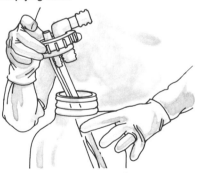

the tubes are clamped. Then turn the pump on, watching for bubbling that indicates a leak in the system, and unclamp the tubes one at a time.

Chest drainage system: air leakage

Detecting problems

Follow these guidelines to locate an air leak in a Thora-Drain III system:

1. Disconnect the tubing from the suction port on the unit. As the patient takes several breaths, observe the water-seal chamber for bubbling. This finding indicates an air leak somewhere in the system.

Water-seal chamber

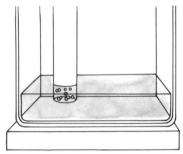

2. To find the leak, first clamp the chest tube near the insertion site (check your hospital's policy on clamping first). Then, as the patient takes several breaths, observe the water-seal chamber for bubbling. If none occurs, the source of the leak is above the clamp, either at the insertion site or inside the patient. Depending on the patient's condition, this finding may be expected or may indicate a complication. (If, for example, he has an unresolved pneumothorax, this finding would be expected.) Remove the clamp and reconnect the tubing to the suction port on the unit. Then resume closed chest drainage and report the leak.

3. If bubbling continues after you clamp the chest tube, the air leak is in the drainage system below the clamp. Move the Kelly clamp about 4″ to 6″ (10 to 15 cm) down the tube, and check the water-seal chamber for bubbling again. Continue to move the clamp down the

C

tube in 4″ to 6″ increments and check for bubbling.

When bubbling in the water-seal chamber stops, you know the leak is between the clamp's present position and its previous position. Try to seal the leak by taping this portion of the tube.

Clamping chest tube

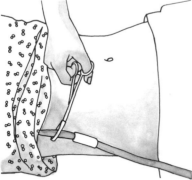

If bubbling continues after you've moved the clamp down the entire length of the tube, the leak is in the Thora-Drain III unit. The unit must be replaced.

Chest drainage system: chamber

Changing the collection chamber

Here's what to do when using a Thora-Drain III system:

1. Obtain a sterile replacement chamber and two padded Kelly clamps. (Make sure your hospital's policy allow you to clamp before proceeding.)

2. Clamp the chest tube close to the insertion site, with the padded Kelly clamps. This will prevent atmospheric air from entering the pleural space.

3. Gently twist the used collection chamber to the left to loosen it. Remove the chamber.

4. Remove the lock cap from the replacement collection chamber.

5. Position the replacement chamber so it's turned to the left.

6. Lock the replacement chamber in place by turning it to the right.

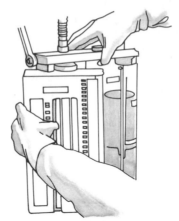

7. Remove the two padded Kelly clamps.

8. Put the lock cap on the used collection chamber and discard it. Check the drainage system for an air leak. (See *Chest drainage system: air leakage.*)

Chest drainage system: management

Good technique

Here's a valuable checklist you can use.
Assessing and teaching the patient
• Evaluate the patient's condition frequently. Report any changes, including rapid, shallow breathing; subcutaneous emphysema; excessive drainage; cyanosis; or chest pain.
• Teach him about his chest drainage system. Instruct him to report any disconnections immediately and to keep the drainage unit below chest level.
Checking chest and drainage tubing
• Check the chest tube connection for signs of an air leak, such as a hissing sound. Check the tube frequently for tears, punctures, and other damage affecting its integrity. (See *Chest drainage system: air leakage.*)

• Make sure the chest tube dressing remains secure.
• Keep the drainage tubing on his bed. Don't permit dependent loops and kinks to form.
• Stripping as ordered. (See *Chest tube stripping.*)
Observing the collection chamber
• Record drainage volume and character hourly. Report increased or decreased volume. Consider more than 100 ml/hour excessive. If drainage stops, check for an obstruction.
• When the collection chamber fills, replace the compartment or unit according to the manufacturer's instructions. (See *Chest drainage system: chamber.*)
Maintaining a water seal
• Listen for hissing sounds, which indicate an air leak.
• Turn off suction control briefly and observe for tidaling (fluctuations in the water-seal chamber as the patient breathes), indicating an intact water seal. If you don't see tidaling, check the tube for patency and report the problem. Tidaling stops when the lung reexpands. Also, you won't see it if the patient has a mediastinal chest tube. (See *Chest drainage system: patency.*)
• Check suction control since some units are hooked up to suction instead of gravity drainage.
• Check for bubbling, which could also indicate an air leak. Expect to see gentle bubbling in this chamber. The doctor may reduce suction if bubbling becomes excessive.

Chest drainage system: patency

Checking the tubing

First, disconnect the tubing from the suction port on the unit. As the patient takes several breaths, observe the water-seal chamber for tidaling (rising and falling of the water in the column). This tells you the system is patent. No tidaling may mean that an obstruction is in the chest tube's eyelets. Report this finding. (See *Chest drainage system: management.*)

Chest drainage system: preparation

Setup procedures

First, gather the following equipment: a sterile Thora-Drain III unit; a container with 1,000 ml of normal saline solution or distilled water; a suction device and tubing; 1-inch occlusive tape; and a padded Kelly clamp.

1. After washing your hands, open the sterile package containing the Thora-Drain III unit. Secure the unit to the patient's bed.

2. Remove the cap from the top of the water-seal chamber. Fill the chamber to the line shown on the front with the saline solution or distilled water. Replace the cap, making certain it's secure. (This cap contains a positive-pressure relief valve.)

Filling water-seal chamber

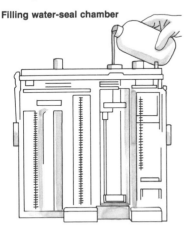

3. Fill the suction-control chamber with the solution or distilled water to the desired level of suction.

4. Clamp the chest tube with the padded Kelly clamp (if your hospital permits you to perform this procedure). Take the protective cover off the distal end of the chest tube. Then remove the protective cover from the connector on the latex tub-

ing attached to the collection chamber. Attach this connector to the chest tube. Make sure the fit is tight.

5. Remove the padded Kelly clamp. Then tape the junction of the latex tubing and the chest tube to secure it.

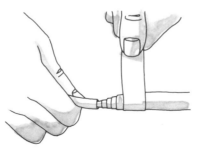

6. Connect the suction device tubing to the suction port.

7. Turn on the device. You should see a mild, continuous bubbling in the suction-control chamber.

Chest pain: assessment

Guidelines to follow

After checking your patient's vital signs, follow these guidelines:

First, assume a myocardial infarction (MI) until your assessment indicates otherwise. *Any* patient can have an MI. Though the chances increase as the risk factors increase, don't let the absence of risk factors lull you into thinking the problem isn't cardiac. (See *MI: emergency intervention.*)

If you conclude that your patient's in trouble, start emergency measures immediately: Administer oxygen; open a vein for medications; call for a portable monitor and ECG; alert the doctor, the respiratory therapist, and the ECG technician; and have resuscitation equipment placed outside the door and ready to go.

The same holds true when your patient's signs and symptoms aren't conclusive but he "just doesn't look right." (See also *Chest pain: diagnosis.*)

Chest pain: diagnosis

Pinpointing the cause

Position your patient properly and check his vital signs. Immediately call the nurses' station and have someone bring you his chart. If you're new to the patient, ask that a nurse who's cared for him be called to his room. Don't hang up the phone or turn off the intercom; you want to keep a line of communication open.

With help on the way, turn your attention to symptom analysis. As you do, keep in mind that symptoms vary so you'll want to be as specific as possible. Here's what you should look for:

• *Location.* Have your patient point to where the pain is and tell you whether it's radiating to other areas. Substernal pain that radiates to the left arm or the neck or jaw usually indicates a cardiac problem. (But remember that cardiac pain can arise anywhere in the precordium and can radiate to outside the thorax, even to the back.)

• *Type.* Is his pain sharp or dull? Did it come on suddenly or gradually? Was he active or resting when it began? Usually—but not always—a dull, sudden pain that's brought on by exertion indicates a cardiac problem. Patients frequently describe this pain as a pressure on the chest.

• *Duration.* How long ago did the pain begin? Has it been steady or intermittent? The longer and steadier the pain, the greater the danger it's a result of a cardiac problem.

• *Associated manifestations.* What other signs and symptoms does your patient have? Besides chest pain, you should check for nausea, fatigue, edema, irregular heartbeats, dyspnea, and cyanosis—any of which could indicate a weak or damaged heart.

• *Pertinent negatives.* What you *don't* find can also be significant. The fewer classic characteristics of cardiac pain and associated mani-

C

festations your patient has, the less chance he's in imminent danger. But don't rely too strongly on pertinent negatives; an MI can easily arrive unannounced.

In conducting your symptom analysis, ask only those questions you can't answer from what your patient's already said or you've already observed. That way, you won't waste precious time. If your patient *is* in obvious distress, limit your questions to those he can answer with "yes" or "no" so you won't tire him unnecessarily. (See also *Chest pain: assessment.*)

Chest physiotherapy

Performing it on an infant

If performing chest physiotherapy on an infant is difficult because your hand is too big, try this. Use the mask from a size 0 or 00 pediatric resuscitation bag. Cover the hole (where the mask usually attaches to the bag) with a piece of gauze. The mask makes a percussor that's just the right size.

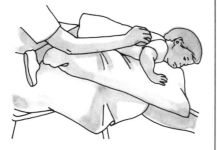

A nipple from a baby bottle also makes a good chest percussor for an infant. But before you begin, put a light blanket or diaper over the infant as a buffer so the nipple won't irritate his skin.

Chest tube insertion

When you're assisting

Here's how to reassure the patient, prepare him for the procedure, as-

sist the doctor, and monitor the patient's recovery:

1. Explain the procedure to the patient and tell him that it will help him breathe more easily.

2. Sedate him, as ordered.

3. Prepare his skin with povidone-iodine solution. Drape the area with sterile towels.

4. Help the patient hold still while the doctor anesthetizes his skin, makes an incision, and inserts the tube. To relieve pneumothorax, the doctor will insert it in the second intercostal space along the midclavicular line. For pleural effusion or hemothorax, he'll insert it in the fourth to sixth intercostal space in the anterior or midaxillary line. (See *Pneumothorax.*)

5. Connect the tube to an underwater-seal chest drainage unit. (See *Chest drainage system: preparation.*) Tape all tube connections securely and apply suction, as ordered, after the doctor has sutured the tube in place and applied petrolatum gauze and a sterile dressing.

6. Secure the unit to the patient's bed.

As part of the follow-up care:
• Prepare the patient for a chest X-ray to check tube placement.
• Administer pain medication, as ordered.
• Secure the tube to the drawsheet with a safety pin, allowing sufficient tubing so that the patient can turn over. Don't leave dangling loops.
• Keep clamps and extra petrolatum gauze at the patient's bedside in case the tubing is accidentally disconnected or pulled out. (See *Chest tube removal.*)

Chest tube placement

Checking for possible problems

Your patient has chest tubes inserted; recalling chest anatomy, you remember chest tubes are placed

in the pleural space, an area of negative pressure.

Are the tubes patent—and doing their job? To answer this, you must take a good look at the tubes. You see a closed system—designed to take air or fluid away from the patient—that involves a series of tubes. Thinking of the system as one continuous tube will help you trace it from the patient to drainage collection device. (See also *Chest drainage system: patency.*)

You see a clear, pliable tube emerging from the patient's chest wall connected externally to about 6' (1.8 m) of tubing. This tubing leads to a drainage collection device at the bedside.

As you know, respiration causes physical changes within the body. In this case, these changes can also be seen as mechanical changes; that is, the fluid in the tubing should fluctuate as the patient breathes.

Your most important question is: How are the patient's respirations? (Is his breathing labored? Recall that chest expansion should be bilateral.)

Move further down the tubing: Are all the connections tight—including the cap on the collection device? Is the tubing tight from collection device to suction source? Does the drainage in the collection device exceed the initial amount of sterile water placed as the underwater seal? Or, is the collection device so filled with drainage that suction force and draining capacity are diminishing?

Any break or loose connection in the system may be an entry for atmospheric air, which would result in lung collapse. (See *Chest drainage system: air leakage.*)

If you've checked all the other variables and a problem remains, you may need to examine the insertion site. If hospital policy permits, change the chest dressing. Can you hear any air escape? Is the tube inserted snugly into the patient's chest? Are the sutures intact? Is the junction between the distal part of the chest tube and drainage tube secure? Can you see any clots impeding outward flow?

Inspect and palpate the skin. Do you see or feel any sign of subcutaneous emphysema (for example, air in subcutaneous tissue)? If so, notify the doctor. (See *Chest drainage system: management.*)

Chest tube removal

When a patient pulls his out

Imagine this scene: You go to your patient's room and find him very restless; in fact, he's pulled off his oxygen mask. His skin feels cool and slightly damp, and he looks pale and dusky around his mouth. His respirations are 24; his pulse, 140; and he has a palpable blood pressure of 100.

When you pull down the sheet to assess his incision, you see that his anterior chest tube dressing has been ripped off, and the tube pulled out. What should you do?

Call for help and ask whoever responds to page the surgeon stat. Replace the patient's oxygen mask. Tell him you know he's having trouble breathing and you've called for his doctor.

Obtain some sterile petrolatum gauze. Tell the patient to take a deep breath. At the peak of his inspiration, place the gauze over the chest tube insertion site to form an airtight seal. Apply firm pressure with your hand. Have another nurse reassess the patient's vital signs and check to see that an I.V. site is available for administration of an antiarrhythmic or vasopressor if needed.

As you maintain pressure, have somone obtain supplies the doctor may need: a chest tube, a chest tube insertion tray or suture tray, sterile gloves and towels, antiseptic skin solution, a local anesthetic, silk suture (if it's not in the tray), and an arterial blood gas (ABG) kit.

When the doctor arrives, describe the patient's condition to him. As he inserts the new chest tube,

assist as necessary, maintaining a sterile field. (See *Chest tube insertion.*) Monitor the patient's vital signs, being especially alert for an irregular pulse and falling blood pressure.

Once the tube is in place, continue to monitor the patient's vital signs and check to see that he's breathing more easily. Call the radiology department for a stat portable chest X-ray to confirm the tube's position. The doctor will probably order an ABG study between 30 and 45 minutes after the new tube is inserted. See that the doctor gets both the X-ray and ABG study results at once—he may need to reposition the chest tube if the X-ray shows incomplete re-expansion of the middle and lower lobes. He may also want to reassess ABG levels if the patient remains hypoxic despite the new tube.

Chest tube stripping

Performing it correctly

Stripping chest tubes is done to keep the tubes open and draining freely.

How to strip chest tubes
Stripping a chest tube mechanically dislodges clots or debris from the tube and pushes them toward the drainage container.

Here's the most common way: Compress and stabilize the tubing (just below the connector joining it to the thoracic catheter) with your thumb and forefinger of one hand. Then, slide your other hand along

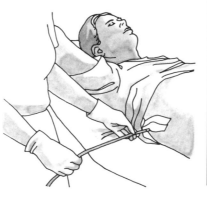

firmly from that point, flattening a section of tubing. Release the hand closest to the patient's chest, grip the tubing just above the sliding hand, and flatten another section of tubing. Continue this action along the entire length of tubing until you reach the drainage container.

You can reduce friction by using hand lotion, an alcohol sponge, or a roller (which is commercially available and helps maintain uniform pressure on the tubing).

Besides mechanically moving the drainage, stripping creates a brief pulse of suction as you release the flattened length of tubing and lets it re-expand. In fact, research has shown that stripping can create high transient negative pressures (suction).

Other ways of stripping chest tubes produce less suction pressure. For example, squeezing hand-over-hand along the tubing produces a pressure of only about -30 cm H_2O—*if* you release the tubing and let it re-expand between squeezes. But if you leave one hand in place until you've gripped the tubing firmly with the other, you'll produce a stair-step buildup of suction.

Another way to strip chest tubes is by fan-folding several layers of tubing and squeezing them with both hands. This creates positive pressure while you squeeze the tubing and suction of about -50 cm H_2O when you release the tubing.

When to strip chest tubes
No hard-and-fast rules exist about when to strip chest tubes—that decision depends on the particular circumstances.

Usually stripping is done if fresh blood or a clot gets in the tubing. You can usually keep the drainage moving by keeping the tubing in a straight line from the patient's chest to the drainage container, and let gravity do the work for you. If necessary, you can squeeze alternately with each hand along the tubing and release in between each squeeze to gently prod the drainage along.

When full-fledged stripping seems indicated, remember that you may generate high levels of suction in the process. Be especially cautious and observant when you're stripping chest tubes in a patient with fragile lung tissue—for instance, a patient with advanced emphysema. Some hospitals still require routine stripping of chest tubes at set intervals. But this practice is changing to one of individualized nursing judgments.

Chest wound, sucking

Managing one

If a sharp object or fragment from a missile penetrated your patient's chest wall, it may have created a sucking chest wound. Such a wound destroys the necessary pressure gradient between the pleural space and outside atmosphere. Unless you can restore this pressure gradient, the patient will quickly develop respiratory failure.

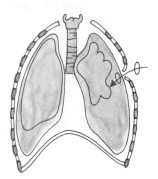

Equipment
You'll need the following:
• nasal cannula, face mask, and oxygen equipment
• petrolatum gauze
• wide tape
• chest tube tray.
Procedure
Here's what to do:
• Monitor your patient closely.
• Administer oxygen through a nasal cannula or a face mask.
• Don't remove any object protruding from your patient's chest—doing so will destroy the pressure gradient even faster and increase bleeding.
• Reassure the patient, then ask him to exhale forcefully. At the moment

of maximum expiration, cover the wound with petrolatum gauze to seal it.
• Secure the gauze with wide tape.
• Monitor the patient closely for signs and symptoms of tension pneumothorax, and notify the doctor if this condition develops. (See *Pneumothorax, tension.*)
• If the doctor decides to insert a chest tube, get the equipment ready and be prepared to assist.
• If the doctor orders surgery, prepare your patient appropriately. (See *Chest tube insertion.*)

Child abuse: legal action

When you suspect it

Most state legislatures have adopted child-abuse statutes to protect children from physical, mental, and sexual abuse. If your work involves children, read the statutes and your hospital's policy on handling possible child-abuse victims.

If you suspect child abuse, you should follow this procedure:
• Contact your local department of social services, protective services, or welfare.
• Report your suspicions of child abuse and ask for assistance in obtaining a court order to hold the child in temporary custody.
• Don't withhold your suspicions for fear of civil or criminal liability. Most statutes provide immunity against such liability to encourage good-faith reports. (See *Child abuse: recognition.*)

Child abuse: recognition

Clues to watch for

Ask yourself the following questions when you suspect child abuse.
How does the child react to touch? If he ducks or flinches, he probably

associates touch with pain. Typically, abused children aren't hugged very often, so they don't associate touch with affection.
Does the child leave his parents without hesitation when he must undergo a painful procedure, such as having a wound sutured? Even an older child will tend to cling to his parents in this situation. A child who walks away from his parents may be eager for a brief escape.
Is it bravery or a conditioned response? If a child undergoes a painful procedure without crying, grimacing, struggling, or holding his breath, he's either extremely ill or accustomed to pain. An abusive parent who observes such passive behavior may say something like, "He knows better than to cry."
How do the parents feel about the child's injury? Abusive parents may say, "I don't know why he's so bad. He never does what I tell him." These parents are probably rationalizing that if the child hadn't misbehaved, he wouldn't have been injured.
Does the child have old injuries that the parents can't explain? Note any suspicious marks on the skin. Ask yourself, for instance, if the marks on an infant's back are really ant bites, as the parents say, or if they look more like cigarette burns. Are the teeth marks on a young child really from his brother? Adult bite marks are surprisingly small.
Do the parents allow the child to answer the questions you ask him? Abusive parents may try to direct the child's response. A statement such as "Tell the nurse how your brother hit you in the face" or "Tell the nurse how you fell over your wagon" may be a signal that the parents want the child to stick to the story they've concocted. Parents who won't allow the child to speak at all may fear what he'll say.
What do the parents expect from the child? Frequently, abusive parents have unreasonable expectations of their child and demand complete obedience. They may, for instance, expect a 5-year-old to sit

quietly for an hour or a 2-year-old to control his bowels when he's under stress and in pain.

How does the child relate to his parents? Note whether he seems afraid or looks guilty when his parents enter the room. Does he look to them for support? If his parents have been abusing him, he'll probably feel guilty because they had to bring him for medical care.

How do the parents interact with each other? Do they support and comfort each other? Or do they argue and blame each other for the incident? Perhaps one accuses the other of neglecting or mistreating the child.

How do the parents react to authority figures? If a policeman happens to be in the emergency department, observe the parents' reaction. Most people are curious; few try to hide their faces. Also note the reaction when you mention the child welfare agency. Hostile or paranoid behavior may indicate that they're anxious because you suspect child abuse. (See *Child abuse: legal action.*)

Childbirth, emergency

When you must assist

If you ever need to assist with an emergency birth outside the hospital, ask someone nearby to gather the following supplies: some newspapers, clean towels, a bulb syringe (or turkey baster), a clean pair of scissors, some strong string, and some sanitary pads. While you're waiting for the supplies, help the woman get into position for delivery. Don't insist that she take the traditional supine position, unless she wants to lie flat. Rather, allow her to choose the most comfortable position. She may want to squat, lie on her side, or sit up with someone supporting her back.

Next, wash your hands, then place a pad of newspapers covered with towels on the bed, under the vaginal opening. Try not to touch the opening, as this would introduce the risk of infection.

When you see crowning, place the palm of your hand on the infant's head and apply gentle pressure. This will prevent an uncontrolled delivery and reduce the likelihood of vaginal tears and rapid pressure changes in the infant's skull. If the woman feels an uncontrollable urge to push, tell her to pant (breathe quick, small puffs of air through her mouth).

Crowning

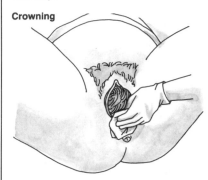

Support the infant's head as it passes through the vaginal opening. To determine if the umbilical cord is wrapped around his neck, feel for it with your finger. If it's wrapped loosely, you may be able to slip it over his head or shoulder.

Normally, you wouldn't want to cut the cord with nonsterile scissors. But if you can't slip the cord from the infant's neck, you may have to. If so, tie it in two places with the string and cut between them.

Clear the infant's mouth and nose, using the bulb syringe. Gently guide

Delivering the shoulders

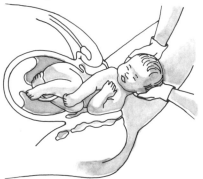

his head down to allow delivery of the first shoulder, then up for delivery of the second shoulder. Since shoulders are the widest part of the infant's body, the rest of the delivery should be easy. But be prepared to hold onto him; he may come out quickly, and he'll be slippery.

When the delivery is completed, ask someone to write down the date and time of birth. Hold the infant at the level of the mother's uterus to prevent hypovolemia or hypervolemia, caused by blood flowing between the infant and the placenta. If he's not breathing, stimulate him by flicking the bottoms of his feet or firmly rubbing his back. Quickly dry and cover him.

If you didn't need to cut the umbilical cord earlier, simply tie it now; let emergency or hospital personnel cut it later. Be sure not to put tension on it, however, as that could tear the cord or placenta, or invert the uterus.

Place the infant on the mother's abdomen while you wait for delivery of the placenta. When it appears, examine it to see if it's intact. Finally, remember to compliment the mother on a job well done.

After the placenta is delivered, massage the woman's abdomen to make the uterus contract. (See *Uterus, postpartum.*) Check the abdomen frequently to make sure it stays firm; lack of firmness could cause uterine hemorrhage. (See *Hemorrhage, postpartum.*) If the mother is going to nurse the infant, place the infant to her breast; nursing will prompt the release of oxytocin, the pituitary hormone that stimulates uterine contraction.

Place one or two sanitary pads (or towels) at the vaginal opening, and keep monitoring for excessive bleeding. Assess the mother's pulse, capillary refill, level of consciousness, skin temperature, and skin color for signs of decreased perfusion. Also assess the infant's respirations and skin temperature.

When the ambulance arrives, give the paramedics both an oral and written report. Include the infant's presentation and position, sex, and appearance. Be sure the placenta goes to the hospital with the woman and her newborn infant.

Childbirth: preterm labor

Emergency intervention

Here's what to do if you're off duty but you're called to assist a woman who's going into preterm labor:

Have the patient lie on her left side; this will increase blood flow to the uterus (decreasing uterine activity), and keep the fetus's weight off the cervix (decreasing cervical dilation). Place a pillow against her back for support, and encourage her to drink two to three glasses of water. (Dehydration is associated with preterm labor.)

In many cases, contractions in preterm labor are painless, so don't assume your patient will feel them when they occur. Assess them yourself by pressing your fingertips firmly against her abdomen. When you can feel the contractions, time them, from the beginning of one to the beginning of the next. Also, look for other signs of preterm labor: fluid leaking from the vagina; menstrual-like cramps; pressure in the lower back, abdomen, or thighs; and intestinal cramps with or without diarrhea.

Have the patient rest for an hour; resist the impulse to rush her to the hospital. This would only increase her anxiety, possibly intensifying the labor. But if the contractions are occurring every 10 minutes or less after an hour's rest, notify the patient's doctor or nurse-midwife and prepare to transport her. Waiting any longer increases the risk of premature delivery.

Report the time the contractions started and how frequently they are occurring to her doctor. Report, too, all other signs you observed.

Children, disabled

Helping them walk

Here's something you can recommend to parents of a handicapped child: Make a set of sturdy, economical parallel bars from wooden dowels and ordinary kitchen chairs. Here's how:

Buy the following at a lumber yard: two 8' (2.4 m) dowels, 1" (3 cm) in diameter. Sand and varnish them and attach a piece of clothesline to each end with a small nail. Then place the dowels over the seats of two kitchen chairs and tie the ends of the dowels to the chair backs. The height and width of the chair seats is just right for a toddler.

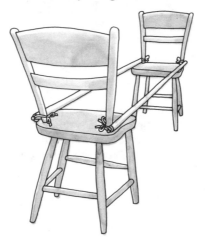

When the bars aren't in use, the child's parents can untie them and put them away.

Cholinergic crisis

Differentiating it from myasthenic crisis

If your patient has myasthenia gravis, you may have to distinguish between two life-threatening situations: myasthenic crisis and cholinergic crisis.

In myasthenic crisis, the patient's muscle weakness becomes acutely exacerbated from insufficient anti-cholinesterase or a worsening of the disease process.

In cholinergic crisis, overmedication of anticholinesterase precipitates acute muscle weakness. Other signs and symptoms include abdominal cramps and diarrhea, nausea and vomiting, pallor, and bradycardia.

Expect the following signs and symptoms with either crisis:
• difficulty breathing, swallowing, chewing, or speaking
• increased salivation, lacrimation, bronchial secretions, and sweating
• apprehension and restlessness.

To distinguish between the two emergencies, perform the Tensilon test: Give a small dose of edrophonium chloride (Tensilon), as ordered. If the patient's condition improves, he's in myasthenic crisis. Immediately administer an oral cholinergic drug, such as neostigmine (Prostigmin), as ordered.

However, if the edrophonium exacerbates his condition, he's in cholinergic crisis. Slowly administer atropine I.V. to counteract his reaction to edrophonium; then reduce anticholinesterase doses, as ordered.

Chvostek's sign

Assessing for hypocalcemia

To elicit this sign, tap the patient's facial nerve just in front of the earlobe and below the zygomatic arch or, alternatively, between the zygomatic arch and the corner of the mouth. A positive response (indicating latent tetany) ranges from simple mouth-corner twitching to

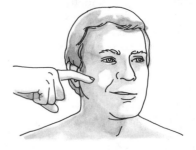

twitching of all facial muscles on the side tested. Simple twitching may be normal in some patients. However, a more pronounced response usually indicates a positive Chvostek's sign. (See also *Trousseau's sign.*)

Clubbed fingers

Assessing for early clubbing

Gently palpate the bases of your patient's fingernails. Normally, they'll feel firm but in early clubbing, they'll feel springy. To evaluate late clubbing, have your patient place the first phalanges of his forefingers together. Normal nail bases are concave and create a small, diamond-shaped space when the first phalanges are opposed. In late

Normal

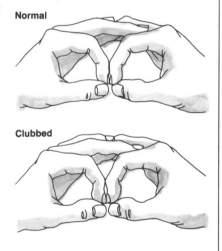

Clubbed

clubbing, however, the now-convex nail bases can touch without leaving a space.

Cocaine addiction: complications

What to watch for

When a patient arrives in the ED because of a cocaine overdose, you'll treat his problems symptomatically. (There's no antidote for cocaine.) The medical complica-

tions of an overdose can be devastating. Watch for seizures, hypertensive crises, myocardial infarctions, angina, dysrhythmias, abnormal respirations (Cheynes-Stokes), and cerebrovascular spasm and hemorrhage.

If you suspect a patient has been using cocaine, ask the doctor to order a toxicology screening. But even if the test shows cocaine metabolites, don't be surprised if he denies that he's using the drug. At this point, you should call a psychiatric liaison nurse or drug abuse counselor. Together, you can try to break through his denial.

You can't force a patient to admit that he uses cocaine. But some nurses have said that hammering away at the denial has worked for them. Point out how his addiction has contributed to his medical, social, or legal problems. Calmly, nonjudgmentally, say to him: "I'm confused. You're saying you don't have a problem with cocaine but you're living on the streets. Six months ago you had a good homelife. Now your family doesn't want you. I think we should talk about this."

Stick with him, even if you feel you aren't getting anywhere. You're showing him that you care about his health and welfare. You won't help him if you withdraw or discuss his abuse in an angry tone. (See also *Cocaine addiction: signs; Cocaine addiction: treatment.*)

Cocaine addiction: signs

Clues to addiction

How can you spot a cocaine addict? His physical, social, and legal problems may give him away. Look for:
• chronic nasal congestion and cold symptoms with snorting. After heavy use, the nasal septum may be perforated.
• unexplained weight loss (30 to 40 lbs [13.5 to 18 kg] in 6 months, for

example). Cocaine kills the user's appetite.
• declining social status or an incongruent economic situation. For example, he may have had a stable job and homelife, but now he's unemployed and homeless.
• recent behavioral changes, including antisocial acts such as stealing, embezzling, prostitution, or selling drugs.
• frequent visits to an ED for depression or suicide threats.
• behavior that's markedly different with each clinical visit or each shift. If he's depressed, lethargic, and apathetic the first time you see him, then elated, energetic, and talkative the next, he may be using cocaine before a clinical visit or during a hospital stay.
• needle tracks that have a pale center, where the needle was inserted, within a large, bruised area. This is caused by severe vasoconstriction when cocaine enters the bloodstream. (See also *Cocaine addiction: complications; Cocaine addiction: treatment.*)

Cocaine addiction: treatment

Helping the addict

A cocaine addict will usually resist treatment. Ideally, you'd like to see him volunteer for treatment without coercion, but realistically, you may need to get others involved. His family may help by putting pressure on him.

The hospital where you work may offer inpatient treatment for cocaine addicts. This approach is controversial, though. Some health care professionals say an inpatient program is unnecessary for someone who is not experiencing life-threatening withdrawal symptoms. The same people are also concerned that as an inpatient, he's removed from situations in which the drug is available and can't practice saying no.

The first goal of treatment, whether inpatient or outpatient, is to help the addict admit that cocaine has hurt him. Then he must acknowledge that he needs to stop using the drug. Rehabilitation should include daily group counseling sessions. There, he'll be taught assertive skills to help him resist taking cocaine. Also, he'll be encouraged to find friends who are "clean." And he'll learn to identify and work through the negative feelings that he sought to relieve by using cocaine.

Drug therapy may help the addict pull through the withdrawal crisis. His doctor may prescribe a tricyclic antidepressant (TCA); even a patient who continues to use cocaine may benefit from a TCA. Research suggests that TCAs reduce the craving for more cocaine and may interfere with the euphoria of the cocaine high. (See also *Cocaine addiction: complications; Cocaine addiction: signs.*)

Collar, Philadelphia

Description and application

The Philadelphia cervical collar is a lightweight molded polyethylene collar designed to hold the neck straight with the chin slightly ele-

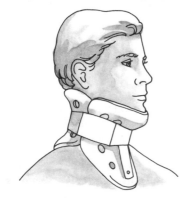

vated and tucked in. It immobilizes the cervical spine, decreases muscle spasms, helps relieve pain, pre-

vents further injury, and promotes healing.

When applying the collar, fit it snugly around the patient's neck and attach the Velcro fasteners or buckles at the back. Be sure to check his airway and neurovascular status to ensure that the collar isn't laced too high in the front, which could hyperextend his neck. If he has a neck sprain, this could cause ligaments to heal in a shortened position. If he has a cervical spine fracture, it could cause serious neurologic damage. (See *Collars, cervical.*)

Collars, cervical

Keeping them clean

When a patient has to wear a cervical collar for a long time, suggest he cover it with a 1-foot (30-cm) piece of stockinette to keep it clean. The stockinette cover will also keep the collar odor-free and can be easily removed for washing. (See *Collar, Philadelphia.*)

Commode

Keeping the lid raised

Do you find that a commode lid has a penchant for slamming shut just as you lower a patient onto the seat? Here's a way to keep the lid raised.

Get a Velcro book latch (usually used to hold large chart pages open). The book latch has two parts: a long tab (A) and a circle (B). (Both parts have adhesive backs that stick to almost any surface.)

Attach the adhesive side of B to the underside of the commode lid. Then attach the adhesive side of A to the commode frame with one end of the tab hanging down. (The tab's Velcro side should face away from the commode.)

Before you help a patient onto the commode, lift the lid. Bring tab A

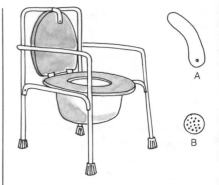

up over the lid and secure it to circle B on the lid. The lid will remain raised until you undo the latch.

Communication: dying patients

Final messages

Listen to the dying with complete attention and also let them *know* you're listening. Here are some techniques:
• Respond in ways that tell them you accept whatever they say or "see."
• Follow up what they say in a gentle way. Ask questions and offer sensitive, probing insights that might encourage them to keep talking.
• Make them repeat statements if necessary. Don't be afraid to say, "I'm not sure I follow you. Can you explain that a little more?"
• Support them. For instance, if they're having difficulty "letting go," don't deny the problem. Acknowledge it and offer to help.

Equally important, however, don't keep pushing. If they don't want to talk, drop it—they have to be ready. But at the same time, reinforce that you're still greatly interested, that they should let you know whenever they want to talk.

Pass on these messages to the family members so that they can share this time and perhaps understand the messages better. (See *Deathbed statements.*)

Communication: elderly patients

Overcoming communication barriers

Common physical problems—such as poor vision and hearing—can create barriers to communication. The trouble is, once you've labeled your elderly patients "confused," you may interpret hearing and visual limitations as still more examples of confusion.

Between 30% and 60% of all elderly people have progressive hearing losses. You can help by adjusting your conversation:
• Speak more slowly than usual and keep your voice pitch normal. Many elderly patients can't discriminate words if you speak quickly or in a high-pitched voice.
• Keep you hands away from your face when you speak. An elderly patient may "hear" you better if he can read your lips.
• Ask the patient to turn off his television or radio before you speak to him, or find another, quieter place to talk. Many elderly patients lose their ability to tune out or interpret distracting noises, so they may have trouble concentrating.
• Wait quietly for an elderly patient to answer your questions. He may be slow to understand the meaning of the words, even if he's heard them clearly.
• Keep explanations brief, and be sure the patient understands you before you go on to something else. (See also *Visually-impaired patients; Communication: hearing impaired.*)

Communication: family

Helping relatives of an acutely ill patient

Family members need ongoing, honest communication about the patient's progress. They also seek realistic hope and reassurance that he's well cared for. Here's how to ensure effective communication.

Personalize your communication
Address family members by name. And when referring to the patient, call him by the name most frequently used by family members—his nickname.

Explain surprising behavior
Acutely ill patients frequently exhibit behaviors unfamiliar to family members. One common—and disturbing—behavior is the failure to recognize the family. The patient who does this may later ask family members why they haven't visited. Such behaviors can burden family members with feelings of sadness and guilt: sadness that their loved one could think such a thing; guilt at leaving his side for any amount of time. This is where you need to step in with explanations and reassurance.

First, give the possible reasons behind such behavior—lack of sleep (see *Sleep deprivation*), fever, or increased intracranial pressure, for example. Second, reassure family members that this behavior is probably temporary and doesn't necessarily have anything to do with the patient's recovery. Third, reassure them that you'll continue to remind the patient of their presence and concern.

Offer effective reorientation
Another thing you can do is to reorient your patient frequently in the family's presence. This will reassure them that his disoriented behavior is being attended to. And they'll learn from you how they can help reorient him. (See *ICU care.*)

Show kindness
You can demonstrate kindness simply by the inflection in your voice or a smile—or by a hug, a warm handshake, or a hand on a shoulder.

Touch is a powerful communicator, both for you and the family. But family members may be afraid to touch the patient because they're overwhelmed by the surrounding equipment or intimidated by the lack of privacy. You need to lead the way—by showing how they can hold the patient's hand without disturbing intravenous lines, for instance. Your example will tell them that touch is a safe, effective, and acceptable means of communication.

Supply hope and cheer
Family members need hope—not easy to maintain when their loved one is seriously ill. Your role is to identify *realistic* hope that reflects the patient's condition.

Realistic hope may not be hope for recovery, but it may be hope for increased comfort or for transfer from a critical care unit to a medical/surgical unit. Be honest with the family; providing false hope sets up distrust.

Cheerfulness can convey hope, so you shouldn't hesitate to share cheerful moments or experiences. Such sharing is a good diversion and reaffirms that life does go on outside a hospital. This is especially important if the patient has been hospitalized for a long time. Collaborate with volunteer services and other support departments to create outlets for the monotony and constraints of long-term hospitalization.

If you ever feel you can't maintain a hopeful outlook, ask your supervisor for a breather. That'll give you time to gain perspective on the patient's case and will help the family receive consistently hopeful care. (See *Grief.*)

Communication: group

Leading a discussion

Sometimes you have to work with groups to get the job done; these tips will help you be more effective. First, begin by setting the right emotional atmosphere. If your group consists of a patient and his wife, set the stage for patient teaching by introducing yourself. Then, address each of them by name and proceed with your teaching.

If you're going to talk to a larger group—the other nurses on your unit, for example—try to create a bond between you and them by making a personal comment to each one before the meeting begins.

To achieve a comfortable atmosphere with a group of people you don't know, welcome each of them as they come in. This is also a good time to set the mood of the gathering. If you'd like the discussion to be informal, keep your own manner informal.

These techniques help each person in the group feel comfortable with you, but you also need to help them feel comfortable with each other—especially if you hope to have an informal group discussion.

You need a plan for what you hope to do and the steps you intend to take—what you plan to say, how you plan to begin group interaction, and the likely progression of the interaction. Frequently, a group will find its *own* way of reaching a decision, but your plans can furnish an alternative and give you the confidence of having a structure to fall back on.

To avoid this common problem, be sure you start every discussion by telling everyone: "Here's what I want to accomplish. And here's how I plan to go about it."

A potential disaster in any discussion—with 3 people or 30—is wandering off track and accomplishing nothing. You can prevent this with seven surefire techniques.

1. Summarize what's been said or decided. Pull all the threads of the discussion together, and tie that to your original goal.

2. Ask the group to restate the main points. Then remind them of your goals and the need to focus on it.

3. To turn a monologue back into a discussion, focus on other members.

4. To avoid having everyone talk but one person, you can't do much and still be subtle about it. Calling attention to the person during the discussion might be threatening or make him angry. The best bet is to wait until after the discussion, then ask him why he didn't participate. That will help you plan your strategy for the next discussion.

5. To cope with a feud—two people with ideas as different as night and day—emphasize the idea of "contrast" rather than "conflict." Then look for shared points of view.

6. To handle angry or painful feelings, here's a rule of thumb: When the feelings aren't interfering with the group's purposes, don't mention them. If they are—or if they're obviously making other people uncomfortable—ask the group what they're feeling and the source of those feelings.

A strong group can usually deal with such a problem, then go back to its discussion.

7. To make progress when the group can't agree, save what you can. You may have to change your goals—set smaller ones, for example, if the group can't resolve a major conflict. You may have to change the group—divide into smaller groups, for example, if the group is too big or too diverse to work together. (See *Staff management: group dynamics.*)

Communication: hearing impaired

Useful techniques

Try the following:
• Get your patient's attention by saying his name loud enough so he can hear you and respond. Don't shout, and don't get his attention by walking up to him and touching his arm—you'll only startle him.
• Make sure his area is well lit.
• Face him when talking to him.

• If he wears glasses, make sure he puts them on when you're speaking to him.
• Keep your mouth clearly visible; don't cover it with your hands.

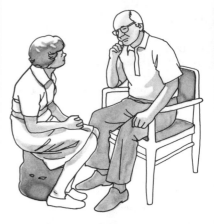

• Speak to him at a slower than normal pace. But not so slow that you make him feel stupid.

Here are some other hints. Make sure the room is as quiet as possible so the patient doesn't have any distractions. When you begin to talk, announce the subject—for example, "I'd like to talk to you about your medications." That's because, to a certain degree, a hearing-impaired person relies on predictability in a conversation. By knowing the subject of the conversation, your patient will recognize words that might otherwise be unclear to him.

If you must use unfamiliar words, such as medical terms, write them down. That way, sounds that are strange to him become visibly understandable. If you have important information for your patient—for example, that he shouldn't get out of bed unassisted—but can't get through to him, enlist the help of a relative or close friend.

Even if your patient denies he has a hearing problem, take steps to communicate better. Try to help him face his problem. You could also say something like, "You know, I had to repeat that several times. Do you think you might have a hearing problem?" Or "I'm sorry; it's obvious you can't hear me. Is it too noisy in here for you?" You could also offer a suggestion: "Would you consider making an appointment with a hearing specialist?" Talk to his doctor or to an audiologist. Also, ask his relatives or close friends to help. Frequently, they can get through to him better than anyone else.

Caring for a hearing-impaired patient means planning to spend more time with him than you normally would. But it's time well spent. (See *Communication: elderly patients.*)

Communication: ICU patients

Effective techniques

In the intensive care unit (ICU), quick communication with a suddenly deteriorating patient may be the deciding factor in his survival. But if you've worked in an ICU, you know that communicating effectively with patients is more difficult there than in almost any other unit because of their physical condition. Here's how you can improve communication:

• The first time a patient awakens in the ICU, make sure he understands where he is and what's happening to him. (If he's connected to life-support equipment, be sure he understands why.) For example, a patient who's had an endotracheal tube inserted for an emergency tracheotomy won't be able to think about communicating with you until he understands why he can't speak.

• Establish a relationship with each ICU patient as soon as possible. That way, you'll quickly establish communication as well.

For example, if you know a patient's going to be admitted to the ICU after surgery, visit him beforehand for some preoperative teaching. Besides becoming a familiar face to the patient and his family, you'll help him relax by giving him some idea of what to expect in the ICU—the environment, the equipment, and the procedures he can expect to undergo.

If preoperative teaching isn't possible, enlist the family members' aid in getting to know the patient after he's admitted. They can tell you what position he likes for sleeping, for example, and what fears and concerns about hospitalization he may have previously communicated to them.

• To reinforce the relationships you've established, ask your head nurse to keep your patient assignments as regular as possible.

• Let each of your ICU patients contribute to his own care plan to the extent that he can. Communicating with you about his care will encourage other types of communication as well.

• If necessary, give the patient communication aids. (See *Communication: respirator patients.*)

• Talk to the patient as much and as often as possible. Even when you aren't sure he can hear you or understand what you're saying, explain to him what you'll be doing and why—*before* you perform any procedure.

Here's another tip: Be careful not to talk about a patient with other ICU nurses or with doctors when he can overhear—and possibly misinterpret—your conversations. (This is particularly likely to happen when you're caring for a patient who's uncommunicative because he's intubated or comatose.)

Also avoid talking about one patient while standing near, or caring for, another—who may assume you're talking about *him*. This kind of communication can only confuse and frighten patients.

Don't underestimate stress or burnout you may feel as a barrier to communication with your ICU patients. Some ICU nurses unconsciously withdraw from patients as a way of coping with extreme stress and avoiding burnout. Others cope by becoming preoccupied with re-cording their observations and performing treatments, so they don't have time to communicate. Still other nurses become so anxious about their ICU responsibilities that they're unable to consider their patients' communication needs.

Communication: illiterate patients

When you're certain your patient can't read

When you're fairly sure your patient has difficulty reading, or worse, can't read at all, how can you help him? You've got to work within his defense mechanisms.

You might ask him if some of the words he reads get mixed up sometimes, or if once in a while the things he reads don't make sense. You can tell him it happens to a lot of people—which it does. If he answers you with a shy nod or a surprised "How did you know?" you have all the information you'll need to use alternate patient-teaching methods.

The first method to try is making drawings of what you want the patient to do *as* you tell him. Illustrate the most important points. For example, he needs to remember to take his medicine once a day, not that the medicine is a cardiac glycoside. Don't worry about technical expertise in the illustration. On the other hand, don't draw as you would for a child, such as with stick figures. This patient is very sensitive about his problem, and you don't want to insult him.

Another method is tape-recording your instructions. This way the patient can play them back and memorize them.

If you have good rapport with the patient, you may want to try a variation of a technique used in basic reading classes. Start by orally teaching the patient what you want him to know, for example, a particular procedure. Then have him re-

C

peat it back to you. Remember throughout to speak in a normal voice—you don't have to shout. The patient isn't deaf—he just can't read.

Communication, nonverbal

Interpreting messages

Assessing a patient's nonverbal behavior at the onset of any conversation can tell you a lot. Here's what to look for.

Appearance
Observe the patient's appearance and note it on the chart. A person who's not feeling well may neglect his appearance; for example, not combing his hair or shaving. By observing his appearance, you can later measure whether he's getting better or worse.

Kinesics
Observe how he moves; it can clue you in to whether he's scared, confident, or in pain. Although entering a hospital can make any patient nervous and awkward, his walk can still clue you in to whether he's scared or confident. Some people's walks announce, "Here comes somebody." Others' seem to say, "Don't mind me. I'm not much."

Eye contact
Notice whether he maintains eye contact. Lack of eye contact may signal low self-esteem (perhaps stemming from his lack of caring for himself).

Posture
Notice his posture. The way he sits or lies on the bed can tell you something about his emotional or physical state. Usually someone who sits with his shoulders slumped, head hung low, and eyes cast down has a low self-image—or he may be in pain. A straight but relaxed posture suggests more self-assurance—or freedom from pain.

Facial expression
Learn to read the expression on a patient's face. His expression may reveal an array of feelings—such as pain, fear, or worry.

Gestures
Watch a patient's gestures. They may indicate nervousness or impatience. In some cases, gestures are the *only* means of conversation. Can you imagine carrying on a two-way conversation with a patient on a ventilator without using gestures? For example, if he wants to be suctioned he might snap his fingers to signal "come here," then point to the tracheostomy and suction equipment to indicate suctioning.

Touch
Pay attention to the way your patient uses touch. Some may use touch as a way of reaching out to you—for attention or maybe just for human warmth. Others may not feel comfortable with touching and are determined to keep their sense of "personal space."

Paralanguage
Note your patient's voice quality and nonlanguage vocalizations, including the tone of voice, inflection, spacing of words, stressing of certain words, and pauses between speaking. Sobbing, laughing, and grunting are also elements of paralanguage. Observing paralanguage in your patient may help you recognize if he's upset or worried, or any other feeling he might be experiencing.

Environment
Look at the patient's surroundings. His environment can tell you a lot about him which will help you gear your patient teaching.

During the initial admission interview, his hospital room is basically devoid of personality. With a few days' accumulation of get-well cards, gifts, and flowers, his room begins to reveal more about him. What types of books, family pictures, or handiwork are there—and what do they tell you about his hobbies or interests?

As we said, by looking at what the patient is telling you nonverbally as well as listening to what he says verbally, you can better understand his needs. And that means you can better plan to meet those needs.

Communication: respirator patients

Using visual aids

Every ICU should have a set of simple communication aids for patients who can't communicate verbally. Scan the following list:
• *Paper, clipboard, and felt-tip pen.* Attach the pen to the clipboard with a ribbon or string so it can't fall out of the patient's reach.

• *Magic Slates.* These resemble flip charts with a clear plastic sheet stapled to a waxed black surface. They are especially useful for patients who want to communicate brief messages that won't need to be saved.
• *Alphabet board.* If a patient's poor eyesight impairs his handwriting ability, or if he doesn't have the strength or coordination to write legibly, he may be able to communicate by pointing to the letters of the alphabet that spell his message. Try printing the alphabet on a piece of cardboard and asking him to point out letters that create his words: This method is faster (but

may be more difficult to comprehend) than using movable magnetic letters.

• *Word cards.* On each page of a 4″ × 6″ cardboard flip chart, write a common word or phrase the patient may want to use. (Here's where your knowledge of the patient and his condition becomes a true bridge to communication.) For example, use phrases like "I'm in pain," "Please turn me," or "I need the bedpan." Or print several phrases on a large piece of cardboard so the patient can point to the appropriate ones.

• *Foreign language cards.* These can make a critical difference when you're caring for patients who don't speak English well—or at all. Available commercially, the cards display common medical terms and phrases (with phonetic pronunciation guides) as well as their English translations. If your unit doesn't have funds to purchase these cards, you can make some for each patient. (Consult his family for help with understanding his language.) (See *Communication: ICU patients.*)

Communication: stroke patients

Helping them express their needs

Set up a simple way for your stroke patient to express his basic needs. If he can write, give him a Magic Slate; if he can't write but can still move his fingers, try an alphabet board.

Phrase your questions by asking yes-or-no questions whenever possible so he'll be able to answer easily. If you must repeat questions do so quietly and calmly, using gestures and facial expressions to reinforce the message you're trying to convey. Resist the impulse to talk to him like a deaf person or a child.

If he's dysphasic, try not to embarrass him by correcting his speech.

Most important, show him that you understand the nature of his condition through your words and actions. For example, you might say: "I know that you know what you want to say." In this way, you make it clear you don't suspect him of being unintelligent, that you realize his mind is working clearly. This will help his self-esteem. (See *Communication: respirator patients; Stroke patients.*)

Compartment syndrome

Causes and interventions

Suppose your patient develops compartment syndrome, a neuromuscular compression within a muscle group caused by tissue swelling. Intervene as follows:

• Quickly decrease the edema-ischemia cycle by elevating the patient's affected limb, applying cold packs, and removing anything constricting the limb—such as an elastic bandage or a tight dressing.

• Immediately notify the doctor.

• Expect to assist with measuring the compartment pressure.

• Administer an analgesic for pain, as ordered.

Cross section of mid-lower leg

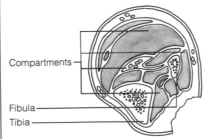

Compartments

Fibula

Tibia

• Anticipate that the doctor will perform emergency fasciotomy if initial interventions don't provide relief within 30 minutes. Fasciotomy is a surgical procedure to incise the fascia enclosing the muscle, allowing it

to swell beyond its compartment. The incision may be left open to heal by granulation. Later, split-thickness skin grafts will be applied.

Confidential information

Keeping it to yourself

First, check your hospital's policy on what information must be charted and what may be withheld as confidential. If you disagree with the policy, discuss your reservations with your hospital director or supervisor. Make sure you know what's expected of you—and that you can ethically comply.

Next, you can explain the policy to each of your patients when you feel it's appropriate. If the policy calls for charting almost all information, you could describe how it protects the patient by limiting access to the charts. After you've explained the policy, follow it consistently.

Will you risk losing your patients' trust? (See *Patients' trust.*) By telling your patients in advance what sort of information you must pass on to others, you won't be caught in the trap of having to betray confidences.

Will patients start to "bottle up" their problems? Again, experienced nurses say no. Most patients will open up to you if you've developed a good relationship with them.

If some patients try to manipulate you by threatening to withhold information unless you swear to keep it confidential, refuse. Chances are they'll talk to you anyway. If they don't, they probably are not ready to be helped. Just remember: If patients make you choose between being a friend and being a professional, you have to choose the latter. (See *Confidentiality; Confidentiality and co-workers.*)

C

Confidentiality
Knowing when to breach it

How should you handle a situation where ensuring a patient's right to privacy would jeopardize public welfare and safety? State laws *require* you and other health professionals to violate your patients' right to privacy when you discover:
• any injury that seems to have been caused by a dangerous weapon or by a criminal act (even if the patient denies the apparent cause of his injury)
• suspected child abuse
• animal bites; poisoning; and certain communicable diseases, such as sexually transmitted diseases and tuberculosis
• certain congenital or hereditary conditions, such as ophthalmia neonatorum or phenylketonuria.

In such cases, report your findings to state agencies or to your hospital administrators who will make the official report. (See *Confidential information.*)

Confidentiality and co-workers
When a co-worker violates a patient's trust

If a co-worker consistently discusses "interesting cases," mentioning names and intimate details about care, talk to her. You've probably heard the old saying, "Loose lips sink ships." Well, your chatty co-worker is sailing into dangerous waters both ethically and legally.

Ethically? The American Nurses' Association's *Code for Nurses* says this: "The nurse safeguards the client's right to privacy by judiciously protecting information of a confidential nature." Legally? Nurses who violate patient privacy risk lawsuits.

Suggest using a bit of common sense. Talking about work is natural. But it should never be done in public places like elevators, visitors' lounges, and cafeterias.

Discuss your co-worker's loose talk privately with her, pointing out the ethical and legal risks. Recommend that she restrict her discussions to the nurses' lounge or a private office—and that she limit her "audience" to co-workers directly involved in the case.

If she shrugs off this advice, ask the supervisor to speak to her. A warning from higher up just might make this nurse more careful about what she says and where she says it. (See *Confidential information; Confidentiality; Patients' trust.*)

Conflict management
Developing flexibility

Conflict doesn't inevitably mean flaring tempers and damaged relationships. Instead, you can control potentially explosive situations. How? By developing flexibility in the use of conflict-management techniques.

Each technique represents a different balance—between the outcome you want and the outcome the other person wants. How can you tell which technique to use? That depends on the answer to questions such as:
• How much power do I have, compared with the other person, to influence the outcome of this conflict?
• How much do I value my relationship with the other person?
• How much time is available to resolve this conflict?

Accommodation
When you respond to conflict by accommodating, you're basically putting your own concerns aside and letting the other person have her way. Although you won't want to do this frequently, accommodation may be the best action to take at times.

Accommodating is more cooperative than assertive. It may be your best response when:
• a conflict would create a serious

disruption, such as arguing with a colleague in front of a patient.
• the person you're in conflict with has the power to resolve the conflict unilaterally—for example, when your boss wants one thing and you want another.
• you realize that what you want to do is wrong or won't solve the problem. Admitting this earns a special dividend: the other person's respect.
Avoidance
Avoiding conflict only protects you from an upsetting confrontation. At times, however, that may be enough. For instance, it's probably best when you alone don't have an impact on "the system"—such as when you'd prefer primary nursing but the hospital uses team nursing.

Avoiding conflict is unassertive because you're not dealing with the problem. But it may be your best choice when:
• you'd have to pay too high a price to get what you want.
• what you want isn't worth the trouble of working through the conflict.
• you need to gather more information before you form an opinion or present your side of the issue.
• someone else is in a better position than you to resolve the conflict.
• tempers flare and you need a cooling off period.
• the conflict is a symptom of a deeper issue.
Collaboration
Collaborating is mutual problem-solving that ends with full agreement on a solution. This takes more time than the other techniques, so it isn't always possible (such as during an emergency). It's not practical either; trivial issues often aren't worth the effort used to resolve them. Consider collaborating when:
• you can learn something from exploring the other person's point of view.
• you can gain commitment from others.
• you need to work through feelings left over from an earlier conflict or some resulting from this one.

Competition

Typically, you can only use competition to resolve conflict when you have more power than the other person in the situation and when you're willing to sacrifice some of the quality of your relationship with her. Basically, it's telling her to do things your way or else.

Obviously, you won't often choose this way to resolve conflict. Despite the fact that it's aggressive and uncooperative, competition can be appropriate when:
• minutes count in an emergency and you're certain you know what quick, decisive action to take.
• the other person may take unfair advantage of you unless you act quickly. For example, aggressive people may impose upon your rights.

Compromise

When you and another person give up part of what you each want to resolve a conflict, that's compromise. It's not as satisfying as collaboration because you each get less than you wanted. But it usually provides a good balance of assertiveness and cooperation. Also, it may be the only way you can get at least part of what you want if you don't have the power or time to try for more.

Consider using compromise when:
• you can't come up with a solution that's more satisfactory in meeting both your needs.
• you've tried competing with someone more powerful than you, and compromise is the next best choice.
• the issue is too important for you to accommodate or avoid.
• you're willing to trade off some of what you want so that the conflict is resolved quickly, or to end it before you risk damaging your relationship with the other person.

Next time you're involved in a conflict—stop, think, and then try one of these techniques. If it doesn't work, try another technique, always aiming to balance what you want with what the other person wants. You won't always get your own way, of course, but you will get respect from the people you deal with daily. That's something everyone wants.

Conflicts

A three-step approach

Here's a three-step approach to dealing with conflict.

Step 1
Make sure you perceive the problem accurately. Without enough facts, people tend to manufacture fantasies about what's going on. Don't fantasize—find out.

Step 2
Decide if the battle's worth fighting. You have to examine your own philosophy and values. What really matters to you? How sure are you that you're right? How far are you willing to go to win? Whenever you're angry, you have a choice between staying angry or letting go. There are plenty of things in the world to be angry about, but you can't stay angry about all of them. Learn to let go of anger over trivial matters.

Step 3
Use your anger to resolve conflict, not exacerbate it. Don't accuse, attack, or call people names. Instead, enlist others' help by saying, "Look, I think we have a problem, and I'd like to discuss it with you. I'd like to know what we can do about it." (See *Conflict management.*)

Conflict with family members

Managing it adeptly

Conflicts can arise over almost anything in the hospital setting. Family members frequently complain about the quality of care. They focus on:
• how often the patient is visited
• how friendly the nurses are
• how well hospital services are coordinated
• how flexible the hospital is in letting family members spend the night or stay beyond visiting hours.

To prevent conflicts, make sure your unit has a strong commitment to nursing education for all staff, a firm adherence to all hospital policies, efficient supervision, and openness in evaluating your services.

If a conflict develops despite such measures, look for deeper problems, such as a lack of mutual respect between nurse and family, poor staff morale, or general depression in the complaining family member.

Conflicts commonly develop between nurses and the parents of hospitalized children when the treatments ordered aren't those the parents want.

Two guidelines help in such conflicts. First, don't get into a fight defending doctor's orders or trying to establish your own superiority in knowing what's best for the child. And second, don't give in.

Recognize that the true issue is rarely the treatment decision itself. More often it's the parents' wanting the power to decide what's right for their child.

To handle such conflicts, clarify the orders and tell the parents you must carry them out unless the parents want to negotiate with the doctor themselves about changing the orders.

Conflicts may also arise from such issues as the presence of family members during procedures and the extent of their involvement in the patient's care. Usually, the real issue is the family's need to feel significant and adequate in meeting the patient's needs.

Generally speaking, you'll meet the patient's needs best by supporting family involvement. If the family members want to take over for the patient—thus increasing his dependency—help them identify a role for themselves in supporting and encouraging the patient rather than actually providing his care. This technique is particularly useful with the parents of hospitalized children who need to assume increased self-care.

Conflicts may develop when nurses are displeased by the way parents care for their children in the hospital. Looking down on already discouraged parents will make the situation worse. Instead, get the parents involved in care areas that will help them feel adequate. Help them meet other parents and discuss parenting techniques. Share some of your own techniques.

When the staff fails to consistently enforce hospital policies, patients and family members will take advantage of the inconsistencies. Common areas of manipulation are no-smoking rules, visiting hours, and use of hospital supplies.

To prevent such conflicts, be sure each shift notifies other shifts of any manipulation attempts. Then the whole staff can quickly restore policy standards. (See *Conflict management; Conflicts.*)

Congestive heart failure, acute

Helping your patient through the crisis

In the acute phase, your patient may have pulmonary or systemic congestion. Watch for unusual fatigue, dyspnea, coughing, ankle edema, weight gain, cyanosis, pulmonary congestion, distended neck veins, pain, anxiety, and fear.

Keep the patient's movement to a minimum. Turn him and massage his skin and pressure points at least every 2 hours. Explain the danger

of holding his breath (Valsalva's maneuver) when being turned.

Auscultate his lungs for breath sounds and crackles. Watch for pulmonary congestion that may lead to pulmonary edema. Administer oxygen to help him breathe easier and to make him more comfortable.

Right-sided failure

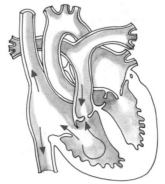

Remember four major goals as you care for your patient: Reduce his circulatory impairment, administer medications properly (probably digitalis and a diuretic), help regulate his fluid and electrolyte balance, and help allay his anxiety.

To reduce his circulatory impairment, decrease the venous return to his heart by placing him in a semi-Fowler's position. When he's allowed, have him sit on the side of the bed with his feet on a chair and his arms resting on an overbed table. Make sure he understands that he must rest to reduce his cardiac work load (a day of complete rest saves the heart about 25,000 contractions). As he improves, he may increase his activity.

To maintain a proper fluid and electrolyte balance, the patient will also need to restrict his sodium intake. Weigh him daily at the same time and with the same scale. Observe and chart any edema.

Finally, acknowledge and try to alleviate the patient's anxiety. Tell him that fears of dying, choking, and being disabled and dependent are normal for someone in his con-

dition. Emphasize signs of recovery, such as improved vital signs and decreased edema, but don't give false assurances. (See *Congestive heart failure: fear.*)

Congestive heart failure: complications

Preventing problems

Cardiac deterioration may result from inadequate gas exchange and impaired arterial and venous peripheral circulation. With this diagnosis, your goal in planning interventions is to prevent complications: pulmonary and systemic congestion, infection, and cardiogenic shock. Be sure to:

1. Prevent pulmonary and systemic congestion. Check for fluid retention and weigh the patient daily. If his weight increases more than 1 lb (0.5 kg) a day, promptly notify the doctor. Monitor fluid intake and output and test urine specific gravity every 2 hours. To minimize fluid retention, avoid rapid or excessive hydration. When administering I.V. fluids or drugs, use a microdrip system or infusion pump. Give oxygen as needed and evaluate the patient's response to it by monitoring his arterial blood gases.

2. Monitor drug therapy. Systemic congestion may inhibit drug metabolism and even low doses may cause toxic effects, so be especially alert for signs of effectiveness or drug toxicity. If a drug doesn't seem to be achieving its desired effect, discuss with the doctor the possible need for an increased dose. Watch carefully for adverse reactions that affect fluid balance. If the patient retains fluid, give diuretics as ordered, but observe for hypokalemia. If the patient is taking digitalis and develops hypokalemia, observe closely for signs of digitalis toxicity. Give potassium supplements for hypokalemia, as ordered. (See also *Hypokalemia management.*)

3. Try to prevent cardiogenic shock. Observe for signs of cardiogenic shock, particularly if the patient is more than 65 years old or has had a previous myocardial infarction with congestive heart failure. These signs include altered mental status, decreased urine output (less than 20 ml/hour), hypotension, and respiratory distress. Report any of these signs immediately. (See *Cardiogenic shock care.*)

Congestive heart failure: fear

Reducing your patient's anxiety

The patient may experience fear of heart failure, life-style changes, powerlessness or death; may express anger and hostility as a result of his illness; or may lack the knowledge necessary for full compliance. If you see these problems, your goal is to reduce the patient's anxiety level. This is essential since anxiety produces vasoconstriction; increases arterial pressure, heart rate, and respirations; and, according to some evidence, reduces urine output. Teach the patient relaxation techniques, and play soft music or read to him. (See *Relaxation techniques.*) Encourage the patient and his family to verbalize their fears. Make sure you:

1. Teach the patient about his treatment. Begin your teaching on the day of admission. Tell the patient to stay in bed most of the time at first, getting up just to use the bathroom and to sit in a chair for meals. Advise him to change positions slowly to prevent dizziness. Explain that you'll perform passive range-of-motion exercises three times a day and evaluate the effects of these exercises on his respirations, heart rate, and energy level.

Explain any dietary and fluid restrictions. Tell him that you'll record his intake and output and weigh him once daily.

2. Help the patient accept realistic limitations. The patient with congestive heart failure (CHF) frequently feels torn between what he wants to do and what his weakened heart allows him to do. In resolving this dilemma, the patient can easily overreact: The cautious patient may restrict activity unnecessarily, whereas the stoic patient may overexert himself. Help your patient steer clear of these extremes by giving him a thorough explanation of CHF and the specific limitations that are appropriate for his condition.

Discuss specific changes in lifestyle, but avoid frightening him. Negotiate changes that don't involve his self-image. If he objects strongly to eliminating an activity, explore the reasons with him. When possible, suggest that he continue a favorite activity at a less strenuous level.

Before discharge, assess the patient's ability to comply with treatment and make referrals for follow-up care as needed. If the patient fails to understand his treatment regimen, clarify his role. Also, refer him to the American Heart Association for information and, if necessary, to psychological and social services to promote and ease necessary adjustments in life-style. (See *Congestive heart failure, acute.*)

Congestive heart failure: history

Getting all the details

Your first aim in history-taking is to define the progression of congestive heart failure (CHF) in a detailed interview. However, you'll have to modify the interview according to the patient's condition. If the patient's in distress during admission, keep the initial history brief and to the point; avoid repeating questions the doctor's already asked. If you can't complete a satisfactory interview at admission, continue it later, when the patient's more comfortable.

Be sure to ask the patient these questions:

"Have you had a previous myocardial infarction or dysrhythmia, recent hemorrhage, anemia, respiratory infection, chronic respiratory disease, pulmonary embolism, thyrotoxicosis, fever, hypoxia, or any other problem that could cause or aggravate CHF?

"What drugs are you currently taking? Have you taken medications according to the prescribed schedule?

"Have you recently experienced shortness of breath?" (Try to pinpoint when.) "Do you become breathless with slight exertion, with heavy exertion, or at night?

"Have you recently experienced fatigue, muscle weakness, decreased urination, weight gain, anorexia, bloated feelings, depression, or anxiety?" (For each reported symptom, determine its severity, onset, and duration.)

"Have you recently experienced any stressful events?

"Have you ever been treated for CHF with medication or any dietary, fluid, and activity restrictions?" (If so, has he followed the prescribed treatment?)

"What effect does CHF have on your life-style? What support systems do you have?"

During your interview, form an overall impression. Does he appear edematous? Is he overweight? Is he breathless when he speaks?

Contact lens insertion

Inserting a soft lens

Follow these steps:

1. Position the patient comfortably, having him either sit or lie down.

2. Obtain the wetting solutions recommended or approved by the manufacturer.

C

3. Wash and rinse your hands. Dry them on a paper towel, because it's less likely to leave lint on your fingers. To minimize the risk of injuring his eye or damaging the lens, make sure your fingernails are short.

4. Remove the lens from its container of sterile solution, and examine it closely. Never put a torn lens in your patient's eye. Don't insert a lens if it looks cloudy or has specks of lint on it. If necessary, rinse debris from the lens using the approved wetting solution. If it still looks dirty after rinsing, or if it's cloudy or damaged in any way, don't insert it. Instead, notify your patient's eye care professional.

5. Place the lens on the tip of your finger and make sure it's not inside out.

6. Check the lens by gently squeezing it between two fingers. If it's positioned correctly, the edges will point inward. If not, the edges will turn slightly outward.

7. Gently turn the lens to its correct position if inside out. Make sure the lens is fully wet. It dries quickly after you remove it from the solution. If necessary, rewet with the approved wetting solution.

8. Position the lens on the index finger of your dominant hand. Use your other index finger to raise your patient's upper eyelid, and instruct

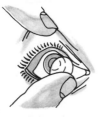

him to look straight ahead. While gently applying downward pressure on the lower lid, move the lens toward his cornea. Place the lens di-

rectly over the pupil and iris, and remove your finger.

9. Release the patient's upper eyelid and gently massage it to expel any air bubbles that may be trapped under the lens. Ask him if he can see clearly, and if he feels any discomfort. If he can't see clearly, look closely to see if the lens is positioned properly. (If it isn't, hold his eyelids apart. Ask him to look straight ahead and gently center the lens with your finger.)

10. If the lens feels uncomfortable, it may have a speck of dust or lint trapped beneath it. You'll have to remove the lens, rinse it with the approved wetting solution, and try again. (See *Contact lens removal.*) Never leave a lens in place if the patient complains of discomfort.

If your patient complains of blurred vision, and he wears a lens in each eye, you may have mixed up the lenses.

A hard contact lens is inserted the same way as a soft lens, but the lens can't be inverted and the eyelid shouldn't be massaged.

Contact lens removal

How to do it properly

Suppose a patient who wears contact lenses comes to the emergency department with facial injuries. Or a patient has chemical irritants or foreign bodies trapped under his contact lenses. You'll need to remove the lenses before you can care for him further. Here's how.
Suction bulb removal (hard and soft lenses)
Gently place the cup end against the contact lens, then pull the bulb

Suction bulb removal

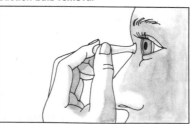

away from the eye in a straight line. (Make sure you don't touch the cornea with the suction bulb. Doing so may cause permanent damage.)
Manual removal (soft lens)
Place your index finger directly on the lens, then slide the lens gently

Manual removal (soft lens)

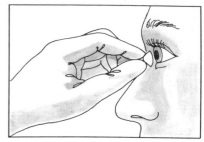

down and away from the cornea. Pinch the lens between your thumb and index fingers, and lift it out.
Manual removal (hard lens)
Pull the eyelids apart to completely expose the contact lens. Press down

Manual removal (hard lens)

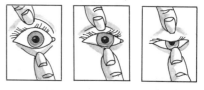

with your right thumb, tipping the lens forward. Then gently pinch the patient's eyelids together to expel the lens.

To help prevent complications, such as infection or corneal abrasion, remember these nursing considerations:
- Make sure your hands are clean and dry before removing a lens.
- Never use force to remove a lens. If you have difficulty, slide the lens onto the sclera, then call the doctor.
- Look for "lost" lenses in the upper cul-de-sac of the eye—their most common hiding place.
- Preserve each lens in a separate sterile container (marked *left* or *right*) filled with sterile saline solution.
- Don't ask a patient to replace a lens until an ophthalmologist has examined him. Before replacement,

clean the lens and the patient's eye with appropriate solutions. (See *Contact lens insertion.*)

Continent intestinal reservoir

Nursing responsibilities

A major nursing responsibility in managing a continent intestinal reservoir (CIR) is maintaining continuous pouch decompression to prevent excess pressure on suture lines. To decompress the pouch, insert a #28 French indwelling catheter. Then connect the catheter to low intermittent suction and irrigate it frequently with normal saline solution. Reducing pressure in the pouch also helps to keep the valve from slipping, a common problem.

Before the patient is discharged, show him how to intubate the pouch for drainage, using a #30 Medena plastic catheter. During his first week at home, he'll drain the pouch every 2 hours. Gradually, as the pouch enlarges and holds more waste, the patient empties it every 3 or 4 hours.

Initially, the pouch can hold about 75 ml of waste. After about a year, its capacity expands to 300 to 400 ml requiring emptying only two to three times a day.

The liquid nature of the small-bowel waste makes it easy to drain. If drainage is hampered by unusually thick waste, advise your patient to drink more fluids, especially grape juice. At least once daily, he should irrigate the pouch with a total of 150 to 200 ml of tap water, instilling 2 to 3 ounces at a time.

Because the stoma secretes mucus, the patient must wear a small absorbent dressing or patch over it when the pouch is not being drained. The amount of mucus secreted varies with each patient; it will decrease as the stoma shrinks. A CIR may be used safely by a patient who's pregnant. She may need to empty the pouch more frequently, however, because of pressure from her expanding uterus.

Continuing education courses

Choosing the best ones

Brochures or announcements about high-quality continuing education (CE) offerings will include several items: the course title, purpose, target audience, objectives, content, teaching methods, faculty, and fee. This information can help you decide if the course meets *your* needs.

The course title should pique your interest and make you want to learn more about the course.

The purpose statement will give you a description of the course and may explain what you'll learn or why you should attend. It may also identify the target audience, which might be narrow, such as critical care nurses with at least 2 years' experience, or broad, such as nurses who want to manage their time better.

All CE courses should list objectives that identify what you'll learn. Review them carefully, considering your background and experience.

Look for CE programs that list measurable objectives so you'll know what you're supposed to learn.

Delving deeper

If an agenda or course outline is provided, compare the content with the objectives to be sure they correspond. Then review the time allotted for the course to be sure you'll have enough time to achieve the objectives.

Next, consider the teaching methods. Will there be small-group activities? Case studies? Filmstrips? Lectures? Discussions? A combination of these? Think about what you want to learn; for example, if the purpose of a workshop is to teach you to perform a physical examination, you should have the time and opportunity to perform that exam.

Also find out who teaches the course. What are her qualifications? Is she an expert? If the topic is preventing postoperative complications, does the instructor have current clinical experience with perioperative patients? Has she spoken, written, conducted research, or made other presentations about the topic? Check with colleagues, and scan articles the instructor has written.

And what about the sponsor? Is the sponsoring hospital or institution well-known in the area discussed? Is the offering approved? Professional organizations such as the American Association of Critical-Care Nurses have guidelines that help ensure the quality of the program.

The course brochure should also answer other critical questions: What's the registration fee and what does it include? Does it cover only the cost of a workshop or all materials and lunch? Is advance registration required? What's the refund policy? If you register for a conference and can't attend at the last minute, will you get your money back? If so, how much? Can a colleague go in your place?

Worth the effort

After you complete a program, you should receive a certificate of completion, including your name, title of the offering, sponsor, name of the organization that approves the program, and number of continuing education units (CEUs) awarded. (See *Continuing education reimbursement; Continuing education units.*)

Continuing education reimbursement

Getting your employer to pay

Most hospitals offer some financial assistance for continuing education. If yours doesn't, try to negotiate for assistance by following these steps:

• Find out all important program information—course content, cost, location, and time.

• Put your request for financial assistance in a memo to your supervisor. Be specific and emphasize how your patients and colleagues will benefit from what you'll learn.

• Present your proposal as early as possible so schedules and paperwork can be arranged.

• Anticipate your supervisor's possible objections and develop an alternate plan: Can a colleague substitute for you at work? Can you attend another program instead?

• After you complete the program, write another memo to your supervisor about what you learned, and express your appreciation for the hospital's cooperation and support.

• Offer to share program information with interested colleagues. (See *Continuing education courses; Continuing education units.*)

Continuing education units

Avoiding problems with the state licensing board

Because various states have different requirements for continuing education units (CEU), you need to be careful in keeping track of how many CEUs you've earned. You may become licensed in two states with differing CEU requirements. So, when you attend courses and seminars or complete any approved continuing education offering, the provider should give you a certificate granting a specific number of contract hours. Make sure it does, and keep it in your records.

In some states, such as New Mexico, you must list your CEUs on the state board's license renewal form and attach photocopies of the certificates. In Colorado, you just list your CEUs on the back of the re-

newal form. Then, if you're included in the state board's random post-renewal audit, you'll have to send in photocopies of your certificates for approval. (See *Continuing education courses; Continuing education reimbursement.*)

Contrast dyes

Your role during diagnostic testing

Because contrast dyes can sometimes trigger severe allergic reactions, carefully explore your patient's allergy history before he undergoes testing. Ask specifically about allergies to iodine or iodine-containing food, such as shellfish; many imaging dyes contain iodine. If he has had an imaging test before, find out if he experienced a reaction. Keep in mind that even a patient with no allergy history can have a reaction to contrast dye. Because reactions can be delayed, keep emergency resuscitation equipment nearby both during and after the test.

Further minimize his risk by having his accurate weight on the chart before the procedure because contrast dye dosages are weight-related.

Closely monitor him for complications after the test. Signs and symptoms of a mild reaction may include itching, watery eyes, flushing, hives, nausea, vomiting, and diarrhea. With a moderate reaction, he may also experience swelling in his hands and feet and mild breathing problems. Anaphylaxis is a severe reaction causing hypotension, laryngospasm, and bronchospasm; shock and respiratory arrest can quickly follow. (See *Anaphylaxis: emergency care.*)

After the test, encourage him to drink plenty of fluids. Contrast dyes are nephrotoxic; fluids dilute them and flush them through the kidneys faster. If ordered, administer diuretics.

COPD and allergens

Home care tips

Patients who are allergic to pets are really allergic to pet dander—scales from the animal's skin, fur, or feathers. A COPD patient who doesn't have a pet should be advised against getting one. A patient who already has a pet—especially a cat—might be willing to give it away for 3 to 4 months (the time needed to rid his home completely of the dander). If his symptoms improve during this trial separation, he should consider giving the pet away permanently. If he can't part with the pet—and many people can't—advise him to keep it outside as much as possible and to never let it in the bedroom.

If your patient's allergic to wool, suggest he replace wool carpets and blankets with synthetic ones. He should also replace old rug pads, which can contain animal hair, with foam rubber ones.

Advise your patient to remove flowers and flowering plants, especially those with strong scents. Advise him to avoid dark or damp places, such as attics or basements, which are conducive to mold growth. (Mold throws irritating spores into the air.) And advise him not to use aerosol sprays.

Your patient should avoid painting and using chemicals with strong odors. He shouldn't smoke or allow anyone to smoke in his home. And he should avoid places where people smoke, even if this means curtailing his social activities.

Suggest that he replace feather pillows, feather or horsehair mattresses, and down comforters with those made of hypoallergenic materials, such as cotton, polyester, or foam rubber.

Also suggest that he install an exhaust fan to remove cooking fumes and odors. Advise him to avoid scented toilet items, such as soap, shaving cream, toilet paper, makeup, or talcum powder. If steam makes breathing difficult for him, advise him to take cooler showers or baths, use an exhaust fan, or keep the bathroom door ajar so the steam escapes. (See also *COPD and climate control.*)

COPD and climate control

Teaching about temperature and humidity

Air that's too hot or too dry can irritate mucous membranes. Air that's too cold can precipitate bronchospasm. Advise your COPD patient to keep the temperature in his home at about 70° F. (21° C.) during the day and about 65° F. (18° C.) at night. An individually controlled zone heating system with radiant or baseboard heaters is best for COPD patients.

Forced-air heating systems and air conditioners have filters that should be cleaned or replaced regularly. Humidifiers, though helpful, are an excellent breeding ground for mold; they should be cleaned and the water and pad changed regularly. Dehumidifiers reduce the conditions conducive to mold growth, so they're ideal for damp areas, such as the basement, and they too should be cleaned regularly.

Warn patients against using fireplaces and wood- or coal-burning stoves—they're sources of indoor air pollution. If he must use them, tell him to make sure the stove is the correct size for the area to be heated and that the stove and chimney are cleaned regularly. Remind him, too, that hardwood burns cleaner than softwood. (See also *COPD and allergens.*)

COPD and coughing

Teaching the double-cough

The double-cough technique can help dislodge pulmonary secre-

tions. Follow these guidelines:
• Seat your patient in an upright position.
• Have him inhale slowly and deeply through his nose, using his diaphragm.
• Tell him to open his mouth and, using his abdominal muscles, cough twice. He may find that sticking out his tongue helps him cough.

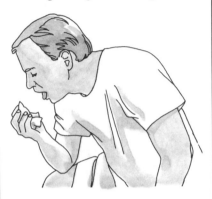

• Instruct him to inhale gently through his nose, without gasping for air through his mouth.
• Have him repeat the procedure, if necessary, after resting.

Cough technique

Teaching the huff cough

If your patient isn't coughing adequately enough to mobilize secretions, he may experience complications that can lengthen his hospital stay. To prevent this, consider teaching him *huff* coughing. First, have him force an exhalation, which releases a burst of air through an open glottis. Then, tell him to make a huffing sound. Repeated huffing may move the secretions enough to stimulate a more normal cough.

CPR: aftercare

Assessment guidelines

After CPR, assess the victim's cardiovascular status immediately. (See also *CPR: technique.*) Use an

ECG machine to determine his heart rate and rhythm, which will help you estimate cardiac output. Review the actions of any drugs he's taking that affect heart rate and rhythm. And look for changes in his condition that could require additional drugs. If he has a pacemaker, make sure it's working properly; if it's not, see what adjustments need to be made.

Also monitor his blood pressure. If he's receiving adrenergic drugs to maintain an adequate blood pressure, make sure the dosage is sufficient, but be alert for adverse reactions to these drugs, such as nausea and vomiting.

Next, assess his peripheral perfusion, which reflects his cardiovascular status.

Auscultate his heart to obtain more information about his cardiovascular status and fluid balance. (See *Heart sounds: abnormalities; Heart sounds: diagnosis.*)

Invasive hemodynamic monitoring is another way to assess cardiovascular status in the patient who's survived a code. Pulmonary artery pressure monitoring, in particular, provides valuable information on left heart functioning and fluid balance. Assess the patient's response to therapy by watching for changes in subsequent pressure readings. A thermodilution pulmonary artery catheter provides helpful cardiac output readings.

Of course, you'll want to study the results of all laboratory tests, especially serum electrolyte and enzyme values.

Monitoring urine output serves a twofold purpose: It reflects cardiovascular status and renal status. About 25% of cardiac output perfuses the kidneys, so when cardiac output decreases, urine output decreases, too.

Assess pulmonary status. If the patient's breathing spontaneously, estimate tidal volume by observing his chest movements. Monitor results of his arterial blood gas and pulmonary function studies. If he's intubated, make sure his airway's

C

patent and his endotracheal tube is positioned correctly.

Finally, assess neurologic status. (See *Neurologic exam: assessment.*) This is particularly important in the patient who has survived a code, because the cerebral anoxia and edema associated with resuscitation efforts may produce neurologic deficits. Evaluate his level of consciousness, pupillary response, and movement of his extremities. Look for prolonged unresponsiveness, nonreactive and dilated pupils, and decerebrate or decorticate posturing. (See *Posturing; Pupillary reaction.*)

CPR: chest compression

Positioning your hands correctly

Before beginning chest compressions, position your hands at the correct location. Follow these steps:
• With the middle and index fingers of the hand closer to the victim's legs, locate the rib cage's lower margin.
• Next, run these two fingers up the rib cage to the notch where the ribs meet the sternum.
• Put your middle finger on this notch, and place your index finger next to it. Then place the heel of

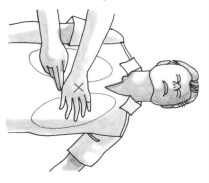

your opposite hand next to the index finger, on the long axis of the sternum.

• Now place your first hand on top of the other, so both hands are parallel and the fingers point away from

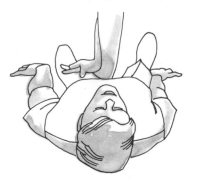

you. Extend or interlace your fingers, and begin compressions. (See *CPR: technique.*)

CPR: technique

Essential steps

Follow these steps when you discover a patient who's collapsed:
1. Gently shake his shoulder and shout, "Are you okay?" If he doesn't respond, call a code. Position him on his back. Support his head and neck and move his body as one unit. If he's in bed, place a backboard under him.
2. Use the head-tilt/chin-lift maneuver to open his airway. Place one hand on his forehead and tilt his head back by applying firm pressure with your palm. Then put the fingers (not the thumb) of your other hand under the lower jaw's bony portion and bring the jaw forward, as shown. Important: If the patient has a cervical spine injury, open the airway with the jaw-thrust maneuver. (See *Jaw-thrust maneuver.*)
3. To determine breathlessness, place your ear over the victim's mouth and watch his chest. Look, listen, and feel for breathing for 3 to 5 seconds.
4. If he's not breathing, seal his mouth and nose and ventilate twice (1 to 1½ seconds for each ventilation). Watch for his chest to rise.
    Important: Give the lungs time to deflate between ventilations.

5. Determine pulselessness by feeling for the carotid pulse on the side closer to you. Check for 5 to 10 seconds while you keep the airway open.
6. Position your hands for chest compression. (See *CPR: chest compression.*) Compress the victim's sternum 1½ to 2 inches (4 to 5 cm). During the upstroke, keep your hands in position on the sternum and allow the chest to relax. Deliver four cycles of 15 compressions (compressing and relaxing evenly) and two ventilations (compression rate: 80 to 100/minute; ventilation duration, 1 to 1½ seconds each).
7. After delivering four cycles, check for pulse and spontaneous breathing. If they're still absent, resume CPR by delivering two ventilations and 15 compressions; deliver four such ventilation/compression cycles.
8. When a second health care professional arrives, she should position herself to deliver either chest compressions or ventilations at the end of a cycle.

If she delivers chest compressions, she should follow this procedure: complete the cycle, then open the airway and check for a pulse. While you're checking for a pulse, make sure the other nurse positions her hands for chest compression. If you don't detect a pulse or breathing, say, "No pulse. Continue CPR."

Under the new guidelines, only professionals will learn two-rescuer CPR. If a nonprofessional trained in one-rescuer CPR arrives to help in a nonhospital situation, she should relieve you with one-person CPR when you get tired.
9. Open the airway and deliver one ventilation. The second rescuer then delivers five compressions in 3 to 4 seconds (compression rate: 80 to 100/minute). Ventilate the patient once for every five compressions. To maintain rhythm, the second rescuer should say, "One-and-two-and-three-and-four-and-

five, pause, vent." Between ventilations, check the patient's pulse to determine effectiveness of the compressions.

Two-rescuer CPR

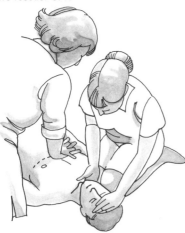

10. When the second rescuer tires, she should say, "Change-one-and-two-and-three-and-four-and-five." Immediately after the ventilation, you and the second rescuer change position simultaneously.

The second rescuer should now open the airway and perform a 5-second pulse check. If she fails to detect a pulse, she says, "No pulse. continue CPR." Then she delivers one ventilation.

Resume compression/ventilation cycles. (See *CPR: aftercare.*)

CPR and children: airway

Emergency intervention outside the hospital

Here's what to do:

1. Assess the injury's severity. To find out if the child is unconscious, gently shake his shoulder and shout at him. If he's conscious and having trouble breathing, get him to an emergency department immediately. Sometimes, a child will find the position that allows him to breathe most easily. Help him maintain this position. If he's uncon-

scious or in acute distress and you're alone with him, call out for help.

2. Place him in a supine position on a hard, flat surface. When moving him, support his head and neck and roll his head and torso as one unit. If you suspect a head or neck injury, take special care to support his head and neck when moving him.

3. A child's small airway can easily be blocked by his tongue. When this happens, you may be able to clear the obstruction simply by opening the airway. This action will move the tongue away from the back of the airway and may allow the victim to breathe.

If the child doesn't have a neck injury, use the *head-tilt/chin-lift maneuver* to open the airway: Kneel next to him at shoulder level. Then place your hand that's closer to his head on his forehead. As you gently tilt his head back, put the fingers of your other hand on his lower jaw and lift the chin up.

Don't place your fingers on the soft tissue of the neck because you may block the airway. And make sure the child's mouth doesn't close completely.

If you suspect a neck injury, use the *jaw-thrust maneuver* to open the airway. (See *Jaw-thrust maneuver.*)

CPR and children: breathing

What to do after opening the airway

Follow these steps:

1. Place your ear over his mouth so you can listen for and feel air being exhaled. Look for movement of his chest and abdomen. If he's breathing, keep the airway open and monitor his respirations.

2. If he *isn't* breathing, pinch his nostrils closed with your thumb and index finger. Take a breath and place your mouth over his mouth to form a tight seal. Give a slow breath for 1 to 1½ seconds, pause to take a

breath yourself, then give another slow breath of 1 to 1½ seconds. (Ventilation rate is 15 breaths/minute.) Air entering a clear airway will make his chest rise.

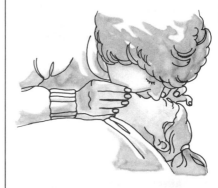

If the first ventilation isn't successful, reposition his head and try again. If you're still not successful, he may have a foreign-body airway obstruction. (See *Airway obstruction: adults; Airway obstruction: unconscious victim.*)

CPR and children: circulation

Assessing it

Follow these guidelines:

1. Call for help. Keep the child's head tilted with one hand as you assess circulation with the other. Locate the carotid artery on the side of the neck, in the groove between the trachea and the sternocleidomastoid muscle. Palpate the artery for 5 to 10 seconds. If the child has a pulse, continue resuscitation breathing by giving one breath every 4 seconds (or 15 breaths per minute). If someone has responded to your call for help, tell him to call an ambulance.

2. If the child has no pulse, kneel next to his chest so you can start giving chest compressions. Using the hand closer to his feet, locate the lower border of the rib cage on the side nearer you. Then hold your middle and index fingers together

C

and move them up the rib cage to the notch where the ribs and sternum join.

3. Put your middle finger on the notch and your index finger next to it. Note the position of your index finger.

4. Lift your hand and place the heel just above the spot where the index finger was. The heel of your hand should be aligned with the long axis of the sternum.

5. Using the heel of one hand only, compress the chest 1 to 1½ inches (3 to 4 cm). Deliver five compressions at a rate of 80 to 100/minute, allowing the chest wall to relax after each compression. To prevent an internal injury, keep your hand in place on the sternum and keep your fingers off the child's ribs.

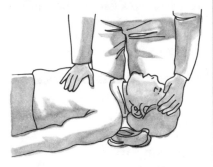

Leave one hand on the sternum to deliver compressions and the other on the forehead to maintain the head-tilt position. For a child, each CPR cycle consists of five compressions and one ventilation. Count "one and two and three and four and five" as you perform the chest compressions. Pause after your fifth compression and give one ventilation. Give CPR for 10 cycles or 1 minute, then check again for breathing and a pulse. If he isn't breathing or has no pulse, continue CPR. If someone has gone for help, check for breathing and a pulse every few minutes. If you're alone with the child, perform CPR for another minute, check his respirations and pulse, and try to get help. Return as quickly as possible and resume CPR.

Cranial nerve assessment

Performing it expertly

Follow these steps when you do a cranial nerve assessment:

• *I-Olfactory (sensory)*. Have the patient close his eyes. Occlude one nostril with your finger, and ask him to identify nonirritating odors, such as coffee, tea, cloves, soap, chewing gum, and peppermint. Repeat the test on the other nostril.

• *II-Optic (sensory)*. Assess visual acuity with a Snellen chart or newspaper. Or ask the patient to count how many fingers you're holding up. Check visual fields by confrontation. Have the patient sit directly in front of you and stare at your nose. Slowly move your finger from the periphery toward the center until the patient says he can see it. Check color vision by asking the patient to name the color of several nearby objects.

• *III-Oculomotor (motor), IV-Trochlear (motor), VI-Abducens (motor)*. The motor functions of these nerves overlap, so test them together. First, inspect the eyelids for ptosis. Then assess ocular movements and note any eye deviation. Test accommodation and direct and consensual light reflexes. (See *Pupillary reaction*.)

III, IV, and VI

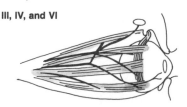

• *V-Trigeminal (both)*. To test motor function, ask the patient to close his jaws tightly. Then try to separate his clenched jaw. Also test the corneal reflex. (See *Reflex, corneal*.) To check sensory function, ask the patient to close his eyes. Then lightly touch his forehead, cheeks,

and chin. Can he feel the touch equally on both sides?

V

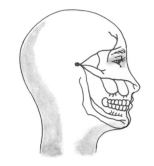

• *VII-Facial (both)*. Have the patient show his teeth, attempt to close his eyes against resistance, and puff out his cheeks. Then dab sugar, salt, or vinegar on the front of his tongue. Have the patient identify these substances by their taste.

• *VIII-Acoustic (sensory)*. Rub a few strands of hair between your fingers next to the patient's ear while his eyes are closed. Then have him identify which ear you selected. Also check his ability to hear a watch ticking or a whisper. Observe the patient's balance. Does he sway when walking or standing? Perform a Romberg test, if indicated. (See *Hearing tests*.)

• *IX-Glossopharyngeal (both) and X-Vagus (both)*. First, have the patient identify tastes at the back of his tongue. Then inspect the soft palate. Observe for symmetrical elevation when the patient says "aah." Touch the soft palate's mucous membrane with a cotton-tipped applicator to elicit the palatal reflex. Touch the posterior pharyngeal wall with a tongue depressor to elicit the gag reflex.

• *XI-Spinal accessory*. Palpate and inspect the sternocleidomastoid muscle as the patient pushes his chin against your hand. Palpate and inspect the trapezius muscle as the patient shrugs his shoulders against your resistance. Also have the patient stretch out his hands toward you.

• *XII-Hypoglossal*. Observe the tongue for asymmetry, atrophy, deviation to one side, and fasciculations. Ask the patient to push his tongue against a tongue depressor. Then have him move his tongue rapidly in and out and from side to side. (See *Cranial nerve function.*)

Cranial nerve function

Assembling a test kit

Make a kit using a plastic basket with a handle (similar to an I.V. tray) containing cotton, safety pins, pennies, keys, peppermint, reflex hammer, tuning fork, pencil, tongue depressors, and an ophthalmoscope. For added convenience, mark each item with the name of the cranial nerve function it tests. This tote kit saves time when a neurosurgical test is required. (See *Cranial nerve assessment.*)

Craniotomy patients

Postop positioning

The first thing you need to know is what type of craniotomy your patient has had.

Craniotomies are classified as supratentorial and infratentorial. If your patient has had a *supratentorial* craniotomy, elevate the head of his bed 30 to 45 degrees. (You can place a pillow under his head and shoulders.) This position will help promote venous drainage from the brain, minimizing cerebral edema. Also, place the patient in neutral alignment—that is, with his head and torso in a straight line. The reason: A flexed neck would hamper drainage through the jugular veins, increasing intracranial pressure.

Elevating the head of his bed 30 to 45 degrees and maintaining neutral alignment serve two other purposes: reducing the risk of cerebral bleeding and helping improve cerebrospinal fluid circulation.

After an *infratentorial* craniotomy, keep the patient lying flat with a small pillow under the nape of his

neck. This position will minimize pressure from the cerebrum on the cerebellum and brain stem. Keep head and body alignment neutral to promote venous drainage and prevent tearing of the suture line.

Crash cart

How it should be stocked

A typical crash cart is stocked with equipment, drugs, tray sets, and other supplies needed to manage common emergencies.

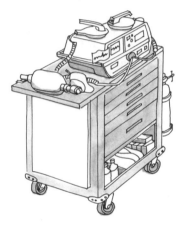

As you're probably aware, crash cart contents vary from hospital to hospital and from unit to unit. Be sure you're familiar with your unit's crash cart. Check it at least once every shift, and after each emergency, to restock supplies and to test the defibrillator/monitor unit. Also check the drugs' expiration dates, and stock the cart with fresh drugs if necessary.

Creatinine clearance

Obtaining accurate test results

To determine accurate creatinine clearance results, use the following guidelines:
• Have the patient empty his bladder and discard the first specimen, while you record the exact time he voided it.

• When he must void again, start accumulating his urine specimens for 24 hours. Then, send the accumulated specimens to the laboratory.
• Have a lab technician obtain a blood sample and send it to the laboratory for serum creatinine study.

Credé's maneuver

Teaching it to help patients void

Credé's maneuver is a simple exercise that can help start a stream of urine. Here's what to tell the patient:

"While sitting on the toilet, place your hands flat on your abdomen, just below the navel. Firmly stroke downward about six times. This will put pressure on your bladder and stimulate your urge to void. (Women can increase pressure further by bending forward at the hips.)

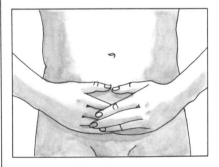

"Now place one hand on top of the other above your pubic area, as shown. Then, press firmly inward and downward. This will compress the bladder and expel urine."

Crepitation, subcutaneous

Initial detection and management

Subcutaneous crepitation occurs when air or gas bubbles escape into tissues. It may signal life-threatening rupture of an air-filled or gas-

C

producing organ or may indicate sepsis from a fulminating anaerobic infection.

Look for signs of respiratory distress—such as severe dyspnea, tachypnea, accessory muscle use, nasal flaring, air hunger, or tachycardia. If these signs exist, have another nurse notify the doctor while you quickly test for Hamman's sign to detect trapped air bubbles in the mediastinum. (See *Hamman's sign.*)

If the patient has an open wound with a foul odor and local swelling and discoloration, have another nurse immediately notify the doctor. Then, take the patient's vital signs, checking especially for fever, tachycardia, hypotension, and tachypnea. Next, start an I.V. to administer fluids and medication, provide supplemental oxygen, and be prepared to assist with emergency surgery to drain and debride the wound. If the patient's condition is life-threatening, you may need to prepare him for transfer to a facility with a hyperbaric chamber.

Crisis intervention

How to help the family

Like a storm that hits hard and fast, a crisis leaves the family floundering. But you can help smooth the troubled waters. Your intervention will have two phases: planning and action. In planning, determine how disrupted the family is and consider all the possible coping methods.

Prior to planning, follow these guidelines to assess the crisis:
• Find out how the family perceives the problem—why the event provoked a crisis. Families aren't always aware of the relationship between a previous situation and their current stress.
• Find out what support systems are available to the family.
• Find out how the family coped in the past with stress. Note any suicidal or homicidal tendencies and make psychiatric referrals if necessary.

Now you're ready to start planning. First, see if the family is continuing their daily functioning of work, school, housework, and child care. How are other family members being affected? Are they also in crisis? Are the children receiving adequate emotional and physical care? Are they upset? You may find that a woman is so stressed by the care of her physically disabled child that she no longer cares for herself, the house, or the child. She'll require immediate intervention for child care and housework.

Consider the options
Next, investigate options open to the family to restore balance. These are usually methods they've used in the past. For example, the mother who feels like abusing her colicky baby might propose that she share the child's care with others until the colic passes. Or parents who feel their premature baby may die might choose to be told the exact status of their child and perhaps give help in his care to alleviate some of their anxiety.

After you explore the possible options, put them to work. Your goals are:
• to help family members understand why they're in crisis
• to help them air feelings they've suppressed
• to explore new ways of coping
• to restore family functioning.
These goals are especially important if the family hasn't seen the relationship between the precipitating event and the crisis.

Of course, you can reduce tension by providing an opportunity for the family to express their feelings. Many people suppress their emotions of hate, grief, and guilt. This is especially true of parents who have a physically disabled child. They characteristically feel shock, denial, shame, envy, bitterness, and rejection. These feelings aren't readily admitted in our society, but they're real and must be acknowledged to reduce anxiety. You might begin a conversation such as this, by saying: "People

sometimes have difficulty accepting something like this. Many parents are angry (or bitter, shocked, envious, and so on). Do you feel that way?" Listen supportively and be prepared for the feelings that might be expressed.

Test the coping methods
Try to evaluate each coping method after it's tried. If it wasn't successful, explore other options. For example, if a baby who fails to thrive makes his mother anxious because he doesn't respond to a specific formula, have her try another formula, nipple, or method of handling him during feeding.

If a thorough assessment and adequate intervention are carried out, the coping methods tried during this phase may well be successful. And the family may then be more open to ideas about preventing future crises.

Resolve and reinforce
When the family in crisis realistically examines the problem, has adequate support, and can use old or new ways of coping, the crisis should be resolved within 6 weeks after the event. Evaluate at that time whether the family is beginning to function normally again. Look for a positive mood and a decrease in psychosocial symptoms such as depression, insomnia, crying, and headaches.

Finally, reinforce the family members' coping mechanisms by reviewing the experience and their actions. Let them feel satisfaction in resolving the crisis.

And take personal satisfaction, too, for you've helped calm their storm and have made them better able to cope in the future.

Criticism and assertiveness

Reacting more positively

Criticisms are common in a high-pressure profession like nursing. Few nurses are skilled at handling them. Many nurses have developed ineffective people-pleasing responses to criticism, such as withdrawing from the situation. Other nurses interpret all criticism as a personal attack and become short-tempered with everyone. And others, who try to control their anger, find it seeps out as sarcasm. They tend to punish their critics by behaving coldly to them. They don't get mad—they get even.

None of these responses are effective. And if you've used any of them, you know how your self-esteem, personal satisfaction, and working relationships can suffer because of them. If you want to break away from such ineffective, destructive responses, start by not taking criticism so personally.

The first step in dealing with criticism is managing your internal dialogue after someone criticizes you. Nurses who handle criticism will have a dialogue that consists of pep talks to themselves; telling themselves to "relax and handle the situation."

After you've learned to manage your internal dialogue, you're ready to analyze and manage your interaction with your critic. You'll need to do the following:
• Ask for specifics.
• Listen to his emotions.
• Show him you heard him by reflecting his feelings back to him.
• Resolve the situation by either dismissing the criticism if it doesn't involve you or acknowledging the critic's concern by reflecting his feelings.
• Apologize if it was your fault and change your behavior if you see fit. Then attempt to put your relationship back on track as soon as possible. (See also *Assertiveness; Criticism technique.*)

Criticism technique

Effective methods

No one likes to be criticized, but criticism is inevitable. To help you handle it gracefully, try these tips:
• Be honest with yourself and admit that you have faults. If you stay humble, criticism won't jar you so much.
• Put yourself in your critic's place. Would you have had the same reaction?
• If you think the criticism is unfair, discuss it with your critic. Get your feelings out in the open. Don't harbor resentment because it'll surely come out later.
• Don't apologize excessively or unnecessarily.
• If you're being criticized, hold your tongue whenever you feel your stress level rising. Think before you respond.
• Disarm your critic by asking for helpful advice—on how you might have done the job better, for example.
• Finally, listen carefully to justified criticism. (See also *Criticism and assertiveness.*)

Criticizing others

Giving constructive advice

Follow this advice for making criticism less painful for you and your staff:
• Choose an appropriate time and place for your discussion. Don't criticize a person in front of other staff members or visitors or in the middle of an emergency.
• To begin, use "I" statements—they're less threatening and have a more positive impact on the person you're criticizing. For example, say "I've noticed there's a problem in getting patients to the operating room on time," not "You haven't been doing your job."
• Discuss solutions to the problem with her, encouraging her to suggest some of her own. Be sure to listen carefully.
• Discuss possible incentives for change. How would changing her behavior help both of you and help resolve the situation?
• Ask her for feedback to make sure she understands your criticism and the proposed solutions.
• Don't avoid her or treat her differently after the confrontation. Remember, you criticized her behavior, not her.

Crying

Responding to your distraught patient

Stay quietly with him at first, unless you sense that he prefers to be alone. If you're unsure of his wishes, ask him, "Is it all right if I stay with you? You really seem upset right now." Just by offering him a choice, you give him some control over his situation; this, in turn, can make him more responsive and open. Provide privacy by closing the door or drawing the curtains around his bed.

Don't urge him to stop; crying is therapeutic.

Use touch if and when you feel the situation allows.

Offer a cold facecloth or a warm drink. These small gestures not only convey your caring but also provide a bit of physical comfort as well.

Ask "What would you like me to do?" or say even more positively, "Tell me how I can help." You might be able to remedy the small situations, even though you cannot remedy the larger threats of disease and emotional trauma.

When the patient stops crying, talk about his crying. Sometimes a patient will feel embarrassed afterward and will withdraw—particularly if he is a man. To keep such a patient from retreating in embarrassment, you could say something like, "I'm glad you felt able to cry with me in the room," or "You were wise to let yourself go. You really needed to cry." Don't give him false reassurances. For example, don't say, "I'm sure you'll feel better."

C

CT scanning

Understanding the high-dose delayed method

Here is a suggested description to give your patient:

"Because you'll be receiving a contrast dye, we need to know if you have any allergies or if you've ever had any bad reactions to dyes. Also, the dye may cause nausea and vomiting, so don't eat or drink anything for at least 3 to 4 hours before the test.

"An I.V. line will be inserted in your arm, and the doctor will give you a test dose of dye. If you don't react to it, the rest of the dye will be infused rapidly. This will take about 2 to 3 minutes. You may feel a warm, flushing sensation throughout your body and notice a metallic, salty taste in your mouth. These effects will last only a minute. The doctor will stay with you while the dye is being infused.

"After an hour or so, you'll be taken to the CT scanner—a large X-ray machine that takes three-dimensional pictures of your brain. The I.V. will remain in your arm. You'll receive a radiation dose that equals no more than a series of regular X-rays.

"You'll be helped onto a special table that's concave and hard; you may feel a little uncomfortable until you settle into it. You'll be wrapped snugly in a sheet, and your head will be positioned in a cradle with a foam support for your neck. A wide rubber strap will be wrapped around your forehead to keep your head still during the test.

"Next, the table will move slowly until your head enters the scanner's large, round opening. You may feel confined at this point. You'll hear clicking sounds and gears turning and may see a tiny light. Just be sure to lie very still. After the scanning is completed, you'll be transported back to your room." (See *Contrast dyes; Diagnostic studies.*)

Cullen's sign

What to look for

If you see irregular, bluish hemorrhagic patches on the skin around the umbilicus or (occasionally) around abdominal scars, suspect Cullen's sign. It indicates massive hemorrhage after trauma or rupture in such disorders as duodenal ulcer, ectopic pregnancy, abdominal aneurysm, gallbladder or common bile duct obstruction, or acute hemorrhagic pancreatitis. Usually, Cullen's sign appears gradually; blood travels from a retroperitoneal organ or structure to the periumbilical area,

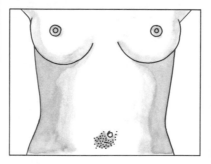

where it diffuses through subcutaneous tissues. It may be difficult to detect in a dark-skinned patient. The extent of discoloration depends on the extent of bleeding. In time, the bluish discoloration fades to greenish yellow and then yellow before disappearing. (See *Aortic dissection; Pregnancy, ectopic.*)

Cystostomy tubes

Caring for a suprapubic catheter

Here are some nursing considerations:
• Check catheter patency frequently to prevent kinks in tubing that could block urine flow.
• Notify the doctor if the catheter doesn't drain properly. He may pull out the catheter 1" (3 cm) at a time until urine flows. Be prepared to irrigate the catheter as ordered (usu-

ally with 50 ml of sterile normal saline solution).
• Tape the drainage tube to the side of the patient's abdomen.
• Cover the catheter area with sterile dressing.
• Change the insertion site dressings at least every 24 hours, noting the color, character, and amount of drainage. (See also *Drains, postoperative; Drains: preparation.*)
• Cleanse the incision site with povidone-iodine solution, as ordered.

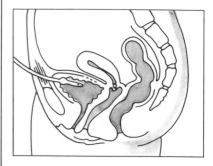

• Inspect the incision for redness, warmth, swelling, or purulent drainage.
• If required, perform a voiding trial by clamping the catheter for 4 hours, asking the patient to try urinating, then unclamping the catheter and measuring residual urine.

Cytomegalovirus

Preventing infection

Cytomegalovirus (CMV) is transmitted by direct contact with infected urine, saliva, breast milk, cervical secretions, semen, blood, or donor organs. An infected child can transmit CMV for up to 4 years.

Any neonate who has a birth defect and flulike symptoms should be suspected of having CMV and be treated accordingly. Many doctors routinely test for CMV in all neonates who have birth defects. (In adults, CMV infection can resemble mononucleosis or be so mild that it goes unnoticed. Once the initial infection is over, the virus can become latent and be reactivated at any time—no one knows why. About half the women of childbearing age have had a CMV infection.)

The greatest risk of CMV infection is to a fetus, especially in the second and third trimesters and at birth. The virus can cause congenital defects, such as mental retardation, motor disabilities, hearing loss, and chronic liver disease. These defects are usually more severe when the mother has a primary CMV infection, rather than a reactivated latent virus.

Protect yourself by avoiding direct contact with the urine and respiratory secretions of children who have CMV. This means that besides washing your hands, you should wear gloves whenever you change a diaper and dispose of the soiled diaper as you would any contaminated material. Also, don't kiss an infected child.

If you are pregnant or planning to become pregnant, avoid working in this high-risk setting. If that's not possible, following the above precautions will substantially reduce your chance of contracting a CMV infection. The precautions won't eliminate the chance entirely, but neither will changing your workplace; because CMV is so widespread, it can be contracted anywhere. (See also *Infection control; Pregnant nurse: infection risks.*)

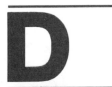

Day care for adults

An alternative to a nursing home

As you may know, adult day care is a special program for elderly patients available in some communi-

ties. Its purpose: to help the elderly remain independent by providing them with health care, rehabilitation therapy, and social contact with their peers.

If the patient is not bedridden and not dangerous to others, he may be a good candidate for adult day care.

Arrange a visit to an adult day-care center. A nurse at the center will interview your patient and his caretakers to evaluate his health needs, psychosocial status, and family support.

The nurse will also observe the relationship between the patient and his caretakers. After the interview, your patient and his caretakers will meet the staff, watch some group activities, and ask questions about the program. Transportation shouldn't be a problem; the center usually provides it.

Before your patient can be formally admitted to the center, his doctor must send a medical report there. The report should include a list of prescribed medications and other pertinent information about your patient's therapy.

The center's multidisciplinary team develops care plans for new patients. This team includes a doctor, nutritionist, social worker, podiatrist, dentist, therapist (physical, speech, and occupational), and a registered nurse who coordinates the program.

Besides coordinating the services of the multidisciplinary team, nurses at adult day-care centers often lead orientation, discussion, and support groups. They also teach and counsel patients and of course, give hands-on care.

Sometimes a nurse from the center will visit the patient's home to see if it's safe. She might recommend changes, such as installing bathtub and toilet support bars or getting rid of throw rugs.

One benefit of adult day care is that family members get a respite from giving direct care. Yet they remain involved with the patient's

program. Frequent phone calls and meetings give family members the opportunity to review the patient's care plan and discuss problems with home care.

Adult day programs offer an innovative and economical alternative to other forms of ambulatory care. With the elderly population burgeoning and public health care funds shrinking, you can expect to see quite a few patients participating in them. Keep it in mind during your discharge planning. (See *Home health care planning.*)

Death

Offering support to the family

After the doctor pronounces death, ask the patient's family to leave the room for a short time. Explain that a nurse will make the patient look as much as possible the way he had in life. Then the family can come back and see him.

Families usually leave willingly. If they insist on staying, delay the postmortem care until after they leave.

When the family members leave, find a private room for them to go to. Most families also need help in making plans for the next 24 hours. To offer such help, you should know:
• your hospital's policy and requirement for discharging bodies
• the procedure for contacting a funeral home
• your hospital's procedure for autopsy and organ donation
• any religious requirements regarding handling of the body.

As other relatives arrive, be prepared to answer these questions:
• Was he in pain?
• Was he alone?
• What time did he die?
• What did he die of? (Keep your explanation simple.) (See *Grief.*)

D

Death: child

Helping a family deal with their child's death

Here's how to handle the family.

1. *Don't keep the family in the business office signing papers.* Families' despair and grief intensify when they can't be with their child. Such paperwork may make them feel that the hospital cares more about money and administrative concerns than about their child.

2. *Escort them to a private room.* If no room is available, take them to an office. Give them the privacy they need to display their grief when they hear about their child.

3. *Insist that the doctor tell them the cause of death as soon as possible.* Families need the doctor's assurance that they weren't responsible for their child's death.

4. *Say—and show—that you're sorry.* If you don't know what to say, a simple "I'm so sorry" will help. And don't tell parents you know what they're going through unless you've lost a child.

5. *Let family members be with their child.* Many parents suffer needless guilt because they couldn't be with their child during his last minutes. But don't expect them to ask if they can be with him—offer them the opportunity. If they *can't* be with their child, explain why. Don't pull family members away from their child's body or let friends and relatives intervene. Families need to adjust to the death—in their own way.

6. *Give the family instructions.* Families need answers to many questions right after the child's death: Who calls the funeral home? When do I go home? Do I wait here until the funeral home picks up the body? Where can I go to be alone? Can I stay with my child's body? Is this the last chance I'll have to hold him? Can I get his clothes and personal items?

7. *Keep in touch with the family if you can.* The family needs you more than ever 4 to 6 weeks after their child's death. Ask how they're coping. Explain that many people develop emotional and physical symptoms with their grief. Explain that not all family members grieve in the same way. Ask what symptoms they're suffering, and refer them to counseling sources if they'd like help. (See *Grief.*)

Death and staff support

When a co-worker is angry and upset

Let the co-worker decide whether she wants help. Some grieving co-workers will be too angry to accept your offer of help. Then do the following:

1. *Find a private spot*—for example, a quiet table in the corner of the cafeteria. If none exists, look for another quiet place to talk—for example, a bathroom, lounge, or stairway.

2. *Use touch for support.* You'll have to use your judgment about touching. Most people draw strength from a touch on the shoulder or arm during a crisis, but some can't handle the intimacy. If the person withdraws from your touch, don't persist.

3. *Listen—don't talk.* Start the conversation with a general supportive comment like, "I'm so sorry for your loss. I'm here to listen if you want to talk." Then listen. You can help even with silence if the person wants a few minutes of quiet companionship.

Don't break the silence with advice. Grieving people don't expect you to tell them the meaning of life or how to cope. They simply want understanding and your attention.

4. *Encourage the person to talk.* If you think the other person is uncomfortable with the silence, but unable to break it, you can help her express her feelings through non-threatening, gentle probing.

Ask, "What's making you cry?" or "What are you thinking?" Avoid questions that start with "why" ("Why are you crying?") because they sound threatening. And avoid questions that elicit yes-or-no answers. They won't give the person a chance to express her feelings.

Above all, don't push or try to force an answer. Let the other person choose to ignore your questions. She may feel comforted enough by your presence and understanding that she'll want to get back to work without ever talking about the death.

5. *Continue your attention.* Whether your initial efforts are accepted or not, talk to the person again several days later.

If someone continues to reject help and seems unable to resolve her emotions, ask your hospital's pastoral care services for advice; they're usually available to help staff as well as patients. With support for their own grief, staff members can reach out to patients and their families and help them handle theirs.

Deathbed statements

Witnessing your patient's last words

If you witness a dying patient's oral statement—a declaration or oral will—remember to follow these legal safeguards:

• Document the statement word for word.

• Record other witnesses' names and the patient's physical and mental condition.

• Take careful notes. They could be used in court to probate a will, resolve creditors' claims, prosecute the patient's assailants, or help refresh your memory if you're called to testify.

• Make a copy of the statement; if possible, get the patient and other witnesses to sign it. Then record that you did this in your notes.

• Advise your supervisor and the patient's doctor of the witnessing so they know there's an important legal document in the patient's medical record. (See *Communication: dying patients.*)

Decisions

Making intelligent ones

Here's a method that will help you analyze problems systematically, then reach the best decision.

1. *Define the problem.* Resist the impulse to jump ahead of yourself. Define the problem by comparing the situation that exists (what is) with the situation that might or should exist (what could be).

2. *Analyze the situation and set goals.* To find out why the existing situation is creating a problem, ask yourself: *What's* happening (or not happening)? *Where* is it happening (or not happening)? *When* is it happening (or not happening)? *What* are my goals? These questions all require *objective* answers to help you identify the situation and its effect on your own goals. Never ask yourself *why* the situation has developed until you've collected all the facts. Doing so will bring you to a premature—and probably incorrect—conclusion.

3. *Generate alternate ways to achieve your goals.* Sometimes you may have only one reasonable course of action. (For example, if a patient's blood pressure drops to a dangerous level, you know your goal is to raise his pressure. If the doctor has prescribed a drug for that purpose, you have a clear course of action.) But usually, situations involve many more alternatives— none of them perfect and all involving some risk. In such uncertain situations, you can only try for the best choice.

4. *Develop criteria to weigh alternatives.* The alternative that seems ideal for meeting your goals may not be feasible because of some inflexible, real-world constraints. Are you limited by a budget? By time? By

your patient's safety needs? List these constraints, so you can evaluate each alternative later.

5. *Compare alternatives against these criteria and your goals.* Start by ruling out any alternatives that don't meet all criteria. Then evaluate how well each solution meets your goals.

6. *Select the most effective solution.* If you have trouble choosing, go back to Step 3 and try to develop more alternatives.

7. *Implement your solution.* Try it out. For example, in the case described in Step 3 where your patient's blood pressure drops to a dangerous level, what can you do if the doctor won't prescribe a drug until he sees the patient? Maybe you could obtain permission to start an I.V. of normal saline solution.

8. *Evaluate the outcome.* Not all your decisions will be effective. But you can increase the success rate percentage by analyzing your results. If your decision was effective, you'll know that you should solve the same problem that way again. If your decision was ineffective, analyze the outcome and try to understand why. If you can't correct the mistake at once, you can at least make a mental note to handle the situation differently next time.

Defibrillation technique

How to do it properly

Suppose you're at the nurses' station when you hear a cardiac monitor alarm go off. Your patient is in ventricular fibrillation. Calling for help, you run into his room.

Quickly check his bedside monitor to verify fibrillation, and assess his responsiveness, airway, breathing, and pulse. He is unresponsive, isn't breathing, and has no pulse. Call a code and begin cardiopulmonary resuscitation (CPR). (See *CPR: technique.*)

As you perform CPR, the nurse who brings in the crash cart should immediately plug the defibrillator into a grounded electrical outlet. The other nurse should then turn on the power by pressing the POWER button.

Next, have the other nurse select the current charge by turning the ENERGY SELECT dial. If a doctor isn't present to give you a specific current charge, set the dial at 200 joules.

Verify that the defibrillator is in the nonsynchronized mode setting (the SYNC button should *not* be lit), and turn on the bedside monitor's recorder so you'll get an ECG readout.

Tell the other nurse to press the CHARGE button to activate the machine. The button will flash while charging. When it stops flashing, the machine is charged.

8. While the defibrillator is being prepared, apply gel pads to the patient's chest (or conductive jelly to the paddles). The conductive material will prevent burns and decrease the skin's resistance to the electric current. (Never use alcohol pads; they're poor conductors and can burn the patient.)

Place the paddles on the patient's chest: the paddle labeled STERNUM just to the right of the upper sternum and below the clavicle, and the paddle labeled APEX to the left of the left nipple, centered over the midclavicular line. Apply the paddles with firm pressure (about 25 lb) to attach them securely to the

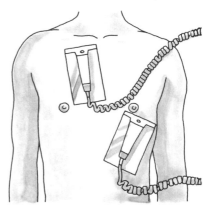

D

patient's chest. Make sure both paddles are flat against his skin and more than 2″ apart. You can also use anterior-posterior paddles for defibrillation, although they're more commonly used for elective cardioversion. Place the flat, posterior paddle under the patient's left scapula, behind the heart. Place the anterior paddle directly over the left precordium. Press the DISCHARGE button on the anterior paddle.

Stand clear of the patient and bed, and tell the other nurse to do the same. Take a quick look at the monitor to verify that the patient is still in ventricular fibrillation. Then simultaneously press the black DISCHARGE buttons on the front of each paddle's handle.

Have the other nurse record on the ECG strip the patient's name, the date and time, and the number of joules delivered.

Check the monitor. If the patient remains in ventricular fibrillation, verify it by checking his pulse, then continue CPR. Increase the charge as ordered, and try again. To recharge the machine, press the amber button on the side of the APEX paddle.

When you've completed the procedure, turn off the defibrillator. Use a damp cloth or alcohol pads to clean the paddles. Clean the patient, and make sure the crash cart is restocked by the appropriate personnel. Then document your actions.

Delusions

Responding therapeutically

Delusions are unfounded or false beliefs with no basis in reality and not correctable by logic, reason, or argument. Delusions exist to satisfy an emotional need. That's why a patient's fears, desires, and past experiences play an important role in the type of delusion he experiences. Here's how to respond therapeutically:
• Explore the delusion with the patient.

• Set the delusion in a time frame.
• Find out if the patient's under exaggerated stress, perhaps because of financial, family, or job difficulties.
• Try to pinpoint what triggered the delusion. Two common triggers are medication and a change in the patient's ability to control his life.
• Don't see the delusion first and the patient second.
• Always address the patient by his last name unless he asks you to use his first name.
• Always state your own name, your title, and the purpose of your visit.
• Give a brief explanation before doing anything new to the patient.
• Don't confuse him by using abbreviations. Use plain English so he won't misunderstand and make up his own meanings.
• Don't whisper outside his room.

Find out whether your patient's delusion is fixed or fleeting. This will determine whether you'll be able to break through his delusion in the short time you're caring for him. *Fixed* delusions have endured for a long time and have been repeatedly reinforced. (A paranoid schizophrenic patient interprets a minor auto accident as proof that someone's trying to kill him.) These delusions are impossible to correct without long-term therapy. *Fleeting* delusions are recent and usually arise from conditions or situations that can be corrected. (See also *Hallucinations; Illusions; Psychotic patients*.)

Deposition

How to give one

Before a lawsuit goes to trial, both parties in the suit are given the "right of discovery"—the right to question the witnesses about matters in the suit. Their answers are called a deposition. This is given under oath, recorded, and used as evidence at the trial.

A deposition is supposed to diminish the possibility of surprise in

a trial. It's a preview of the witnesses' versions of the story. This way, both parties are prepared to counter or corroborate those versions at the actual trial.

Many nurses have been unnerved by the fast pace and unfamiliarity of the pretrial deposition because they weren't properly prepared. To make sure that doesn't happen to you, get the charts (and any other documents pertaining to the lawsuit) from your hospital's records. Go over these documents line by line to jog your memory of what happened and to help organize your thinking. Then get a lawyer. (If the hospital's lawyer or your malpractice insurance carrier's lawyer can't help you, get one of your own—it's worth it.)

Here are some other pointers:
• Don't be antagonistic toward the cross-examining lawyer, but don't let him intimidate you.
• Explain yourself simply and honestly without any dramatization. Be organized in your thinking and speaking.
• Never deny discussing your case with your lawyer.
• Ask the lawyers to repeat questions that you didn't hear or understand.
• Don't show any signs of displeasure if you disagree with some testimony. (See *Testifying: expert witness; Testifying: preparation; Witnessing, expert*.)

Depressed patients

Precautions to take

When you have a depressed patient, remember to do the following:
• Allow him to express his feelings. This may help him get in touch with his feelings and understand his current stress. It can also give *you* a chance to suggest available resources and help him sort out his options.

• Tell the doctor and other staff members that the patient's depressed. This will help you revise his care plan as needed to address his problem. Make sure you document your conversation with the doctor, along with what you did for the patient. If he attempts suicide and his family sues you, you'll need to prove you recognized his problem and took steps to treat it.

• Ask for a clinical nurse specialist/liaison consultation. This can provide an objective assessment of the patient and staff situation. A clinical nurse specialist has the expertise in depression that is needed.

• Assess each depressed patient for suicide risk on an ongoing basis. This will help you stay alert for self-destructive behaviors and provide for your patient's safety.

• Don't ignore or avoid a patient whose signs and symptoms indicate depression (for example, sadness, crying, change in appetite, or apathy). If you do, you'll increase his feelings of isolation and low self-esteem and his potential for suicide.

• Don't allow a history of substance abuse to interfere with assessing for depression. Biased reactions can interfere with your ability to provide objective patient care and may further alienate the patient. (See *Crying; Suicidal teenagers: warning signs.*)

Diabetes, juvenile

Body tracings for patient teaching

Make body tracings for young diabetic patients to teach them proper rotation of insulin injection sites.

Trace the child's body outline on a brown wrapping paper as large as the child's body. The two sides of the paper represent the front and back of his body. After each injection, help the child find and date the site on the paper.

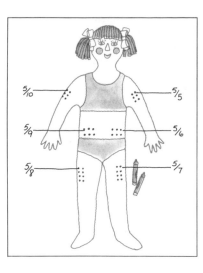

Children can decorate the tracing with yarn and felt-tip pens. (See also *Diabetic patients.*)

Diabetic ketoacidosis

Emergency actions

The patient with high blood glucose levels, with or without ketones, needs I.V. fluids and insulin.

First, give your patient normal saline solution 1,000 ml/hour until the blood pressure is stable and a significant urine output is established. Once the circulating volume is satisfactory, you can give hypotonic (0.45%) sodium chloride and decrease the rate. As soon as the I.V. has been started, obtain an arterial blood sample for blood gas studies. (See *Arterial puncture.*) You'll also need to get a venous blood sample for electrolyte studies. The patient will have lost not only excessive sodium through the urine but also potassium and other electrolytes. As soon as his kidney function is adequately established, these electrolytes must be replaced.

Monitor his vital signs, blood glucose level, and fluid intake and output to help the doctor in his treatment. Although acidosis exists, the patient won't be given sodium bicarbonate unless his pH falls below 7.2. (See *Acidosis, metabolic.*)

Along with fluids, give your patient insulin—usually low doses to prevent hypoglycemia. For example, 10 to 30 units of insulin may be given I.V. as a loading dose; the amounts will vary with institutional practice as well as with the patient's weight and the degree of his acidosis. Some hospitals use 0.15 units/kg of body weight. The first dose may be followed by an infusion of 4 to 8 units/hour.

Once the patient's glucose level drops to 250 mg/dl, notify the doctor. He'll probably want to add dextrose 5% solution to the I.V. If the patient's glucose level reaches 200 mg/dl, the doctor may even want to hold the level there for a while. Too rapid a reduction can lead to cerebral edema, though this occurs more often in children than in adults. When adequate renal function is established, potassium will also be added to the I.V.

Diabetic patients

Teaching them self-injection

If your patient's extremely anxious, try to gain his confidence by offering to let him watch you give *yourself* an injection. But don't make the offer if you're not willing to do it.

The best way to teach self-injection is to talk the patient through one. Here's how:

• Tell him, "I'll help you give yourself an injection now." But immediately reassure him that you'll guide him every step of the way and that the whole thing will be over in less than a minute.

• As you're telling him he's going to inject himself, fill the syringe. If he's due for an injection, use insulin; if not, use normal saline solution. Don't use water; it's not physiologically compatible with tissue fluids and may hurt when injected.

• Place the syringe in his dominant hand and an alcohol swab in his other. Tell him to wipe the injection site, preferably on his thigh, in an outward, circular motion.

• Tell him to pinch the skin around the site. Help him position the needle at a 90-degree angle over it, ready for immediate penetration.

• Tell him to penetrate the skin with the needle, but add, "Leave it there, and I'll tell you what to do next." This will stop him from withdrawing the needle prematurely. (Be ready to steady his hand after he penetrates the skin, but don't let on that you're ready or you'll risk undermining his confidence.)

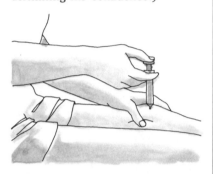

• Tell him to inject the solution.

• Tell him to withdraw the needle and apply pressure to the injection site with an alcohol sponge.

• Now congratulate him: "You've just given yourself an injection." Give him a minute for the realization to sink in. (See also *Diabetes, juvenile; Insulin preparation.*)

Diabetic shock: intervention

Responding quickly and effectively

Let's suppose that during your rounds, you find that you can't rouse a patient who was admitted yesterday with uncontrolled diabetes. His respirations and apical rate are somewhat rapid; he looks pale, and his skin is cool and clammy. You recall that he didn't eat well at breakfast or lunch, but he did take his normal dose of regular and NPH insulin at 8 a.m. Is this a diabetic patient experiencing hypoglycemia? To find out, quickly obtain a drop of blood by finger stick and

test it with a visually read glucose reagent strip. (See *Glucose monitoring.*) His blood glucose level is below 40 mg/dl. This indicates your patient is in diabetic shock and has lost consciousness. If his blood glucose level isn't raised immediately, he could suffer brain damage, become comatose, or die.

Take immediate action. Place the patient in a supine position. Continue to check his airway and pulse as you establish an I.V. line and prepare an infusion of dextrose 50% solution (D_{50}) if the doctor orders it. Give 25 to 50 ml of D_{50} slowly by I.V. push. Because D_{50} is a hypertonic solution, it can sclerose tissue if it infiltrates. So check for a blood return after every 5 to 10 ml is infused. The patient should respond within minutes.

An alternative to D_{50} is glucagon. Combine the powder with the supplied diluent and administer 1 mg of the solution subcutaneously or intramuscularly. If the patient doesn't respond within 10 to 15 minutes, repeat the dose.

If two doses of glucagon fail to raise his consciousness, give D_{50}. He may have no glycogen stores to mobilize, rendering glucagon useless.

If you can't get a stat blood glucose reading and you don't know whether the patient's experiencing hypoglycemia or hyperglycemia, assume that it's hypoglycemia and administer glucose. The brain can tolerate an extremely high blood glucose level longer than it can tolerate a low blood glucose level.

When the patient is alert and able to swallow, give him carbohydrates. If you used D_{50}, give him 20 g of a simple carbohydrate, such as 8 oz (240 ml) of orange juice.

Don't add a packet of sugar to the juice unless you need to limit fluid intake—for example, if he has end-stage renal disease (ESRD). In this case, the sugar plus 4 oz of juice will provide a total of 20 g of simple carbohydrates. (Remember to give juice that's low in potassium to ESRD patients.)

If you used glucagon to restore the patient's consciousness, give him 60 g of combined simple and complex carbohydrates. Glucagon depletes glycogen stores, which the carbohydrates will replenish. Some equivalents: 4 oz (120 ml) of orange juice is 10 g of a simple carbohydrate, whereas six Saltines are 15 g of a complex carbohydrate. An 8-oz carton of skim milk provides 12 g of a simple carbohydrate and 8 g of protein.

After eating these foods, the patient should resume his normal meal pattern. Remind him to finish each meal. He should be given replacements for any carbohydrates he doesn't want to eat.

Because the patient's likely to be cold after experiencing diabetic shock, remember to cover him with a blanket and offer him a warm drink. Check his blood glucose level every 2 hours and his vital signs as needed for the next 12 to 24 hours.

Consider also suggesting a change in his insulin dosage or meal plan. Individualizing his care plan should help to prevent diabetic shock in the future. (See *Diabetic shock: patient teaching; Diabetic shock: prevention; Hypoglycemia.*)

Diabetic shock: patient teaching

Guidelines to give your patient

Successful prevention of diabetic shock starts with patient teaching. Tell him:

"Follow your medication schedule exactly, eating all meals and snacks at the prescribed times and in the prescribed amounts. Don't change your eating patterns without first checking with your health care team about a corresponding change in your medication schedule.

"Always keep in mind that your medications and the food you eat work together in preventing episodes of hypoglycemia.

- "Monitor your exercise, trying to maintain a consistent day-to-day level of activity and exercising when your blood glucose level is naturally highest. (This is usually 1 to 2 hours after meals.) If possible, don't inject insulin into an extremity that you'll be exercising in the next few hours.

"Eat extra food to compensate for extra exercise. Remember that if you exercise more than usual, you'll use up more glucose. And your medication will lower your blood glucose level even more. This may cause diabetic shock.

"Exercise only with someone who knows the signs and symptoms of diabetic shock.
- "Always carry a source of fast-acting carbohydrate—such as hard candy or packets of sugar—with you for emergency use.
- "Be sure you, your family members, and your close friends know all the possible signs and symptoms of diabetic shock and how to help you if they occur. If you typically don't have *any* early signs and symptoms but instead become unconscious immediately, your family and friends must always be prepared to give you glucagon. (Your doctor or nurse can demonstrate how to do this. Ask if you can receive subcutaneous glucagon injections; that way, you and those who give you injections will need to learn only one type of injection technique.)
- "Always wear or carry some form of identification (like a Medic Alert bracelet or a card in your wallet) that states you're diabetic, as well as what actions a person who finds you in diabetic shock should take.
- "Identify the signs and symptoms that, for you, typically signal the onset of hypoglycemia. That way, you'll learn to recognize when it may be occurring—and you may be able to prevent it from becoming extreme.
- "Refrain from drinking alcoholic beverages: they enhance the action of insulin. If you do drink alcoholic beverages, be sure your health care team tells you what your limit should be.

- "Avoid jeopardizing the success of your treatment regimen: check with the health care team treating your diabetes whenever any other health care practitioner prescribes treatment for a condition—especially if he prescribes medication.
- "If you do have an occurrence of hypoglycemia, write down exactly what happens and what's done for you. If you don't call the doctor right away, share the information at your next appointment.
- "Immediately report to your doctor any hypoglycemic episode that doesn't subside after you eat something or that subsides but recurs soon afterward. Your doctor may advise you to report any hypoglycemic episode, especially if you're elderly." (See *Diabetic shock: intervention; Diabetic shock: prevention; Hypoglycemia.*)

Diabetic shock: prevention

Priorities to follow

With every patient who's at risk for diabetic shock, your *first prevention priority* is to identify his lowest "normal" blood glucose level—the lowest level he can tolerate without experiencing hypoglycemic signs and symptoms. Although sometimes broadly defined as an absolute blood glucose level below 50 mg/dl, this level actually varies greatly from patient to patient.

If you can't obtain this information from the patient, find out what your hospital's guidelines are and use them instead. Then, if the patient becomes hypoglycemic, monitor his blood glucose level carefully as it approaches normal to identify his lower limit.

Your *second prevention priority* is to identify times when specific patients are at high risk for hypoglycemia. These times relate to:
- the duration of action and the half-life (interval needed for excretion of

50% of the drug) of oral antidiabetic agents
- the time of onset, duration of action, and peak activity of insulin.

Using these factors, you can identify priority times for checking a patient's blood glucose level and giving extra nutrients if necessary.

Your *third prevention priority* is to center each assessment of a diabetic patient on seven major risk factors associated with the occurrence of hypoglycemia and diabetic shock.

Risk factor 1: Alteration in the amount or timing of food intake with no alteration in the drug regimen.

Risk factor 2: Increase in exercise above normal level with no alteration in food intake or drug regimen.

Risk factor 3: Excessive doses of insulin or an oral antidiabetic agent with no increase in food intake.

Risk factor 4: Alteration in absorption of insulin from the subcutaneous injection site.

Risk factor 5: Alteration in drug metabolism, prolonging the action of insulin or oral antidiabetic agents.

Risk factor 6: Ingestion of drugs that enhance the action of insulin or oral antidiabetic agents.

Risk factor 7: Onset of illness associated with endogenous hypoglycemia. (See also *Diabetic shock: intervention; Diabetic shock: patient teaching; Glucose monitoring.*)

Diagnostic studies

Patient teaching to reduce stress

To help minimize stress during diagnostic testing, teach your patient and his family about each test, including:
- its proper name (don't use abbreviations)
- why the doctor ordered it
- who will perform it
- where and when it will be done

D

- how long it will take
- how the patient will be prepared for the test, and why
- what he can expect to happen during the test
- how much pain or discomfort he can expect (if any)
- what will be done after the test, and why.

Diarrhea

Preventing skin irritation

Suggest that your patient use a peri bottle (the kind given to new mothers for perineal care during the postpartum period). Tell him to clean his perineum with fluid from the bottle instead of wiping with tissues.

To use the bottle, he simply fills it with warm water (and some soap, if desired) and directs the water over his anus and perineum. Then he can blot the skin dry.

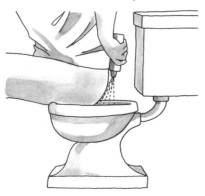

Tell him to store the bottle with the cap off to discourage bacterial growth between uses.

Difficult doctors

Preventing possible problems

Here are some guidelines to head off problems before they start and to handle the difficult doctor if you run into him.

Try to prevent difficult situations by establishing a relationship with

a doctor early on. Discuss clinical situations in a postive way with him. Here are a few tricks for doing so:
- Approach him with a problem before he discovers it.
- Have a written list of two or three questions to ask him.
- Go with him to the patient's bedside. Let him look over the chart and the patient in his own way before you ask your questions. When he seems to have answered his own immediate questions, find out if he's ready for yours with a quick, courteous, "Ready for questions?"
- Keep the conversation objective and factual.
- Don't leave as soon as your questions are answered. Wait and leave the bedside with the doctor. This will tell the doctor and the patient that you're a team. (See also *Doctors; Doctors' orders.*)

Difficult patients

Coping with your reactions to them

Recognizing how you feel about a patient—and why you feel that way—is a big step toward resolving your problem with him. The next step is to accept your feelings as legitimate. Anger, for instance, is a normal defense against anxiety and depression; it can be healthy and helpful. So don't deny your feelings. But do control your *behavior* stemming from them. Your response to a patient who provokes negative feelings must be open and assertive—not defensive and unproductive.

To deal openly with your feelings, talk to someone who can help. Depending on the circumstances, talking directly to a patient can help, but usually you should turn to a trusted colleague for support. Or you may write down your feelings to sort them out. Sometimes opening up the discussion to all nurses caring for a patient can help them deal with their feelings. But you must be careful about how such a discussion is handled. Make sure

everyone has the same goal in mind: coping with negative feelings, not reinforcing them.

Usually, you'll want to examine your feelings, accept them, and ensure that they don't affect your behavior. But sometimes you may realize that you must change your feelings toward a patient to provide better care.

Digitalis toxicity

Recognizing it

Digitalis' therapeutic range is narrow—in some patients, even a therapeutic dose may be toxic. This is why toxicity from digitalis glycosides is relatively common in patients taking these drugs.

Patients taking digitalis preparations who are also taking certain other drugs, or who have certain disorders, are at particularly high risk for developing toxicity. Examples include:
- the patient with reduced renal function taking digoxin
- the patient with reduced hepatic function taking digitoxin
- the patient with electrolyte imbalances, myocardial infarction, pulmonary disease, or hypothyroidism
- the patient on quinidine or verapamil therapy.

If you suspect your patient's developing toxicity, discontinue digitalis and notify the doctor. He may order antiarrhythmic drugs and a temporary pacemaker. He may also discontinue diuretics, which contribute to potassium loss (hypokalemia), and take action to correct electrolyte imbalances.

Expect the doctor to discontinue the digitalis or to readjust the dosage. If you suspect an intentional overdose, assess the patient's mental status—his disease may be causing suicidal depression.

Watch your patient for signs and symptoms of digitalis toxicity. The most common signs and symptoms include anorexia, nausea, vomiting, malaise, headache, ventricular ectopic beats, premature ventricular contractions, and bradycardia. Less common signs and symptoms are blurred vision, headache, halos around lights, disorientation, diarrhea, ventricular tachycardia, sinoatrial and atrioventricular block, and ventricular fibrillations. Digitalis toxicity affects the cardiovascular system and other body systems. So nausea, vomiting, and anorexia commonly accompany toxicity—especially in elderly patients. But digitalis-induced dysrhythmias may occur *without* any other signs and symptoms.

Diplomacy

Using it to your advantage

If your supervisor doesn't offer support, tell her you need it. But don't expect her to solve all your problems for you. When you go to your supervisor, present both the problem and possible solutions.

Here are a few more tips:

1. *Be direct.* Don't be afraid to get right to the point, even with unpleasant information. Trying to soften the blow with unrelated comments may confuse your supervisor and get the conversation started in the wrong direction.

2. *Be objective.* Tell the whole story when you're asking for advice. Don't stack the deck by telling only the side that supports the action you want to take—then blame your supervisor for agreeing to an imprudent solution.

3. *Be the bearer of good news as well as bad.* If you go to your supervisor only with problems, she may think you don't have any successes. Tell her about some, especially if they're the outcome of decisions she helped you make.

4. *Take your supervisor's suggestions seriously.* If you want advice, listen to it, ask questions about it, discuss it, and try it. If you just need someone to listen, say so. Don't ask

for advice then ignore it. You might not get a sympathetic ear the next time. (See also *Supervisors.*)

Dislocation, leg

Assessment and intervention

Your first priorities are to keep the patient's dislocated joint immobilized, to administer analgesics as ordered, and to initiate cold-pack treatment. Make sure his splint is tight enough to keep the joint immobilized but loose enough to ensure adequate circulation to the leg. You'll have to assess your patient's neurovascular status carefully because extreme swelling can lead to nerve and vessel compression that can cause ischemia and further neurovascular injury. This degree of impingement on major arteries can result in compartment syndrome and possibly in amputation of the leg. (See *Compartment syndrome.*)

Knee and patella dislocation

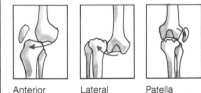

Anterior   Lateral   Patella

Perform a thorough baseline assessment of your patient's neurovascular status. Check his *tibial* and *peroneal* nerve function. If he has *sciatic* nerve damage (common in patients with posterior hip dislocation), he'll have a combination of motor and sensory loss (tibial and peroneal nerves) and pain on knee extension when his hip is flexed. (See *Nerve damage, peripheral.*)

A deficit in motor function—or loss of sensation in these areas—indicates nerve damage. Notify the doctor if you see these signs; he'll want to do an immediate reduction of the dislocation.

Next, check your patient's circulatory status distal to the dislocation. Check all his distal pulses, the color and temperature of the leg, and his capillary refill time. Swelling can cause compression, resulting in vessel damage unless it's treated promptly.

When you're assessing a patient with a dislocated knee, remember that a pedal pulse doesn't necessarily mean that no arterial damage is present. If the popliteal artery is damaged, the collateral circulation around the knee will initially produce an effective pedal pulse. However, it won't be sufficient to prevent eventual circulatory compromise secondary to swelling. Expect to prepare your patient for an arteriogram if the doctor suspects popliteal artery damage. (Some doctors will order an arteriogram for *every* patient with a knee dislocation.)

Doctors

Handling rude behavior

What can you do when a doctor's overbearing behavior threatens to turn your shift into an endurance test? Seething in silence or fighting back won't help. So how can you get things back under control?

You need to take immediate action—do something to calm things down quickly. You'll also need a long-range plan. After all, you'll probably have to work with each other again.

Immediate action

You might feel embarrassed and angry if a doctor reprimands you—especially in front of a patient and his visitors. But don't strike back with a statement like "If I changed your patient's dressing and he got an infection, you'd be the first to blame me." He may only become defensive—and more aggressive.

In such a case, you need to confront the situation promptly and deal with the doctor directly. For example, you might say: "Doctor, I'd like to talk to you. Obviously, you

D

were angry when you first came on the floor. But I don't appreciate taking the brunt of your anger when I haven't done anything wrong. The dressing wasn't changed because I'm following hospital policy."

This technique will work because it will call the doctor's attention to a behavior he may not be aware of and point out that his behavior is inappropriate.

Here's another way to take immediate action with rude doctors: Disarm them with humor. Ever get bawled out for awakening a doctor to come and see a patient in the middle of the night? Instead of listening to his tirade, try saying: "I'll see you when you come in." Then when he comes in, smile pleasantly, and say, "Tell me, doctor, how can you be such a lion on the phone and such a pussycat in person?" He may feel embarrassed and commiserate after that.

Long-range plan

When a doctor's rude to everyone, everyone has to work together to change his behavior. So you'll need your staff's help for an effective long-range plan. If a doctor lashes out at one nurse, she could reply in a matter-of-fact tone, "Excuse me, doctor," then walk away. If he begins the same lecture with another, she should politely excuse herself. And any of you could say: "Doctor, I'll be glad to talk to you when you address me professionally." (See also *Difficult doctors; Doctors' orders.*)

Doctors' orders

Challenging them

When a doctor's order is inappropriate or outside your scope of practice, you must challenge it to protect your patient and yourself.

1. Talk it over. Ask the doctor to clarify his order. Perhaps he's unaware it's inappropriate. If it is appropriate, he can explain his rationale. If the doctor insists you carry it out, and you're still not con-

vinced you should, tell him why your nursing judgment (or Nurse Practice Act) says you can't.

2. Document the incident. Include all details and the names of any witnesses.

3. Report the incident to your supervisor. Don't wait. She may have some suggestions for handling the problem. Moreover, the doctor may respond better if a nursing administrator steps in.

Even if you and the doctor resolve the problem yourselves, inform your supervisor anyway. The doctor may agree with you at the time but complain to your supervisor later.

4. Follow the chain of command. Most medical staffs have a chain of command or a committee to deal with such conflicts. Once you've informed your supervisor about the problem, she should initiate the investigative process. If she doesn't, you must do so. Document each step and continue up the chain until the problem is resolved.

Your hospital's system for handling professional disagreements should support you in challenging a doctor's order. If it doesn't, get advice from an attorney, preferably one experienced in employees' rights. You then can safeguard your interests while protecting your patient's welfare. (See *Difficult doctors; Doctors; Legal risks: doctors' orders.*)

Documentation

Keeping good notes to protect yourself

The primary purpose of nurses' notes is to communicate your assessment of the patient and the problem-solving measures taken. But nurses' notes also protect you from charges of negligence or other forms of malpractice. They serve as legal evidence of the care you gave, and they're valuable tools to refresh your memory if you're brought to

court. Your notes should comply with these rules of good charting.

1. Follow hospital policy regarding notes, and supplement that policy with sound professional judgment.

2. Record only on the proper forms. Enter the date and time of each note.

3. Sign your first initial, last name, and the initials of your title: RN, SN, or whatever. Write legibly and precisely.

4. Chart in chronologic order, recording on every line.

5. Don't erase or write between the lines. If you inadvertently omit a note, write the time you record the note and the time you delivered the care. If you make a mistake, draw a line through it, write "error" or "mistaken entry," and sign your initials. Then write the correct note and time.

6. Record information as close as possible to the time you deliver care. Don't document in advance. And don't leave important notations until the end of the shift. The higher the risk situation, the greater the effort you should make to record as soon as possible. Avoid block charting (for example, writing 7 a.m. - 3 p.m.); put the time that you are actually writing the note.

7. Write notes only for patients *you've* cared for. Don't let someone else document your assessment or intervention; such notes may be inadmissible in court. (An exception is an emergency, such as cardiopulmonary resuscitation, where one nurse may record the care others deliver. This is acceptable because the recording nurse is also involved in the procedure and therefore has personal knowledge of it.)

8. Record perceived data—what you can see, hear, smell, and touch. Stick to facts.

9. Eliminate bias from your notes. Prejudging or labeling a patient can impair patient care and charting. In one such situation, nurses caring for a teenager with chest pain labeled her as spoiled and demanding, which

made them miss the cues to her pulmonary embolism.

10. Don't generalize. If the patient has a sleep problem, avoid vague terms such as "Had a bad night." Be specific. Chart: "Slept from 0100 hours to 0400 hours." For the patient with a bowel disturbance, don't chart "moderate distention." Instead, write down the actual measurement of the girth and note any increase from the previous measurement.

11. Document the patient's baseline assessment (nursing history and physical exam) on the chart. It's part of the permanent record.

12. Include a written nursing care plan that outlines nursing problems and nursing orders. (See *Care plans.*)

13. Include a narrative recording of progress notes to deal with problems identified in the nursing care plan.

14. Use flow sheets to chart routine care. If possible, keep them in the patient's room, so you can record immediately after you carry out the treatment. The flow sheet is also part of the permanent record.

15. Use a problem-oriented approach. Identify and describe the problem, the therapy used to resolve it, and the patient's response.

16. Record all teaching performed.

17. Ensure continuity. Note problems as they occur, the resolution used, and any changes in the patient's status.

18. Record your patient assessment before and after you administer certain medications, such as analgesics.

19. Record the time, date, and pertinent information when you report something to the patient's doctor.

20. Note on the chart if you've raised your patient's bed rails.

21. Write down on the medication record when you gave a drug and how much you gave.

22. Use only hospital-approved or standard abbreviations. Don't repeat data that is stated elsewhere

in the chart—vital signs, medications, and intake or output.

23. Don't label a patient's behavior without describing it.

24. Document whether your patient is giving you a hard time or is noncompliant. Also note if your patient is verbally abusive.

25. Prepare a discharge plan that lists instructions for the patient and for the follow-up community service. Send a copy of the plan home with the patient and keep a copy in the record. (See also *Documentation, computerized.*)

Documentation, computerized

Minimizing your legal risks

When you work with a computerized medical record, your legal liabilities are the same as with a manual system: You're liable for any patient injuries associated with your charting errors.

Here's how to minimize the legal risks:
• Always double-check all patient information you enter.
• Never tell anyone your signature code.
• Tell your supervisor if you suspect someone is using your code.
• Indicate whether the doctor's order is written or oral (in person or by telephone) when you enter it. Also, verify the doctor's orders entered by the unit secretary to ensure accuracy.
• Know your institution's rules and regulations on patient privacy. (See also *Documentation.*)

Doll's eye sign

Testing for an absent sign

To evaluate the patient's oculocephalogyric reflex, hold his upper eyelids open and quickly (but gently) turn his head from side to

side. Note the patient's eye movements with each head turn.

In absent doll's eye sign, the eyes remain fixed in midposition. In an unconscious patient without brain stem dysfunction, the eyes usually move laterally toward the side opposite the direction in which the patient's head is turned.

Drains: fastening

Securing abdominal drains

Even a drain that's been sutured in place may be inadvertently pulled out. Once displaced, it can't be reinserted easily, and the patient may have to return to surgery. So use extra caution when changing the dressing on a drain or repositioning the patient. Always check the placement of a drain both before and after these procedures to make sure it hasn't been displaced. (See *Drains: observation.*)

Certain types of drains must be secured in special ways. A long drainage tube should be "flag taped" to create some slack, but don't make a loop that can get caught on something. A Penrose drain usually has a safety pin attached to it so that it doesn't recede into the abdomen. If you don't see a pin, tell the doctor.

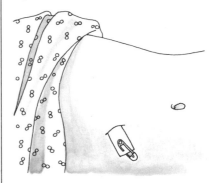

You also have to check drains carefully to make sure they're working properly; they can kink, causing drainage to back up inside the tube and ooze out around the insertion site. Inspect all drains for patency every 4 hours. To ensure effective suction, remember to check such devices periodically for clogged tubing, a full container, or a container that's been turned off. (See also *Drains: guidelines.*)

Drains: guidelines

How abdominal drains are used

When an abdominal drain is used, it's usually inserted through a separate incision rather than through the primary surgical incision, which would make it harder for the wound to heal properly or might even cause dehiscence. If your patient has a drain inserted through the primary incision, be alert for infection and dehiscence. The drain provides bacteria with a portal of entry to the wound.

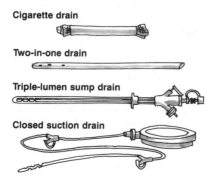

Cigarette drain

Two-in-one drain

Triple-lumen sump drain

Closed suction drain

If your patient has a drain in place, chart its exact location and purpose. Include a sketch showing the location of the drain in relation to the four abdominal quadrants; this helps especially when the patient has more than one drain. Ask the doctor to clarify his postoperative notes if the location and purpose of the drain aren't clear to you. (See *Drains: observation.*)

Drains, head wound

Checking patency

Imagine that your patient has had a craniotomy, and you see a Jack-son-Pratt drain coming through the middle of a dry scalp dressing. Already you've made your first validation: You've discovered the dressing around the tube is dry.

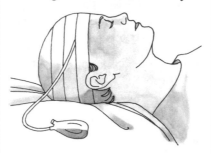

Since excess fluids need to be drained from an area where bony encasement, such as the skull, prevents any expansion, you know this head drain is a postoperative exit drain.

Of course, the big question remains: Is the tube patent? The drain's collection container should be in the aspirating position, exerting a gentle suction force that gradually diminishes as the container fills with fluid. If its sides have expanded and it resembles a lemon-shaped ball, the container's losing its suction force. You'd then empty and decompress the container.

Drains: observation

What to look for when managing abdominal drains

Closely observe the abdominal drainage's color, consistency, and amount at least once every shift. Record your observations in the nurses' notes and report significant changes immediately. A sudden increase in bile drainage from a T tube, for example, may mean the common bile duct is blocked below the tube's insertion site. (See *T tube: nursing measures.*)

Some drains, such as the Penrose, drain directly into a dressing. If your patient has one of these drains, you'll need to record the number of dressing changes and characteristics of the drainage on each dressing.

If the drainage seems excessive, indicating possible hemorrhage and hypovolemia, weigh the dressing to get a more accurate measurement. Note your finding on the patient's intake and output record and report it to the doctor. To monitor lesser amounts of drainage, use a pen to outline the drainage on the dressing. Then record the date and time. (See also *Drains: guidelines; Drains, postoperative.*)

Drains: patients' concerns

Allaying common fears about abdominal drains

Bear in mind that when your patient awakens after abdominal surgery, he may be alarmed by the sight of one or more drains sticking out of his abdomen. To allay his anxiety:
• Reassure him that the drain is only temporary and eventually will be removed.
• Explain why the drain has been inserted, where it's draining from, and what it's draining. (See *Drains: guidelines.*)
• Tell him how often you'll be changing the dressing.
• Keep him informed of how his wound is healing. When possible, point out signs of healing, such as decreasing drainage, fewer particles in the drainage, and a clear color to the drainage.

If the doctor wants the drain advanced periodically, explain to the patient that the purpose of this procedure is to remove internal pockets of fluid.

Provide complete self-care instructions to the patient who is discharged with a drain still in place. You may also need to teach a family member how to care for the drain properly.

Drains, postoperative

Proper management of abdominal drains

Your patient has had abdominal surgery, and his doctor has placed a drain and connected it to a Hemovac. On the second postoperative day, you notice the Hemovac drainage amount has markedly decreased during the last 8 hours. Is the tubing clogged? Or is this decrease normal? You should check some variables before you make any assumptions.

Inspect the patient's abdomen. Is the Hemovac in its aspirating position? Has the abdomen increased in girth since yesterday? (See *Blood loss measurement.*)

Next, look at the tubing's Y connector. If you suspect the tube isn't patent, finger pressure here should make the fluid in the tube fluctuate, much the same way respirations cause fluctuations in chest tubes.

Press the connector, with full force, between your thumb and index finger. Sometimes this gentle assist can start the drainage's forward flow.

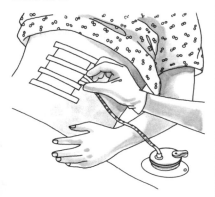

If finger pressure doesn't cause fluctuations, suspect clots in the tubing. Remove the dressings. What do you see and what do you hear? If the tube is patent, the drainage ports at the insertion site shouldn't be outside the patient's skin, and you shouldn't hear air escape.

If all variables check out and the system still isn't draining, you have two alternatives. Perhaps the surgical area has stopped draining or particles have clogged the tube's indwelling portion. If you suspect the tube is clogged, either—according to the hospital's policy—disconnect the tube at the Y junction and gently irrigate with 5 ml of sterile water or notify the doctor. (See also *Drains: guidelines; Drains: observation.*)

Drains: preparation

Cleaning the insertion site for an abdominal drain

Abdominal drainage tends to be serous and sticky, providing an excellent medium for bacterial growth. To maintain skin integrity and patient comfort, clean and dry the drain insertion site every time you change the dressing. You can use a sterile 4″ × 4″ gauze pad or a cotton-tipped applicator soaked in sterile saline solution or in a weak hydrogen peroxide solution (no more than 0.5% peroxide).

Gently clean the area around the drain first, then work outward. If the area around the drain begins to redden, apply a small amount of protective ointment as a skin barrier. Keep in mind, though, that you don't want to manipulate the insertion site any more than necessary. This area is very tender, especially if the drain has been sutured in place.

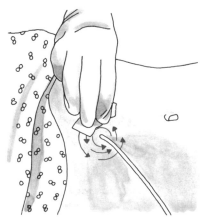

Here's a tip for reducing patient discomfort: Create a bridge under the drain with a folded 4″ × 4″ gauze pad. This will reduce pulling on the insertion site. Of course, monitoring the patient's overall condition and administering medication as ordered will alleviate discomfort, too.

Draping

When your patient's in the lithotomy position

To drape a patient in the lithotomy position, fold a drawsheet in half lengthwise, then fold it in half the other way. The sheet will now be folded in quarters.

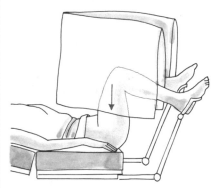

Hold the sheet where all the folds meet, and place it at her waist. Drape each of the two long folds over each of her legs. The drape will resemble the front half of a pair of pants—and cover her effectively.

Dressings

Changing them after nose surgery

To ease the pain of dressing changes for patients who have had nose surgery, cut a piece of 1″ wide Kerlix gauze about 25″ long, and tape the ends together. Then twist it in the middle, making a large figure eight, and place a 2″ × 2″ gauze pad in the middle.

D

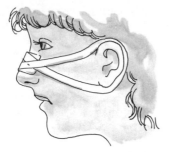

To apply the dressing, hook one loop around each of the patient's ears and center the gauze on his nose. Changing the dressing is simple—just unhook one loop and replace the gauze. No tape touches the patient's sensitive skin.

Dying patients: nutrition

Helping your patient eat

For the dying person, the act of eating is no longer a nutritional goal; it's a social one. We all associate eating with living. But take cancer, for example. Cancer eats everything the patient puts into his system. Malignant cells require calories. Even patients who eat continue to lose weight. So you can no longer measure nutritional success by calories or protein intake. What can you do? Here are some tips.
• Allow patients to choose not only their food but also the size of their portions.
• If you cut the quantity of food in half and place it on a salad plate instead of a dinner platter, the patient may not feel so overwhelmed. Remember, we eat with our eyes, then with our mouths. Imagine a terminally ill patient's satisfaction when he's eaten everything on his plate. And make sure his tray has only one or two dishes on it, again to give the appearance of an achievable goal.
• Present an array of desserts on a cart, just like in a fancy restaurant. Again, serve small portions and allow the patient to take his time in choosing something appealing.
• For patients who require pureed food because dentures no longer fit or a tumor of the mouth prevents chewing, consider a method known as "reforming," which takes solid food, such as a pork chop, and puts it through a food processor. This method helps maintain the dignity of a patient who thinks eating pureed food is demeaning.

And instead of serving an institutional scoop of mashed potatoes, have them molded into the empty skin of a baked potato. That gives the sense of original form and substance while providing nutrition and an appetizing presentation.

Dysphagia: assessment

Recognizing the cues

Elderly patients are particularly prone to swallowing problems because of diminished taste perception and saliva production. Look for the following cues:
• *Reflexes.* First, check for a swallowing reflex. To do this, assess laryngeal elevation by placing your finger along the thyroid notch and asking the patient to swallow. If he can, you'll feel his larynx rise; if he can't, you may be able to stimulate swallowing by gently pushing up his larynx with your fingers or having him flex his head forward.

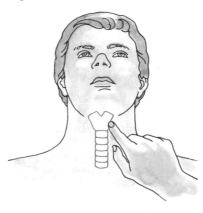

Next, check the patient's cough reflex. Coughing is a protective mechanism—it clears food and fluids from the airway so they don't enter the upper respiratory tract. Ask the patient to cough, but if he can't, don't try to stimulate the reflex. Anyone who can't cough voluntarily or effectively enough to move secretions to the front of his mouth should not be fed orally because the risk of aspiration is too great.

You might also want to check the patient's gag reflex, although this check has drawbacks. For one thing, some patients with overactive gag reflexes have trouble swallowing. But more important, this check can be dangerous if not done with extreme care. Don't assess the gag reflex unless the patient can either swallow or cough on his own—otherwise he won't be able to clear his mouth if he vomits. To stimulate a gag reflex, use a tongue depressor or cotton-tipped applicator to touch the back of the tongue, the right and left sides of the uvula, and the oropharynx. And be sure to keep suctioning equipment and an artificial airway by the patient's bedside in case of emergency.
• *Speech and voice.* When assessing for swallowing problems, don't forget to listen to the patient, too. Speech problems can signal potential swallowing problems. For example, a stroke-related speech disorder such as aphasia (inability to speak), dysphasia (inability to speak coherently), or dysarthria (inability to articulate clearly), is likely to be accompanied by weakness of facial and throat muscles and impaired lip, tongue, and pharynx control. A voice that's hypernasal, slurred, hoarse, or breathy may also signal muscle weakness, so listen for any abnormalities in voice or speech—they could be significant cues to potential swallowing problems.
• *Secretions.* Oral secretions can also be a cue to swallowing difficulties, so check your patient's mouth carefully. Be especially alert

to patients who have very dry mouths—they can choke on food easily because they don't produce enough saliva.

On the other hand, patients who have excessive or thick, sticky secretions can choke or gag on their saliva. These patients tend to drool or dribble much of what they're eating or drinking.

• *Supporting muscles.* A patient whose facial or mouth muscles are weakened won't be able to control food or fluids in his mouth, chew properly, or swallow. So assess overall facial muscle tone, noting any drooping or flaccidity.

If the patient can't close his lips completely, he'll have trouble keeping food in his mouth.

Tongue strength affects the patient's ability to move a bolus of food to the back of the pharynx. To assess tongue strength, ask the patient to press his tongue against one side of his mouth and then the other while you feel it through his cheek.

• *Orientation and neglect.* Disoriented patients may actually forget they have food in their mouths and forget to swallow. Similarly, a stroke patient who's paralyzed on one side may not be aware that food is collecting in that side of his mouth, won't receive the stimulus to chew, and might choke or aspirate.

If you've done a thorough assessment and still feel undecided about whether the patient is at risk for dysphagia, do one last check: Have the patient swallow a small amount of water or chew and swallow a few ice chips. If he can't manage these, he surely can't manage solid food.

A similar check for a patient with a tracheostomy is to mix some edible dye into sterile water and have the patient swallow a small amount. If the colored water seeps around the stoma, it's going into the trachea instead of the esophagus, indicating that the patient has swallowing problems. (See *Cranial nerve assessment; Dysphagia: nutrition; Stroke patients.*)

Dysphagia: nutrition

Helping your patient eat safely

If your assessment shows that a patient has dysphagia and is at risk for choking, you need to find ways to help him eat and drink safely.

An upright position is safest for eating, so if your patient can't support himself, elevate the head of his bed and support his arms with pillows. This will allow gravity to assist the passage of food into the stomach and will help prevent choking and aspiration. If your patient hyperextends his neck when he puts food in his mouth, show him how to flex his neck forward slightly, keeping his chin at midline. This will decrease the possibility of aspiration into the trachea.

Encouraging your patient to think or talk about food just before mealtimes helps stimulate saliva flow and aids in the chewing process. For patients with very dry oral cavities, try these extra measures. Since tart or sour foods are most likely to encourage saliva production, put a lemon slice or dill pickle on the patient's tray. Even if he doesn't care to eat the lemon or pickle, just the sight and smell of it may help to stimulate salivation. Providing mouth care before and after a meal can also stimulate saliva production and can enhance taste perception by freshening the patient's mouth and removing thick or dried secretions.

To stimulate the process of chewing and swallowing, enlist the help of the dietary department in making up meals that contain foods with different temperatures and textures.

If your patient has trouble closing his lips around a spoon or fork or can't keep food in his mouth, help him strengthen his mouth muscles. Have him practice licking jelly from his lips, puckering them, humming, or whistling. If he clamps his lips shut when you try to feed him, press

his chin lightly with your finger to encourage mouth opening. Or if he extends his tongue when you're feeding him, try putting the food on the back of his tongue.

Minimize distractions by removing unnecessary items from the tray and by placing one dish at a time in front of the patient. Serving the meal in a quiet, private place also helps, especially if the patient lacks muscle control and is embarrassed by his eating difficulties. Although we usually think of pleasant conversation as an aid to appetite and digestion, for these patients, it's just another distraction. So keep mealtime talk to a minimum, restricting it to simple instructions, and explain to the patient that you'll chat after the meal.

Patients with left cerebral hemisphere damage may have trouble understanding instructions, so demonstrate biting into a piece of food, chewing, and swallowing. Patients with right cerebral hemisphere damage who have spatial-perceptual deficits can often be talked through the process of eating.

Since a liquid doesn't provide as strong a stimulus as a bolus of solid food, drinking is usually harder for patients to manage. Separate liquids from solids, and be sure the patient has cleared his mouth and pharynx of any solid food before drinking. Don't let a patient try to compensate for loss of saliva by drinking liquids between bites of food. Foods and liquids together create confusing stimuli in the mouth, increasing the likelihood of choking and aspiration. You can, however, start the meal by letting the patient take a few sips of fluid to lubricate his mouth and throat.

What your patient eats may be just as important to his safety as how he eats. With the help of the dietary department, choose various foods that will encourage your patient to chew and swallow and give him better mouth and tongue control.

As mentioned before, foods with distinct temperatures and textures

D

best stimulate salivation, chewing, and swallowing, especially with elderly patients whose senses are diminished. Moistening food with small amounts of liquid—for instance, adding gravy to meat or mashed potatoes or dipping toast or crackers in tea or juice— also helps patients with decreased saliva production.

Because milk increases mucus production in some patients, it's better tolerated when boiled or as an ingredient in cooked foods. Cooking alters the protein in milk and alleviates the problem. Sticky foods, such as soft white bread, bananas, and peanut butter, can adhere to the palate, so steer clear of them, too. (See *Dysphagia: assessment; Stroke patients.*)

Dysplasia, hip

Detecting congenital causes

When assessing the newborn infant, attempt to elicit Ortolani's sign to detect congenital hip dysplasia. Begin by placing the infant supine with his knees and hips flexed. Observe for symmetry.

Place your hands on the infant's knees, with your index fingers along his lateral thighs. Then raise his knees to a 90-degree angle with his back.

Abduct the infant's thighs so that the lateral aspect of his knees lies almost flat on the table. If he has a

Abducting the thighs

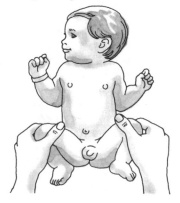

dislocated hip, you'll feel and perhaps hear a click or popping sensation (Ortolani's sign) as the head of the femur moves out of the acetabulum. He may also give a sudden cry of pain.

If you elicit a positive Ortolani's sign, look for other signs of congenital hip dysplasia.
• Observe for asymmetry of the infant's gluteal or thigh folds.
• Flex the infant's hips to detect limited abduction.
• Flex the infant's knees, and observe for apparent shortening of the femur.

Dyspnea

Nursing interventions

If a patient complains of shortness of breath, quickly assess for signs of respiratory distress, such as tachypnea, cyanosis, restlessness, and accessory muscle use. If you detect any of these signs, notify the doctor immediately. Elevate the head of the bed. Prepare to administer oxygen by nasal cannula, mask, or endotracheal tube. Start an I.V. infusion and begin cardiac monitoring to detect dysrhythmias, as ordered. Expect to assist with chest tube insertion for severe pneumothorax. (See *Chest tube insertion.*)

If the patient can answer questions without increasing his distress, take a complete history.

During the physical examination, look for signs of chronic dyspnea, such as accessory muscle hypertrophy (especially in the shoulders and neck). Also look for pursed-lip exhalation, clubbing, peripheral edema, barrel chest, diaphoresis, and distended neck veins. Check blood pressure and auscultate for crackles, abnormal heart sounds or rhythms, egophony, bronchophony, and whispered pectoriloquy. Finally, palpate the abdomen for hepatomegaly.

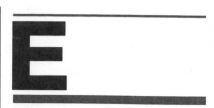

Ear irrigation

Irrigating a child's ear

Next time you irrigate a child's ear, try this: Use a 20-ml syringe with an I.V. plastic cannula instead of the traditional irrigating syringe. This smaller syringe is softer, more pliable, and less frightening to your patient.

To absorb leakage and keep the patient's shirt dry while you're irrigating his ear, try this: Wrap the long edge of a disposable diaper around the patient's neck—absorbent side up—and fasten it with the tape tab.

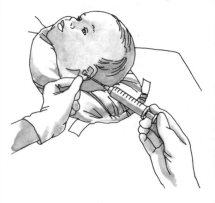

Curve up the outer edge to catch any solution the diaper doesn't absorb. You can use whatever size diaper fits your patient's neck.

ECG, single channel

Equipment operation

Here's what to do:
1. Bring to the patient's bedside the following equipment and supplies: the ECG machine (including five lead wires, four limb electrodes with rubber straps, one suction cup chest electrode, and recording paper), conduction paste, gauze pads, and alcohol sponges. Check the date

of the machine's last inspection; don't use it if the period of authorized use has elapsed.

2. Explain the procedure and answer the patient's questions. Tell him it's painless and will take only about 15 minutes.

3. Connect the appropriate lead wires to their corresponding limb electrodes by inserting the wire prong into the terminal post and tightening the screw.

4. Apply conduction paste to the inside of the patient's right ankle. Place the ground electrode on top of the paste over an area of minimal muscle. Secure it with its strap, being careful not to pull too tight. Follow the same procedure for the patient's left ankle. Be sure to position each leg electrode with its connector end pointing up his leg so the lead wire won't be bent.

5. Then apply conduction paste and place the appropriate limb electrodes on the inside of the patient's forearms. Tell him to relax and breathe normally, and ask him not to talk while the machine is running because that could distort the recordings.

6. Turn on the ECG machine and set the lead selector to the STANDARD (STD) setting to warm up the stylus. Set the paper-speed selector to the standard 25 mm/second or as ordered.

7. Turn the power switch to RUN. The stylus should draw a straight, centered baseline. If it doesn't, adjust the stylus with the POSITION knob.

8. Next, with the lead selector still set to STD, quickly tap the STD button to calibrate the machine. The stylus should record a wave pattern that's about the height of one large box on the recording paper.

9. Set the lead selector to the position for lead 1. Record a minimum of six beats if the rhythm is regular (12 to 16 beats if it appears irregular), then turn the selector to a neutral position to stop the paper from running. Label the lead po-

sition on the paper by pressing the MARK button.

Repeat the procedure for each of the remaining limb leads, moving the lead selector to the appropriate setting for each. Be sure to calibrate the machine before recording each lead to ensure consistency. After recording the last limb lead, turn the lead selector to a neutral position.

10. Tell the patient you're going to run the chest leads now. Locate the first position by finding the first intercostal space on the right sternal border and counting down to the fourth intercostal space. If serial ECGs are ordered, use a felt-tip pen to mark the six positions where you'll place the chest electrodes. This will ensure that subsequent measurements are taken at precisely the same places.

Positions for chest electrodes

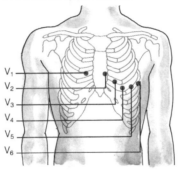

11. Place a small amount of conduction paste at each position where you'll place the electrode. Then attach the chest lead wire to the chest electrode.

12. Squeeze the rubber bulb, place the electrode over the paste at the first position (V_1), and release the bulb. Suction will hold the electrode in place.

13. Set the lead selector to V_1, then record the impulse as you did for the limb leads. Remember to mark the strip.

Move the lead selector to a neutral position and recalibrate the machine. Then move the chest electrode to the V_1 position, return the selector to the V setting, record, and mark. Repeat this procedure for the remaining positions.

14. When you've finished recording all 12 leads, run enough paper through the machine so that when you tear it off, all of the last recording is shown.

15. Write the patient's name and age, doctor's name, and date and time of test on the ECG paper. Note whether the patient experienced any chest pain during the procedure. (If the strip will be interpreted immediately, keep the lead in place in case the procedure needs to be repeated.)

16. After removing the electrodes and disconnecting the lead wires, clean the paste from the patient's skin. Then clean the electrodes—the limb electrodes with alcohol sponges and the chest electrode by holding it under running water.

Eclampsia

Nursing priorities

You have three priorities with this patient:
• to prevent seizures from developing or to control them if present
• to reduce maternal blood pressure
• to prolong the pregnancy as long as you can safely do so.

To prevent or control seizures, the doctor will ask you to give your patient magnesium sulfate or diazepam. Both drugs decrease hyperreflexia, relieve cerebral vasospasm, decrease blood pressure, and increase urine output. Keep her on complete bed rest and decrease stimuli—bright lights, noises, and drafts. As a precaution, raise the bed's padded side rails, and keep the following emergency and seizure equipment nearby:
• an oral airway
• oxygen
• intubation and respiratory equipment
• suction equipment
• diazepam (Valium)
• magnesium sulfate (and its antidote, calcium gluconate), plus other emergency medications

E

• I.V. equipment. (See also *Seizures, generalized motor; Seizures: precautions.*)

Complete bed rest will reduce your patient's blood pressure and cardiac work load, enhancing the effect of the magnesium sulfate or diazepam. If your patient's diastolic pressure stays above 110 mm Hg, the doctor may order an antihypertensive, such as hydralazine.

Monitor the patient's blood pressure, and remember that *changes* in blood pressure, indicating a trend, are more significant than individual readings. Monitor her intake and output, and obtain a urine sample for an albumin test and urinalysis to rule out other causes of proteinuria (for example, infection.)

Reducing your patient's blood pressure and keeping her calm and quiet will help you meet your third priority—to stabilize the fetus. Check fetal heart tones, using an external monitor. (See *Fetal monitoring, external electronic.*) At the first sign of fetal distress, notify the doctor and prepare the patient for an emergency cesarean section.

Edema, angioneurotic

Recognizing it

Angioneurotic edema frequently results from an allergic reaction. It's characterized by rapid onset of painless, nonpitting, subcutaneous swelling, usually in the lips, eyelids,

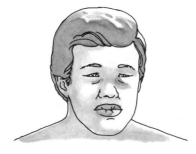

and tongue. It usually resolves in 1 to 2 days. This edema may also involve the hands, feet, genitalia, and viscera; laryngeal edema may cause life-threatening airway obstruction.

Edema, pitting

Assessing for it

Press firmly for 5 to 10 seconds with your fingertips over a bony surface, such as the subcutaneous part of the tibia, fibula, sacrum, or sternum. Then remove your finger and note how long the depression remains. Document your observation on a scale ranging from +1 (barely detectable) to +4 (a persistent pit as deep as 1″ [3 cm]).

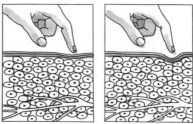

+1 pitting edema   +4 pitting edema

In severe edema (caused, for example, by a lymphatic obstruction), tissue swells so much that fluid can't be displaced, making pitting impossible. The surface feels rockhard, and subcutaneous tissue becomes fibrotic.

Edema, pulmonary

Emergency intervention

If your patient's heart failure deteriorates to pulmonary edema, intervene quickly and efficiently, according to these guidelines:
• Call for help. Notify the doctor at once and get a crash cart.
• Assess and ensure airway patency and oxygenation. Maintain proper airway position. Encourage coughing if it's productive. Suction only if absolutely necessary to avoid further decreasing oxygen levels. Administer oxygen by mask or nasal cannula. Prepare for intermittent positive-pressure breathing treatment, if ordered, and for drawing of arterial blood gas samples. (See *Arterial puncture.*)

• Position the patient so as to decrease his venous return. If possible, place him in high-Fowler's position, letting his legs dangle to further decrease venous return. Monitor his blood pressure closely.
• Assess his vital signs frequently until his condition stabilizes.
• Start an I.V. infusion. Choose an insertion site unaffected by position changes.
• Attach the patient to a cardiac monitor. Observe closely for dysrhythmias.
• Administer medications, as ordered. Prepare to give furosemide, morphine, digoxin I.V., nitroglycerin, nitroprusside, and dobutamine, as ordered.
• Strictly calculate fluid intake and output. Be prepared to insert an indwelling (Foley) catheter, if ordered, to monitor intake and output. Restrict fluids.
• Prepare resuscitation equipment. Have advanced life-support equipment on hand and keep intubation supplies in the patient's room. (See *Crash cart.*)
• Provide emotional support. Maintain a calm, caring attitude. Reassure the patient and his family. Remain with him as much as possible, and provide the family with a quiet waiting area.

Elbow protectors

How to make them

Have your patient make them himself. Tell him to cut the tops and toes off an old pair of socks. He can then place a sanitary pad (with an adhesive strip) inside each sock,

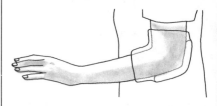

lengthwise over the heel. This makes a pair of comfortable, inexpensive elbow (or heel) protectors.

Elderly patients: bathing

Home care tips

As a person gets older, he doesn't need to bathe as often. A good rule of thumb is that an elderly patient should bathe an average of one to three times a week, depending on his preference, hygiene needs, and skin condition.

Because an elderly patient is susceptible to hypothermia, he should bathe quickly. Be sure the water is tepid and the soap super-fatted, not a harsh deodorant soap. Timing is important, too. Your patient may benefit from a relaxing bath at bedtime.

Bath oils can prevent dry skin, but they can also make the tub slippery. Make sure you help the patient into and out of the tub. Don't use heavily perfumed products; they'll just irritate the skin and the lining of the vagina and urethra. Mineral oil is a good, inexpensive bath oil.

After the bath, gently dry the patient with a towel. Vigorous toweling will remove water from the stratum corneum, causing pruritus. Apply a mild, nonperfumed emollient to the patient's skin—especially his feet—several times a day. Vegetable oil is a good emollient.

Complete baths should be supplemented with partial baths during which only the patient's hands, face, and perineum are cleaned. The elderly patient also needs a nutritious diet, adequate fluids, and a humidified environment to keep his skin healthy. (See also *Elderly patients: care.*)

Elderly patients: care

Improving their quality of life

Help your patient function independently by teaching him how to cope with the changes in his physical and mental capabilities, sensory acuteness, appetite and elimination, and physical appearance.

If he bathes in the morning, suggest that he bathe in the evening. Warm water on his peripheral blood vessels may decrease cerebral blood flow, leading to confusion.

Caution him that alcohol abuse can lead to confusion and slow reflexes. And sedatives, hypnotics, and depressants can lower blood pressure, interfering with neurovascular reflexes.

Help him adjust to aging's impact on his senses by suggesting ways of improving his ability to see, hear, and communicate. Be sure his vision is appropriately tested and corrected. Make sure he gets a thorough hearing evaluation; in many cases, hearing aids can help. Recommend telephone attachments that increase the volume of telephone voices and create a lower, louder ring.

Incontinence is the most distressing indignity of old age. Advise him to avoid long-acting sedatives and hypnotics because he won't awaken in response to the signal that his bladder is nearing capacity. He might limit his fluid intake after 7 or 8 p.m.

Osteoporosis will make his bones structurally weaker and prone to breaking. Encourage your patient to use the ramps in public buildings and at street corners rather than risk the stress of stair climbing.

Osteoarthritis may affect the knees, hips, spine, and distal finger joints. Tell your patient that rest usually relieves the discomfort of osteoarthritis, and using a cane may prevent the pain. Tell him to take plain or enteric-coated aspirin to relieve pain.

Advise him to rise to a standing position slowly to prevent dizziness and falling.

An elderly patient's skin can become abraded just from the friction of moving across bed linens. If bedclothes are irritating, tell him to dust his bottom sheet with cornstarch to help decrease friction between his skin and the sheet or to use sheepskins. Caution him however, that the sheepskins must be kept dry. In fact, all linens that come in contact with his skin should be dry because moisture macerates the skin. (See *Arthritis aids; Elderly patients: bathing.*)

Elderly patients: discharge planning

Preparation pointers

Discharge planning for elderly patients should start as soon as possible after admission. The sooner you start, the better the chances that the patient will comply with your discharge instructions.

Plan short, slow-paced teaching sessions that allow plenty of time for repetition of important points. Each session should last no more than 30 minutes. Before the sessions, ask the patient what he'd like to know and what he already knows about the points you'll be discussing. This will allow you to correct any misconceptions and build on his knowledge.

Try to relate your teaching points to the patient's own experience, so they'll be more meaningful to him. If you'll be explaining a newly diagnosed disease, for example, you might start by asking if he has a friend or family member with the same disease. Make sure he understands all the terms you're using, too. Write out any new terms, with definitions, for him.

Demonstrate all procedures he (or a family member) will have to perform at home. For a procedure such as insulin administration, demonstrate the *exact* technique he will be using at home, not a variation of it. Repeat your demonstrations as often as necessary.

During these teaching sessions, keep in mind the sensory changes brought on by aging. For example, since many elderly persons lose the ability to hear high-pitched sounds, give your instructions in a low-pitched voice. Charts and posters should have large print and vivid, contrasting colors.

Whenever possible, try to work *with* the elderly patient's habits—the habits of a lifetime, remember—rather than trying to change them. This will greatly improve the chances of compliance.

Finally, write down or tape-record all instructions so the patient can review them at home. Plan for appropriate follow-up after discharge.

Elderly patients: emotions

Dealing with confusion and agitation

Confusion and agitation are not inevitable consequences of the aging process, but they may occur in many elderly persons when they're hospitalized. Illness, fear, and feelings of helplessness may provoke uncharacteristically aggressive responses. And invasions of privacy may trigger combative behavior—even in persons who are usually gentle.

To counteract these tendencies, try to keep your elderly patient from getting bored. If he's confined to bed 24 hours a day with little sensory stimulation, he's more likely to become confused. Listening to the radio or watching some television can help keep him occupied. Companionship will help, too, so encourage family members to visit as often as possible. At the same time, the elderly patient should avoid overstimulation. He may be placed in a double room, but he should *not* be put in a small, crowded room. Frequent transfers should also be avoided if possible.

To help minimize confusion and agitation, make sure he doesn't get too hungry or thirsty. Offer him fluids every hour. If he must be re-

strained in bed, keep his food and water within easy reach.

Remember, an elderly patient may strike out with his hands or arms when frightened. This is a normal defensive response. If you approach him from behind, be careful not to come up on him too suddenly. Always avoid quick movements or gestures that might startle him.

If your elderly patient remains agitated or combative, try distraction: Divert his attention from whatever is upsetting him to something more pleasant. For example, you might bring up the subject of his grandchildren or the lovely flowers that his daughter sent him.

Another alternative is to let him have a few minutes to himself in a quiet, dimly lit "time out" room. Relaxation techniques can also be beneficial. (See *Relaxation techniques.*) If they don't work, consider providing him with a cassette player, headphones, and relaxation tapes or familiar music.

Use restraints only as a last resort. Always try alternative ways of calming the patient first. (See *Restraints: precautions.*) Also, give appropriate skin care.

Once you do get an elderly patient calmed down, spend some time with him talking about what upset him. Let him know that your feelings toward him haven't changed. He'll need reassurance at this time, especially after a violent incident. (See *Elderly patients: orientation.*)

Elderly patients: infection

Minimizing risks

Elderly patients run an especially high risk of contracting an infection during a hospital stay. Among patients over age 70, the incidence of these infections is twice as high as it is among patients under age 70. The two most common nosocomial infections are respiratory tract infections and urinary tract infec-

tions. So when your hospitalized elderly patient develops a fever, he should have a chest X-ray, a urine culture, and sensitivity tests.

To detect infection, you may have to look for more than the classic signs and symptoms, such as fever and chills. Look for unusual, insidious signs and symptoms—hypotension, confusion, and agitation, for example—in response to infection.

To prevent infection in elderly patients, most hospitals have strict infection-control procedures concerning catheterizations, catheter care, wound and skin care, urinary tract infections, and influenza. Frequent hand washing will help prevent cross-infections. (See *Foley catheter techniques; Wound care dressings: changes.*)

Make sure the patient receives a nutritious diet, with lots of vitamins A and C, protein, and trace minerals. Elderly persons tend to be particular about what they eat because they have established lifelong eating habits. So if hospital food doesn't appeal to an elderly patient, don't hesitate to ask family members to bring in some of the patient's favorite foods.

An elderly postop patient with impaired circulation presents a special problem. His wound needs an adequate blood supply to heal properly. You can help by keeping his room warm (about 75° F. [24° C.]) to promote vasodilation. Also, encourage him to drink at least 2,000 ml of fluid a day, unless contraindicated. Check the dressing frequently to make sure it isn't causing vasoconstriction. Use hot and cold compresses cautiously because elderly patients don't adapt well to temperature changes.

One last note about preventing infection: If your elderly patient hasn't received immunization shots, urge him to do so. The three most important are influenza, pneumococcal, and diphtheria and tetanus toxoid vaccines.

Elderly patients: orientation

Keeping them oriented

When an elderly patient will be hospitalized for a week or longer, put a clock and calendar at his bedside to help keep him oriented to time. But don't use an ordinary calendar. Instead, personalize a month-at-a-time calendar for each patient.

Mark special dates (such as Father's Day or Christmas) and events ("Aunt Sophie visited today," "discharge date," and so on). Include reminders for self-care activities (such as "do range-of-motion exercises while watching TV," or "physical therapy today"). Even draw comic characters with colored markers on the calendar where appropriate.

Keep several blank calendars on hand so you can make one up when needed. Many patients save them as a "diary" of their hospitalization.

You can also make calendar/time boards for patients who can't remember the mealtime schedule. For each board, cover a 22" × 18" (55 cm × 45 cm) piece of sturdy cardboard with light-colored cloth. Staple three cardboard pockets across the top of the board and staple the labels "month," "day," and "year" above the pockets.

In the pockets, place felt cutouts of all the months and dates. Each day, take out the right date and pin it to the pocket. Change the month and year, as necessary.

Across the bottom of the board, staple three cardboard clock faces, indicating mealtimes, and staple the labels "breakfast," "lunch," and "dinner" above the clock faces. Hang the board at eye level on the wall facing the patient's bed. These boards—with the patient's own clock—help orient him to time and day. (See also *ICU care.*)

Elderly patients: sleep

Helping them sleep better

During sleep, the body secretes a growth hormone that promotes protein anabolism and wound healing.

To help your elderly patient get the sleep he needs, encourage him to engage in some light physical activity during the day, if he can. Just make sure he stops the activity several hours before bedtime, and offer him a protein and dairy food snack, such as warm milk and custard.

At bedtime, try giving him a rhythmic back rub, using an unperfumed lotion to avoid pruritus.

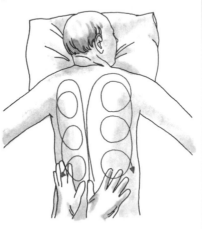

Or provide a warm tub bath to relax skeletal muscles and soothe aching joints. (See *Elderly patients: bathing; Elderly patients: care.*)

Chronic use of sedatives and hypnotics by elderly patients should be avoided; it can lead to drowsiness, delirium, night terrors, agitation, and incontinence.

A better idea is to offer your elderly patient a nightcap of 30 to 60 ml of wine or sherry, if not contraindicated. Sometimes, just one or two tablets of acetaminophen can promote restful sleep by relieving stiffness or discomfort. Beverages containing caffeine should be avoided just before bedtime.

Elderly patients: tests

Minimizing risks during diagnostic testing

Being elderly and in a weakened state, the patient could quickly develop fluid and electrolyte imbalances and could become confused from all the tests. Or he could fall or develop orthostatic hypotension after diagnostic tests. So take precautions with any elderly patient undergoing diagnostic tests. Make sure you monitor his vital signs before and after every test—and during the test, too, if you're present. Check his fluid and electrolyte status frequently, more often than you would with a younger patient. If he's not permitted anything by mouth, he should receive I.V. fluids and be returned to his regular diet as soon as possible.

To prevent falls, keep his bed low and the side rails up. For at least 24 hours after a diagnostic test, don't let him get in or out of bed or try to walk without assistance. (See also *Diagnostic studies; Patient falls.*)

Electrical hazards

Precautions to take

Follow these precautions:
• Keep your patient as dry as possible.
• Use only grounded electrical equipment within 6' (1.8 m) of his bed.

E

• Use only equipment that's been tested and approved by the hospital's engineering department. Tell them of any malfunctions promptly.
• Use green grounding cords whenever possible for an added margin of safety.
• Don't use extension cords except in extreme emergencies.
• For a patient who has an indwelling catheter from an external pacemaker, insulate the connectors to the catheter with electrical tape or other insulating material.
• Inspect all cords for exposed wires.
• Report loose or broken receptacles to the engineering department.
• Don't let patients use their own electrical equipment (such as AC-powered radios or portable TVs) in the hospital without approval by the engineering department.
• Don't touch the bed, patient, or any device attached to the patient when plugging in electrical equipment.
• Make sure your hands and feet are dry before plugging in electrical equipment.
• Inspect the plug for bent, broken, or loose prongs. Make sure the grounding post is present. (See also *Electric shock.*)

Electric shock

When you find a nurse lying on the floor

What if a nurse on your unit receives a severe electric shock and you find her holding a cord, lying in a puddle of I.V. solution?

First, shout for help; tell whoever replies to call a code. Then pause for a moment to assess the situation before acting; you can't help the victim if you yourself receive an electric shock.

To handle this emergency, you have two choices. The safer choice is to cut off the electric current to the unit unless you have patients using lifesaving equipment on your unit. Send someone to the unit's circuit breaker box. When the current is cut off, quickly move the victim away from the puddle and cord, pull the plug, then have the current restored. As you tend to the victim, someone must immediately check and reset (as necessary) all electrical equipment on the unit, starting with the ventilators.

The *less* safe choice is to pull the plug without first cutting off the current. Place several dry pillows on the floor next to the outlet, away from the victim and puddle. Wad some dry, nonconductive material in your hand (for example, a towel or pillowcase), then stand on the pillows and pull the plug.

Assess the victim's airway, breathing, and circulation. If necessary, begin CPR. (See *CPR: technique.*) Insert an artificial airway and administer 100% oxygen with a bag-valve-mask device while someone else continues the chest compressions, periodically checking for a pulse. (See *Breathing devices.*)

Start an I.V. line (but not in the arm that was holding the cord), and begin administering lactated Ringer's solution, normal saline solution, or albumin. Because a victim of electric shock is also a burn victim, fluid replacement is essential.

Begin cardiac monitoring as soon as possible, and convert any dysrhythmias with countershock or drugs, as indicated. Be prepared to give sodium bicarbonate, dopamine, isoproterenol, and other drugs, as ordered.

When the victim's heart rate and blood pressure are stable, assess the parts of her body where the electric current entered and exited. If these entrance and exit wounds are large, gaping, or located over a body cavity, cover them with saline-soaked sterile dressings. Continue to monitor her vital signs until she's transferred to the intensive care unit.

If the electric shock *didn't* cause cardiac arrest, the victim may just be dazed. After safely removing her from danger, help her quietly walk away. Have her lie down while you check her vital and neurologic signs. Start an I.V. line with lactated Ringer's or normal saline solution, and check her skin for entrance and exit wounds. Cover small burned areas with dry sterile dressings to prevent the deeper burns from becoming contaminated. Stay with the victim until help arrives. (See *Electrical hazards.*)

Electroconductive alteration

Maintaining electrophysical stability

When your congestive heart failure patient is diagnosed as having electroconductive alteration, your goal is to maintain electrophysical stability. If needed, continuously monitor the patient's electrocardiogram. Also, check the pulse for atrial fibrillation, a common dysrhythmia in congestive heart failure. This dysrhythmia may result from atrial dilation and distention or from digitalis toxicity. (The administration of digitalis, the drug of choice for atrial fibrillation, and emergency cardioversion are contraindicated if the patient shows signs of digitalis toxicity.) Report any dysrhythmias immediately—the patient's systems are already being stressed, so a dysrhythmia can quickly become life-threatening. Be prepared to respond quickly.

Electrodes

Placing them correctly

If you're using a three-electrode monitor, here's where to position the electrodes for the most commonly ordered monitoring leads.
Lead I
• *Positive* (+): left shoulder, below clavicular hollow
• *Negative* (−): right shoulder, below clavicular hollow

• *Ground* (G) left side of chest, below lowest palpable rib, midclavicular line

Lead I

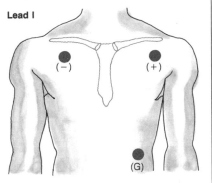

Lead II

• *Positive* (+) left side of chest, below lowest palpable rib, midclavicular line
• *Negative* (−): right shoulder, below clavicular hollow
• *Ground* (G): left shoulder, below clavicular hollow

Lead II

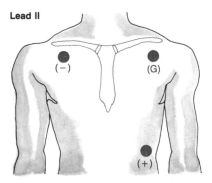

MCL₁

• *Positive* (+): fourth intercostal space, right sternal border
• *Negative* (−): left shoulder, below clavicular hollow
• *Ground* (G): right shoulder, below clavicular hollow

MCL₁

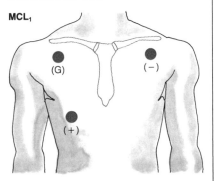

MCL₆

• *Positive* (+): left side of chest, fifth intercostal space, midaxillary line

MCL₆

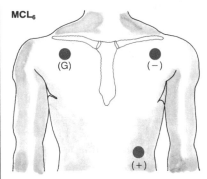

• *Negative* (−): left shoulder, below clavicular hollow
• *Ground* (G): right shoulder, below clavicular hollow

Embolism, pulmonary

Intervening quickly

Your patient has nonspecific respiratory symptoms, including chest pain and dyspnea. He's tachycardic and cyanotic, and his jugular veins are distended with the head of the bed raised 90 degrees. These signs and symptoms strongly suggest pulmonary embolism.

Embolus

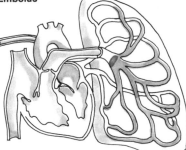

Prompt intervention is especially important to help minimize the life-threatening effects of pulmonary embolism, which may include pulmonary hemorrhage, pulmonary infarct, pulmonary hypertension, acute cor pulmonale with heart failure, and dysrhythmias.

Administer 100% oxygen at 15 liters/minute, using a nonrebreather mask. (See *Oxygen-delivery systems.*) Keep the head of the patient's bed at a 90-degree angle to help him breathe, and connect him to a cardiac monitor.

To treat pulmonary embolism, a doctor will most likely order anticoagulant or thrombolytic therapy. For anticoagulant therapy, you'll administer an initial I.V. bolus dose of 10,000 to 20,000 units of heparin. If the doctor chooses thrombolytic therapy, you'll administer the heparin first, then 250,000 units of streptokinase or urokinase—also in an I.V. bolus dose—followed by another dose of heparin. (Thrombolytic therapy is contraindicated if the patient's had recent surgery or a cerebrovascular accident within the last 2 months, or has endocarditis or septic thrombophlebitis.)

If your patient receives anticoagulant therapy, monitor his partial thromboplastin time every 4 to 6 hours to maintain a control value of 1.5 to 2.5. (You'd do this during thrombolytic therapy, too.) While he's undergoing heparin therapy, watch closely for unusual bleeding, such as petechiae, ecchymoses, bleeding gums, or nosebleeds. Continue to monitor his cardiac and respiratory status hourly.

Embolus, fat

Assessing for it

One of the most serious complications of long bone fractures is fat emboli syndrome (FES), which may occur 24 to 72 hours after the patient's injury. If FES isn't treated quickly, it can cause acute respiratory distress and death. So notify the doctor immediately if you detect the development of FES.

Watch your patient for the following signs and symptoms of FES, and

be prepared to intervene as appropriate:
- altered level of consciousness (in early FES stages)
- chest pain on inspiration
- changes in ECG waveforms from chemical irritation (prominent S waves, T-wave inversions, multiple dysrhythmias, right bundle-branch block)
- cardiovascular collapse
- gradually increasing tachypnea and tachycardia, crackles, and wheezing
- arterial blood gas measurements showing respiratory alkalosis, hypoxemia, or pulmonary shunt
- petechiae (lasting 4 to 6 hours) over the patient's torso, in his axillary folds, in his conjunctival sacs and retina, and on the mucosa of his soft palate
- fever
- localized muscle weakness, spasticity, and rigidity from muscle irritation.

Nursing interventions
Here's what to do if your patient has FES:
- Administer fluids to prevent shock and to dilute free fatty acids.
- Administer corticosteroids, as ordered, to counteract the inflammatory response to free fatty acids.
- Administer digoxin, as ordered, to increase the patient's cardiac output.
- Reassure the patient. He may be frightened or anxious as a result of the hypoxemia.

Emergency, nonhospital

When there's one in your neighborhood

When you're summoned to aid an unconscious person, do the following.

Ask the victim's family or friends the following questions:
- How long has the victim been unconscious?
- What medications was he taking?

- What allergies does he have?
- When did he last eat? What did he eat?
- Does he have any illnesses?
- Did he complain of nausea, vomiting, indigestion, or pain?
- What was he doing just before he lost consciousness?
- Did he complain about any pain or funny feelings just before this happened?

Look for:
- Medic Alert tags indicating epilepsy, diabetes, and so on. Check for them on a bracelet, necklace, or card in wallet.
- Food wrappers, drug bottles, street-drug paraphernalia, and alcoholic beverages.
- Subtle signs of response from the victim. Perhaps a cerebrovascular accident has left the victim with only an eye-blink movement. Perhaps he's only fainted—with a thready pulse and shallow respirations that seem almost nonexistent—so take a full 10 seconds to assess his pulse.
- Characteristic diagnostic signs—for example, the sweet or fruity odor that accompanies diabetic coma; the muscle rigidity, twitching, or aura of unresponsiveness that sometimes follows seizures; the pale, cool, clammy skin associated with shock; a visible bump, depression, or ecchymosis on the head that may indicate intracranial bleeding.

When calling an ambulance:
- Describe the exact nature of the emergency.
- Give a complete address, instructions on how to get there, and the number *you're* calling from.
- Don't hang up until the dispatcher does; he may need more information from you.
- Call the ambulance before calling the victim's doctor if time is critical (for example, if he's stopped breathing or is bleeding severely).

If possible:
- Have someone watch for the ambulance and flag it down when it arrives.

- Gather any medications the victim takes routinely and put them in a bag for the emergency squad. Jot down any allergies and the name of his doctor and attach the note to the bag.

Emergency assessment

Checklist of essentials

Use this guide:
Vital signs
- Auscultate or palpate blood pressure in both arms.
- Note the rate, depth, pattern, and symmetry of respirations.
- Palpate the radial pulse and note its rate, rhythm, and strength.
- Take the patient's temperature.

Neurologic
- Determine the level of consciousness.
- Inspect pupils for size, symmetry, and reaction to light.
- Observe for abnormal posture (decerebrate or decorticate) and facial symmetry, and listen for slurred speech.
- Inspect and palpate the scalp for trauma or deformities.
- Assess deep tendon reflexes, and sensory and motor responses of each affected body part. (See *Neurologic exam: assessment.*)

Eyes, ears, nose, and throat
- Inspect and palpate the face and eyes, ears, nose, and throat for burns, trauma, or deformities.
- Assess gross visual acuity and eye movements.
- Assess speech for dysphonia or aphonia.
- Inspect ears and nose for bleeding, drainage, and foreign objects; oral mucosa for color, hydration, inflammation, and bleeding; and oropharynx for signs of burns from ingestion of caustic agents.
- Inspect and palpate the thyroid gland for tenderness and enlargement. (See *Thyroid assessment.*)

Respiratory

• Observe for use of accessory muscles, paradoxical chest movements, and respiratory distress.
• Inspect the chest for contour, symmetry, and deformities or trauma.
• Auscultate the lungs for adventitious sounds and increased or decreased breath sounds assessment (See *Respiratory exam: auscultation.*)
• Palpate the chest for tenderness, pain, and crepitation.

Cardiovascular

• Palpate peripheral pulses for rate, rhythm, quality, and symmetry.
• Inspect for jugular venous distention.
• Inspect and palpate extremities for edema, mottling and cyanosis, and temperature change.
• Auscultate heart sounds for timing, intensity, pitch, and quality, noting the presence of murmurs, rubs, or extra sounds. (See *Heart exam: auscultation.*)

Gastrointestinal

• Inspect the abdomen for obvious signs of trauma or distention.
• Inspect any vomitus or stool for amount, color, presence of blood, and consistency.
• Auscultate the abdomen for bowel sounds.
• Palpate the abdomen for pain, rebound tenderness, or rigidity; percuss for ascites. (See *Abdominal exam: palpation.*)

Genitourinary

• Inspect the external genitalia for bleeding, ecchymoses, edema, or hematoma.
• Palpate the abdomen for suprapubic pain and the external genitalia for pain and tenderness.
• Palpate for costovertebral angle tenderness.

Musculoskeletal

• Inspect the body for trauma and deformities; the skin for ecchymoses, pigmentation, discoloration, and needle marks.
• Palpate the cervical spine for tenderness and deformities; the pulses distal to any injury; and the area of suspected injury for tenderness, pain, and edema.

• Assess for motor and sensory responses and for nuchal rigidity.
• Observe the range of motion of the injured body part.

Emergency tapes

Helping patients who can't speak

Here's a helpful—perhaps lifesaving—hint for a patient who's unable to speak. Have one of his relatives or friends tape-record several "emergency" phone messages that can be played over the phone to the fire company, police department, ambulance service, or doctor.

The doctor's message might say: "My name is *(patient's name)*, I live at *(patient's address)*. I'm a laryngectomy patient and need *(doctor's name)* assistance at *(repeat address)*. Please notify *(name of friend or relative)* at *(phone number).*"

Tell patients to mark all tapes clearly (only one message should be recorded on each side of a tape) and to keep the tapes, a tape recorder, and the emergency phone numbers by their phones.

The messages allow patients who are alone for long periods of time to be independent and be confident that they can get help if needed.

Employee relations

Improving staff relations

If your relationship with your staff is strained, try these tips:
• Initiate contact with others. Say "Hello" first, using the person's name. Use small talk to start conversations.
• Share your ideas with others on your staff.
• Try to read a person's feelings about important issues; study body language and become an active listener.
• Don't carry grudges. Force yourself to say "Good morning" to

someone you didn't get along with yesterday.
• Bolster others' self-esteem by supporting their objectives and asking how you can help.
• To build trust, be open about admitting mistakes. This lets others know that they can make an occasional mistake—and admit it.

Endoscopy

Assisting with the upper GI procedure

You may be asked to assist with emergency upper GI endoscopy if the doctor suspects an upper GI disorder. This procedure allows the doctor to visualize the patient's esophageal and gastric mucosa and his upper duodenum. It also allows him to instill blood-clotting agents through the tube if bleeding is a problem. Here's a review of this procedure and your role in it.

Equipment:
• local anesthetic and lubricant
• mouthpiece
• flexible fiberoptic endoscope
• suction machine
• narcotic antagonists
• syringes, needles, specimen bottles, gauze, and alcohol.

Before the procedure:
• Notify the doctor if your patient has eaten in the past 6 hours and document this.
• Explain the procedure to your patient.
• Obtain his baseline vital signs.
• Administer sedatives, as ordered.
• Remove dentures, if present.
• Insert an I.V. line, as ordered.
• Spray his throat with the local anesthetic, as ordered, to minimize gagging.
• Keep suction and CPR equipment on hand.

During the procedure:
• Place your patient in a sitting position for scope passage, then on his left side for the examination. (*Don't* have him sit up if he's in shock.)
• Tilt his chin toward his chest, keeping his head in midline.

E

• Tell him to let saliva drain from the side of his mouth and not to swallow it.
• Insert the mouthpiece; the doctor may ask you to hold it in place.
• Tell the patient to breathe deeply; this will help relax his abdominal muscles.

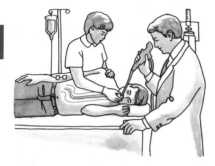

• Label any specimens and send them to the laboratory for analysis, as ordered.

After the procedure:
• Continue to monitor the patient's vital signs.
• Tell him to remain lying down until the sedative has worn off, and restrict his food and fluid intake until his gag reflex returns.
• Be alert for bleeding, dysphagia, fever, tachycardia, cyanosis, diaphoresis, hypotension, and neck, chest, or abdominal pain—these may indicate esophageal, gastric, or duodenal perforation. Notify the doctor if you note any of these signs or symptoms.
• Document all specimens collected, assessment findings, and interventions.

Endotracheal tubes: discomfort

Relieving it

Some intubated patients experience discomfort from the weight of the ventilator tubing on their endotracheal tube. To correct this problem, put a rolled bath towel under the

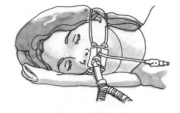

ventilator tubing near the endotracheal tube. This will also help keep the tube in position.

Endotracheal tubes: insertion

Assisting with the procedure

When the doctor orders emergency endotracheal intubation, be prepared to assist with tube insertion or to insert the tube yourself if your hospital's protocol allows. Just follow these essential steps:
• Gather the necessary equipment. If it's ordered, have a respiratory technician or another nurse set up the mechanical ventilator.
• Explain to the patient what you're going to do and why.
• Place him flat on his back with a small blanket or pillow under his head. This position will align the axes of his oropharynx, posterior pharynx, and trachea.
• Check the cuff on the endotracheal tube for leaks.

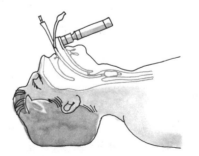

• After intubation, inflate the cuff.
• Check tube placement by auscultating for bilateral breath sounds; observe for chest expansion and feel for warm exhalations at the endotracheal tube's opening.

• Insert an oral airway or bite block.
• Secure the tube and airway with tape applied to skin treated with compound tincture of benzoin.
• Suction secretions from the endotracheal tube and mouth as needed. (See *Endotracheal tubes: suctioning.*)
• Administer oxygen and initiate mechanical ventilation, as ordered.
• After the patient's intubated, suction secretions at least every 2 hours. Prepare the patient for chest X-rays to check tube placement, and restrain and reassure him as needed.

Endotracheal tubes: suctioning

Pointers for success

Follow these steps:
1. Collect your equipment and wash your hands. You'll need a suction kit containing a sterile suction catheter (usually a #12 or #14 French), a sterile cup for saline solution, and a sterile glove; sterile normal saline solution; and a means of mechanical ventilation (either a manual resuscitation bag or the sigh setting on the ventilator). If you're going to instill sterile normal saline solution, obtain an alcohol sponge, a sterile syringe, and a vial of the sterile normal saline solution.

At the patient's bedside, you should have an oxygen flowmeter, suction apparatus, connecting tubing, a collection bottle, and a plastic bag for used supplies.
2. Tell the patient what you're going to do. Unless contraindicated, elevate the head of his bed 45 degrees. This will allow maximum movement of his diaphragm, promoting deep breathing and effective coughing.
3. Open the suction kit. Maintaining sterile technique, place the glove on your dominant hand. (Hospital policy may require you to wear gloves on both hands.)

4. Set up the cup for the solution to rinse and lubricate the catheter and to test it.

5. With your ungloved hand, pour the sterile solution into the cup. Then remove the catheter from its plastic wrapper, being careful to maintain sterility.

6. To lessen the risk of contamination, wrap the catheter around the fingers of your gloved hand. Insert it into the connecting tubing in your ungloved hand.

7. Occlude the lumen of the catheter by pinching it between your fingers. Place the thumb of your ungloved hand over the suction port to apply suction, then look at the gauge on the suction apparatus. It should read between 80 and 120 mm Hg. Adjust the suction pressure accordingly, but be sure to release and reapply suction between test adjustments.

8. Before suctioning, have your assistant hyperinflate the patient's lungs and give him extra oxygen. To hyperinflate his lungs, your assistant should use either a manual resuscitation bag attached to a 100% oxygen source or the sigh setting on the ventilator. If she uses the ventilator, she should set the oxygen control at 100%. Before administering manual sighs, she should check the sigh volume control to see that it's set higher than twice the patient's tidal volume, and the pressure limit control to see that it's set properly for the patient's condition.

9. Lubricate the catheter and check its patency: Apply suction and draw up the solution through the catheter and connecting tubing until you see it in the collection bottle.

10. Tell the patient he may feel short of breath, then open the adapter's suction port. Advance the catheter gently. Don't suction or jab it up and down when you're advancing it, or you may damage mucosa. Stop advancing the catheter when it touches the carina—you'll feel resistance and the patient will usually cough.

11. Withdraw the catheter about ½" (1 cm) from the carina, then

apply suction. While suctioning, rotate the catheter and withdraw it from the airway in one smooth, continuous motion. Don't suction for more than 10 seconds. The entire procedure—from catheter insertion to withdrawal—should take no more than 15 seconds.

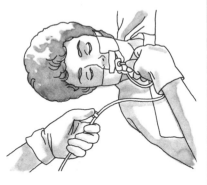

12. Remove the catheter completely and close the adapter's port. Give the patient several breaths or sighs to reinflate and oxygenate his lungs. Note his reaction to the procedure by assessing his color, heart rate and rhythm, and breath sounds.

13. Rinse secretions through the catheter and tubing to the collection bottle by placing the catheter tip in the sterile saline solution and aspirating. Then suction the patient again if necessary.

14. Rinse the catheter, then suction the patient's mouth to remove excess saliva produced during the procedure. Then rinse the catheter and connecting tubing, and disconnect the catheter from the connecting tubing.

15. Wrap the catheter around your gloved finger.

16. Pull off the glove so the catheter is inside it. Discard the catheter and glove into the plastic bag.

17. Evaluate the patient's condition. Assess his breath sounds and heart rate and rhythm, and compare your findings to the baseline assessments. Then check the ventilator controls to be sure they're reset properly, and make the patient comfortable.

Document your findings.

Esophageal tubes

Patient care pointers

Here's how to manage them:
• Test the balloons for leaks before insertion.
• Aspirate from the gastric aspiration tube to verify correct tube placement.
• To maintain proper pressure, double-clamp balloon ports after the balloon pressure's been established.
• Maintain tension on the tube to ensure a snug fit between the balloons and the esophagogastric junction. Use a sponge nasal guard.
• Keep scissors at the patient's bedside to cut balloon ports if airway obstruction occurs.
• Use a Y connector attached to the esophageal balloon lumen, a mercury manometer, and a manometer inflation bulb to inflate the esophageal balloon and determine its pressure.

Make sure you're familiar with the three tubes described below.

Sengstaken-Blakemore tube

A *Sengstaken-Blakemore tube* is a triple lumen tube with gastric and esophageal balloons). Its functions include:
• gastric balloon inflation (about 200 to 250 cc air capacity)
• esophageal balloon inflation (about 30 to 45 mm Hg pressure capacity)
• gastric aspiration.

Sengstaken-Blakemore tube

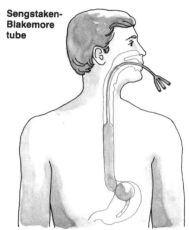

E.

E

The patient may need a nasogastric tube to aspirate secretions that collect above the esophageal balloon. Don't keep the esophageal balloon inflated more than 24 hours after bleeding stops. Then, as ordered, deflate the balloon, release traction, and leave tube in place for another 24 to 36 hours. If gastric aspirate then appears clear, remove the tube, as ordered.

Linton tube

A *Linton tube* is a triple-lumen tube with a gastric balloon. Its functions include:
• gastric balloon inflation (about 700 to 800 cc air capacity)
• gastric aspiration
• esophageal aspiration.

Linton tube

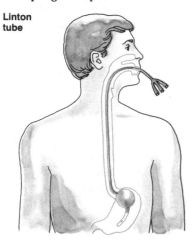

Don't use the tube more than 40 hours, or it may cause cardioesophageal junction necrosis.

Minnesota tube

A *Minnesota tube* is a quad-lumen tube with gastric and esophageal balloons. Its functions include:
• gastric balloon inflation (about 450 to 500 cc air capacity) with adjacent gastric balloon pressure monitoring port
• esophageal balloon inflation with adjacent esophageal pressure monitoring port
• gastric aspiration
• esophageal aspiration.

Don't keep the esophageal balloon inflated more than 24 hours. Keep the gastric balloon inflated for 24 hours after bleeding stops. Then,

Minnesota tube

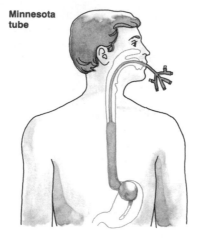

as ordered, deflate the balloon, release traction, and leave the tube in place for another 24 to 36 hours. If gastric aspirate then appears clear, remove the tube, as ordered.

Esophageal varices

When they rupture

Quickly maintain the patient's airway by slightly elevating his head and turning it to the side to prevent aspiration. Call for help and keep the intercom open. Ask whoever responds to page a doctor stat and call for the crash cart. Have someone set up oxygen and suctioning equipment.

Start an infusion of lactated Ringer's or normal saline solution. When you perform the venipuncture, obtain blood samples and send them to the laboratory for typing and cross matching, a complete blood count, coagulation studies, and a liver profile. Tell the unit secretary to alert the blood bank that type O negative blood may be needed. Start the transfusion as soon as the blood arrives. (See *Blood transfusion technique.*)

Begin administering oxygen through a nasal cannula at 4 to 6 liters/minute, and prepare the patient for cardiac monitoring. If they're not already available, have someone obtain a nasogastric tube,

an irrigation tray, and sterile saline solution. Also see that supplies are available for endoscopy and endotracheal intubation.

When the doctor arrives, he'll first want gastric lavage performed through the nasogastric tube. Elevate the head of the bed to Fowler's position and insert the tube. Then irrigate it with saline solution until the return solution is clear. Next, the doctor will perform an endoscopy to provide a definitive diagnosis. Tell the patient what's going to be done, and administer 5 to 10 mg of I.V. diazepam, as ordered, to sedate him. (See *Endoscopy.*)

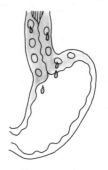

When the presence of bleeding varices is confirmed, the doctor will choose one or a combination of these treatments to stop the bleeding: sclerotherapy, administration of vasopressin, or esophagogastric double-balloon intubation.

If he can get an unobstructed view of the bleeding varices during endoscopy, he may choose sclerotherapy—injecting a sclerosing agent directly into the varices. Once the endoscope is removed, you'll need to monitor the patient for signs of aspiration or airway obstruction; inserting and removing the endoscope could rupture the esophagus.

Vasopressin temporarily stops bleeding by lowering portal vein pressure. If ordered, dilute 200 units in 500 ml of dextrose 5% in water and administer it I.V. through an infusion pump at 0.2 to 0.4 units/minute. Observe the patient's heart rate and rhythm, and be alert for signs of chest pain.

An esophagogastric double-balloon tube (for example, a Sengstaken-Blakemore tube) can temporarily control bleeding by applying pressure directly to the varices. Before the doctor inserts this tube, test its two balloons for leaks. Once the tube's in place, the doctor will inflate first the gastric balloon with 200 to 250 cc of air, then the esophageal balloon with 40 to 60 cc. Apply traction to the tube, attach its aspiration port to a suction device, and have an X-ray taken to confirm that it's positioned properly. (See *Esophageal tubes*.)

Monitor the patient's breathing during and after the insertion. Improper positioning of the esophageal balloon or accidental deflation of the gastric balloon can cause airway obstruction. Check balloon pressures every 20 minutes, and keep scissors at the patient's bedside so you can quickly cut and remove the tube if obstruction occurs.

Exercises, Berger's

Improving circulation in legs

To help stimulate circulation in her legs, have the patient perform these exercises as part of her regular exercise program—four times a day or as often as the doctor specifies. Give her the following instructions:

"Begin by lying flat on your back. Then raise your legs straight up and hold this position for 2 minutes.

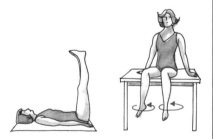

"Now sit on the edge of a table or any flat surface that's high enough so your legs don't touch the floor. Dangle your legs and swirl them in circles for 2 minutes.

"Finally, lie flat for 2 minutes; then repeat the sequence twice."

Eyedrops: administration

Instilling them in infants' eyes

Giving eyedrops to a squirming infant is never easy, but it's especially difficult for a mother who must do it without help. Here's a tip for her:

Tell her to sit on the floor with her legs apart and to lay the baby between them with his head toward her. Then she should place his right arm under her right thigh and his left arm under her left thigh. She should hold his head firmly but gently between her thighs. Then she can administer the drops with both her hands while keeping his head immobilized.

Eyedrops: patient teaching

Pointers for instillation

To make sure your patient instills eyedrops correctly, give her this advice:
• "Tilt your head back.
• "Place your finger just below your lower eyelid and pull it down gently.
• "Hold the eyedropper horizontally above your eye.
• "Look up with both eyes and instill one drop. This way, the tip of the eyedropper won't damage your eye if you jerk suddenly. And it won't contaminate the eyedropper if you blink suddenly.

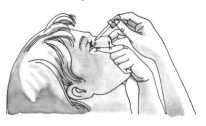

• "If the drops have more than just a local effect, press gently against the inner corner of your eye for about 30 seconds."

If your patient's hands are shaky, tell her to instill drops this way:
• "Hold the eyedropper between your thumb and forefinger.
• "Brace your hand by resting your thumb on your nose and your forefinger on your forehead. (The dropper tip should be directly opposite the center of your eye.)
• "Pull the lower lid down gently.
• "Tilt your head back and look up.
• "Squeeze one drop between your eye and lower lid.
• "Close your eye gently.
• "If the drops have more than just a local effect, press gently against the inner corner of your eye for about 30 seconds." (See also *Eyedrops: administration*.)

Eye exam: external eye

Examining it

For the patient with ocular symptoms, examination of the external eye forms an important part of ocular assessment. Here's how to do it:

First, inspect his eyelids for ptosis and incomplete closure. Also observe his eyelids for edema, erythema, cyanosis, hematoma, and masses. Are they everted or inverted? Do the eyelashes turn inward? Have some of them been lost? Do the lashes adhere to one another or contain discharge? Next, examine the eyelid margins, noting especially any debris, scaling, lesions, or unusual secretions. Also watch for eyelid spasms.

Now gently retract the eyelid with your thumb and forefinger, and assess the conjunctiva for redness, cloudiness, follicles, and blisters or other lesions. Check for chemosis by pressing the lower lid against the eyeball and noting any bulging above this compression point. Observe the sclera, noting any changes from its normal white color.

Next, shine a light across the cornea to detect scars, abrasions, or ulcers. Note any color changes, dots, or opaque or cloudy areas. Also assess the anterior eye chamber, which should be clean, deep, shadow-free, and filled with clear aqueous humor.

Inspect the color, shape, texture, and pattern of the iris. Then assess the pupils' size, shape, and equality. Finally, evaluate their response to light. Are they sluggish, fixed, or unresponsive? Does pupil dilation or constriction occur only on one side?

Document your findings. (See *Pupil size; Pupillary reaction.*)

Eye exam: extraocular muscles

Evaluating them

The coordinated action of six muscles controls eyeball movements. To test the function of each muscle and the cranial nerve that innervates it, ask the patient to look in the direction controlled by that muscle. The six directions you can test make up the cardinal fields of gaze. The patient's inability to turn

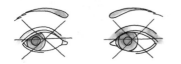

the eye in the designated direction indicates muscle weakness or paralysis. Document your findings.

Eye irrigation

Dealing with a chemical burn or foreign body

To care for a chemical burn or remove a foreign body from your patient's eye, perform eye irrigation immediately and continue it as long

as necessary. Here's how to perform eye irrigation using I.V. tubing and normal saline solution. (An alternative—and less common—method involves inserting a special contact lens, attached to I.V. tubing, into the patient's eye. This allows continuous irrigation.) (See also *Burns: chemical.*)

You'll need the following equipment:
• towels
• eyelid retractor
• cotton balls or dry tissues
• topical anesthetic (such as proparacaine hydrochloride)
• normal saline solution (1,000 ml) at room temperature
• I.V. infusion set without needle
• plastic trash bag
• trash can.

Here's what to do:
• Explain the procedure to your patient to ease his anxiety.
• Wash your hands.
• Place your patient in the supine position, with his head turned so the solution won't flow into the nonirrigated eye.
• Place towels so they'll soak up the irrigating solution. Or place a plastic trash bag under the patient's head, then drape it off the bed and into a trash can that will catch the solution.
• Evert the patient's eyelid and instill a topical anesthetic, as ordered, to ease his discomfort during irrigation.
• Holding the patient's eyelids open with your fingers, ask him to rotate his eyes clockwise during irrigation. Then hold the tubing at a 45-degree angle and irrigate the lower cul-de-sac and the superior fornix. (A lid retractor may help you irrigate the superior fornix.) Make sure

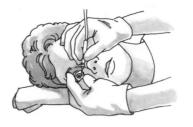

the solution flows across the cornea to the outer canthus.
• To irrigate both eyes, alternate between them, moving the flow of solution from the inner to the outer canthus of each eye. To prevent cross contamination, don't touch the tubing to either eye.
• When you're irrigating a chemically burned eye, use litmus paper—after irrigating for 10 minutes—to test the pH of the palpebral conjunctiva. If the pH isn't neutral, continue irrigating until it is. If you don't have litmus paper, irrigate for at least 10 minutes with 1,000 ml of normal saline solution.
• When you've finished irrigating, dry the patient's eyelids with cotton balls (so he won't feel the urge to rub his eyes). Wipe from the inner to the outer canthus, using a new cotton ball for each wipe.

Eye ointments

The best technique for applying them

Before cataract surgery, the doctor may order drops and ointment for your patient's lower conjunctival sac.

Before applying the ointment, gather the equipment you'll need: the ordered medication, dry cotton balls or tissue, and cotton balls moistened with sterile normal saline solution for cleaning the patient's eyelids and lashes. Then thoroughly wash and dry your hands.

Explain the procedure and answer any questions. Inform the patient that the ointment will temporarily blur his vision. Ask him to hold still while you apply the ointment, to reduce the risk of injuring his eye or contaminating the tube's tip.

Position him so he's sitting with his head tilted slightly back or lying on his back (whichever is more comfortable). Clean his eyelids and canthus areas with a moist cotton ball.

Remove the cap from the ointment tube, and lay the cap down on its side on a clean surface. Ask the patient to look up and focus on a specific object. With one hand, place your index finger on his upper eyelid to help keep his eye open. Then, with your other hand, gently pull down on his skin to expose the conjunctival sac.

Starting at the inner canthus, squeeze a thin ribbon of ointment along the lower conjunctival sac. As you approach the outer canthus, rotate the tube to detach the ointment. Take care not to touch his eye, eyelid, or eyelashes with the tube's tip.

Ask him to gently blink his eyes several times so that the ointment is spread and absorbed. As he blinks, use a clean, dry cotton ball or tissue to gently press on his inner canthus, to prevent possible systemic absorption through the tear duct. Replace the tube's cap, and wash your hands.

If you have to apply ointment to his other eye, consider waiting a short time; the patient may become disoriented if his vision's blurred in both eyes at once.

Properly store the medication. Document the procedure on his medication administration record and note any observations in your nurses' notes. Use this tube of ointment for this patient only. If you contaminate the tube's tip during the procedure, discard the tube and use a new one for future applications.

Eye pain

Assessment

If the patient's eye pain results from a chemical burn, have another nurse notify the doctor immediately. Remove contact lenses, if present, and irrigate the eye. (See *Eye irrigation*.)

If the patient's eye pain doesn't result from a chemical burn, take a complete history.

During the physical examination, don't manipulate the eye if you sus-

pect trauma. Carefully assess the lids and conjunctiva for redness, inflammation, and swelling. Then examine the eyes for ptosis or exophthalmos. Finally, test visual acuity with correction (if possible) and without, and assess extraocular movements. Characterize any discharge: white, clear, or bloody. (See also *Eye exam: external eye*.)

Facial discoloration

Recognizing "raccoon eyes"

Usually, it's easy to differentiate "raccoon eyes" from "black eyes" associated with facial trauma. "Raccoon eyes" are always bilateral.

Raccoon eyes

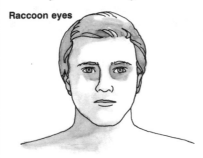

They develop 2 to 3 days after a closed head injury that results in basilar skull fracture. In contrast, the periorbital ecchymosis that occurs with facial trauma can affect one eye or both. It usually develops within hours of injury. (See *Facial trauma*.)

Facial injuries

Cleaning a patient's beard

If a bearded patient suffers a facial injury, his beard may need to be shaved. If it's left on, try this suggestion for cleaning dried blood and debris from it.

Gently scrub the beard with a toothbrush and a solution of warm water and hydrogen peroxide. The warm solution will soften the encrusted material, and the toothbrush will allow you to scrub without applying too much pressure.

Facial trauma

When your patient's in respiratory distress

Imagine you're in the ED and see a young girl who's been in an auto accident. Damage to her soft tissue has caused facial edema, which is starting to obstruct her upper airway. She's in respiratory distress, resulting in hypoxia. You need to take immediate action.

Call for help. Tell the first nurse who responds to page a surgeon, an anesthesiologist, and a respiratory therapist stat. Ask another nurse to get a nasopharyngeal and an oropharyngeal airway (see *Airway, oropharyngeal*), plus emergency airway trays with endotracheal and tracheostomy tubes. Make sure the room's suctioning apparatus is ready to use.

Try to calm the patient; anxiety will further constrict her airway. Explain that you know she's having trouble breathing and you're going to help her. Begin administering humidified oxygen. Place her in the high-Fowler's position to facilitate breathing and relieve edema. Tilt her head forward. This pulls her tongue forward, preventing airway occlusion and allowing mucus, blood, or any foreign objects to drain out of her mouth. Manually check her mouth for dentures or broken teeth. Be prepared to suction secretions and establish an I.V. line if necessary.

Before resorting to an oropharyngeal or a nasopharyngeal airway, work with the patient to improve her breathing. Besides being calm and reassuring, ask her to try to match her breathing with yours. This will buy you some time until a doctor or the respiratory therapist arrives. Remember that inserting an oropharyngeal or a nasopharyngeal airway remains an option, but it would be difficult to do. You'd be hampered by both edema and facial injuries and by the patient's resistance. Use your judgment.

While you're performing these interventions, the other nurse should be continually assessing the patient's vital signs and the quality of her respirations. Be sure to have equipment ready for endotracheal intubation or tracheotomy.

Finally, document what happened. Update your care plan accordingly. (See *Facial discoloration.*)

Fecal incontinence

History taking and physical assessment

Ask the patient with fecal incontinence about its onset, duration, severity, and any discernible pattern—for instance, at night or with diarrhea. Note the frequency, consistency, and volume of stool passed within the last 24 hours and obtain a stool sample. Focus your history taking on GI, neurologic, and psychological disorders.

Let the patient's history guide your physical assessment. If you suspect a brain or spinal cord lesion, perform a complete neurologic examination. If a GI disturbance seems likely, inspect the patient's abdomen for distention, auscultate for bowel sounds, percuss, and palpate for a mass. Inspect the anal area for signs of excoriation or infection. If not contraindicated, check for fecal impaction, which may be associated with incontinence. (See *Rectal exam.*)

Feeding tube: aspiration

When a patient's tube becomes dislodged

If a patient's feeding tube dislodges, he can aspirate the feeding solution and begin choking. Here's what to do if this happens:

Call for help, and remove the feeding tube. (Don't try to replace it—this would waste valuable time, and you could inadvertently place it in his trachea.) Next, lower the head of his bed and place him on his left side. Because the left bronchus is less vertical than the right, this position will decrease the likelihood of feeding solution moving further down into his lungs.

Now suction his mouth and pharynx. Use a tonsil (Yankauer) suction catheter if it is readily available. Otherwise, use a regular suction catheter. The rigid tonsil catheter is better because you can easily slide it into the patient's pharynx.

Begin administering oxygen through a mask. Be sure there's a manual resuscitation bag ready to use if he stops breathing.

After you've suctioned his upper airway and started oxygen administration, reassess the patient's condition. Is he breathing more easily? Has his color improved? If so, he probably aspirated the solution only into his pharynx and upper trachea. But if his condition is unchanged, the solution has most likely entered his lungs.

If the patient's condition doesn't improve, page his doctor. Prepare to call for a portable chest X-ray and to draw a sample for an arterial blood gas (ABG) study, as ordered. The patient will also need deep-tracheal suctioning. (See *Nasotracheal tube: suctioning.*)

After his trachea is suctioned, continue to administer oxygen and monitor his vital signs. Be prepared to call a code; he may still become

bradycardic or severely hypotensive or he may stop breathing.

If his condition remains unchanged or if the ABG study shows severe hypoxemia or hypercapnia, he'll need to be intubated. Set up the supplies and drugs, according to hospital procedures, and assist as needed.

If the patient is transferred to the ICU, inform the nurses there of his condition. He'll need to be closely watched during the next 48 hours for signs of pneumonia. (See *Feeding tube: complications; Feeding tube: insertion.*)

Feeding tube: complications

Avoiding them

If feedings aren't given properly, complications can occur, ranging from nausea to gastric rupture. Follow these guidelines to avoid complications:

• Check the feeding tube's position. Instill 5 to 10 cc of air through the tube and listen with a stethoscope over the patient's stomach or aspirate a small amount of gastric fluid before feeding. (See *Feeding tube: insertion.*)

Checking tube placement

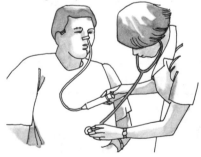

• Suction stomach contents. Do this to check for retained feedings (not indicated for patients with small-bore tubes.)
• Make sure the feeding solution is at room temperature.

• Make sure the feeding tube is patent. Instill a small amount of water.
• Position the patient properly. His head should be elevated 30 to 35 degrees to prevent aspiration.
• Start continuous feedings slowly. Begin the feeding at 25 to 30 ml/hour, using a half-strength solution so you can watch for adverse reactions.
• Split up intermittent feedings. A single feeding shouldn't be more than 300 ml.
• Watch for signs of intolerance, including diarrhea, cramping, abdominal distention, vomiting, and glycosuria. (See *Feeding tube: diarrhea.*)
• If nausea occurs, stop the feeding.
• If diarrhea occurs, lower the rate.
• Use a time tape or a pump for continuous feedings.
• Monitor intake and output.
• Give water when necessary.
• Watch for hypernatremia, hyponatremia, and other electrolyte imbalances.
• Flush the tubing after intermittent feedings with 20 to 50 ml of lukewarm water. (See *Feeding tube, enteral.*)
• Give good mouth care.
• Give good skin care around the feeding tube insertion site.
• Remember the risk of gastric rupture. Watch for abdominal distention that results from excessive tube feedings.

Feeding tube: diarrhea

Prevention guidelines

Bacterial contamination is one of the most frequent causes of diarrhea. But you can prevent it by washing your hands and maintaining strict aseptic technique when you prepare the formula.

Gather the equipment and utensils you need to prepare the solution and wash them in an automatic dishwasher, or wash them with hot, soapy water and rinse thoroughly in boiling water. Place upside down to dry. Rinse the feeding equipment with water before you use it.

Administer the formula as soon as you open it. Don't add newly opened formula to formula that's already in the feeding bag. Unused formula should be stored in the refrigerator in a tightly covered, dated container. Use it within the next 24 hours or as recommended by the manufacturer.

Replace the feeding bag and tubing every 24 hours. Don't let continuous-drip formulas hang at room temperature longer than 6 hours or "homemade" blenderized formulas any longer than 4 hours.

Sometimes the volume of the feeding itself causes diarrhea. Decrease it to a level the patient can tolerate, then gradually increase it according to the patient's tolerance. You can also try feeding the patient smaller amounts more frequently or switching to a continuous-drip method.

When giving a hypertonic formula, administer the first few feedings by continuous drip at one-third to one-half strength for at least 8 hours. Then increase the amount gradually to give the patient time to adjust. Don't increase the rate and strength simultaneously. If the patient develops diarrhea, switch to an isotonic solution.

Lactose intolerance can also cause diarrhea. If the patient has this intolerance, switch to a lactose-free formula. (See *Feeding tube: complications.*)

Feeding tube, enteral

Preventing clogging

Small-diameter enteral feeding tubes often get clogged from the feeding formula residue. To prevent this residue buildup, flush the tubes every 4 hours (and each time the feeding is interrupted or discontin-ued) with 20 ml of cranberry juice, followed by 10 ml of water.

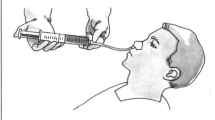

The acidic cranberry juice breaks up the formula's residue, and the water rinses away the juice, preventing sugar from crystallizing in the tube.

Feeding tube: insertion

Good technique

First, wash your hands and bring the following supplies to the patient's bedside: feeding tube and stylet (you'll usually need a #8 French); 50-ml Luer-Lok syringe; clean, small basin filled with tap water; stethoscope; penlight; tongue depressor; clean gloves; cup of ice chips or water; drinking straw; tincture of benzoin; and tape or adhesive dressing. If the patient will need suctioning, obtain suctioning equipment.

1. Explain what you're about to do. Work out a "wait a minute" signal the patient can use during insertion to tell you to stop and let him rest a moment.

2. Have him sit up so you can examine his nostrils and oropharynx for any obstructions or deformities. Ask him if he's ever had a broken nose or nasal surgery. Then choose the nostril with the most open passage to insert the tube. Be sure to ask him to swallow so you can assess his gag reflex. Put on your gloves. If necessary, suction him.

3. To estimate how far to insert the tube, use it to measure the dis-

tance from the tip of his nose to his earlobe, then from the earlobe to the base of the xiphoid process. This measurement is usually at the tube's 50-cm mark.

Estimating tube length

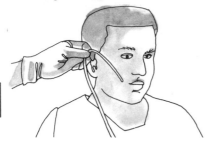

4. If the tube has a lubricant to help with stylet insertion, irrigate the tube with 5 ml of water from the 50-ml syringe to activate it. (Always use a large syringe to irrigate a feeding tube.)

5. Insert the stylet into the tube, making certain it's securely positioned against the weighted top and both Luer-Lok connections snugly fit together.

6. Moisten the outside of the tube with water.

7. Ask the patient to tip his head back slightly. Gently insert the tube into the nostril you've chosen. Slowly direct the tube down the nasal passage toward the ear.

Inserting the tube

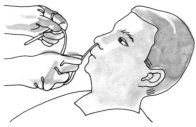

8. As you pass the tube through the nasopharynx, have him bend his head forward as far as he can to help close the epiglottis and open the esophagus. If he starts to gag or choke, stop advancing the tube and check his mouth and throat with your penlight; the tube may be coiled there. If it's not, try pulling

the tube back a bit to see if it has entered the airway.

Let the patient rest and encourage him to take several deep breaths before you go on. Continue passing the tube a few centimeters at a time until you reach the premeasured distance.

9. Determine if the tube's correctly positioned in the stomach by injecting 10 to 20 cc of air through the tube as you auscultate the left upper abdominal quadrant for a loud whooshing sound. The air should pass without resistance, and you should hear the sound immediately.

If you hear a muffled or faint sound—and the patient has a poor gag reflex—the tube may have passed into the lung and the air may be echoing back from there. Inject another 10 to 20 cc of air and auscultate the lungs. If you can hear the sound more clearly, the tube's probably in the lung. Pull it out and pass it again.

If the patient's obese, the sound may be very faint; you may have to inject air two or three times. If so, be sure to aspirate the air after you've confirmed the tube's placement so the patient won't become uncomfortable.

10. Now try to aspirate gastric contents. Note, however, that the small lumen of this feeding tube may make aspiration difficult or impossible. So if the patient is intubated or lacks a gag reflex and you have any doubt at all that the tube's not in the stomach, obtain an X-ray to confirm placement.

11. When the tube's placement is confirmed, take off your gloves and gently remove the stylet. Never try to reinsert a partially or fully removed stylet while the feeding tube is in place; the stylet may perforate the tube and seriously injure the patient.

12. Tape the tube securely in place. Use a little tincture of benzoin on the tip of the patient's nose and the tube to make the tape adhere better. (See *Nasogastric tube: fastening.*)

13. Document the procedure and your patient's response in your nurses' notes. (See also *Feeding tube: complications.*)

Fetal monitoring, external electronic

Proper technique

Ultrasound is a noninvasive technique for monitoring contractions and fetal heart rate *before* or *after* the membranes rupture. To prepare your patient for ultrasound monitoring, lubricate her abdomen and place the pressure transducer on the area of the fundus where the contractions are strongest. Adjust the transducer strap to fit snugly around the patient's abdomen. (This transducer converts the uterine contraction's pressure into an electronic signal and records it on graph paper.) To measure the fetal heart rate, reposition the ultrasound transducer over the spot where the fetal heart sounds are clearest. Remember that, although ultrasound is the easiest method to use, it needs frequent adjustments. (See also *Fetal monitoring, internal electronic.*)

Fetal monitoring, internal electronic

Doing it correctly during labor

This type of monitoring monitors contractions and fetal heart rate when the mother has ruptured membranes and a dilated cervix (2 to 3 cm), with the fetus' presenting part positioned at its opening. To perform this procedure, first help the doctor insert a saline-filled catheter into the mother's uterus, then connect the catheter to an external transducer. As contractions raise the catheter's fluid pressure, the transducer converts the pressure into an electronic signal recorded on graph paper as a curved line. Next, to measure the fetal heart rate, assist the doctor in inserting a spiral electrode into the skin of the fetus' presenting part.

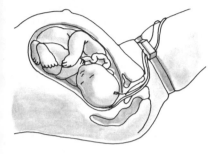

This will chart the heart rate instantly via a cardiotachometer and record it on graph paper. Internal fetal monitoring is the most accurate way to check fetal heart rate and uterine contractions, because the mother's movements don't affect the readings. However, it's an invasive procedure requiring sterile conditions and caution when placing the electrode. (See also *Fetal monitoring, external electronic.*)

Fire

When there's one in your hospital

Are you prepared for a fire in your hospital? Know your hospital's fire plan, your role in it, and what procedures to follow. Be familiar with the location and use of all fire equipment on your unit.

Do not open windows. Closing them—along with all doors and vertical openings (laundry chutes, for example)—will contain the smoke or flames in one area. The firemen will open them when necessary. The security or maintenance staff may also be assigned this duty. The fire marshal will direct this procedure.

Know your hospital's evacuation plans. Here are some general guidelines:
• Except for patients in immediate danger, evacuate ambulatory ones first. This will reduce confusion and give you more room to evacuate nonambulatory patients.

• Learn several transfer techniques you can use when evacuating patients.
• Unless the fire is a major one—consisting of extensive flames and smoke—move patients to a safe area on the same floor (horizontal evacuation).
• Don't move patients to a higher floor unless absolutely necessary.
• Always move patients toward an exit.
• Never use elevators during a fire.
• Always touch a closed door before opening it to enter or leave a room. Never open it if it's hot.

Fixation devices, external

Nursing considerations

To prepare your patient, tell him that an external fixation device, once in place, doesn't hurt. Explain that it will decrease possible swelling, muscle atrophy, and stiffness, and thereby hasten mobility. Take these steps:
• Elevate the immobilized limb to reduce swelling.
• If the patient has a tibial fracture, make sure a sling or foot board is in place to prevent ankle joint deformity.

Universal day frame

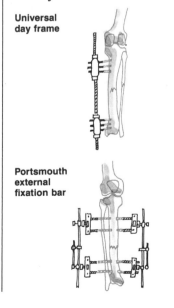

Portsmouth external fixation bar

Hoffman external fixation system

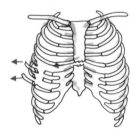

• Monitor the patient's neurovascular signs frequently.
• Watch for inflammation and drainage at the pin insertion sites, as well as for loosening of the pins.
• Give pin care, as ordered.
• Teach the patient to do isometric and active exercises, as ordered. (See *Pin care.*)

Flail chest

What you need to do

When your patient develops flail chest, it's important to act quickly.

1. Assess the patient's airway, breathing, and circulation, and intervene as necessary.
2. Stabilize the chest wall with manual pressure or sandbags.
3. Place him on a cardiac monitor.
4. Start I.V. fluids and administer oxygen.
5. Prepare him for intubation and ventilation with positive end-expiratory pressure. (See *Endotracheal tubes: insertion.*)
6. Assess for signs of pneumothorax or myocardial contusion. (See *Pneumothorax; Myocardial contusion.*)
7. Obtain a blood sample for arterial blood gas studies.
8. Administer pain medication, as ordered.

Fluid imbalance assessment

Doing it properly

Any patient can suffer from fluid imbalance. But infants, young children, elderly patients, and anyone with reduced or absent thirst sensation are especially susceptible.

To help prevent fluid imbalance, ask the patient about his normal drinking and voiding patterns, his estimated daily fluid intake and output, his weight stability, and his medication history.

During your nursing care, be sure to document his fluid intake and output and weigh him daily—at the same time, on the same scale.

Physical changes

Check for the following indications of fluid imbalance:

• *blood pressure changes.* With dehydration, blood pressure drops and orthostatic hypotension may develop. With overhydration, blood pressure rises until the heart can't pump effectively; then, blood pressure drops and venous congestion occurs. *Jugular venous pressure* can be used to assess increased or decreased volume. Distended veins indicate hypervolemia or volume overload. (See *Jugular venous pressure.*) *Central venous pressure* measures pressure in the superior vena cava or right atrium; a high pressure indicates hypervolemia.

• *pulse rate changes.* A weak, rapid, thready pulse signals dehydration. A full, bounding pulse suggests overhydration.

• *level of consciousness changes.* Confusion, disorientation, and lethargy accompany overhydration. A markedly reduced level of consciousness may accompany severe dehydration.

• *muscle tone and reflex changes.* Muscle weakness and decreased deep tendon reflexes may signal overhydration and hyponatremia.

• *GI changes.* Overhydration and hyponatremia impair GI motility, causing decreased bowel sounds. (With dehydration, bowel sounds usually remain normal unless compensatory sympathetic nervous system mechanisms reduce peristalsis.)

• *urine output changes.* Dehydration reduces urine output; overhydration increases it.

• *respiratory changes.* Adventitious lung sounds (gurgles, wheezes, and crackles) may occur with overhydration (from excess body fluid). Dehydration causes thick, tenacious secretions; overhydration leads to copius liquid secretions.

• *integumentary changes.* Moist skin may signal overhydration; dry, scaly skin and poor skin turgor may mean dehydration. (See *Skin turgor.*) Edema in dependent body parts indicates overhydration. (See *Edema, pitting.*)

Laboratory changes

Check for the following:

• *hematocrit (HCT).* HCT shows the relation between the number of red blood cells and the volume of plasma. A low HCT can result from dilution of the blood. An elevated HCT points to fluid deficit (but it will be low if the patient is actually bleeding.) Serial values showing trends will be the most useful.

• *sodium.* If only water is lost, serum sodium levels will be elevated. If only water is gained (or less water is lost than sodium), sodium levels will be low. When both are lost or gained in the same proportion, a fluid deficit can exist despite a normal serum sodium level.

Cardiac changes

An S_3 gallop, heard with your stethoscope bell at the heart's apex and sounding like "Ken-*tuck*-y," is caused by rapid ventricular filling, and it's an early sign of congestive heart failure with its accompanying fluid overload. This lower-pitched S_3 is often louder on inspiration or when the patient lies on his left side.

Weight

Increased weight indicates overhydration. A decrease in weight indicates dehydration. (See *Fluid imbalance care.*)

Fluid imbalance care

Essentials

Fluid homeostasis can go topsy-turvy in someone hospitalized for surgery, illness, or trauma.

Rather than dealing with a deficit or excess of water or a deficit or excess of sodium, you're frequently dealing with patients who have a deficit or excess of both. It's confusing, but breaking it down into the four responsible factors may give us a better handle on the situation.

The best nursing care for water deficit is, of course, prevention. Identify the patients at risk, monitor their intake and output, and provide liquids for those who can't meet their own needs (including older people and those receiving high-protein tube feedings). Evaluate their water needs carefully. (See *Fluid intake: adults; Fluid intake: children.*)

For water intoxication, routinely determine urine specific gravity. When the kidney's concentrating functions are suspect, urine and serum osmolality measurements may be indicated. Scrupulous intake and output records, daily weighing, and protection of edematous skin from the trauma of heat, cold, or prolonged pressure are necessities. You'll probably have the patient on fluid restriction and may be administering small infusions of hypertonic saline solution.

When treating the patient with a sodium deficit (hyponatremia), prepare to replace fluid and electrolyte losses to restore osmolality and to pull fluid back out of the cells. The patient in shock needs such replacement rapidly. If a patient is on fluid restriction, be prepared to explain the need for it and start appropriate comfort measures, such as keeping the mouth moist.

If your patient's on an I.V., be sure to check the I.V. fluid delivery rate. If a patient's infusion falls behind, evaluate his status before trying to catch up on the rate—especially if he has cardiac, renal, or neurologic problems.

In a patient with an excess of sodium (hypernatremia), you can expect his treatment to consist of water replacement, sodium restriction, and possibly diuretics. Be sure to monitor possible fluid overload by meticulous intake and output records and by careful daily weighing. And watch those patients taking diuretics for potassium deficiency. (See *Fluid imbalance assessment.*)

Fluid intake: adults

Promoting drinking

Helping a weak or debilitated patient drink can be frustrating. Holding a cup to his mouth may get more fluid *on* him than *in* him.

Instead, put a flexible straw upside down in his cup, so the short end is in the fluid; the flexible, ridged section rests on the rim of the cup; and the long end points down, outside the cup.

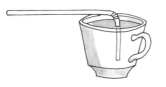

By sucking slightly on the end of the straw, your patient can siphon the fluid into his mouth. He can easily regulate the flow of fluid with his tongue.

For a patient who needs fluids and would like to have a soda but can't tolerate its carbonation, try stirring about ¼ teaspoon of sugar into the soda. The sugar will neutralize the carbonation. Patients who've had throat surgery or radiation therapy, as well as ulcer patients, will appreciate this help.

Fluid intake: children

Increasing intake

A patient sometimes balks at drinking all the fluids his doctor orders; this is especially true if the patient is a child. As an incentive, give him an animal picture (cut from magazines and children's books) each time he drinks the prescribed amount of fluid. He can then paste the picture on a poster board attached to his bed or bulletin board.

He'll be proud when visitors and staff note how many animals he's accumulated on his poster. And the poster will remind everyone to encourage the child to drink more fluids.

You can also devise an attractive "scorecard." Draw on a sheet of paper various sketches representing fluids: soda bottles, Popsicles, ice cream, gelatin, milk, and water. After the child drinks the fluid, he should color the appropriate symbol on his scorecard.

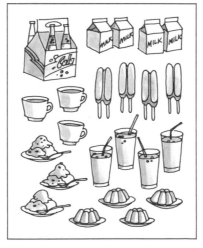

How about getting the patients to help you decorate their straws? Glue or tape name cards, pictures of happy faces, or animals onto the straws. With such an incentive,

children will be more interested in finishing their fluids. (See *Fluid intake: adults.*)

Fluorescein staining

How it works

Fluorescein staining of a patient's eye helps the doctor detect foreign bodies, corneal abrasions, or other corneal injuries.

Fluorescein dye, applied to the patient's palpebral conjunctiva, temporarily turns the sclera orange. Then, when the doctor shines a cobalt blue light on the eye, damaged epithelium shows up as bright green, indicating a corneal injury.

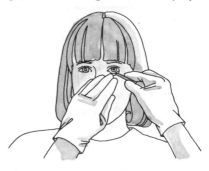

If you perform this procedure, always use fluorescein strips instead of drops, which can easily become contaminated with *Pseudomonas.* Insert the strips just above the patient's lower eyelid. Have your patient gently roll her eyes, with her lids closed, so the dye spreads over her cornea. After the examination, irrigate her eye with normal saline solution to remove the excess dye. (See also *Eye exam: external eye; Eye irrigation; Eye pain.*)

Foley catheter and bathing

Precautions

Most patients with indwelling catheters take showers rather than baths. But if for some reason, your

F

patient is unable to shower and must bathe, have him take the following precautions:

• Avoid traction on the catheter.

• Pass as much urine as possible from the tubing into the drainage bag before getting into the tub.

• Try to keep the drainage bag and tubing lower than the bladder to prevent backflow of urine into the tubing. A reflux valve will usually prevent this, but if a small amount of urine flows back from the bag into the tubing, this isn't likely to be a problem.

Foley catheter and leg bag

Securing the tube

A patient with an indwelling urinary catheter and leg bag may be hypersensitive to the tape that secures the tubing to his leg. So don't use tape—use a sanitary napkin belt instead.

Put some tape around the teeth of the belt's front hook and cut off the back hook. Tape the catheter tubing to the front hook, and the tubing will stay in place securely. (See also *Foley catheter fastening*.)

Foley catheter assessment

Checking patency

Imagine your patient has a Foley catheter. As you know, this frequently used tubing device is inserted into the patient's bladder to drain urine away from the body into a leg bag or a bedside collection device.

Patent catheter tubing is essential. Any obstruction of urine output—or of an externally introduced genitourinary irrigant—will increase the volume beyond the bladder's stretching capacity. If unchecked, the added volume will reflux into the ureters and, in turn, back up into the kidneys, possibly causing infection and damaging the kidneys.

Your main questions when assessing a Foley catheter should be: Is urine draining? If not, why? Is the catheter obstructed by its position or by sediment? Are the kidneys failing to produce urine?

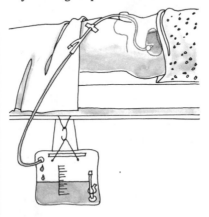

To answer these questions, you'd first check the catheter's position.

If the catheter should move downward, its drainage ports may come into the bladder neck area. In this position, the catheter may become wedged so firmly that it acts as a cork rather than as an open pathway for drainage.

Next, ask yourself: Could the ports be blocked with sediment or mucus? Irrigating with 20 ml of normal saline solution (per doctor's order) may correct this problem.

Roll the Foley catheter between your thumb and forefinger: Does the tube have a gritty, sandy feeling? If so, urine chemicals may be forming crystals at the tip of the catheter, and you should remove and replace the catheter.

If, after checking these variables, you instill the irrigant but it doesn't return, consider anuria. At this point, you should notify the patient's doctor, since you've already eliminated the readily correctable variables.

Foley catheter fastening

Securing one properly

It's important to secure a catheter to a patient's leg to avoid tension on the urethra. However, taping it to your patient's leg can irritate his skin. Your patient may need a catheter for an extended period of time, or he may be allergic to tape. So, use these improvisations for securing the catheter.

Wrap a long piece of Kling bandage around the patient's thigh. Be sure it's tight enough to stay up but loose enough to avoid constriction. Tape the bandage to itself and loop a rubber band around the catheter. Insert an open safety pin into the loop and attach the pin to the bandage.

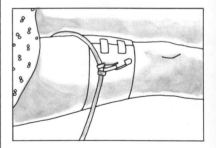

Another suggestion is to tie a long piece of umbilical tape or gauze to the balloon port of the catheter. Then tie the rest of the tape (or gauze) around the patient's thigh. With the catheter secured this way, the patient can move about freely without the discomfort of sticky tape on his skin.

Another solution is to take a long piece of gauze and wrap it once around the patient's thigh. Lay the tubing over the gauze, then wrap the rest of the gauze around his thigh over the tubing and tape the gauze to itself. Now the tubing is sandwiched between two layers of gauze. To be doubly sure the tubing is secure, tape it to the gauze. (See also *Foley catheter and leg bag.*)

Foley catheter problems

Some good solutions

Preventing kinks in Foley catheter tubing is a daily challenge, especially with restless patients. If the tubing kinks, the patient can develop urine reflux, leakage, or a urinary tract infection. Next time, try wrapping a coiled telephone cord

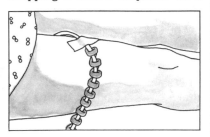

around the tubing. Even if the patient twists and turns, the tubing won't kink.

Foley catheter techniques

Preventing urinary tract infections

When a patient needs an indwelling catheter, try to protect him from infection. Here are some basic guidelines for safe catheter care.

First, consider the catheter's size. Many practitioners believe that the larger the catheter, the better. But that's not usually the case. As long as the urine is free of sediment, a #14 or #16 French catheter will do. Of course, a patient who develops clots or has heavy debris in his urine—a postoperative urologic patient, for instance—would need a larger catheter.

Some practitioners contend that if the catheter is too small, urine may bypass it. Actually, this problem can occur when the catheter is too large—and thus irritates the bladder, producing bladder spasms

that cause urine leakage. The practice of removing a catheter after urine has bypassed it and inserting a larger one simply perpetuates the problem. The large catheter causes more spasms, and leakage, and it may also dilate the urethra.

Before choosing an indwelling catheter, consider the patient's needs. Then, use the smallest catheter capable of doing the job.

For a patient with an indwelling catheter, the typical order at many institutions used to be "provide meatal care b.i.d." Frequently, this care included applying an antimicrobial ointment. The rationale was the ointment would stop bacteria from entering the bladder. But studies have shown that ointment doesn't significantly decrease the rate or urinary tract infections. In fact, covering the warm, moist environment of the meatus with ointment may actually promote bacterial growth.

You want to keep the meatus clean and free of incrustations and secretions. The best way to accomplish this is by having the patient practice good hygiene, especially after bowel movements. If he can take care of himself, that will reduce the risk of cross-infection because fewer people will be handling the catheter. If he can't take care of himself, wash around the catheter at the meatus and perineal area with soap and water, and towel it dry.

Provide meatal care once a day. The Centers for Disease Control doesn't endorse the practice of b.i.d. meatal care.

Maintain a closed drainage system. If you must open the system, use strict aseptic technique. Use a sterile needle and syringe to withdraw the specimen from the catheter. Keep the drainage bag below the base of the bladder to prevent reflux of urine back into the bladder. Change a catheter only if it's not patent, instead of at set intervals.

The only foolproof way to prevent a UTI, of course, is to simply avoid using an indwelling catheter when

possible. But when your patient needs one, follow the guidelines here to minimize the risk of infection. (See also *Foley catheter and bathing; Foley catheter assessment.*)

Fracture, hip

Assessing it

Different types of hip fractures can occur. The classic hip fracture is an extracapsular fracture, one outside the hip joint capsule, such as in the intertrochanteric region. The affected leg is shortened, bruised, adducted, externally rotated 90 degrees, and slightly flexed. And the patient feels pain in the hip.

With an intracapsular fracture, the joint capsule itself limits rotation to only 45 degrees. The upper thigh is more likely to be swollen than the area below it. With a displaced intracapsular fracture, the leg is shortened and externally rotated because of muscle spasm and displacement at the fracture site.

Not all patients with a fractured hip are in pain. A patient with an impacted intracapsular fracture is usually pain-free at first. He may even walk into the emergency department, having tolerated the fractured hip for days before increasing discomfort finally caused him to seek medical attention. He may have only a slight limp; the leg may not be shortened and may be properly aligned. Although the leg doesn't look deformed, he may have a knock-kneed deformity. And forcing his hip slightly into internal rotation will cause pain. This patient can lift his foot off the bed; the patient with a displaced fracture can't.

Subtrochanteric fractures are usually sustained by young patients during severe hip trauma. Whether open or closed, such a fracture causes extensive bleeding into soft tissue. The affected leg is shortened and may be rotated anteriorly and laterally. The line of pull and the strength of the hip and thigh muscles markedly displace bone fragments. The iliopsoas and other powerful short muscles pull on the neck of the femur fragment and flex and rotate the proximal fragment.

While examining the patient with a hip fracture, assess the neurovascular status of the entire leg below the injury. Check pulses, capillary refill time, skin color and temperature, and both sensory motor nerve functions. Note any edema. (See also *Fracture assessment; Neurologic exam: assessment.*)

Fracture assessment

Confirming your suspicions

If you suspect a patient has a fractured femur, hip, or pelvis, here's how to immediately confirm or refute it. This technique is especially helpful for nurses who work in nursing homes or on geriatric units and need to assess a patient immediately after a fall.

Place your stethoscope on the patient's symphysis pubis and percuss each patella with your finger or a pen. On the side of the fracture, you'll hear a sound lower in volume and pitch than you'll hear on the unaffected side. (The reason is simple: The break in the bone interferes with the sound's conduction and decreases its frequency.)

Likewise, you can detect a fractured humerus, clavicle, or scapula

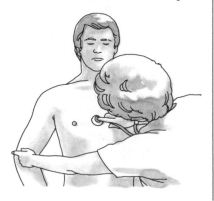

by placing your stethoscope on the patient's sternum and percussing both funny bones (the back of the elbows where the ulnar nerve rests against a prominence of the humerus). (See *Fracture care.*)

Fracture care

Emergency procedures

What do you do when you arrive at a scene and the victim has a bone protruding through the skin of his ankle? You learn he's fallen from rocks while rock climbing.

He's awake, alert, and in extreme pain. The wound is bleeding profusely. You know you must take swift action because if the bleeding isn't controlled, the man may become hypotensive, go into hypovolemic shock, and then cardiac arrest.

Have an assistant apply direct pressure to the wound with a clean cloth, while you quickly assess the victim's airway, breathing, and circulation, and check him for other injuries. Remember that because he's fallen, he may have suffered a neck or back injury.

Now concentrate on controlling the bleeding. If the open fracture makes it difficult to apply steady and direct pressure to the wound, press firmly on an arterial pressure point. The femoral artery is located one third of the way across the groin. To find it, feel for the underlying pulsation.

If direct, firm pressure on the femoral point for 10 to 15 minutes doesn't slow the bleeding, consider applying a tourniquet. If you *must* apply a tourniquet, apply it above the knee and closely monitor the leg's neurovascular status. Never apply a tourniquet below the knee; this can irreparably damage nerves and arteries. Remember, tourniquets are dangerous, even lethal, and should be used only as a last resort. (See *Tourniquets.*)

While applying pressure, assess the victim for signs and symptoms of shock: cold and clammy skin, dull eyes, dilated pupils, and weak pulses. If you detect these signs, you can improve the victim's circulation by elevating his feet (after splinting his injured leg). Cover the victim to conserve warmth, and make him as comfortable as possible. Reassure him that a doctor is coming.

Splinting the victim's injured leg should help ease his pain. By immobilizing the bone fragments, you'll also prevent further injury to the bone, soft tissue, nerves, and blood vessels.

Before splinting, protect the wound from contamination by covering it with clean gauze. All protruding material itself is contaminated, so don't try to place soft tissue or bone back into the wound. Besides risking contamination, this will produce unnecessary pain and could increase bleeding.

Next, gather baseline data on the leg's neurovascular status. Are pulses present, decreased, or absent? Is sensation present or absent, or does the victim report a tingling feeling?

Splint the entire lower leg, including the joints above and below the injury—in this case, the knee and ankle joints. When you're done, reassess the leg's neurovascular status, comparing your findings with the baseline data.

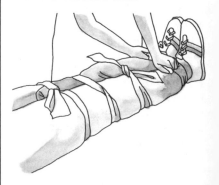

Remember that a splint applied too tightly can produce a tourniquet effect. Check the leg periodically to make sure circulation isn't restricted.

Continue to reassure the victim and reassess his vital signs and the leg's status until the doctor arrives. When he does, give a full report of the accident, your interventions, and your assessment of the victim's current condition. (See *Fracture assessment.*)

Frostbite

Patient care

Begin thawing the patient's frostbitten area *immediately* and *rapidly*—most cellular damage occurs during the freezing and thawing processes, so you want to avoid slow thawing.

Immerse the frostbitten part in a warm water bath (100° to 108° F. [37.7° to 42.2° C.]), preferably with a whirlpool. (If your patient's face or ears are affected, pour warm water over the area or apply warm, moist soaks. Change soaks frequently to maintain the desired temperature.) Handle the affected part gently, and protect it from friction and pressure. *Don't massage it*—this can cause tissue damage. If the patient's clothes are frozen to the area, don't try to remove them until after the area's thawed.

Your patient will experience considerable pain as the affected area thaws. Expect to administer an analgesic and a sedative, such as intramuscular or I.V. morphine or meperidine (Demerol), as ordered.

As the area thaws, a pink flush will appear and (on an extremity) will progress distally until the area's flushed to the tip. Keep the area immersed until the area is flushed, is warm to your touch, blanches when you press it, and stays flushed when you remove it from the water bath. Don't apply any dressings to the area. If the patient's fingers or toes are affected, place sterile cotton between the digits to minimize friction. Check the color of the flush

after you rewarm the area, because it may help indicate the severity of the injury: it may be mottled blue or purple if your patient has superficial frostbite, and blue, violet, or gray if he has deep frostbite. If his frostbite is extremely severe, the affected area may remain gray and cold even after it's completely thawed, and won't regain function.

Check your patient's neurovascular status as soon as the affected area's completely thawed. The area may appear transiently cyanotic, but this should disappear unless the patient has an underlying injury (such as a fracture or sprain) or severe frostbite. You should be able to feel pulses in the affected area—if they're weak or absent, this may indicate thrombus formation. Report your findings to the doctor *immediately*—he may ask you to give low-molecular-weight dextran I.V. to reverse intravascular red blood cell aggregation and to improve microcirculation.

Expect to give tetanus prophlaxis, as ordered.

Fundal height

Measuring it

You usually measure a pregnant woman's fundal height to estimate the number of weeks of gestation. The fundus reaches the umbilicus at 20 weeks' gestation, and from then on the number of centimeters of fundal height roughly equals the number of weeks of gestation.

Before the procedure have your patient empty her bladder. Help her lie on her back. If her condition permits, elevate her head and knees to relax her abdominal muscles.

During the procedure place your hands along her sides and move them toward her head, gently pressing on the abdomen until you've located the fundus. Draw a line with a ballpoint pen, marking the tip of the fundus. Measure the distance

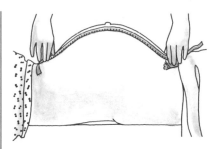

from the top of the symphysis pubis to the top of the fundus. This is the fundal height.

Gavage, antacid

Proper procedure

Antacid gavages are usually prescribed to maintain the patient's gastric pH level at 4.5 or higher (normal is 1.1 to 2.4). The antacids most often prescribed are Amphojel, Maalox, Mylanta, and Riopan. The usual dose is 60 to 90 ml, instilled through a nasogastric (NG) tube. (See *Medication, nasogastric.*) You'll clamp the tube for 15 to 20 minutes, then aspirate the stomach contents and recheck the gastric pH. If it's below the desired level, repeat the gavage. For some patients, the doctor may increase the amount of antacid to be instilled to maintain gastric pH at a neutral level (7.0 to 7.5).

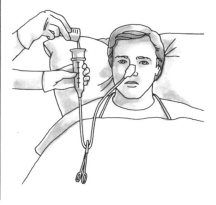

Once you achieve the desired level, you can decrease the frequency of the gavages, repeating the procedure every 60 minutes or as necessary. Raise the head of the bed at least 30 degrees to prevent gastric reflux, since aspiration of antacids can cause serious pulmonary complications.

Some doctors might order the NG tube attached to low intermittent suction after GI bleeding has been controlled and antacid gavage discontinued. Others, believing the tube itself is an irritant and possible cause of GI bleeding, might want the tube removed. So, check the doctor's orders before proceeding.

If the NG tube remains inserted, your responsibilites include checking the tube frequently for patency and recording the patient's hourly intake and output. Record any fluids or antacids instilled through the tube as part of the patient's intake; any fluids or antacids aspirated through the tube as output. Observe the aspirate carefully and notify the doctor immediately if bleeding recurs. (See also *Nasogastric tube: patient care.*)

GI bleeding

Keeping your patient comfortable

The patient with GI bleeding will need his gown and bedsheets changed frequently. If the patient has melena or hematochezia, administer scrupulous skin care. This would include applying an ointment that's not water-soluble (such as Desitin or A and D Ointment) to the perianal area.

A room deodorizer will help mask the foul odor of blood mixed with gastric fluid or stool. Here's a tip: Put a few drops of peppermint oil on a gauze pad and leave it in the patient's room.

Blood irritates the oral mucosa as well as the skin, so all patients with upper GI bleeding, even those without a nasogastric (NG) tube,

require meticulous oral hygiene. Help the patient brush his teeth and have him use mouthwash to remove blood or debris from his mouth and to stimulate salivation.

If the patient has a NG tube, tape it so it doesn't exert pressure on his nares. Use an anesthetic spray or offer the patient lozenges to alleviate soreness in the back of his throat caused by the tube. (See *Nasogastric tube: fastening; Nasogastric tube: patient care.*)

Arrange your care so the patient has plenty of time to rest between nursing procedures. This will help him relax, both physically and mentally. Besides the stressful factors that may have contributed to his GI bleeding, he has even more to worry about now: fear of death, separation from family and friends, feelings of guilt, and so forth. Use your time in the patient's room to encourage him to express his concerns. Listen attentively and provide emotional support.

Glasgow Coma Scale

Using it to assess level of consciousness

Use this scale when checking your patient's consciousness. Add up the response from each of the three categories. The lower the numbers, the lower the level of consciousness. The total will range from 3 to 15. A score of 7 or less indicates coma.
- *Best eye-opening response*
  —Purposeful and spontaneous: 4
  —To voice: 3
  —To pain: 2
  —No response: 1
  —Untestable: U
- *Best verbal response*
  —Oriented: 5
  —Disoriented: 4
  —Inappropriate words: 3
  —Incomprehensible sounds: 2
  —No response: 1
  —Untestable: U

- *Best motor response*
  —Obeys commands: 6
  —Localizes pain: 5
  —Withdraws to pain: 4
  —Flexion to pain: 3
  —Extension to pain: 2
  —No response: 1
  —Untestable: U

Glaucoma

Assessment and intervention

Once acute closed-angle glaucoma has been diagnosed, the first medical priority is to reduce the patient's intraocular pressure (IOP). The doctor will order topical therapy first—timolol (Timoptic) and miotic eye drops. Once you've administered these medications, you'll probably start an I.V. line to administer a carbonic anhydrase inhibitor or a hyperosmotic agent. This medication will decrease formation of aqueous humor and so decrease the patient's IOP.

Assess the patient's vital signs; then, to relieve his pain, expect to administer analgesics, such as Demerol (meperidine) or morphine sulphate intramuscularly. If the patient's pain persists, continue to administer analgesics as ordered. To control the patient's nausea and vomiting, the doctor may ask you to administer an antiemetic, such as prochlorperazine or trimethobenzamide hydrochloride, by suppository or intramuscularly. Provide continuous emotional support because your patient's impaired vision and pain will make him anxious and frightened.

As the patient's IOP falls, his peripheral vision and visual acuity should progressively improve. Check your patient's vision periodically. The doctor will also monitor the patient's IOP, adjusting the amount and frequency of his medication accordingly.

Although some of the drugs the patient receives will increase his thirst, give the patient nothing by mouth. This is because he may need surgery. To provide some relief, periodically let him suck on a water-moistened gauze sponge.

Remember, the patient's depth perception is distorted, so he's vulnerable to injury. Keep the side rails of his bed up all times and explain the need for this precaution. (See *Visually impaired patients.*)

Glucose monitoring

Effective techniques

Blood or urine glucose testing monitors glucose levels in the patient with diabetes mellitus. Blood glucose tests, considered more reliable than urine tests, include reagent strips, glucose meters, and glycohemoglobin tests.

Reagent strips used to determine blood glucose levels include the Chemstrip bG and Visidex. To use a reagent strip, the patient draws a blood droplet—usually by fingertip puncture with a manual device such as the Monolet lancet or a mechanical device such as the Autolet, the Hemalet, the Penlet, or the Monojector. Tell the patient to follow the package instructions carefully.

Reagent strip monitoring

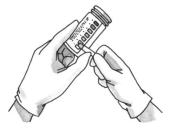

The glucose meter, such as the Glucometer II, Glucoscan II, or Accu-Chek bG, offers more precise blood glucose measurement than the patient can get with visual testing. However, it's more expensive. Before using a meter, the patient may need to complete its calibration and control procedures. Calibration checks only the meter's accuracy. The control procedure checks the accuracy of the entire system: the meter, reagent strips, and the user's technique (timing, flushing, and strip blotting). Instruct the patient to follow the manufacturer's instructions.

Glucose meter monitoring

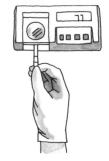

Urine glucose tests include Clinitest tablets, reagent strips, and paper tape. Clinitest tablets detect glycosuria. If your patient's using these tablets, tell him to follow these important guidelines:
• Use only freshly voided urine.
• Place 2 or 5 urine drops (or as indicated) and 10 water drops in a clean test tube, then add 1 Clinitest tablet. (Use only fresh whole tablets that dissolve completely and always use the Clinitest dropper.)
• Don't shake the tube during the reaction.
• About 15 seconds after the reaction stops, compare urine color to the proper color chart.

Because the Clinitest depends on copper reduction of sugars (including glucose), other urine sugars can cause false-positive results. So can large doses of vitamin C or aspirin (more than six tablets daily), and use of such drugs as sulfisoxazole, levodopa, probenecid, and isoniazid. Cephalosporins may cause color reactions that make Clinitest results difficult to read.

Reagent strips and paper tape methods include such tests as Diastix, Keto-Diastix, Clinistix, and Tes-Tape. These tests—specific for glucose—show urine glucose-oxidase reactions. If your patient's using either type, tell him to dip the strip or paper tape quickly in and out of urine, then hold it in the air to read

it. Use of ascorbic acid, phenazopyridine, salicylates, and levodopa can alter test results.

Good Samaritan acts

How they protect you

Never has a nurse been found liable for negligence while giving emergency care at the scene of an accident. Good Samaritan statutes in nearly every state and province encourage doctors and nurses to offer emergency aid by relieving them from liability in such situations.

Although the Good Samaritan laws vary, most provide immunity from liability if you:
• give the care during an emergency
• act in good faith without knowingly or intentionally harming the victim
• give care without expecting payment for your interventions
• have no special obligation (such as a lifeguard or a policeman would) to help the victim.

Gowers' sign

Checking for it

To check for Gowers' sign, place the patient supine and ask him to rise. A positive Gowers' sign—an inability to lift the trunk without using the hands and arms to brace and push—

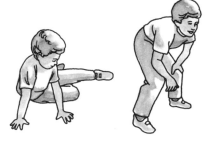

indicates pelvic muscle weakness, as occurs in muscular dystrophy and spinal muscle atrophy.

Graves' disease

Teaching about treatment and restrictions

Instruct your patient to restrict physical activity, because exertion will only increase his metabolic rate and exacerbate his irritability. Encourage him to switch to activities that require minimal physical exertion—reading, for example—and to rest frequently. Reassure him that he'll be able to resume his customary activities when his metabolic rate returns to normal.

Urge following the prescribed diet to prevent nutritional deficiencies. Advise him to eat well-balanced meals each day, plus snacks, so that his caloric intake can keep up with the rapid expenditure of calories caused by hypermetabolism. (Once he's regained the weight he lost, he should cut his caloric intake back to normal.) Caution him to avoid caffeine, yellow and red food dyes, and artificial preservatives because these substances will make him more irritable. If necessary, arrange for nutritional counseling.

Teach the patient about thyroid hormone antagonists if they're prescribed. Also provide instructions about other prescribed drugs, such as propranolol, to control cardiac effects and tranquilizers to control irritability and hyperactivity. Warn against taking aspirin and any aspirin-containing drugs, because they increase the metabolic rate.

Advise your patient and his family to avoid stressful situations. Environmental stimulation should be kept to a minimum. For example, he should avoid watching television programs or movies that may cause him to become excited or upset. Reassure him and his family that behavioral changes, such as irritability, anxiety, lack of concentration, and fatigue, are related to hyperthyroidism and will subside with treatment.

If ophthalmopathy is present, teach the essentials of good eye care, and advise the patient to wear sunglasses and avoid irritating his eyes. If eyedrops are ordered, show him how to instill them. (See *Eyedrops: patient teaching.*) Instruct him to limit his fluid and salt intake to minimize fluid retention, which would make his eyeballs protrude even farther.

Suggest that he sleep with his head elevated to aid drainage, thereby preventing fluid from accumulating behind his eyes. Tell him to notify his doctor at once if visual changes, such as blurring, occur. Urge him to see an ophthalmologist regularly. (See also *Thyroid crisis.*)

Grief

Helping the family adjust to sudden illness

First, understand that family members will have different needs at different stages. For example, first they'll require:
• basic medical information about the patient's illness and condition
• emotional support to help them realize, and cope with, the seriousness of the illness
• help with putting what they see and hear in perspective.

Then as the illness progresses, they'll need:
• more specific information about the patient's condition
• reassurance that the staff really cares about the patient.

If the patient dies, they'll need:
• help with adjusting to *that* reality
• reassurance that the staff really cares about *them*.

When you meet the family, encourage them to express their anxieties and fears. Give emotional support and promise information. Assess their perception of the reality of his illness. Give hope while stressing the seriousness of the patient's illness.

As you can imagine, not being able to see the patient adds to the family members' fear and interferes with their ability to accept and cope with changes in his condition. During this waiting period, you can provide information and reassurance by:
• giving continuing emotional support
• giving frequent updates on the patient's condition
• giving the family members a feeling of control by offering to let them make any available choices and offering to take messages to the patient
• mobilizing support systems that have helped the family through previous crises.

As eager as they are to see the patient, family members will be frightened. Ease their fears by describing, before their first visit, what they can expect to see and experience there.

After the visit, the family members are likely to need even more emotional support, because they're beginning to understand how close to death their loved one is. Offer support by sitting quietly with them, indicating your understanding of their feelings, and—if they welcome it—by touching them.

In the days following a patient's admission, try to be there during visiting hours to give the family members frequent updates and to ask how they're doing. If the patient's condition deteriorates, the family typically asks for support to face the likely outcome. (See *Communication: family; Death; Death: child.*)

Hallucinations

When your patient experiences them

Several conditions can cause hallucinations: local disease of a sensory organ, mental or emotional exhaustion, certain drugs and poisons, and psychotic illnesses. Hallucinations can also arise from anxieties and unmet psychological needs. Here are several things you should listen for when dealing with a hallucinating patient:

• the content of the hallucination
• how real or vivid the hallucination seems to the patient
• its association with emotions, ideas, or feelings
• when it occurs, how frequently, and whether others are present
• whether it's related to sleep
• how much the patient recognizes that the hallucination isn't real
• how much the hallucination affects the patient's judgment
• how the patient responds to the hallucination—for example, by harming himself or others.

Caring for a patient who's hallucinating involves these interventions:

• Establish contact with reality by stating your name.
• Acknowledge that the patient is having a hallucination and state that you're not experiencing it.
• Explore the hallucination with the patient.
• Don't challenge the hallucination as unreal or inconsistent.
• Don't leave the patient alone during or just after a hallucination; sometimes just your presence can dissipate it.
• Keep the patient occupied with reality.
• Foster the patient's trust in you and the staff.

Here are some additional tips:

• Interrupt auditory hallucinations by getting the patient to look at you and talk to you.
• If the hallucination's tactile (for example, crawling insects or a burning sensation), touch the patient, but *tell him first that you're going to touch him.* If he has a crawling sensation, use a firm touch. If he has a burning sensation, use a gentle touch and tell him your hands are cool.
• If possible, put the patient in a room with one or more other patients.
• Avoid giving him unnecessary sleep medications. (See *Delusions; Illusions; Psychotic patients.*)

Halo vests

Managing traction

Halo vest traction is a type of skeletal traction used to immobilize the patient's head and neck after cervical spine injury. It allows greater mobility than skull tongs and carries less risk of infection.

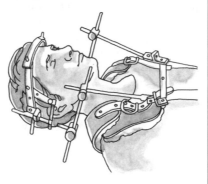

Here's how to care for your patient:

• Reassure him and explain the procedure to him.
• Assess his neurologic signs, as ordered, with particular emphasis on his motor function.
• Notify the doctor immediately if the patient experiences decreased sensation or increased loss of motor function; this may indicate spinal cord trauma.
• Check the pin sites and use cleansing procedures, as ordered. (See *Pin care.*)
• Obtain an order for an analgesic if your patient complains of headache after the doctor retightens the pins.
• Never lift the patient using the device's bars. (See *Shampooing: patient with halo vest; Traction patients.*)

Hamman's sign

Testing procedure

To test for Hamman's sign, help the patient assume a left-lateral recumbent position. Then, place your stethoscope over the precordium. If

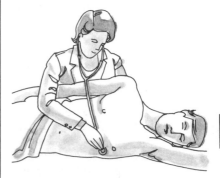

you hear a loud crunching sound that synchronizes with his heartbeat, the patient has a positive Hamman's sign. Depending on which organ is ruptured, be prepared to assist with endotracheal intubation, emergency tracheotomy, or chest tube insertion. Immediately start administering supplemental oxygen. Start an I.V. to administer fluids and medication, and connect the patient to a cardiac monitor. (See also *Chest tube insertion; Endotracheal tube: insertion.*)

Head injury

Nursing role in closed injuries

Don't move the patient. Assume that he has a spinal injury until you can rule it out. Immobilize his head and neck. Ask someone to call for an ambulance. Taking care not to hyperextend his neck, make sure he has an open airway; do a jaw-thrust maneuver to keep his tongue from obstructing his airway. Be prepared to start CPR if necessary.

Continually assess his respiratory rate, the quality of his peripheral pulses, pupil responses, and level of consciousness. Look for

H

signs of cerebral hemorrhage, such as blood or a clear, odorless fluid coming from his ears and nose. (See *Cerebrospinal fluid.*) Try to orient him if he regains consciousness, and tell him to stay still. If he's combative, ask his friends to hold him down.

Examine his skull for abrasions or swelling. Talk to him as you assess him. If he's unconscious, remind others around you that he might hear what's being said.

To check for fractures, inspect his arms and legs. Feel for misaligned bones and crepitus (listen for crepitus, too). Try to move him as little as possible to prevent further trauma. (See *Fracture assessment.*)

After you've assessed his condition, gather other pertinent data. Ask his friends or family members about his medical history and allergies, and ask if he's taking any medications or been using drugs or alcohol. Find out when he last ate. You'll need to give emergency personnel a complete report of how events progressed.

Later, after the ambulance arrives, give emergency personnel a concise report of the injury, your assessment findings, and the progression of events until the ambulance arrived. Assist emergency personnel as they place a cervical brace around his neck and get him onto a spinal board. (See *Head trauma: postop care; Head trauma care.*)

Head trauma: postop care

Nursing responsibilities

After surgery, the head trauma patient will probably receive diazepam (Valium) and pancuronium bromide (Pavulon) to control his posturing and occasional spontaneous rapid respirations. (See *Pancuronium therapy.*) Both reactions can elevate intracranial pressure (ICP) by increasing metabolic de-

mands, oxygen consumption, and cerebral blood flow. If the patient develops a fever, which will increase ICP, respond promptly by using a hypothermia blanket to bring down his temperature. Also administer broad-spectrum antibiotics prophylactically. (See *Intracranial pressure: care.*)

Once the patient's arterial blood gas measurements have stabilized within normal limits, wean him from the ventilator and extubate him. Suctioning and chest physiotherapy will remove large amounts of tracheobronchial secretions. A tracheotomy may be performed.

Nutrition is another concern. Start the patient on total parenteral nutrition (TPN) and lipids within a few days of admission. Use a Dobbhoff nasogastric tube to deliver supplemental feedings. (See *Feeding tubes: complications; TPN: administration.*)

If the patient's lungs become congested, suction him two times per shift and change his position frequently. A productive cough will help remove secretions.

When he can be taken off TPN and lipids, add more water to the feeding solution to ensure adequate fluid intake. Also add Propac, a protein supplement, to provide additional calories. Physical therapy will be started sometime during the recovery phase.

About a month after admission, the patient may enter the agitated phase of recovery from head injury. To make sure he doesn't hurt himself or anyone else, pad the side rails of his bed, use soft wrist restraints, and orient the patient frequently to his environment.

The combined efforts of the speech therapist and the nursing staff will result in a significant improvement in the patient's ability to swallow. At this time, decrease tube feedings during the night. You will also need to work with the patient on bowel and bladder control. Administer the laxative bisacodyl (Dulcolax), as needed, during the evenings. Remove the Foley cathe-

ter and replace it with an external catheter.

Head trauma care

Managing a patient with a subdural hematoma

When a head trauma patient arrives in the ED, contact other departments—respiratory therapy, X-ray, CT scanning, and surgery—to prepare for his arrival. The doctor will notify a neurosurgeon.

Subdural hematoma

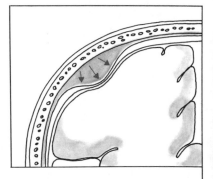

Assess the patient's airway, breathing, and circulation. A respiratory therapist may be needed to maintain a patent airway and to promote adequate oxygenation (this helps decrease his intracranial pressure).

The ED doctor may insert an endotracheal tube to further stabilize the patient's respiratory status. A chest X-ray will confirm that the tube has been placed correctly.

Using both cardiac and blood pressure monitors, assess the patient's vital signs continuously. Watch for Cushing's triad—decreased heart rate, increased blood pressure, and widened pulse pressure.

Start two large-bore I.V. lines immediately to administer fluids and medications. Avoid using D_5W or lactated Ringer's solution because the free water in these solutions will exacerbate cerebral edema in head trauma. To counteract cerebral edema, administer mannitol, an osmotic diuretic. Then insert an indwelling (Foley) catheter so that intake and output can be closely monitored and the patient's renal function assessed continuously. (See *Head injury; Head trauma: postop care.*)

Hearing tests

Evaluating your patient's hearing loss

The Weber and Rinne tests can help determine if your patient's hearing loss is conductive or sensorineural. The Weber test evaluates bone conduction; the Rinne test, bone and air conduction. Using a 512 Hz tuning fork, perform these preliminary tests as described below:

Weber test. Place the base of a vibrating tuning fork firmly against the midline of the patient's skull at the forehead. Ask him if he hears the tone equally well in both ears. If he does, the Weber test is graded midline—a normal finding. In an abnormal Weber test (graded right or left), sound is louder in one ear, suggesting a conductive hearing loss in that ear or a sensorineural loss in the opposite ear.

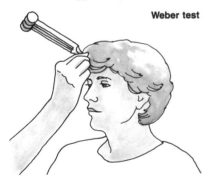

Weber test

Rinne test. Hold the base of a vibrating tuning fork against the patient's mastoid process until he can no longer hear the sound to test bone conduction. Then quickly move the vibrating fork in front of his ear canal to test air conduction. Ask him to tell you which location has the louder or longer sound. Repeat the procedure for the other ear. The normal finding is that air con-

Rinne test

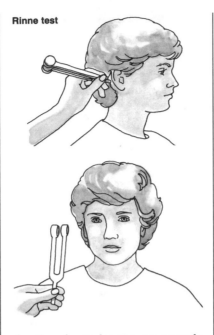

duction lasts longer or sounds louder than bone conduction. In an abnormal finding, bone conduction lasts longer or sounds louder than air conduction.

Heart exam: auscultation

Normal findings

Sounds from the *mitral valve* are heard best at the fifth intercostal space at the midclavicular line. Sounds from the *tricuspid valve* are heard best at the fourth or fifth intercostal space at the left sternal border. Sounds from the *aortic valve* are heard best at the second intercostal space at the right sternal border. Sounds from the *pulmonic valve*

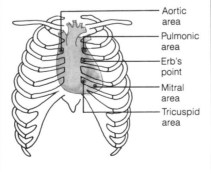

- Aortic area
- Pulmonic area
- Erb's point
- Mitral area
- Tricuspid area

are heard best at the second intercostal space at the left sternal border.

Listen for S_1 (the "lub" of "lub-dub") at the mitral area because the mitral valve makes a louder sound than the tricuspid valve. At the mitral area, the "lub" is lower-pitched, longer, and duller than the "dub."

Listen for S_2 (the "dub" of "lub-dub") at the aortic area because the aortic valve (on the left side) makes a louder sound than the pulmonic valve (on the right side). At the aortic area, S_2 is louder than S_1; at any site, S_2 is higher-pitched, shorter, and snappier than S_1.

A normal split S_1 is best heard at the triscuid area, where the weaker component of the tricupsid sound is loudest. Listen for "T-lub-dub."

A normal split S_2 is best heard at the pulmonic area, where the weaker component of the pulmonic sound is loudest. Listen for "lub-T-dub." The normal split S_2 becomes louder during inspiration and disappears during expiration. (See *Heart exam: palpation; Heart sounds: abnormalities; Heart sounds: diagnosis.*)

Heart exam: palpation

Palpating the four valve areas

Begin by making sure the patient is lying on his back, with the head of his bed raised 30 to 45 degrees. This is a good position, especially for the patient who's had a myocardial infarction, because it eases the work load on his heart.

When palpating the four valve areas, follow any sequence you like. But to ensure consistency, use the same sequence for palpation and auscultation.

The mitral valve area is also the point of maximal impulse. It should be ½″ to ¾″ (1 to 2 cm) in diameter, or roughly the size of a quarter. Using your palm, palpate this area for thrills—palpable murmurs that indicate turbulent blood flow. If you've ever put your hand on a purring cat, you know just what a thrill feels like. Next, use your finger pads to palpate the mitral valve area for pulsations, which feel similar to a bounding pulse. This finding may indicate increased blood volume or pressure.

Move on to the other three valve areas, palpating in the same manner. At each stop, use your palms to feel for thrills, then use your finger pads to feel for pulsations.

Heart sounds: abnormalities

Detection guidelines

Listen for the extra heart sounds, S_3 and S_4. An S_3 gallop is one of the earliest signs of left ventricular failure. It occurs early in diastole, immediately after S_2, during rapid ventricular filling. (It sounds like "Ken-tuck-y," with the first two syllables being S_1 and S_2.) In heart failure, blood rushes through the open atrioventricular valve into the damaged ventricle and strikes a distended, incompetent wall, creating the S_3 sound. (Remember, though, that an S_3 may be normal in children and young adults.)

The atrial gallop, S_4, occurs during the late diastolic phase when the atria contract to force their blood into the ventricles, so you'll always hear it before S_1. It sounds like "Tennes-see," with the second and third syllables representing S_1 and S_2.

This extra heart sound inevitably means that one ventricle or the other is distended. Yet that distention may not mean ventricular failure, because S_4 also may occur after a myocardial infarction or in hypertension, coronary artery disease, cardiomyopathy, or aortic stenosis. (See also *Heart exam: auscultation; Heart sounds: diagnosis.*)

Heart sounds: diagnosis

Distinguishing friction rub from murmur

Is the sound you hear a pericardial friction rub or a murmur? The classic pericardial friction rub has three sound components, which are related to the phases of the cardiac cycle. In some patients, however, the rub's presystolic and early diastolic sounds may be inaudible, causing it to resemble the murmur of mitral insufficiency or aortic stenosis and regurgitation.

If you don't detect the classic three-component sounds, you can distinguish a pericardial friction rub from a murmur by auscultating again and asking yourself these questions:
• *How deep is the sound?* A pericardial friction rub usually sounds superficial; a murmur sounds deeper in the chest.
• *Does the sound radiate?* A pericardial friction rub usually doesn't radiate; a murmur may radiate widely.
• *Does the sound vary with inspiration or change in patient position?* A pericardial friction rub is usually loudest during inspiration and is best heard when the patient leans forward. A murmur varies in timing and duration with both factors. (See *Heart exam: auscultation; Heart sounds: abnormalities.*)

Heart exhaustion: cooling

What complications to look for

Your patient may start shivering violently after you initiate cooling measures. Take steps to control this (as ordered) because shivering increases your patient's metabolic rate and heat production. Watch his cardiac monitor to detect shivering. If he starts to shiver, anticipate giving chlorpromazine (Thorazine) I.V., which decreases shivering and metabolic oxygen consumption and dilates cutaneous blood vessels. (Use chlorpromazine with caution and monitor your patient's blood pressure carefully because the drug may cause a marked decrease in your patient's blood pressure.) Or the doctor may ask you to give barbiturates. These drugs have effects similar to chlorpromazine's, but keep in mind that they may mask your patient's neurologic status. If the patient's shivering is severe, the doctor may give him sodium thiopental.

Your patient's uncontrolled shivering may progress to frank seizures. If this occurs, expect to administer I.V. diazepam (Valium) or phenobarbital. Although you might expect the doctor to order phenytoin sodium (Dilantin) because it's commonly used to control seizures, in this situation he probably won't. It's been reported ineffective in patients with heat-related illnesses.

Check your patient's fluid status once cooling is underway. If you haven't already done so, draw blood for laboratory tests to determine the degree of his dehydration. His blood urea nitrogren, hematocrit, serum sodium, and serum protein levels will probably be elevated. The doctor will probably insert a central venous pressure line to assess the patient's hydration status and heart function and to allow rapid fluid administration. (If the patient is severely hypotensive, the doctor may insert a Swan-Ganz catheter instead.) Expect to insert an indwelling (Foley) catheter and to administer I.V. fluids rapidly. (See *Foley catheter fastening.*) The doctor will probably order normal saline solution, one-half strength normal saline solution, or dextrose 5% in one-half strength normal saline solution—depending on the results of your patient's laboratory tests. (See *Heat exhaustion: management.*)

Heat exhaustion: management

Nursing priorities

Initially, you may not be able to tell whether your patient has heat exhaustion or heat stroke. Signs and symptoms of both often overlap, and sometimes only frank central nervous system disturbances and grossly elevated AST (SGOT), LDH, and CPK values in heat stroke distinguish the two disorders. But you won't have the results of laboratory tests immediately, and you may not even have time to draw blood. So start rapid cooling and fluid replacement if you have any reason to suspect heat stroke.

Insert a rectal thermistor probe to monitor your patient's temperature (glass thermometers are dangerous if your patient develops seizures, and they're not usually adequate for measuring extremely elevated temperatures). If a thermometer's all that's available, measure the patient's rectal temperature every 5 to 10 minutes.

Continue surface cooling measures, as ordered:
• Cover the naked patient with sheets or towels soaked with a slurry of ice chips and water. Change them frequently to maintain the cooling effect.
• Apply ice packs to areas of maximum heat transfer (axillae and inguinal areas) or apply a hypothermia blanket to his thorax. These

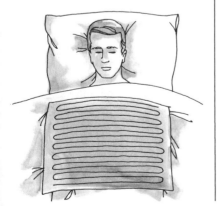

provide cooling while avoiding cutaneous vasoconstriction.
• Spray the patient's body with warm water and then direct *dry* air over him with a fan, which maximizes evaporative cooling. (If air in the treatment area is humid, this method won't work as well.) If you use this method, make sure you provide a *rapid* air flow.

While you provide surface cooling measures, massage your patient as necessary to reduce the cutaneous vasoconstriction that may occur if his skin temperature drops below 82.4° F. (28° C.) Keep in mind that maximimum vaporization depends on a high skin-to-air temperature gradient as well as an adequate cutaneous blood flow.

Besides these surface cooling measures, the doctor may also ask you to give cold I.V. fluids and cold enemas, and he may start a cold gastric or peritoneal lavage. These methods provide only a small fraction of the cooling necessary, but they may be useful if your patient's temperature is extremely elevated and he doesn't respond quickly to surface cooling measures. (See *Heat exhaustion: cooling.*)

Hemoptysis

What to do when it occurs

If your patient coughs up copious amounts of blood, prepare to assist with endotracheal intubation and suction the patient frequently to remove blood. (See *Endotracheal tube: insertion.*) Remember, massive hemoptysis can cause airway obstruction and asphyxiation. Insert an I.V. line to allow for fluid replacement, drug administration, and blood transfusion, if needed. Also be prepared to assist with emergency bronchoscopy to identify the bleeding site. Monitor blood pressure and pulse to detect hypotension and tachycardia, and draw an arterial blood gas sample for laboratory analysis to monitor respiratory status.

After taking a brief history, take the patient's vital signs and examine his nose, mouth, and pharynx for sources of bleeding. Inspect the configuration of his chest and look for abnormal movement during breathing, use of accessory muscles, or retractions. Observe his respiratory rate, depth, and rhythm. Finally, examine his skin for lesions.

Next, perform a heart exam, auscultating for heart murmurs, bruits, and pleural friction rubs. (See *Heart sounds: abnormalities; Heart sounds: diagnosis.*)

Obtain a sputum sample and examine it for overall quantity, for the amount of blood it contains, and for its color, odor, and consistency.

Hemorrhage, postpartum

Emergency intervention

Suppose your postpartum patient begins to bleed uncontrollably. If you don't act quickly to stop the bleeding, she may become hypovolemic, which could lead to shock and, ultimately, cardiac arrest. So take the following actions:

Lower the head of your patient's bed. Call another nurse and ask her to contact the doctor. Continue monitoring the patient's vital signs (at least once every 15 minutes) and massage her fundus to try to control the bleeding. If her fundus starts to firm up, stop massaging. Check her every 15 minutes for the first hour, then every 30 to 60 minutes for 2 to 3 hours after the first hour, depending on the severity of bleeding and the firmness of her fundus. (See *Uterus, postpartum.*)

Palpate her abdomen for a distended bladder, which could interfere with uterine contractions. If her bladder is full, ask the other nurse to catheterize her. (See *Bladder assessment.*)

Your patient will require fluids, medication, or blood to increase her circulating volume. If she came to

H

the postpartum unit with an I.V., simply increase the infusion rate to compensate for her decreased blood volume. Otherwise, insert a large-bore (18-gauge) angiocatheter and start an infusion of normal saline solution with oxytocin (Pitocin) to stimulate uterine contractions.

You should have a standing order to add 20 units (two ampules) of Pitocin to 1,000 ml of normal saline solution for a 20 milliunits/ml solution. Administer the drug at 20 to 40 milliunits/minute, as needed.

Draw blood for a complete blood count and possible typing and cross matching (if she needs blood). Calmly explain your actions and concerns to your patient.

If you can't control the bleeding, the doctor may decide to do a dilation and curettage to remove placental fragments. As you prepare your patient for surgery, continue to monitor her vital signs, fundus, and bleeding.

Heparin injection

Reducing pain

To reduce pain, irritation, and ecchymosis at the site of a subcutaneous heparin injection, place an ice pack on the injection site for 3 to 5 minutes before and after the injection. This will help most patients.

Hernia, hiatal

Medical management

For a hiatal hernia patient with little or no esophagitis and minimal symptoms, medical management would be preferable to surgery. Medical management includes frequent small, bland feedings; avoidance of caffeine, alcohol, spices, and smoking—all of which stimulate gastric acid; and ingestion of antacids (for example, Gelusil or Maalox) 45 to 60 minutes after meals

and at bedtime. Obese patients need weight reduction along with low-fat intake. Avoiding constipation is necessary because straining intensifies intra-abdominal pressure. Tight clothing also increases intra-abdominal pressure; so does lifting objects by bending at the hips (rather than at the knees).

A hiatal hernia patient should elevate the head of his bed on 6″ (15 cm) blocks to minimize regurgitation of stomach contents and to prevent their aspiration. And he shouldn't lie down for several hours after eating, to give food time to pass out of the stomach. Metoclopramide (Reglan, Maxeran), 10 mg given three times a day and at bedtime, enhances pressure in the lower esophageal sphincter and hastens gastric emptying.

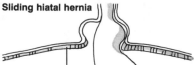

Sliding hiatal hernia

Diaphragm

Stomach

All these measures may adequately control symptoms of hiatal hernia. But other patients need surgery: those with moderate to severe esophagitis, for example, with or without peptic stricture; those who suffer frequent aspiration of gastric reflux; those whose hernias are associated with scleroderma; and those for whom medical management fails to control symptoms.

HHNK

What to do

Because the patient with hyperglycemic hyperosmolar nonketotic coma (HHNK) sometimes has a blood glucose level as high as 2,800 mg/dl, he can become more dehydrated than the patient with dia-

betic ketoacidosis (DKA). But usually there's little or no ketosis, and no acidosis.

In HHNK, dehydration from osmotic diuresis can become so severe that you can lift up the patient's skin from his forehead. With dehydration posing the worst threat to the untreated DKA patient, you can imagine how much more severe its penalties could be for the even more dehydrated HHNK patient.

The treatment, then, is rehydration. In fact, medical and nursing interventions for HHNK are basically the same as those for DKA, except that, despite the higher blood glucose level, the insulin dose is smaller. (These patients appear to be more sensitive to insulin.) Treatment consists of fluid and electrolyte replacement and low-dose insulin therapy, sometimes with heparin therapy.

Because the patient in HHNK is usually more severely dehydrated than the patient in DKA, a larger total volume of fluid needs to be replaced. And because he's usually older, he's likely to have cardiac or renal disease. That means the strength of the saline solution infused must be tailored to each person's specific problems.

Rapid fluid replacement can also be potentially hazardous to a patient with an already compromised cardiac staus. Observe your patient closely for signs and symptoms of fluid overload. Follow his urine output carefully, check for edema, and listen to his lungs for the moist crackles that alert you to fluid there. Don't neglect monitoring the vital signs. Watch for a rising blood pressure and bounding pulse.

Also, check the patient's blood glucose level frequently.

Most HHNK patients will be transferred to the intensive care unit. But a skillful assessment and an understanding of HHNK can often help you prevent this problem from progressing to frank coma. (See *Diabetic ketoacidosis.*)

Hickman catheter: direct method

Drawing blood by direct method

Obtain a syringe with 2.5 ml of normal saline solution, a syringe with 2.5 ml of heparin solution (100 units/ml), two specimen tubes, a 21-gauge butterfly needle, and a Vacutainer Luer adapter. This adapter has a Luer fitting at one end and a needle covered by a rubber sheath at the other end.

Label one of the specimen tubes with the word "discard." Then attach the adapter to the butterfly needle tubing and insert the butterfly needle into the injection cap.

Now insert the adapter needle into the specimen tube marked "discard." When you do this, the needle will pierce the rubber sheath.

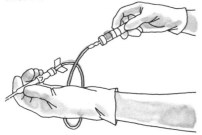

After the specimen tube fills, remove and discard it. The sheath will slide back over the needle, preventing blood leakage. Attach the other specimen tube and obtain a laboratory specimen. After removing the butterfly needle, flush the catheter with normal saline solution and the heparin solution. Then reclamp it.

Hickman catheter: patient teaching

Guidelines

Start teaching your patient to care for his Hickman catheter from the moment it's inserted. This way, he'll have more time to practice his new skills and will feel more confident about caring for the catheter after he's discharged. If possible, include a family member in your teaching.

What will your patient need to know? How to prevent complications, and how to recognize them if they do occur; how to re-dress the catheter insertion site; how to heparinize the catheter; and how to replace the catheter cap.

Avoiding complications

Besides teaching your patient how to prevent complications, also explain how to recognize them early and what to do if they occur.

• *Infection.* Your patient should know that a Hickman catheter puts him at risk for infection—either at the catheter insertion site or in his bloodstream. So stress the importance of good hand washing and clean technique whenever he handles the catheter. Tell him to look for signs and symptoms of infection around the insertion site—redness, tenderness, or drainage—whenever he re-dresses it.

Also explain that he can avoid contracting a blood infection by using sterile technique when he heparinizes his catheter line or handles I.V. solutions or tubings and by caring for an infected insertion site promptly. Fever, weakness, muscle aches, fatigue, poor appetite, and chills—all these may indicate blood infection.

Of course, remind him to call his doctor or home care nurse immediately if he experiences any signs or symptoms of infection.

• *Air embolism.* Tell your patient that whenever he connects or disconnects the catheter from the tubing or removes the cap, air can enter his vein, travel to his heart, lungs, or brain, and cause serious problems. If air does enter the catheter, he or someone else should call his doctor immediately. Until the doctor gives instructions, the patient should lie on his left side with his head lower than the rest of his body.

To avoid problems from air embolism, tell your patient to remember the three "C"s: Clamped, Connected, or Capped. His catheter should always be *clamped* with a clamp or rubber-tipped hemostat, *connected* to I.V. tubing or syringe, or *capped* with a sterile catheter cap.

• *Catheter obstruction.* If your patient doesn't heparinize his catheter daily or before and after each fluid administration, blood may clot and block the catheter.

If the catheter becomes blocked, tell him to flush the blood by heparinizing the catheter. Stress the importance of *gentle* flushing because force-flushing the catheter could push a clot into his bloodstream.

Performing procedures

Also explain and demonstrate these procedures for your patient:

• *Re-dressing the catheter insertion site.* After showing him correct hand-washing technique, explain how to re-dress the catheter insertion site. He should do this twice a week unless the dressing becomes opened, wet, or soiled. If that happens, he should re-dress the site immediately.

• *Heparinizing the catheter.* He should heparinize his catheter at least once a day (or more often if he's receiving I.V. fluids intermittently) to keep the I.V. line patent.

Show him how to withdraw solution from the vial, then inject it into the catheter's rubber cap. If he contaminates the solution while withdrawing it, he should discard it. If he feels any resistance when heparinizing the catheter, he should stop the procedure and call his doctor or home care nurse immediately.

• *Changing the catheter cap.* Your patient should change the catheter cap at least once a week. Stress the importance of keeping the catheter clamped when he's changing the cap.

Finally, to make sure your patient has correctly learned the skills you've taught him, ask him to demonstrate each technique for you.

H

Hickman catheter: syringe

Drawing blood using a syringe

First, you'll need to gather these supplies: a syringe with 2.5 ml of normal saline solution, a syringe with 2.5 ml of heparin solution (100 units/ml), a new injection cap, two empty 10-ml syringes, a specimen tube, and a 21-gauge needle. Don't substitute a smaller needle; it may cause hemolysis.

Begin by removing the injection cap from the end of the clamped Hickman catheter and attaching a 10-ml syringe to it. Then, after unclamping the catheter, draw about 6 ml of blood into the syringe. If you can't obtain blood from the catheter, have your patient take a deep breath, cough, raise one or both arms, or change position. If these measures don't work, notify the patient's doctor.

Once you've drawn blood into the syringe, reclamp the catheter. This blood will contain some heparin from the last time the catheter was flushed. And because heparin in a blood sample would make the test results inaccurate, you must discard this first syringe.

Connect the second 10-ml syringe to the catheter. Again, unclamp the catheter and draw blood. (The amount you draw will depend on the size of the specimen tube.) After reclamping the catheter, disconnect the syringe. Now, attach the needle to this syringe and slowly inject the blood into the specimen tube. Then flush the catheter, first with the 2.5 ml of normal saline solution, then with the 2.5 ml of heparin solution. Put the new injection cap on the catheter.

As an alternative, you can draw a sample without removing the injection cap. To do this, you'll need two 21-gauge needles, instead of just one. First, attach a needle to one of the 10-ml syringes. Then,

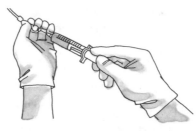

insert this needle into the cap and draw blood. Discard the syringe and needle. Now, obtain the blood specimen for the laboratory, using the second 10-ml syringe and needle. But don't draw or inject the specimen too quickly or forcefully, or else you could cause hemolysis.

Hickman catheter: tubing protection

Effective method

To protect a patient's Hickman catheter tubing against tugs or pulls at the catheter exit site, secure the tubing this way: Loop a rubber band around the tubing and pin the rubber band to the patient's gown or pajama top. If the tubing is inadvertently pulled, the rubber band—rather than the catheter or patient—absorbs the pull.

Hip replacement

Preventing complications

To increase your patient's understanding of possible postoperative complications, explain the hip replacement procedure to him beforehand.

Be sure he understands that it involves a complete replacement of the hip joint—both the ball and the socket. Explain that a metal prosthesis will replace the ball of his hip joint, and a high-density plastic cup will replace the socket. Also tell him which type of procedure his surgeon will perform—one that uses bone cement to hold the artificial parts in place or one that

allows the bone to grow into pores in the metal prosthesis, eliminating the need for cement.

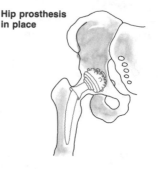

Hip prosthesis in place

Teach him postop exercises

Any patient who's had total hip replacement surgery needs to perform exercises to maintain adequate circulation to strengthen his hip muscles and prepare him for walking with crutches.

When you show him how to do these exercises before surgery, stress their importance in regaining mobility, strength, and muscle tone, in maintaining circulation, and in improving lung aeration. Ask him to demonstrate the exercises so you're sure he's doing them correctly.

• *Ankle exercises.* Tell him to point his toes up, then down—as if he's pressing on the gas pedal of a car. He should perform this exercise from 10 to 15 times every hour.

• *Quadriceps and gluteal muscle setting exercises.* Tell him to push the back of his knee down into the bed while squeezing his buttock muscles together; this will help tighten his thigh muscles. He should hold this positon for 5 seconds before relaxing. Make sure he knows he should exercise *both* legs, either together or separately.

• *Arm-strengthening exercises.* After surgery, your patient will have a trapeze overhead to help him move around in bed. Tell him that using it to pull himself up will improve circulation in his gluteal area.

• *Deep breathing, coughing, and incentive spirometry.* Show him how to perform these exercises, which he should repeat several times every hour. These exercises will expand his lungs and help clear his air passages.

Discuss proper positioning

Explain that, after surgery, the head of his bed may be elevated to a 45-degree angle and the foot of the bed may be elevated slightly. Depending on his doctor's orders, he may have to lie on his unaffected side for a specific amount of time. Assure him that you'll help position him.

Also, explain that traction, an abduction splint, or pillows placed between his legs may be used for correct hip positioning. Be sure he knows that maintaining correct position during the early recovery phase is *essential* for preventing dislocation and promoting healing.

Abduction pillow

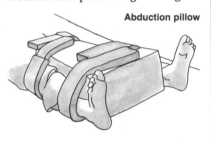

Let him know, too, that you and the physical therapist will teach him proper positioning for getting in and out of bed, using the trapeze.

Prepare him for discharge

On the third to fifth postoperative day (depending on the doctor's orders), he may begin walking. He'll probably learn this activity with a physical therapist's help, but you'll need to assist him, too.

You'll also need to teach him the following signs and symptoms of prosthesis dislocation:
• sudden, sharp pain, with a clicking or popping sound at the joint
• hip edema
• shortened leg, with the foot in external rotation
• loss of control over leg motion or complete loss of leg motion.

Stress that, if he suspects prosthesis dislocation, he should contact his doctor immediately or go to the hospital emergency department.

Discuss the recuperation process

Stress that he'll need help with any activities that require hip flexion—putting on shoes and socks, for example. And tell him to avoid activities that abduct the hip, such as crossing his legs.

Also, explain how adequate fluid intake and a well-balanced diet (with vitamin supplementation if needed) can help promote healing.

Finally, tell him to expect, not instant improvement, but a period of recovery that may last up to 6 months. During this time, he may continue to experience pain and to have problems with mobility.

Holter monitor: connection

Doing it properly

A Holter monitor lets an ambulatory patient go about his daily activities while undergoing continuous electrocardiography.

Preparing the electrode sites

These sites are:
• the junction of the right clavicle and first costosternal border
• the junction of the left clavicle and first costosternal border
• the fifth intercostal space at the right midclavicular line
• the fifth intercostal space at the left midclavicular line
• midsternum at the nipple line. (This is for the ground wire, which may be placed elsewhere on the chest.)

Clean each site with alcohol. Then shave any hair from the sites, using water and a razor. (The electrodes won't stick securely to the skin if you use soap or a cleanser.) With an abrasive pad or liquid, rub briskly to roughen the skin at each site. This will ensure good contact between the skin and the electrodes. Finally, reclean the sites thoroughly with alcohol and let the skin dry.

Placing the electrodes

Connect an electrode to each of the five lead wires. Never connect these wires *after* placing the electrodes on the patient; this may cause bruises or soft tissue damage.

Attach the electrodes to the five sites described above. To match the lead wires to the appropriate sites, follow the color code or other designations on the monitor.

Securing other connections

Once the electrodes are in place, make 2″ (5 cm) tension loops in the lead wires and tape them to the patient's chest. An accidental tug will then open the loop instead of disconnecting the electrode.

Now tape the junction box, where the lead wires connect to the patient's cable, to a flat part of the patient's abdomen. Have the patient dress. The cable should extend through an opening in his or her clothing near the waist.

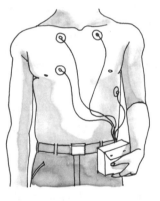

Insert a cassette and a 9-volt battery into the tape recorder. Slip the recorder into its carrying case and show the patient how to wear it on his shoulder or belt. Explain that the recorder is lightweight, so it shouldn't cause any discomfort. (See *Holter monitor: patient teaching.*)

Holter monitor: patient teaching

The importance of keeping a diary

A key part of your instructions to a patient with a Holter monitor is explaining the diary that the patient must keep. He should note the time of all daily activities, especially physical ones, such as walking, climbing stairs, having a bowel movement, or having sex. Before engaging in these activities, he should push the "event" button on the tape recorder. This will create a highlighted area on the electro-cardiogram (ECG) tracing for the next 5 minutes.

Instruct him to also record symptoms, such as palpitations, chills, and dizziness, as well as any pain in his chest, jaw, shoulder, or neck. He should note the symptom and the time, and push the "event" button when the symptom occurs.

After 24 hours, the patient will return the monitor and diary to the outpatient clinic. Disconnect the monitor, but don't remove the electrodes unless ordered otherwise. Instead, tell him to do this at home while taking a shower because water will help loosen electrodes without causing pain. (See *Holter monitor: connection.*)

Homans' sign

Eliciting it

First, support the patient's thigh with one hand and his foot with the other. Bend his leg slightly at the knee, then firmly and abruptly dorsiflex his ankle. Deep calf pain indicates a positive Homans' sign.

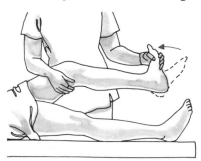

(The patient may also resist ankle dorsiflexion or flex the knee involuntarily if Homans' sign is positive.)

Home health care planning

Helping your patient prepare

To advise your patient, ask what resources exist at home and what kinds of outside help he'll require.

Briefly inquire about the layout of his home. Are rooms and doorways large enough or adaptable to any special equipment he might need, such as a hospital bed or a wheelchair? If he must avoid steps, can a ground-floor dining room temporarily be converted to his room? Are toilet and bathing facilities nearby? You'll know from daily care whether handrails or a bedside commode will be necessary, so advise the family accordingly.

If the general layout seems adaptable for home care, briefly assess the relative who'll be the principal caregiver. Does he have the time, ability, willingness, emotional and physical stamina, and knowledge to give care? You and the home health care nurse may have to teach him and other relatives what the patient will need, so add this to your list of responsibilities.

What's the attitude of the rest of the family members? Can they adjust to the demands of patient care and how those demands will change their lives, even if only temporarily?

Expand your examination of "people" resources by inquiring about friends or neighbors who can pitch in if necessary. Help the family make a list of people who can pick up supplies if needed.

How about emergency procedures? Can the family have a call bell or phone rigged up within the patient's reach? Other emergency precautions depend upon the patient's condition, such as having a written protocol for what to do if an I.V. line is accidentally pulled out or who to call if there's a sudden, critical change in the patient's respirations.

Take a look at the need for and feasibility of safety measures. Will the patient need a ventilator? If so, he'll also need a portable generator in case the power fails.

Finally, what kind of special services will the patient need? If additional outside help is needed, precisely what kind and how much can the family afford? Does the patient qualify for Medicare or Medicaid? Or does he have private insurance that covers home health care?

Once you've helped your patient plan the kind of care he needs, determine what's available. Begin by checking with the patient to find out whether he has used some form of home health care in the past or whether his doctor has recommended a particular service.

Next, ask for referrals from community health agencies and community nurses, your hospital's social service department, and your local community information service. Other sources of information include local chapters of such national organizations as the American Cancer Society, the American Diabetes Association, the Arthritis Foundation, and so on.

The goal here is to avoid calling home health care agencies or services and nurses at random from the Yellow Pages, so use every resource at your disposal. For example, call your county's Office on Aging to see if your community has special programs for senior citizens.

You'll also want to make a list of local medical-surgical supply centers and oxygen therapy services, along with their costs, hours, and procedures. (See also *Day care for adults; Home health care services.*)

Home health care services

What to ask

When your patient needs home health care but doesn't qualify for

Medicare or needs more than intermittent care, his alternative is a private home health care service. You or your patient should ask for referrals and thoroughly investigate the services you're interested in—asking these questions:

1. Is there a supervising RN or director of nursing services, and is she licensed to practice in your state? (Some private home health care services are part of a national chain with administrative nursing staff in a headquarters office. A director of nursing 1,000 miles away isn't going to do your patient much good, so be sure there's a qualified supervisor on the premises.)

2. What's the background of the administrative and supervisory staff? Do they have education and experience in home health care and administration?

3. Is an initial in-depth nursing assessment of the patient made by an RN? Does the same nurse prepare an equally in-depth nursing care plan that takes into account all the patient's needs and problems and involves both the patient and the family in setting goals? (Only an RN is qualified to do a nursing assessment and a care plan; the same nurse should do both to ensure continuity and greater understanding of the situation.)

4. How does the service select its nursing personnel? Have they been screened by personal interview, careful reference checks, and skill inventory? Are they kept up to date with orientation and staff development programs offered through the service?

5. On what basis are nursing personnel assigned to individual patients? By availability only? Or is an effort made to match the patient's needs with the caregiver's experience and qualifications? Is compatibility considered?

6. Once on the job, do nurse's aides and homemakers write daily nursing notes that are reviewed regularly by the supervising RN or director of nursing services?

7. Does the service regularly collaborate with other members of the health care team—doctor, social worker, and therapist—so their efforts are coordinated?

8. Does the service request and obtain written doctor's orders and update them at least every 60 days?

9. Does a supervising RN visit routinely to evaluate patient progress and nursing care?

10. Is there a supervising RN on call to all levels of nursing personnel around the clock, 7 days a week?

11. Is there evidence of continuity of care through nursing assessments, nursing care plans, patient care conferences, nurses' notes, and nursing supervisor evaluations?

12. Is the service an employer—rather than just an employment agency? (The question here is who has to take care of withholding tax, workers' compensation, unemployment and liability insurance, Social Security, and employer quarterly reports. Be absolutely clear about this, or your patient may be in for a lot of tedious paperwork and unexpected expenses.)

13. What are the fees for the various levels of nursing personnel, and how are the fees billed? What do the rates include? What is extra, and how much does it cost? (See also *Home health care planning.*)

Hospice philosophy

Using it in the hospital

If a patient is terminally ill and you've done all you can for him medically, try to make him as peaceful and comfortable as possible. He probably needs a friend to talk to. Anytime a patient or family member wants to talk, try to stop what you're doing and listen. If they need to talk with you for 20 or 30 minutes, do so. A colleague will probably be more than willing to cover your other patients for you, and the other staff is likely to understand and help you.

Honesty is another need patients have. Those with cancer usually ask their doctor how well their treatment is working. If they aren't responding to treatment, the doctor will probably tell them. Even so, they're apt to ask the nurse the hard question: "Am I going to die?"

Never tell patients they're dying or say anything to take away all hope. They rarely need an answer; they just want a caring listener who won't try to change the subject or deny their fears.

Some patients *can't* express their fears. Or they won't feel comfortable talking to you. When you have a patient like this, spend extra time sitting with him just to give him the comfort of having someone nearby. Sometimes a reticent patient will talk during his bath. He knows he has the nurse's undivided attention for a block of time, and that gives him courage.

If he clearly doesn't want to talk, or if he wants to be alone, respect that wish, although it might be very hard.

Encouraging independence

Independence is as important to sick people as to well ones—maybe even more important, since their disease itself reflects a loss of control. So try to give patients control, even if it makes your own job more difficult. That includes control of pain with regular, sufficient doses of medication around the clock and control of dietary needs.

Control extends beyond the patient's physical needs. Accept each patient as a person and a family member, not just a set of symptoms. Sometimes this means providing personal services for patients.

If you can, go out of your way to visit patients on your day off, take their laundry home, or bring in special foods. Acknowledge the patient's role as a family member, and provide cots so spouses can spend the night. Encourage children to visit, even small ones, unless they've recently been exposed to communicable diseases. Or sometimes "family" includes a pet. Allow the pet in the room for an hour or so.

Put an emphasis on living by celebrating holidays, birthdays, and other special days with the patient and his family. This philosopy will help each patient experience the best possible quality of life while he's in the unit. (See also *Communication: dying patients.*)

Hoyer lift

Making the seat more comfortable

When you use a Hoyer lift to transfer a patient from his wheelchair to the toilet, leave the lift's canvas seat (which has a hole in it) under him. However, some patients may complain that the canvas is scratchy.

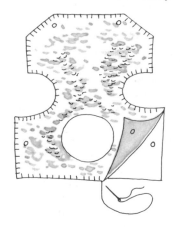

To make the seat more comfortable, sew a piece of sheepskin (with a hole cut in the middle) to the canvas seat. The patients appreciate the soft seat, and the entire seat—canvas and sheepskin—can easily be taken off the lift and laundered.

Humor

How it can help you

Laughing not only preserves your sanity, but also improves your health, outlook on life, and ability to communicate. Next time you feel frustration pile up, try playing it for laughs. Here are some suggestions:

1. Develop your sense of humor. How you view life, talk to yourself, and let events affect you— positively or negatively—are indicators of how well developed your sense of humor is. If yours could use a boost, start by identifying the petty, negative things that grind you down every day; then, brainstorm some possible solutions—ranging from the practical to the ridiculous.

This approach can yield some surprisingly effective solutions.

2. Remember that humor often grows from painful memories soothed by time and distance. We can all recall embarrassing moments that became hilarious only in retrospect.

The paradoxical relationship between the humorous and the painful helps explain why humor can sometimes defuse anxious or frustrating moments.

3. Don't wait for inspiration—plan ahead. At one time or another you've probably found yourself tongue-tied in a situation with someone who really irritated you.

One way to avoid this is to keep a list of situations that commonly occur with people who upset you. Then, when you have time to be creative, think of some salty responses to make. Write them down. Or, when you hear a clever comeback, write it down and think how you could use it.

4. Don't ignore other people's preferences. What's funny varies considerably from one group or person to another.

Don't risk using humor with anyone you don't know well. Many people who are proud of their ethnic heritage don't appreciate ethnic jokes. Some people dislike puns. If you regularly use a style of humor that offends or annoys others, you'll fall flat on your face and create tensions instead of easing them.

5. Share a laugh with your co-workers. Showcasing humor can help ease the daily tensions we all feel. Encourage co-workers to exchange examples of their own brand of humor on the unit's bulletin board.

Using humor with your patients
When used appropriately, and with loving care, humor is useful when dealing with patients, if they seem receptive to it. Sometimes even difficult patients or dying patients appreciate humor. Humor is a part of the process that can help you develop a comforting, healing relationship with your patients.

Hyperkalemia: prevention

Safeguards to follow

When managing the patient with hyperkalemia:
• Frequently monitor serum potassium and other electrolyte levels, and carefully record intake and output.
• Administer Kayexalate (sodium polystyrene sulfonate) orally, or rectally by retention enema. Watch for signs of hypokalemia with prolonged use of this medication. Also watch for clinical effects of hypoglycemia (muscle weakness, syncope, hunger, and diaphoresis) with repeated insulin and glucose treatments.
• Look for signs of hyperkalemia in predisposed patients, especially those with poor urine output or those receiving potassium supplements orally or intravenously. Administer no more than 10 to 20 mEq/liter of potassium chloride/hour; check the I.V. infusion site for phlebitis or infiltration of potassium. Also, before giving a blood transfusion, check to see how long ago the blood was donated; hemolysis of older blood cells releases potassium. Infuse only fresh blood to patients with average to high serum potassium levels.
• Monitor for and report cardiac dysrhythmias.

Hypertension, severe

Steps to take

Not every patient with severely elevated blood pressure is in hypertensive crisis. When you get a very high reading, follow these steps:

1. Remeasure the patient's blood pressure, taking it in both arms.

2. Take his history. Besides the usual questions, ask specifically about headaches, nausea, vomiting, blurred vision, drowsiness, numbness or tingling, chest pain, shortness of breath, ankle swelling, and changes in urine output. For each symptom reported, determine its severity, onset, and duration. Ask about previous diagnoses and treatments for hypertension, including past and present medications.

3. Assess his physical condition. Look for signs of neurologic dysfunction, retinal damage, congestive heart failure, pulmonary edema, and renal failure.

4. Have your patient lie down in a comfortable position and, if possible, away from any commotion.

At this point, report your findings to the doctor. While awaiting his diagnosis, continue with the following steps:

5. Prepare to obtain a chest X-ray and an electrocardiogram.

6. Prepare to collect blood and urine samples for laboratory studies. Blood studies usually include a complete blood count, creatinine level, electrolyte profile, and plasma catecholamine value. Urine studies usually require a single sample to test for red blood cells, protein, and metanephrine, plus a sample collected over 24 hours to measure vanillylmandelic acid.

7. Continue monitoring your patient and recording all your findings. (His blood pressure will probably decrease somewhat with rest).

8. If he needs nitroprusside (Nipride) therapy, prepare to transfer him to an ICU.

9. If he's not going to an ICU, prepare to start an I.V. line for other antihypertensive drugs and be sure these drugs are available. Also have ready an infusion pump or a microdrip unit for accurate dose titration. (See also *Hypertension detection.*)

Hypertension detection

Recognizing labile hypertension

Many of the patients you meet in your daily practice may be diagnosed hypertensives. Others may be undiagnosed with the only clue being a family history. To detect the undiagnosed or uncontrolled hypertensive patient and reinforce teaching for the diagnosed patient, follow these guidelines when taking patient histories and conducting routine assessments:

• Encourage all patients to have their blood pressure checked at least once every 2 years, or more frequently if possible.

• Before taking a patient's blood pressure reading, have him rest in a seated position for a few minutes. Take two or more readings, then calculate the average. This should eliminate the risk of obtaining an aberrently high first reading.

• Keep a log of the patient's blood pressure readings for his checkups. Refer a patient with an average diastolic reading greater than 90 mm Hg to his doctor.

• Work with newly diagnosed patients as they adjust to the changed life-style necessary for controlling their blood pressure. Use all support measures and materials available to help them maintain these changes.

• When medication is prescribed, the patient will need his serum lipid level checked before starting treatment, then rechecked periodically.

• Encourage the patient to ask about his medication. Verify that he thoroughly understands what each drug is supposed to do, how and when to take it, what precautions to follow, what adverse effects may occur, and what to do about such effects.

• Reinforce the importance of taking medications as prescribed. Remind the patient who is experiencing adverse effects that he doesn't have to suffer and that other drugs are available. A knowledgeable doctor, pharmacist, or nurse can discuss alternatives.

If a patient takes many medications and has more than one doctor, help him to list all the medications he takes. This list should include both prescription and over-the-counter drugs, as well as those taken intermittently. Advise the patient to keep the list current and show it to all health care providers who care for him. (See *Blood pressure measurement; Hypertension, severe.*)

Hyperthermia, malignant

Emergency intervention

Malignant hyperthermia can develop after anesthesia induction with halothane (Fluothane). Here are critical countermeasures to follow in the CCU.

Arriving with the transfer team, the surgeon will order a second dose of dantrolene (Dantrium), to follow one given in the operating room. Because this drug prevents release of calcium, it will relieve the skeletal muscle contractions.

Dantrolene is usually given in 1 mg/kg doses until the spasms subside. The surgeon may increase the dose to a maximum of 10 mg/kg, but most patients respond after receiving a cumulative dose of about 2.5 mg/kg.

Next, administer sodium bicarbonate and continue 100% hyperventilation to correct metabolic acidosis. To prevent myoglobinuria and resulting renal failure, maintain urine output with I.V. mannitol (Osmitrol) and furosemide (Frusemide, Lasix).

To lower the patient's body temperature—thus decreasing metabolic demands—place him on a cooling blanket and pack his axillae and groin with ice. Rapidly infuse iced normal saline solution.

Obtain blood samples from his arterial line for analysis of arterial blood gases; clotting factors and time; and calcium, potassium, creatine phosphokinase (CPK), and serum myoglobin levels. Also determine his urine myoglobin level.

Constantly monitor his electrocardiogram. Leakage of calcium and potassium from the skeletal muscle could precipitate ventricular ectopia, which might lead to ventricular tachycardia or fibrillation. At the doctor's order, treat ventricular dysrhythmias with procainamide (Pronestyl). (The usual treatment, lidocaine [lignocaine, Xylocaine], is contraindicated in this situation because it may exacerbate the underlying hypermetabolism.)

Also, throughout your interventions, reassure the patient by explaining to him what you're doing.

Once the hyperthermia is controlled, you must still monitor the patient closely—the condition may recur within the next 24 to 48 hours. Continuous rectal temperatures can help you detect the rise in temperature indicating relapse early on.

As the patient's condition improves, explain to the family what happened and why. Because the tendency toward malignant hyperthermia is genetically inherited, suggest that all family members undergo a muscle biopsy to determine their susceptibility.

Finally, recommend a Medic Alert bracelet so he won't be exposed to this life-threatening reaction to anesthesia induction again.

Hypoglycemia

Emergency care

If your patient's responsive, give him a food or beverage containing 10 to 15 g of a simple, fast-acting carbohydrate. Possibilities include:
• ½ cup (4 oz) fruit juice, such as orange or apple juice
• ½ cup nondiet soft drink, such as ginger ale or cola
• ½ cup gelatin dessert
• 4 sugar cubes
• 2 sugar packets
• 2 graham cracker squares
• ¼ cup (2 oz) corn syrup, honey, or grape jelly
• 6 jelly beans
• 10 gumdrops.

If your patient's unresponsive, give medications as ordered. If these aren't available, squeeze a glucose product such as Glutose, Glutol, or Instant Glucose into the patient's mouth, where it can be absorbed through oral tissues or swallowed by reflex (but make sure you don't obstruct the patient's airway). If you can't obtain these products, place some honey on the patient's tongue, or squeeze prepared cake-decorating icing (such as CakeMate) between the patient's gum and cheek. Obtain medical help promptly. (See *Diabetic shock: intervention; Diabetic shock: prevention.*)

Hypokalemia management

Guidelines for safe care

When managing the patient:
• Check serum potassium and other electrolyte levels in patients prone to potassium imbalance and in those requiring potassium replacement.
• Assess intake and output carefully. Remember, kidneys excrete 80% to 90% of ingested potassium. So, never give supplementary potassium to a patient whose urine output is below 600 ml/day. Also, measure GI loss of potassium from suctioning or vomiting.
• Dilute oral potassium solutions in 4 oz (120 ml) or more of water or juice to reduce irritation of gastric and small-bowel mucosa.
• Give I.V. potassium only after it's diluted in solution; potassium is very irritating to vascular, subcutaneous, and fatty tissues, and may cause phlebitis or tissue necrosis if it infiltrates. Infuse slowly to prevent *hyperkalemia*. Never administer by I.V. push or bolus; this may cause cardiac arrest.
• Carefully monitor patients receiving digitalis, because hypokalemia enhances the action of digitalis and may produce signs and symptoms of digitalis toxicity (anorexia, nausea, vomiting, yellow vision, and dysrhythmias). (See *Digitalis toxicity.*)

Hypospadias

Securing the diaper after surgery

Here's a technique for putting on a diaper. Toddlers who've had hypospadias surgery usually have a suprapubic or perineal catheter. But they still need to wear a diaper for bowel movements. To protect the penile operative site or dressing from pressure by the diaper, make the following modification.

Cut an "X" in the front half of a regular disposable diaper. Then cut the bottom from a Styrofoam cup

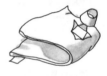

and insert the cup through the "X" until the rim is flush with the inside of the diaper. Tape the cup to the outside of the diaper.

Then fasten the diaper securely around the baby's waist without putting pressure on the penile

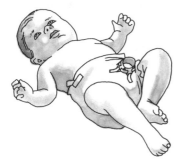

dressing. You can easily check the dressing by looking through the bottom of the cup.

Hypotension, orthostatic

Preambulation exercises

To help minimize the effects of orthostatic hypotension, such as dizziness and blurred vision, when your patient stands up, teach her how to perform these leg exercises before getting out of bed.
• "Lie flat on your back, and flex one knee slightly, keeping your heel on the bed.

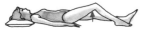

• "Lift your heel off the bed and try to straighten your leg.

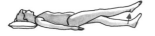

• "Flex your knee again, and lower your heel to the bed.

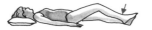

• "Straighten your leg.
• "Repeat the procedure for the other leg. Alternating legs, perform the exercises six times for each leg." (See also *Blood pressure, orthostatic.*)

Hypothermia care

How to help your patient

If you find that your patient's temperature is below 95° F. (35° C.), confirming hypothermia, you'll need to begin rewarming him. Usually, this is done in one of three ways.

Passive external rewarming simply means removing the patient from the cold and wrapping him in warm blankets. This method may be adequate by itself, or it may be a first step for one of the other two methods.

Active external rewarming consists of immersing the patient in a warm water bath, covering him with an electric or hypothermia blanket, or applying hot water bottles. As you'd expect, this method raises the patient's temperature more quickly than passive rewarming. But be cautious: Using water or blankets that are too warm can burn the patient. In fact, even when used correctly, this method can cause serious problems. When peripheral vessels dilate in reponse to the warmth, cold blood is shunted to the heart and the core temperature can drop as much as 3° F. (1.5° C.) or more, leading to ventricular fibrillation and cardiac arrest. Be prepared to begin cardiopulmonary resuscitation or to defibrillate.

Internal rewarming provides warmth directly to the patient's core by means of warmed oxygen inhalation and, when possible, peritoneal lavage or dialysis and extracorporeal blood warming. To warm oxygen, use a humidifier. Usually, you can begin administering the warmed oxygen (104° to 108° F. [40° to 42° C.]) by mask or endotracheal tube, while equipment for the other procedure is being set up. Warmed oxygen inhalation can be used alone to rewarm the patient's core if facilities for the other two treatments aren't available.

The method you choose to rewarm the patient will depend on his initial temperature and correspond-

ing symptoms. Usually, internal rewarming is used only when severe cardiac compromise develops and the patient's core temperature plunges below 89.6° F. (32° C.)

Otherwise, external rewarming is recommended, since it's much slower and thus much safer. External rewarming should be adequate for a core temperature below 89.6° F. (32° C.), if the temperature dropped *rapidly*, because the body hasn't had time to develop dangerous pathophysiologic changes.

Besides using one of these rewarming methods, you'll probably need to start an I.V. line and warm all I.V. fluids before administering them. If the patient has severe vasoconstriction, you may need a central line.

Monitor the patient to ensure that he's rewarming slowly and safely. Check his temperature rectally every 15 minutes to see that it doesn't rise more than 1° F. (.5° C.) an hour. Also, assess his vital signs and level of consciousness and begin cardiac monitoring.

Because the patient's cough reflex is supressed, secretions may build up. So, make sure his airway remains patent. To do this, you may have to suction him frequently. Again, be prepared to begin cardiopulmonary resuscitation or to defibrillate the patient in case he develops ventricular fibrillation. (See also *Hypothermia detection; Hypothermia prevention.*)

Hypothermia detection

When to suspect it in elderly patients

Usually, the hardest thing about detecting hypothermia is knowing when to suspect it. Most victims of hypothermia are not dug out of a snowbank or pulled from a frozen pond. In fact, an elderly victim may be found unconscious in his apartment with the thermostat set in the low 60s. But because he won't have a history of prolonged exposure to severe cold and because his signs and symptoms can be nonspecific, you may not suspect hypothermia—at least not at first.

To make sure you don't overlook hypothermia, always consider it a possibility when you're confronted with an unconscious elderly patient in the ED or on a home visit. Routinely add these steps to your initial assessment: Look for signs and symptoms of hypothermia that mimic other conditions (for example, a pale, puffy face that may be mistaken for myxedema, or confusion that may be mistaken for a sign of hypoglycemia, uremia, or congestive heart failure).

Also, look for subtle clues, such as cold skin on parts of the body that are usually covered (for example, the inner thighs).

If the patient's skin is cool, take his temperature rectally. (An axillary or oral temperature is less reliable.) Make sure you use a thermometer that measures temperatures below 94° F. (34° C.) and to shake it all the way down before using it. (See also *Hypothermia care; Hypothermia prevention.*)

Hypothermia prevention

Keeping a patient warm

To help prevent hypothermia, give your elderly patients these tips on how to protect themselves:
• "Wear multiple layers of clothing when outdoors in cold weather.
• "Use available transportation services, such as buses or subways.
• "Don't overexert yourself.
• "Eat nutritious meals.
• "If you're more than 65 years old, keep your thermostat set above 65.
• "If necessary, seek aid from appropriate government agencies, church groups, or other sources to pay your fuel bills.

• "Take fewer baths to reduce heat loss from evaporation.
• "Sleep in a warm room with the windows closed.
• "Wear socks and a cap to bed. (The cap will decrease heat loss from your head.)
• "Use extra-low-voltage electric blankets."

Hypovolemic shock intervention

Emergency technique

The primary goal with hypovolemic shock is to maintain or restore an adequate circulating volume. First, start an I.V. and get fluids going while you look for the bleeding site. You can start large-bore lines in the upper body or in central veins; you'll need two or more lines to maintain adequate volume replacement.

Ideally, the fluid of choice for replacement should be similar to the fluid lost. The primary I.V. fluids used are crystalloids, plasma expanders, and blood products. Direct blood loss can now be replaced by autotransfusion. (See *Autotransfusion systems.*)

Positioning is an excellent means of redistributing blood volume. A modified Trendelenburg's position (supine with legs slightly elevated) is used to increase venous return. This position is preferred to the traditional Trendelenburg's position because it avoids abdominal pressure against the diaphragm, which can lead to respiratory restriction. The modified Trendelenburg's position also prevents increases in cerebral edema in patients with head injuries.

Circulating blood volume can also be increased by the use of medical antishock trousers, which exert a positive pressure on the lower extremities and abdomen. (See *MAST suit.*) This helps control tamponade or bleeding by direct and indirect pressure and can re-

distribute one to two units of blood to the vital organs.

Direct pressure to a bleeding site may control loss; however, prompt surgical exploration and repair may be indicated.

Two types of drugs may be used as hypovolemic shock progresses: steroids and vasopressors. Steroids may stabilize cellular membranes, but their use is still controversial. Vasopressors can increase cardiac output and peripheral resistance, but they should not be a substitute for adequate volume replacement.

During this fast-paced treatment, try to stay organized. Here are some suggestions:
• Delegate someone to keep a running log of what's going on.
• Save all I.V. bags and drug containers. These will help you do more thorough charting.
• If something—such as a medication dose—doesn't seem right, ask for clarification.
• Keep the room clear of nonessential people.
• Operate on your own strengths. For example, if you're told to start an I.V., but you're not good at it, let another nurse know. You could say, "I'll handle vital signs and meds, while you start the I.V."
• Keep looking at the entire patient. There's a tendency to develop tunnel vision in this situation. For example, while a patient's right femoral artery is pumping blood, everyone might be watching that and forgetting to check whether the patient's breathing.

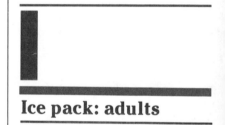

Ice pack: adults

Guidelines

Here's a tidy way to make an ice bag out of a hot water bottle by stuffing crushed ice into it. If a wide-

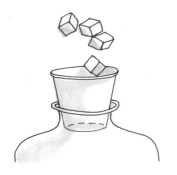

mouth funnel's not available, simply punch out the bottom of a paper cup. Fit it in the neck of the ice bag, and use it as a funnel. The ice will slide in easily, with no mess.

Ice pack: chemotherapy

Methods to use

For patients receiving chemotherapy, an ice pack applied to the scalp is standard procedure to help minimize hair loss. But ice packs are drippy and messy, so you need to modify the procedure.

Place the patient in a high-Fowler's or semi-Fowler's position and gently dampen his hair roots with warm water. Then get three cold gel packs and tape a washcloth around each.

Place the slightly pliable packs around the patient's hairline in a circle, and tape them together to keep them in place. Then put an ice bag on the uncovered crown of the patient's head. To make sure the ice bag and gel packs stay put, secure them with Kerlix or Kling in turban style.

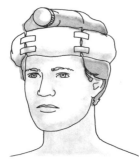

Besides eliminating the drippy mess, this type of ice cap allows the patient to sit up and read or even walk around.

Ice pack: children

Helpful tips

Here's an easy way to make ice packs that pediatric patients can hold on lumps, cuts, and other minor injuries. Take some empty, round, plastic containers (such as medicine cups) and fill them with water. Then freeze them. You'll find these makeshift ice packs are just the right size for little hands to hold.

Ice pack: eyelid

Easy application

When the weight of a regular ice pack on the eyelid is too painful for a patient, make an "icy finger" ice pack instead.

Fill finger cots with water, tie them shut, and freeze them. Place two ice-filled cots inside a piece of 2″ (5 cm) stockinette and pin or tape two pieces of twill tape to the stockinette—one at each end. Place the stockinette over the patient's eyes and tie the twill tape at the back of the patient's head.

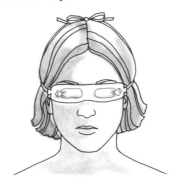

This icy finger pack is lighter than regular ice packs and will stay in place itself so the patient can freely use both hands. Keep a supply of them in the freezer for fast and easy replacement.

ICU care

Orienting patients to time

Intensive care units usually have no windows, so lights are on around the clock. This contributes to the confusion many ICU patients experience. Many patients don't know whether it's day or night. To help orient them, put a card indicating a.m. or p.m. next to the clock on the wall. This will help relieve a bit of their frustration. (See *Elderly patients: orientation*.)

ICU noise

Helping patients sleep

In a busy—and sometimes noisy—intensive care unit, many patients have trouble sleeping. A cassette player with earphones, brought from home, will help drown out the noise for these patients. And when listening to their favorite music, they'll relax and fall asleep easier. (See *Insomnia*.)

IHSS

Instructing the patient

Idiopathic hypertrophic subaortic stenosis (IHSS) is a type of cardiomyopathy characterized by left ventricular septal hypertrophy and interstitial fibrosis. Septal hypertrophy causes malalignment of the cardiac fibers and papillary muscles. This, in turn, can lead to a prolapse in the leaflet valves of the mitral valve, causing an obstruction. Here are special instructions for patients with this disorder:
• Faithfully take prescribed beta blockers and calcium channel blockers. These drugs will reduce cardiac dysrhythmias, myocardial oxygen demand, and contractility.
• Tell your patient to notify other doctors, health care workers, and his dentist that he'll need prophylactic antibiotic therapy with any

invasive procedure. This will help prevent endocarditis.

• Show him how to take his pulse. He'll need to do this before taking his propranolol hydrochloride (Inderal), which will lower his heart rate and thus reduce his heart's work load. Tell your patient not to take Inderal if his pulse rate drops below 50 beats/minute. Instead, he should call his doctor immediately.

• Advise him to stop any activity that causes angina, dizziness, or palpitations—all symptoms of decreased cardiac output. Tell him to call the doctor immediately.

• Warn him not to stand or sit up suddenly. Sudden position changes can decrease venous pooling and dump blood into the heart, increasing the obstruction.

• Remind him not to take any nitroglycerin or vasodilators he may have at home for chest pain. They will deplete blood volume to the left ventricle, making the heart beat more forcefully.

• Also caution him against taking drugs that increase the force of heart contractions—digoxin (Lanoxin) or isoproterenol hydrochloride (Isuprel), for example. The obstruction would worsen because the more forceful cardiac contractions against it would deprive the left ventricle of blood at the end of systole.

Ileal conduit

Healing techniques

A patient who's had an ileal conduit may develop skin breakdown around his stoma. To help repair his skin, use a heat lamp, a paper cup, and cotton balls.

First, push out the bottom of the cup (leaving a smooth edge) and fill the cup with cotton balls. Then have the patient hold the cup tightly over his stoma while you position the heat lamp over the stoma area.

The cotton balls will absorb his urine; as they become saturated, remove the cup and give him a new one. He can stay under the heat lamp comfortably for about 30 minutes. After a few days of this treatment three times a day, his skin should begin to heal. (See *Ostomy: diarrhea.*)

Illusions

Helping the patient who experiences them

Illusions involve a physical or environmental stimulus that the patient misinterprets. He perceives something not for what it actually is, but for what his inner needs or fears tell him it is. Even so, you can usually see a connection between what's actually there and what the patient says is there—for example, between a hissing humidity mask and a menacing snake. Here's how to minimize the chances that your patient experiences an illusion:

• Let the patient have sense-related objects from home whenever it's feasible. Seeing a familiar picture, hearing the familiar tick of a clock, feeling a familiar pillow or blanket—these sensations help anchor him to reality.

• Minimize the number of unfamiliar elements in the patient's surroundings. Provide a night light that doesn't create strange shadows; remove pictures that are ambiguous and can be misinterpreted; explain strange equipment and, if possible, let the patient handle it.

• Involve the patient as much as possible in planning his daily routine.

• Match the patient's surroundings to the sensory level he's used to, either by reducing sensory overload or increasing sensory stimuli. (See also *Hallucinations; Psychotic patients; Sleep deprivation.*)

Immobilizers

Using them

Some musculoskeletal injuries, such as dislocations and sprains, don't require a cast for immobilization. For injuries like these, and for postreduction immobilization of some fractures, the doctor may use an immobilizer. Here's what you should know about the uses and fitting of some types of immobilizers:

• *Wrist immobilizers* immobilize the wrist after a severe sprain or surgery. Check the patient's neurologic and circulatory status frequently.

Wrist immobilizer

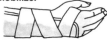

• *Belt-type shoulder immobilizers* immobilize shoulder dislocations and clavicular fractures. Assess the patient's respiratory status frequently to make sure that tight straps don't restrict his breathing.

Belt-type shoulder immobilizer

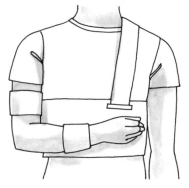

• *Knee immobilizers* immobilize the knee after a severe sprain or strain or after surgery. Measure the patient's thigh and calf circumference and consult the manufacturer's chart to select the correct size. The doctor will specify the length and contour of the immobilizer he wants to use for the patient.

Knee immobilizer

• *Clavicle straps* immobilize clavicular fractures. Make sure the strap doesn't apply excessive pressure under the patient's arms—this could cause nerve damage.

Clavicle strap

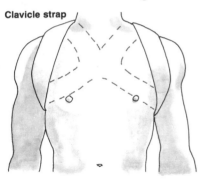

• *Sling and swathe bandages* immobilize shoulder dislocations and some fractures of the humerus and elbow. Remove any rings or bracelets the patient's wearing; swelling may impair circulation. Make sure the sling supports your patient's fingers to the first interphalangeal joints. This will

Sling and swathe bandage

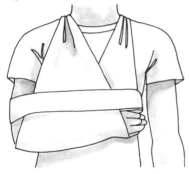

help prevent nerve damage, which can lead to wrist drop. (See also *Fracture care.*)

Incentive spirometry: adults

Encouraging deep breathing

Make sure your patient understands that the spirometer helps him make up for the natural sighing he's not doing now. A respiratory therapist will set the volume goal—the amount of air the patient should take in with each breath. Then teach him these steps to deeper breaths.

1. Help him to sit up in bed or on the edge of the bed. In this position, his abdominal contents won't restrict chest expansion.

2. Tell him to exhale normally, then to put the mouthpiece between his lips and close his mouth tightly around it.

3. Instruct him to inhale slowly and as deeply as possible. If he has difficulty with this step, ask him to suck in as he would with a straw, but to do so more slowly. Inspiring slowly will ensure an even distribution of air to the alveoli.

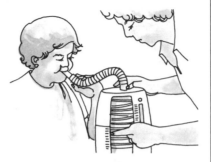

4. Note the maximum volume of air he inhales. This is called his inspiratory capacity. When you're teaching him preoperatively, record his baseline inspiratory capacity. A sudden decrease in this measurement postoperatively could indicate an acute pulmonary problem.

5. Tell him to hold the maximum volume of air he's inhaled for 3 seconds. This will help open alveoli that have collapsed. Make sure he doesn't do Valsalva's maneuver while holding this volume of air.

6. Instruct him to take the mouthpiece out of his mouth and slowly exhale.

He should repeat this exercise postoperatively for five to ten minutes each hour. A 60-second rest between deep breaths should help prevent fatigue and dizziness.

If he has difficulty doing his exercises because of postop pain, encourage him to ask for pain medication and teach him to splint his thorax or abdomen, using a pillow or folded blanket. (See also *Incentive spirometry: children.*)

Incentive spirometery: children

Encouraging use

How do you get a child to use an incentive spirometer? Try this: Make a loop out of one end of a pipe cleaner. Dip the loop into some diluted baby shampoo. Then ask the child to take a deep breath and blow into the loop. He'll love the bubbles—and you'll love his sudden compliance.

Here's another tactic: Use an old-fashioned pinwheel as a substitute for an incentive spirometer. Children love to blow on the pinwheel and watch the colors go round. They can even have contests to see who can blow the hardest. Besides helping the children comply with their respiratory therapy regimen, the pinwheel also promotes social interaction. (See also *Incentive spirometry: adults.*)

Incident report: documentation

What to write

Some hospitals use several different report forms for documenting different types of incidents. However, make sure you do the following when you fill out the form:
• Identify the patient.
• Describe the incident, recording only the facts as you know them, not your opinions or conclusions. Avoid assigning blame or suggesting how the incident could have been prevented.
• Take care to report the incident exactly as you saw it—even if your version conflicts with someone else's. And don't include second-

hand information; each staff member with information about the incident should write a separate incident report.

• Identify all witnesses to the event—including hospital staff, family, visitors, and other patients. If possible, include their addresses.

• Identify by number and manufacturer any equipment and medications you've set aside and labeled according to hospital policy.

• Document the circumstances surrounding the incident.

• Send the report to the appropriate person, according to hospital policy.

If litigation ensues, can the incident report be made available to the plaintiff? That varies from state to state—but the answer shouldn't affect your documentation. At this stage, your only concern is to document the incident as completely and accurately as possible. (See also *Incident report: notification.*)

Incident report: notification

What to do after an incident

No matter what the situation, your first priority is to protect the patient. Call immediately for any help if you need to stabilize a patient's condition. Even if you weren't responsible for the initial injury, you could be drawn into subsequent litigation if your initial response causes additional harm.

If the patient is well enough to speak, ask him to relate what happened. Then call the patient's doctor, so he can give any necessary orders. Except in an emergency, don't consult another doctor just because he happens to be available. Why? Because of the contractual nature of the doctor-patient relationship, seeking advice from another doctor is inappropriate unless the patient's welfare requires it.

Next, notify your manager or an administrator. This gives the hospital notice that an incident has occurred and initiates the incident reporting process. At this point, the hospital becomes responsible for its actions in dealing with the incident as well as for your actions as an employee.

The administrator you contact will help you decide what other staff members to notify. If required by hospital policy, notify the pharmacist whenever a medication is involved so he can help correct the problem and investigate ways to prevent a recurrence.

Not all incidents call for this step; you, the doctor, and an administrator should make this decision.

If notifying the family is appropriate, the next step is to determine who should speak to them. As the patient's nurse, you may be the best choice, assuming that you're familiar with all the circumstances surrounding the incident. But if the incident has upset you, ask the patient's doctor or an administrator to speak to the family.

If you talk to the family, give them a complete, truthful account of the incident, without covering up any facts. But avoid assigning any blame or responsibility for the incident. Explain that the matter is under investigation.

Evaluate the circumstances surrounding the incident. For example, how was the unit staffed? What was happening on the unit at the time? As you may know, the legal standard for evaluating nursing practice is: What would a reasonably prudent nurse have done under the same or similar circumstances?

Keep in mind that nursing actions or omissions that might be considered substandard under ordinary circumstances may be viewed differently in the context of an emergency. For example, one court held that a nurse busy with a complicated delivery was justified in failing to perform a vaginal examination on a new admission because she knew that the patient had just been examined in the doctor's office.

This isn't a time for assigning blame; it's a time for observation and fact-finding while the incident is still fresh in your mind.

Attach a tag to the equipment or medication (including containers and inserts) and follow hospital policy for storing it. Remember, equipment and medications are potential evidence, so make sure the hospital can identify everyone who has access to them. These precautions help prevent alterations or substitutions and maintain each item's credibility as evidence. (See *Legal risks: equipment.*)

But your responsibilities don't end with these steps. You must also document all your findings in the patient's chart, on an incident report form, and—as an extra precaution—in your personal records. (See *Incident report: documentation.*)

Incontinence, urinary

Teaching pelvic-floor exercises

You can help your patient prevent or minimize stress incontinence by instructing her to do simple exercises that will strengthen her pelvic-floor muscles. She can perform them sitting or standing and during various activities, such as reading, watching TV, waiting in a line, and especially while urinating.

Here's what to tell her:

• "Tense the muscles around your anus. This will tighten the posterior muscles of the pelvic floor.

• "While urinating, stop the flow of urine and then restart it. This will tighten the anterior muscles of the pelvic floor.

• "Now that you've identified these muscles, you can exercise them anywhere at any time. As you perform the exercises, slowly tighten each group of muscles and then release them." (See *Sex after childbirth.*)

Incontinence assessment, urinary

Pinpointing the nature and cause

Ask the patient when he first noticed the incontinence and whether it began suddenly or gradually. Have him describe his typical urinary pattern: Does incontinence usually occur during the day or at night? Does he have any urinary control, or is he totally incontinent? If he sometimes urinates with control, ask him the usual times and approximate amounts voided. Determine his normal fluid intake. Ask about other urinary problems, such as hesitancy, frequency, urgency, nocturia, and decreased force or interruption of the urinary stream. Also ask if he's sought treatment for incontinence or found a way to deal with it himself.

Obtain a medical history, especially noting any urinary tract infection, prostate conditions, spinal injury or tumor, cerebrovascular accident, or surgery involving the bladder, prostate, or pelvic floor.

After completing the history, have the patient empty his bladder. Inspect his urinary meatus for obvious inflammation or anatomic defect. Have female patients bear down; note any urine leakage. Gently palpate the abdomen for bladder distention (see *Bladder assessment*), which signals urine retention. Perform a complete neurologic assessment, noting motor and sensory function and obvious muscle atrophy.

Infection control

Recommended precautions

To minimize the risk of contracting or spreading an infection, consider all blood and body fluids as poten-

tially infectious. With *all* patients, use the following precautions recommended by the Centers for Disease Control and American Hospital Association:

• Wash your hands before and after contact with patients, even if you wear gloves. Wash your hands *immediately* if you come in contact with blood or body fluids.

• Wear gloves when you anticipate contact with blood, body fluids, tissues, or contaminated equipment. Change gloves between patients. Wear gloves when handling blood specimens or emptying fluid-filled containers.

• Wear a gown when your clothes are likely to be soiled during patient care and when emptying fluid-filled containers.

• Wear a mask and goggles or eyeglasses if aerosolization or splattering might occur in a nursing or surgical procedure. Wear a mask when caring for a patient with an airborne infection. Private rooms can be used for patients who have airborne infections.

• Place used needle syringe units in a puncture-resistant container located in each patient room. Don't recap needles. (See *I.V. therapy: needle safety.*)

• Bag all linen in a break-resistant bag and tie.

• Treat all laboratory specimens as potentially infectious.

• Report any needlestick injuries to your supervisor and infection control nurse. Go to the emergency department for treatment and fill out an employee incident report.

• When performing CPR, use a disposable mouth-to-mask device for artificial breathing. (See also *AIDS: self-protection.*)

Inhalers

Teaching your patients to use them properly

Inhalers aren't as easy to use as most people think. In fact, a patient may have difficulty using one cor-

rectly unless taught to do so. During an acute attack, his anxiety and shakiness may make using the inhaler nearly impossible.

To make sure your patient knows how to use an inhaler properly, review the following procedure:

• Show him how to assemble the inhaler, then have him assemble it. This way, you can correct his mistakes.

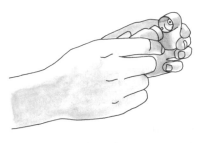

• Remind him to remove loose upper dentures before he uses the inhaler, because loose dentures can fall down and block the sprayed medication.

• Show him how to shake the cartridge to mix the medication.

• Tell him to put the cartridge to his lips and exhale through his nose. Remind him to exhale only enough to get the stale air out of his lungs (so the medication can get in). Forcing air out of his lungs will collapse his airways even further.

• Then, have him press down firmly on the cartridge while taking a deep breath. Stress two points: First, he should breathe slowly and deeply. Rapid breaths will cause the medication to land on the surface of the upper airways; shallow breaths won't carry the medication deep enough into the lungs.

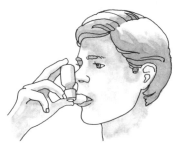

Second, he must press the cartridge when he starts to inhale.

Timing is important. Remind him not to press hard—the dose is predetermined, so only one dose will be released, regardless of the pressure applied.

• Remind him to keep his tongue flat in his mouth. Otherwise, he'll spray medication directly on his tongue.

• After he depresses the cartridge and inhales deeply, tell him to hold his breath and count to 10. This will let the medication settle on the surface of his airways and prevent him from exhaling it immediately.

• Then tell him to exhale slowly with his lips pursed.

• If two inhalations have been prescribed for him, tell him to wait 10 to 15 minutes before inhaling the second time. The first inhalation will open the proximal airways and allow the second inhalation to penetrate deeper into his lungs.

• Encourage him to practice in front of a mirror until he becomes more skilled at using the inhaler. But because practice with actual medication can be dangerous, suggest he either cap the inhaler or practice with an empty cartridge.

• Remind him that all metered-dose inhalers—nonprescription as well as prescription—contain medicine and are potential sources of abuse. Warn him to use the inhaler only as directed and not to use over-the-counter inhalers without his doctor's knowledge. If he finds he needs it more frequently than prescribed, he should notify his doctor.

After the treatment, he should clean the inhaler thoroughly: first remove the metal canister by pulling it up firmly, then rinse the plastic container under warm running water and dry it thoroughly. If the patient takes both a beta-adrenergic bronchodilator (such as Metaproterenol) and a corticosteroid (such as beclomethasone), he should always take the bronchodilator first. This will dilate his airways so he can inhale the corticosteroid more deeply into his lungs.

Injection, intramuscular

Relaxing the muscle

Did you ever notice that a patient usually tightens his gluteal muscles in anticipation of an intramuscular injection? If so, he's in for more discomfort than necessary.

To help divert his attention, ask him to wiggle his toes just before you give the injection. While he's concentrating on his toes, he won't tighten the gluteal muscles, so the injection will be less painful. (See also *Injection, intramuscular deltoid.*)

Injection, intramuscular deltoid

Making it less painful

Use the pinch grasp technique: Grasp the muscle, then pinch it hard enough to cause some initial discomfort. The pressure of the pinch will distract the patient from the injection and therefore reduce the pain he feels. Follow this procedure:

1. Disinfect the deltoid muscle area.

2. Using your left hand, grasp the muscle, then pull it about ½" to 1" (1 to 3 cm) toward you.

3. Apply a pinching pressure hard enough to cause some discomfort. This will make the skin tense and the muscle bulge.

4. Hold the syringe in your right hand, then rest your wrist about 3"

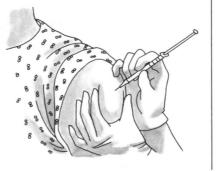

to 4" (7.5 to 10 cm) from the injection site.

5. With the syringe at a 90-degree angle, insert the needle about ½" to 1" into the deltoid muscle.

6. Aspirate the syringe to see if the needle is in a blood vessel. If it isn't, give the injection.

7. Use your left hand to place an alcohol-soaked gauze pad over the injection site as you withdraw the needle with your right hand.

8. Massage the area for 5 to 20 seconds. (See also *Injection, intramuscular.*)

Insomnia

Helping your patient sleep

Here are possible causes of insomnia and ways to counteract them:

• *Acroparesthesia.* Teach your patient to assume a comfortable position in bed, with his limbs unrestricted. If he tends to awaken with a numb leg or arm, teach him to massage and move it until sensation completely returns, and then to assume an unrestricted position.

• *Anxiety.* Encourage your patient to discuss his fears and concerns, and teach him such relaxation techniques as guided imagery and deep breathing. If ordered, administer a mild sedative, such as diazepam, before bedtime. (See *Relaxation techniques.*)

• *Dyspnea.* Elevate the head of your patient's bed, or provide at least two pillows or a reclining chair to help him sleep. Suction his airway when he awakens, and encourage deep breathing every 2 to 4 hours. Also provide supplementary oxygen via nasal cannula.

• *Pain.* Administer pain medication, as ordered, 20 minutes before bedtime. Also teach deep, even, slow breathing to promote relaxation. Help the patient with back pain to lie on his side with his legs flexed. Encourage the patient with epigastric pain to take an antacid before bedtime and to sleep with the head of his bed elevated. (See also *Pain, low back.*)

• *Pruritus.* Wash your patient's skin with a mild soap and water, and dry it thoroughly. Apply moisturizing lotion on dry, unbroken skin and an antipruritic, such as calamine lotion, on itchy areas.

• *Restless leg movement.* Help the patient exercise his legs gently by slowly walking with him around the room and down the hall. If ordered, administer a muscle relaxant, such as diazepam. (See also *ICU noise.*)

Instructions

Writing better ones

Next time you tell someone how to do something, be sure your instructions are clear and helpful. Follow these five guidelines:

1. Don't make step-by-step instructions seem complicated by combining them with a lot of general information. If you need to convey general information as well, write a basic fact sheet for the general information and a separate list of step-by-step instructions.

2. Break the instructions down into specific steps. The more complicated the instructions, the more you need to break them down.

3. Use short, dynamic sentences and imperative verbs; avoid long, confusing sentences. Don't use passive verbs; they can make it difficult to tell who's responsible for the action. For example, if the instructions say, "The injection is to be given at 8 a.m.," the patient wonders, "by whom?"

4. Find a logical order for listing steps that don't have to be performed in order: alphabetical, chronological, simple to complex—but not random.

5. Don't use too many or confusing illustrations. Remember your purpose is to instruct, not decorate. (See also *Elderly patients: discharge planning; Patient-teaching techniques.*)

Insulin preparation

When a patient can use only one hand

How can a diabetic patient, who can only use one hand, prepare his insulin independently? A simple, inexpensive broom clip holder can help.

The clip, available in most hardware stores, holds a standard-size insulin bottle securely and can be mounted on most surfaces with a single screw. It should be put in a convenient place, one that's easy to

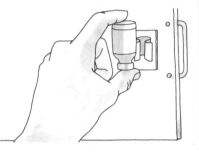

reach: the inside of a kitchen cabinet door usually works well. (Of course, the clip must not interfere with the cabinet door closing.)

Interviewing applicants

Evaluation pointers

A resumé and an employment application tell you a lot about what a nurse says she can do. But they don't tell you what she really *will* do. That's for you to find out during a job interview. Ask yourself these questions about the candidate:

• Are her responses to your questions candid and spontaneous or defensive and guarded? An open and spontaneous person is more likely to be a cooperative co-worker.

• How does she perceive her role as a nurse? Is she merely applying for a job? Or is she motivated by the responsibilities and challenges that define the profession?

• Has her career shown a consistent pattern of achievements? Did she take continuing-education courses on her own? Does she say she wants to enhance her skills in any special area?

Remember, a candidate's qualifications may be dazzling on paper. But unless she can use what she knows, she probably won't be an asset to your staff. (See also *Interviewing technique; Staff management: hiring.*)

Interviewing technique

Asking the right questions

To gather revealing insights from a job applicant, ask questions during the interview that encourage her to talk at length instead of simply answering "yes" or "no." You're inviting a one-word answer when you ask, "Did you like your last job?" You can learn much more about an applicant (and especially about her attitude toward work) by asking an open-ended question, such as "What aspects of your previous job did you like best?" or "What kinds of things bothered you most?"

Here's another open-ended approach: Ask an applicant to discuss her accomplishments. If she's self-assured, she'll probably welcome the chance to discuss them. But if she avoids your questions, she may be revealing either extreme modesty or lack of achievement. Either way, she may not be as assertive as you'd like.

Center your other questions around her reasons for leaving her last job or changing her current position. If her answers seem defensive, she may tend to blame others for her failings rather than take responsibility for failing to improve her performance on the job.

Lastly, check references. Former employers can help confirm or revise your impression of an applicant and, in most cases, can tell you more than you're able to determine from an interview. (See also *Interviewing applicants; Staff management: hiring.*)

Intestinal tubes

How to manage them

When caring for a patient with an intestinal obstruction, you may need to help place an intestinal tube and provide continuing care. Such a tube, used for diagnostic or physiologic studies, most commonly serves to decompress the small bowel. Remember these important points about intestinal tubes:

• Follow hospital policy and doctor's orders regarding tube insertion, care, and withdrawal.

• Place the patient on his right side for tube advancement.

• Advance the tube and change his position, as ordered. Don't anchor the tube firmly until it's reached the desired position.

Miller-Abbott tube

Cantor tube

Harris tube

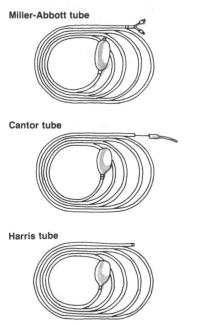

• Drain the tube by gravity during insertion. If drainage stops, inject 10 cc of air.

• Confirm tube placement by X-ray.

• As ordered, attach the suction lumen to intermittent low suction when the tube reaches its mark.

• When withdrawing the tube, remove mercury from the balloon first (if indicated) and remove the tube by 6″ (15 cm) increments each hour or as ordered.

Intracranial pressure: assessment

Correct procedure

Regular and careful neurologic assessment is essential in detecting the early warning signals of intracranial pressure (ICP).

Make sure you always check these five signs during your assessment:

1. *Level of consciousness*. A change in level of consciousness usually is your first clue that your patient's ICP is increasing. Assess his general orientation. (See *Glasgow Coma Scale.*)

2. *Pupillary reactions (direct and consensual)*. Assess your patient's pupils carefully. Keep in mind, however, that about 17% of the general population have unequal pupils since birth; typically, the difference is less than 1 mm. (See *Pupillary reaction.*)

3. *Motor strength and function*. Start by observing the patient's spontaneous movements; then, ask him to follow some simple commands.

Ask the patient to hold your hands and push you away from him; as he does, resist him firmly but without pushing back. Some authorities recommend putting the patient's open palm against yours to prevent misinterpretation of any grasping motion.

To assess his leg strength, place his feet together on the bed, then ask him to push down against your upturned hands—like "stepping on the gas."

If your patient's awake and cooperative and can move all his extremities normally, you don't need

to assess his motor function any further. But if he's unresponsive, try evaluating his response to stimuli.

Start by touching or tickling him before resorting to noxious stimuli. If you must use noxious stimuli, apply direct pressure to his nail beds on each extremity. (Some health care experts recommend firm pressure on the Achilles tendon to test the legs.) Don't use a sharp object to apply nail bed pressure; instead, use a tongue depressor or some other blunt object.

If your patient's responses are normal, he'll either push away the source of the noxious stimulus or pull away from it. If he doesn't, increased ICP may be dulling his brain's ability to respond to stimuli normally.

You don't need to hurt your patient to assess him, so never resort to pinching or sternal rubbing.

If his increased ICP has already caused severe brain compression, your patient may be completely unresponsive to all stimuli. This is also when you may see decorticate or decerebrate posturing.

4. *Vital signs*. Even though increased ICP may be well advanced before it causes changes in your patient's heart rate, blood pressure, or respirations, always include measurements of vital signs in your assessment. For example, you may note decreased heart rate, increased systolic blood pressure, and widened pulse pressure—known together as Cushing's triad. This occurs when other body systems try to do what the brain no longer can: compensate for increased ICP.

Keep in mind that any respiratory pattern irregularity may indicate increased ICP. For example, your patient may be tachypneic at first. But if his ICP continues to increase, he will breathe more slowly and irregularly. These changes result from pressure on the respiratory centers in the brain stem.

5. *Vomiting and headache*. Vomiting (partly due to compression of the vomiting center in the medulla)

and headache (due to increased pressure on pain-sensitive intracranial arteries) are additional clues to increased ICP. (See also *Intracranial pressure: control; Neurologic exam: assessment.*)

Intracranial pressure: care

Preventing an increase during nursing care

Follow these guidelines:
During suctioning
• Maintain the patient's PaO_2 by hyperinflating his lungs with 100% oxygen before suctioning.
• Suction for 15 seconds or less.
• Suction the patient only when necessary.
During positioning
Increased intracranial pressure (ICP) also can occur following patient turning, hip flexion, or positioning against a footboard. Neck flexion, neck extension, and the prone position can increase ICP by obstructing jugular venous drainage. (See *Craniotomy patients; Intracranial pressure: control*)
During other nursing care
Studies show that increased ICP can occur when you touch the patient while manipulating tubing (for example, a nasogastric tube or indwelling [Foley] catheter) or taking his blood pressure. Of course, when you touch him during a painful or invasive nursing procedure (for example, an intramuscular injection), the resulting stress contributes to increased ICP.

You can't help touching the patient, of course—but you can minimize the number and length of times you do so, as follows:
• Keep the blood pressure cuff on the patient's arm and disconnect only the tubing when necessary. Remember not to apply the cuff too tightly.
• Keep intravenous tubing unkinked and supported so it doesn't make the patient uncomfortable.

• Make sure oxygen tubing is long enough to keep it from tugging at the patient's face.
• As much as possible, limit painful procedures, such as multiple venipunctures for blood tests. For example, when you need to obtain frequent arterial blood gas measurements, insert an arterial line.

As a general precaution about touching, always be sure a conscious patient knows you're there before you touch him. But don't forget the enormous value of therapeutic touch in keeping the patient calm—and in reducing his risk of increased ICP. (See also *Intracranial pressure: management.*)

Intracranial pressure: control

Preventive strategies

Patient positioning is your first step in preventing intracranial pressure. Follow these steps:
• Raise the head of the bed 15 to 30 degrees to promote venous drainage from the brain. (A higher head elevation would impair arterial blood flow to the brain.
• Avoid head rotation and neck flexion, which increases intracranial pressure (ICP) by decreasing venous drainage. If necessary, remove the patient's pillow and immobilize his head with sandbags.
• Avoid the use of footboards and hip flexion of more than 90 degrees—both increase ICP.
• Keep the patient as still as possible, without using restraints. (Pulling against restraints may cause him to inadvertently perform the Valsalva's maneuver, which increases ICP.)
• If you must turn him, use the logroll technique to keep his head in a neutral position. Instruct him to exhale while you're turning him to avoid Valsalva's maneuver. (See also *Craniotomy patients; Intracranial pressure: management.*)

Intracranial pressure: management

Minimizing unwanted auditory stimuli

To prevent an increase in intracranial pressure (ICP), be careful what your patient hears. Whether he's unconscious or alert, stress from hearing others talk about his condition can increase his ICP. So can the multitude of strange, even frightening, sounds he hears all around him. Here are some suggestions for minimizing unwanted auditory stimuli:
• Whenever possible and appropriate, speak directly to the patient. Even better, touch him by holding his hand or gently stroking his face. In one research study, these simple procedures actually decreased some patients' ICP.
• Provide as much meaningful auditory input as possible, even for an unconscious patient. Examples include playing soft music (a type the patient's always liked) or having family and friends come to talk or read to him.
• Be sure that any sound-emitting equipment near him is absolutely necessary for his care. If it isn't, ask that the equipment be removed.
• Don't discuss his condition or his care at his bedside, regardless of his level of consciousness. Instead, talk with doctors, other nurses, family members, and friends outside his room or in a private conference room. (See also *Intracranial pressure: care; Intracranial pressure: control.*)

Intracranial pressure: monitoring

What to consider

Your patient's monitoring system will affect the guidelines you'll need to follow. Here are the systems and what to look for with each one.

Intraventricular catheter

• Expect difficult catheter placement if the patient's ventricle is collapsed, swollen, or displaced.

• Monitor patient closely for infections, such as meningitis and ventriculitis.

• Check catheter patency frequently. If catheter becomes occluded with blood or brain tissue, notify the doctor. He may flush it with sterile I.V. saline solution.

• Be sure stopcocks are positioned properly. Incorrect stopcock placement may create excessive cerebrospinal fluid (CSF) drainage, causing a sudden drop in intracranial pressure (ICP) and possible subdural hematoma. (See *Cerebrospinal fluid.*)

• Note any sudden changes in ICP reading. A collapsed ventricle may compress the catheter, causing a false reading.

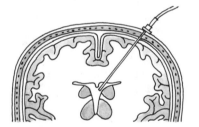

• Recalibrate transducer and monitor frequently.

Subarachnoid screw

• Monitor patient closely for signs of infection.

• Recalibrate the transducer and monitor frequently.

• Check screw patency frequently. If the screw becomes occluded with blood or brain tissue, notify the

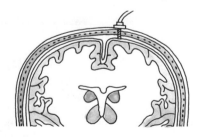

doctor. He may flush it with a small amount of sterile I.V. saline solution.

Epidural probe

• Monitor patient closely for signs of infection.

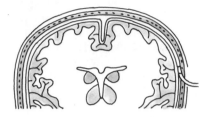

• Be sure the probe's plugged tightly into monitor or pressure module. (See also *Intracranial pressure: control.*)

Itching

Teaching your patient how to control it

Give your patient these guidelines to help reduce itching:

Follow these simple steps:

• "Avoid scratching or rubbing the itchy areas. Ask your family to let you know if you're scratching, because you may be unaware of it. Keep your fingernails short to avoid skin damage from any unconscious scratching.

• "Wear cool, light, loose nightclothes. Avoid wearing rough clothing—particularly wool—over the itchy area.

• "Take tepid baths, using little soap and rinsing thoroughly. Try a skin-soothing oatmeal or cornstarch bath for a change.

• "Apply an emollient lotion after bathing to soften and cool the skin.

• "Apply cold compresses to the itchy area.

• "Use topical ointments and take prescribed medications, as directed.

• "Avoid prolonged exposure to excessive heat and humidity. For maximum comfort, keep room temperatures at 68° to 70° F. (20° to 21.1° C.) and humidity at 30% to 40%.

• "Take up an enjoyable hobby that distracts you from the itching during the day and leaves you tired enough to sleep at night."

I.V. home therapy: screening

Evaluating your patient's suitability

You should be aware of what qualifies and disqualifies a patient for I.V. home therapy. Here are some of the questions you'll have to ask to determine whether your patient is a good candidate:

• Is he medically stable?

• Is your patient or his backup person emotionally stable?

• Does your patient have the motivation to get involved in his own care?

• Will he be able to learn and remember procedures?

• Does he have normal visual acuity and manual dexterity?

• Does he have the appropriate home environment? Is there a clean, dry place to store I.V. supplies? Is the refrigerator large enough to store mixtures? Is the area where he'll do most of the preparation a low-traffic area? Can he move about easily without tripping over something? Are electrical outlets available for hooking up necessary equipment? (See also *I.V. home therapy: start-up; I.V. home therapy: teaching.*)

I.V. home therapy: start-up

Instructions for connecting the admixture

Tell the patient: "You'll need the following equipment: an I.V. bag with medication; I.V. tubing; a 22-gauge needle; a povidone-iodine sponge; and a 1" × 2" (3 cm × 5 cm) strip of tape.

1. "Wash your hands thoroughly and put on gloves.

2. "Hang the I.V. bag on a hook or pole. Remove the blue tab. *Don't allow the I.V. port to touch anything.*

3. "Open the I.V. tubing box and remove the tubing. Slide the roller clamp as near the drip chamber as possible and close the roller clamp.

4. "Carefully open the needle package and remove the protective cover from the I.V. tubing needle adapter. Securely connect the needle to the tubing.

5. "Carefully remove the tubing spike's protective cover. Fully insert the spike into the bag port.

6. "Squeeze the drip chamber. Release the chamber; it should fill halfway with I.V. fluid. (See *I.V. therapy: drip chambers.*)

7. "Open the roller clamp to flush the tubing and needle. Then close the roller clamp.

8. "Open the povidone-iodine sponge and scrub the end of the injection cap for 30 seconds.

9. "Carefully remove the needle's protective cover and insert the needle all the way into the center of the injection cap. If you feel resistance, don't force the needle. Recheck the angle of the needle.

10. "Apply the tape to secure the tubing to your arm. Don't put the tape over the dressing's tape. (See also *I.V. therapy: taping.*)

11. "Begin the infusion."

I.V. home therapy: teaching

Disconnecting the infusion and flushing the catheter

Give the patient these instructions: "You'll need a povidone-iodine sponge and a heparin flush with holder.

"Then do the following:

1. "Wash your hands thoroughly.

2. "Open the povidone-iodine sponge.

3. "Prepare the heparin flush solution; expel air from the unit.

4. "Allow the solution to run down the tubing as far as it will go, until the flow stops.

5. "Close the tubing clamp. Remove the strip of tape that's holding the tubing.

6. "Stabilize the catheter hub while removing the needle and tubing.

7. "While keeping the catheter hub stable, clean the end of the cap with the povidone-iodine sponge for 30 seconds.

8. "Still keeping the catheter hub stable, insert the needle of the heparin flush unit into the center of the cap. If you feel resistance, don't force the needle. Recheck the needle angle.

9. "*Gently* inject the full dose of heparin.

10. "Keep the catheter stable while withdrawing the heparin flush unit from the cap." (See also *I.V. home therapy: screening.*)

I.V. therapy: air removal

Clearing air from the line

Here are the best ways to remove air from an I.V. line.

1. *Tap the I.V tubing.* Pull the air-filled section of the tubing taut. The vibrations will make the bubbles slowly rise into the drip chamber.

2. *Curl the I.V tubing.* Curl it around a pen (or a syringe). Then roll the pen upward toward the drip chamber.

Curling the tubing

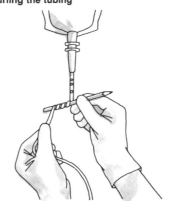

ber. This will force the air up into the drip chamber. Be sure the drip chamber is filled before you remove the pen and release the tubing.

3. *Lower the I.V. bag* below the level of the patient's heart, then open the roller clamp. Blood will flow into the tubing, pushing air into the drip chamber.

4. *Remove air with a needle and syringe.* Attach a small-gauge needle to a 10-ml syringe, then pull back on the plunger a little. Next, use a hemostat to clamp the tubing below the Y connector (and below the air). After cleaning the Y connector, insert the needle. Now, release the roller clamp, allowing fluid and air to flow into the syringe. Remove the syringe first, then the hemostat below the Y connector.

Removing air with a needle and syringe

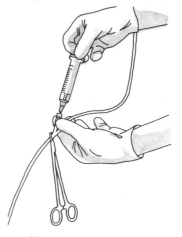

5. *Inject solution into the Y connector.* Attach a small-gauge needle to a 10-ml syringe. Then withdraw 5 to 10 ml of I.V. solution from a port of the hanging I.V. bag. Clamp the tubing below the Y connector and the air. Then clean the Y connector and insert the needle into it. Slowly inject the I.V. solution into the tubing. This will push the air into the drip chamber.

6. *Flush the I.V. tubing.* Put on gloves. Using sterile technique, disconnect the I.V. tubing from the catheter, then immediately attach a heparin lock to the catheter.

Holding the tubing over a receptacle, flush enough fluid to remove the air. Attach a new needle to the tubing. Then insert the needle into the heparin lock and tape it.

I.V. therapy: anesthesia

Injecting a local anesthetic

Although injecting a local anesthetic is controversial, it is recommended, especially if you're inserting a large-bore (20-gauge or larger) needle or if the patient's a child or young adult. A younger, tough-skinned patient is likely to find venipuncture more painful than an elderly patient who has more fragile skin. By anesthetizing the site, you help the patient relax and encourage his cooperation during future venipunctures.

Draw up 0.1 to 0.2 ml of 1% lidocaine hydrochloride (Xylocaine) without epinephrine into an insulin or tuberculin syringe. After making sure the patient isn't allergic to lidocaine, inject the drug subcutaneously beside or over the vein. Inject the anesthetic a little deeper if the vein is deep. Take care to avoid injecting the anesthetic into the vein. Then, perform venipuncture in the middle of the subcutaneous wheal.

If the patient's allergic to lidocaine, administer an intradermal injection of 0.2 ml of normal saline solution. Perform venipuncture into the wheal as soon as it appears, because it shrinks quickly. But remember, a saline injection won't anesthetize the deeper dermis.

I.V. therapy: armboards

Deciding on usage

If you've inserted an I.V. catheter well away from body joints, the patient probably won't need an arm-board. But if it's near a joint, then arm flexion or extension may alter the infusion rate. An armboard will help prevent this.

To test whether your patient needs an armboard, first establish the proper I.V. flow rate. Then, have him perform range-of-motion exercises with that arm. If this makes the infusion rate slow or speed up significantly, apply an armboard. Another way to ensure a uniform infusion rate is to attach the I.V. to an infusion pump.

Use a disposable, lightweight arm-board that's long enough to support both the hand and lower arm, but don't use one that's longer than necessary. To absorb perspiration, cover the armboard with gauze pads or a washcloth. Secure the armboard with two or three strips of double-backed tape covered with a folded 4″ × 4″ gauze pad.

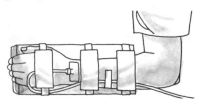

Use as little tape as necessary to hold the armboard in place, and make sure the tape's loose enough to allow blood to circulate freely. Don't tape over the I.V. site. If possible, leave the patient's fingers free.

I.V. therapy: aspiration-irrigation

Doing it properly

Before attempting aspiration-irrigation, try clearing the vein by straightening the patient's arm with the I.V., elevating the I.V. bag and clamping the tubing. Then, firmly squeeze the tubing at a point distal to the I.V. insertion site. This exerts a mild pressure that can promote the flow of fluid through the catheter. If that doesn't work, go ahead with the aspiration-irrigation procedure:

1. Warn the patient that he may feel momentary discomfort at the insertion site when the line clears.

2. Insert a 3- or 5-ml syringe with a 20- or 21-gauge needle into the distal injection port on the I.V. tubing. Clamp the tubing close above the port where the needle and syringe are inserted. Then, after straightening the catheter by stretching the skin area at the I.V.'s insertion site, forcefully aspirate 3 to 5 ml of I.V. fluid into the syringe. Then unclamp the tubing. If the I.V. fluid contains medication, use saline solution instead of I.V. fluid.

3. If blood appears, discard the syringe, then irrigate with a new syringe filled with saline solution. If no blood appears, inject the solution with slight to moderate pressure. Don't force the injection if you feel strong resistance. Try aspirating, then irrigating again. If you still feel resistance, remove the catheter.

4. Reinsert a new catheter if patency isn't established.

An alternative method: Attach a saline-filled syringe (without a needle) directly to the catheter hub, then forcefully aspirate. If bloody material returns, discard the syringe, attach a new saline-filled syringe, and gently irrigate the line.

IV therapy: blood specimen

Avoiding a venipuncture

If you need to draw a blood sample from a patient who has an I.V. line, you can avoid a venipuncture by following this procedure:

1. Use a hemostat to clamp the I.V. line above the injection port for 1 minute.

2. Apply a tourniquet.

3. Insert the needle of a Vacutainer into the injection port and apply a 10-ml vacuum tube.

4. Collect the first 2 ml of blood, then remove and discard the tube.

5. Attach a new tube and collect the pure venous blood that now flows.

If the blood flow is impaired, simply tap the vein at the tip of the I.V. catheter to break the seal between the catheter and vein.

Samples obtained this way can be used for complete blood counts, coagulation studies, cross matching, and most serum chemical determinations. The procedure should not be used to draw blood for glucose or potassium levels if the infusate contains 5% or greater glucose or more than 10 mmol/liter of potassium.

I.V. therapy: catheter embolus prevention

Effective strategies

Review with your staff ways to prevent catheter embolus. For instance, when inserting a through-the-needle catheter, don't pull the catheter back through the needle. If the catheter has a separate hub, make sure it's sutured in place in case the hub becomes disconnected. At each dressing change, check the hub to be sure it's still secured.

Record on the patient's chart the kind of catheter he has, its length, and its composition. (All catheters should be radiopaque.) If it's a through-the-needle catheter, note whether the needle or introducer is still in place; if handled improperly, a needle could sever the catheter, and an introducer could crack. Also, a polyethylene catheter may become stiff and brittle after it's been in place for several weeks, so it should be handled carefully.

If the patient is restless, splint his arm to prevent movement. During dressing changes, be careful not to manipulate the catheter. And when you remove the catheter, measure

it and check the tip to make sure it's intact. (See *I.V. therapy: catheter embolus treatment; I.V. therapy: catheter removal.*)

I.V. therapy: catheter embolus treatment

Emergency guidelines for catheter embolus

What do you do when you remove your patient's I.V catheter and notice that the end is rough and uneven? Also, the patient has just experienced sudden pain at the insertion site and it's edematous and tender to the touch. There's no blood return indicating infiltration. You must remove the embolus immediately to prevent possible death.

Have the patient apply digital pressure on the vein slightly above the insertion site. This may keep the embolus from migrating. At the same time, apply a tourniquet on his arm above his elbow to try to trap the embolus in his arm.

Summon someone to call a doctor while you stay with the patient. Explain to him what has happened, and assure him you are taking care of the problem. Tell him to lie still and especially not to move his arm, so the embolus won't migrate from the site.

Monitor vital signs, arterial blood gas levels, appearance, and specific complaints. Cyanosis, dyspnea, chest pain, hypotension, or tachycardia indicate that the embolus is causing complications—impaired gas exchange, pulmonary artery obstruction, ventricular dysrhythmias, or cardiac tamponade.

Administer oxygen, and start a new I.V. to give fluids and medications as ordered. Have someone call the radiology department to request X-ray films stat. Measure the remainder of the catheter to determine the length of the embolized fragment. Be sure to watch tourniquet time and monitor circulation to the patient's fingers.

When the embolus is located on the X-rays, prepare the patient for its removal by prepping the site and administering ordered medications. Don't give him anything by mouth. If the embolus is still in the patient's arm, it can probably be removed with a loop snare or flexible endoscopy forceps, or by cutdown, requiring only local anesthesia. But if the embolus has migrated to the chest, thoracotomy or mediastinotomy may be necessary, requiring general anesthesia. (See also *I.V. therapy: catheter embolus prevention.*)

I.V. therapy: catheter removal

Proper technique

First, stop the infusion. Moisten the edge of the transparent occlusive dressing with an alcohol sponge to loosen it. Then remove the dressing and adhesive tape.

Next, place a *dry gauze pad* over the insertion site. (An *alcohol sponge* will prolong clotting time.)

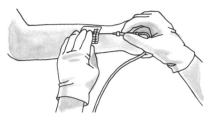

Withdraw the catheter in a steady, straight motion. Apply continuous even pressure until the bleeding stops. Inspect the site for signs of complication. Apply an adhesive bandage strip over the site.

I.V. therapy: clots

Prevention pointers

Here are some helpful hints:
• When starting an I.V., insert the catheter with its tip away from the

arm's flexion and extension areas. This will help prevent catheter kinking and stasis of blood at its tip.

• Use heparin locks instead of slow keep-vein-open I.V.s as much as possible. If your patient must have a keep-vein-open I.V., open the clamp wide for a fast flush—say for 3 to 4 seconds every few hours (providing the increased medication from the I.V. fluid would produce no ill effects).

• Flush I.V. lines or heparin locks with either heparin or saline solution immediately after the infusion of any solution or drug, especially those that tend to precipitate—such as phenytoin sodium (Dilantin), diazepam (Valium), and antibiotics.

• To prevent blood from backing up and clotting in the catheter or tubing, keep the I.V. solution elevated at least 36″ (90 cm) above the insertion site. If your patient is active, he's especially vulnerable to blood backup because activity increases peripheral venous pressure. Also, his movements may cause the catheter tip to lodge against the vein's wall, preventing I.V. flow.

Explain to your patient why he needs to keep his arm well below the level of the I.V. solution and to avoid leaning, lying, or sitting on the tubing.

• Use an I.V. pump or a controller to regulate I.V.s that are difficult to control—in patients with extra-small veins or patients who have frequent blood backups in their I.V. tubings, for example. A controller will alert you to a slowed rate, which could indicate infiltration.

If a controller or pump isn't available, make sure you monitor the flow rate—at least once an hour. This is important for patients whose I.V.s are most likely to lose patency—young adults (who often have strong peripheral venous pressures), patients who have small catheters, and ambulatory patients.

• If the I.V. rate is sluggish despite efforts to improve it, try this: Remove the tape and dressing from the catheter insertion site. Then,

pull the catheter out approximately ¼″ (.5 cm). This helps if the catheter is lodged against a vein wall or located in a valve or narrow section of the vein. Never attempt to push the catheter farther into the vein because that would introduce bacteria into the circulation.

I.V. therapy: complications

Preventing phlebitis and infiltration

The key to preventing phlebitis and infiltration is selecting the proper cannula and the most suitable vein. (See *I.V. therapy: vein selection.*) First, select the smallest cannula capable of delivering the necessary volume of medication. Then select the largest straight vein that's not near a joint.

This smallest cannula and largest vein combination allows maximum blood flow around the cannula, diluting drugs and solutions quickly. And this also prevents the cannula from coming into contact with the vein wall. Selecting a site away from a joint, or course, will ensure that the patient's movement won't cause the cannula to move.

Establish a routine
If phlebitis or infiltration develops despite these precautions, early detection can still protect the patient from serious harm. So, using this routine, begin by checking the level of solution in the container. Then check the flow rate and adjust it if necessary. Next, make sure the tubing isn't kinked or pinched. If a filter is being used, check to see that it's patent and free of trapped air.

Keep in mind that with a gravity controller, the flow rate will change when the patient changes position. So if your patient moves from the bed to a chair, you may need to adjust the drop rate. Of course, phlebitis or infiltration can change the flow rate, too.

Despite what you may have been taught, checking for blood return is not a sure way to determine if the I.V. line is patent or an infiltration is present. (See *I.V. therapy: needle placement.*)

Inspect and palpate the site
Next in your assessment, inspect and palpate the I.V. site. Usually, you don't have to remove the dressing to do so. The first signs of phlebitis or infiltration will develop at the cannula tip, near the edge of the dressing. (If a transparent dressing is used, of course, you can inspect the entire site without disturbing the dressing.) Look for redness, blanching, or swelling. If you see swelling, compare the area on the patient's other arm. Sometimes what appears to be swelling from infiltration is actually dependent edema or even the normal shape of the patient's arm.

One way to determine if swelling results from an infiltration is by using a penlight. Place the light on the swollen area and observe the size of the halo it creates. Then place the light on the same area of the patient's other arm and observe that halo. If the first halo is larger than the second, the swelling indicates an infiltration, because fluid in the tissues causes a greater diffusion of light.

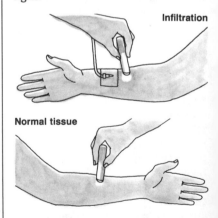

Infiltration

Normal tissue

Next, gently palpate the I.V. site. Pain on palpation is an early sign of phlebitis. Compare skin temperature at the I.V. site to skin temperature of the other arm. Warmth can also indicate phlebitis even before the skin is red or tender. Cool skin, however, may be the earliest sign of infiltration.

In most patients, an infiltration may slow the flow rate, but if a patient has poor skin turgor, it may speed up the rate because resistance is lower in the tissue than in the vein. If you noted earlier that the flow rate has changed, apply pressure to the vein about 1″ to 2″ (3 to 5 cm) distal to the cannula tip. If the I.V. solution continues to flow, an infiltration has developed.

If applying pressure to the vein stops the flow of I.V. solution, this can also be a sign that phlebitis has developed. Usually, though, if phlebitis is severe enough to affect the flow rate, you'll see earlier signs, such as redness and swelling at the I.V. site.

Act quickly

When you detect phlebitis or infiltration, stop the infusion at once, select a new site, and restart the infusion. Then apply warm compresses to the affected area, unless the problem is an infiltration of blood or vesicants. In that case, follow the procedure for the specific fluid that's infiltrated.

I.V. therapy: devices

Various kinds of equipment

Special considerations are necessary with different needle and catheter types. Follow these guidelines:
• *Winged-tip (butterfly) needle.* As a rule, use this steel device only for short-term administration of fluids that aren't highly viscous. (During prolonged I.V. administration, the risk of vein damage and infiltration with this device increases.) Because the winged-tip needle is relatively easy to insert, it may also be a good choice for an infant or child, or for an adult with small veins. But flexible plastic catheters

offer more comfortable and trouble-free I.V. therapy.

Winged-tip needle

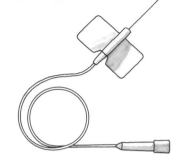

• *Over-the-needle catheter.* This flexible device, capable of delivering any type of I.V. fluid (including blood products), is the best choice for most patients. Available as either a straight or winged-tip catheter, the plastic device is more stable than the steel winged-tip needle and less likely to damage the vein during prolonged therapy.

To minimize discomfort during venipuncture and reduce the risk of complications, use a 22-gauge catheter for most patients. Besides having a small diameter, it's relatively short, so arm movement is less likely to significantly slow the flow rate—particularly when the site is near a flexion area. Use a 24-gauge catheter for infants and for adults with fragile skin or small veins. (You may have trouble inserting such a tiny catheter in older children and adults, who have comparatively tough skin.)

But if the doctor has ordered blood (or any fluid for fast infusion), the patient needs a larger catheter, typically 20- or 18-gauge. Use a 16-gauge catheter for patients being treated for acute trauma, undergoing major surgery, or receiving multiple rapid blood transfusions.

Over-the-needle catheter

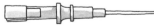

If the patient's I.V. therapy is intermittent rather than continuous, use a heparin lock instead of a keep-vein-open (KVO) line. A heparin lock frees the patient from a con-

tinuous I.V. infusion set and reduces the risk of postinfusion phlebitis as well. (See *I.V. therapy: intermittent devices.*) Don't use a heparin lock with a winged-tip needle because

Short heparin lock

of the risk of infiltration associated with steel needles. Infiltration of the small fluid doses you'd give through

Long heparin lock

a heparin lock may not be detectable until you've given several doses.

I.V. therapy: dressings

Application and removal

Gather the following supplies: an I.V. start pack, extra alcohol sponges, and a transparent occlusive dressing. Then follow these steps.

1. Check the patient's identification bracelet, and explain the procedure to him. Then wash your hands with povidone-iodine soap and put on gloves.

2. Remove the old dressing, and assess the site for tenderness, redness, and swelling.

3. Clean the site with alcohol sponges, starting at the center and wiping outward in a circular motion until the last sponge comes away clean.

4. Repeat this procedure using a povidone-iodine sponge or ampulet (unless the patient is allergic to iodine). Use a gauze pad to blot the excess solution.

5. Apply a small dab of povidone-iodine ointment (unless contraindicated).

6. Check to see that the I.V. device is taped securely.

7. Write the date, time, size and type of I.V. device, and your initials on a transparent occlusive dress-

ing. Then use the tab to peel the dressing halfway from its paper backing. Place half the dressing on one side of the catheter.

8. Pull off the remaining backing while "pinching" the dressing over the catheter. Smooth the rest of the

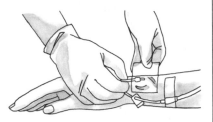

dressing in place. Document the procedure and your assessment of the site in your nurses' notes.

I.V. therapy: drip chambers

Priming them

Two methods enable you to prime a drip chamber and minimize the amount of air entering the tubing—kinking the tubing or inverting the I.V. bag.

To kink the tubing, slide the roller clamp to the distal end of the tubing and close it. This will prevent fluid from entering when you insert the piercing pin into the bag. Kink the tubing immediately below the drip chamber by rolling it back against the chamber. While holding the tubing, insert the piercing pin into the hanging bag. Then, squeeze the drip chamber and release the tubing.

Kinking the tubing

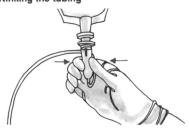

To prime the chamber by inverting the bag, slide the roller clamp to the distal end of the tubing and

close it. Invert the I.V. bag and insert the piercing pin into it. Keeping the bag inverted, squeeze and hold the bottom half of the drip chamber. Turn the bag upright and release the chamber.

Inverting the I.V. bag

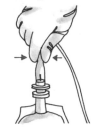

Keep in mind that for some I.V. solution bags (such as the Travenol Viaflex bag), the air inside them must be preserved when the piercing pin is inserted. This air creates a clearer meniscus for reading the fluid level in these bags. To preserve the air, use the steps described for kinking the tubing.

I.V. therapy: drugs

Mixing procedure

To avoid problems and ensure that you have one uniform solution, follow these tips:
• When you add a drug solution to an I.V. solution in a burette or bag, shake the mixture thoroughly to form a new solution. If the drug has a water base, the new solution won't separate. But if the drug has an oil or lipid base—such as paraldehyde—you should shake the solution every 15 to 30 minutes during the infusion. (See *I.V. therapy: volume-control set.*)
• When injecting a drug into a portal site, use a long needle. This helps keep the drug from getting trapped.
• When injecting a dense drug solution into I.V. tubing, keep the patient's arm or hand as level as possible. Also, be sure the tubing doesn't hang below the level of his arm while you're giving the drug. These precautions will prevent drugs from flowing back through

the tubing—a key consideration when using a slow infusion rate.

Next time you mix I.V. drugs, recall these tips. Your patient will receive the right amount of drug at the right time—because you'll have the right solution.

I.V. therapy: flow rates

Calculating them

To calculate the right flow rate for your patient, answer these questions:
• How much solution did the doctor order?
• How much time is allowed for delivery?

Take the amount of solution to be administered and divide it by the delivery time; for example,

$$\frac{1000 \text{ ml}}{8 \text{ hours}} = 125 \text{ ml per hour}$$

Now, decide which type of drip system you're using. If you're delivering a lot of fluid in a short time, use a macrodrip system. The macrodrip, depending on the manufacturer, takes 10, 15, or 20 drops to deliver 1 ml. If you're delivering a small amount of fluid over a long time, use a microdrip system. The microdrip takes 60 drops to deliver 1 ml.

Insert your answers into this formula:

$$\frac{\text{drops per ml}}{60 \text{ minutes per hour}} \times \frac{\text{amount of fluid per hour}}{} = \frac{\text{drops per minute}}{}$$

If you're using a macrodrip system, your equation will look like one of these:

$$\frac{10}{60} \times \frac{125}{1} = \frac{125}{6} = 21 \text{ drops per minute}$$

$$\frac{15}{60} \times \frac{125}{1} = \frac{125}{4} = 31 \text{ drops per minute}$$

$$\frac{20}{60} \times \frac{125}{1} = \frac{125}{3} = 41 \text{ drops per minute}$$

If you're using a microdrip system, your equation will look this:

$$\frac{60}{60} \times \frac{125}{1} = 125 \text{ drops per minute}$$

After you've determined the rate, setting the flow is easy. When you've established your I.V. line, slowly open the clamp to start fluid dripping into the drip chamber. Hold your watch close to the chamber, and time the drips for 1 minute. Open or close the clamp, as needed, to adjust the drip rate. *Remember*: Anytime the clamp slips, for whatever reason, or the patient makes a sudden move, the drip rate may be affected. Be sure to check it periodically, using the method described above. Remind the patient and his family not to tamper with the clamp.

I.V. therapy: flushing the line

Tips on how to do it

When an I.V. infusion slows to less than the desired flow rate, you could spend a lot of time trying to flush it. Instead, try this first: Open and close the roller clamp several times on a section of the tube that hasn't been clamped. This milking action will often return the I.V. to its normal flow rate. Make sure there are no other

Roller clamps

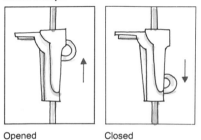

Opened   Closed

signs of infiltration or occlusion before trying this technique. (See *I.V. therapy: clots.*)

I.V. therapy: heparin locks

Patient tips for showering

Cut the fingers (but not the thumb) off a plastic glove. Pull the glove over the patient's hand and wrist,

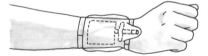

covering the heparin lock with the thumb portion of the glove. Cover the insertions and dressing site with the glove and tape the ends of the glove to the patient's skin. The glove will keep the site dry and will be easier to apply than plastic wrap. (See also *I.V. therapy: intermittent devices.*)

I.V. therapy: infection control

Intravascular device care

The best way to control infection is to wash your hands and put on gloves. Do so before inserting or manipulating any I.V. therapy device.

Use tincture of iodine (3%), iodophor, chlorhexidine, or alcohol to scrub the insertion site for at least 30 seconds. Then let the site dry another 30 seconds before inserting the intravascular device. (Institutional policy may require you to apply an antiseptic ointment to the site immediately after inserting the device.) (See also *I.V therapy: insertion.*)

Unnecessary movement will irritate the insertion site and predispose the patient to infection. To avoid these complications, carefully secure the cannula or needle with sterile gauze and tape or a sterile transparent dressing. Record the date of the insertion and the type and length of the intravascular de-

vice on the tape so that other staff members will know when to change the site. Also, label the tubing and solution container with the date and time.

Maintain a closed system as much as possible. If you must enter the system, disinfect the insertion port first. Avoid flushing or irrigating the system; this can damage the vein or artery and cause clots to break loose in the vasculature. Pressure-monitoring lines are the only exception because they require continuous flushing to maintain patency.

Evaluate the insertion site at least once a shift by palpating around the dressing site for pain. Also, observe the surrounding area for redness and swelling. If the patient complains of pain or tenderness, or if he has a fever, remove the dressing and inspect the site.

Remember that the risk of infection increases after 72 hours. So, change peripheral I.V. sites at least every 72 hours, and even sooner if you detect signs of infiltration, phlebitis, or infection. If you can't change the site because no other site is available, notify the doctor and document your reason for not changing the site. Intravascular devices inserted under nonsterile emergency conditions should be changed as soon as possible.

Change the dressing every 48 to 72 hours. (Total parenteral nutrition dressings should be changed every 24 to 48 hours.) (See also *Central line: dressings; I.V. therapy: dressings.*)

Change the tubing every 48 hours. Also change it after administering whole blood, blood products, or lipid emulsions; cells adhering to the tubing may cause infection.

If you detect signs of purulent thrombophlebitis, cellulitis, or bacteremia caused by the intravascular device, change the *entire system* (including the cannula, tubing, and fluid container) immediately. Use sterile scissors to cut ½" (1 cm) off the cannula, letting the tip fall into a sterile container. Send the tip to the laboratory for culture and sensitivity testing.

Evaluate the patient's vital signs every 4 hours to detect infection. Suspect complications if the patient has a fever or other signs of sepsis. (See *I.V. therapy: complications.*)

I.V. therapy: infusion control devices

Using them effectively

Learning to use an infusion control device (ICD) requires learning how to troubleshoot one. This can help prevent restarts, infiltrations, or equipment failures at a time when your patient needs that infusion. Each ICD should have the manufacturer's operating instructions attached to it. The instructions tell you what causes the alarm to sound and what to do when it does.

Usually, a sounding alarm indicates battery failure, an empty catheter or needle, infiltration, a clogged inline filter, or an improperly placed drop sensor. If you troubleshoot an ICD but still can't stop the alarm, discontinue using that device. Then report the problem to the department that handles equipment repairs or report it directly to the service representative. (See *Legal risks: equipment.*)

When you use an ICD, keep in mind that I.V. bottles and bags are deliberately overfilled to provide for any error. Also, additives increase the volume of the total infusion. So be sure you know the actual volume of fluid to be infused and calculate the flow rate accordingly.

Besides learning to use ICDs yourself, you may need to teach a patient how to use them; ICDs are now available for home use.

I.V. therapy: insertion

Specifics about start-up

Gather the following supplies: an I.V. start pack containing a tourniquet, alcohol sponge, povidone-iodine ampule and ointment, two 2" × 2" gauze pads, tape, adhesive bandage strip, and insertion-site label; an instant hot pack; extra alcohol sponges; an over-the-needle catheter; an extension set; an armboard; and stockinette. Also, obtain the I.V. solution to be infused, hang the container, and attach and prime the tubing and extension set tubing. (See *I.V. therapy: drip chambers.*)

1. Check the patient's identification bracelet against the name on the order and solution bottle. Then explain the procedure to him.

2. Wash your hands and put on gloves. If he's immunocompromised, use povidone-iodine soap.

3. Distend his metacarpal veins by applying the tourniquet about 8" to 10" (20 to 25 cm) above the approximate site. If his veins don't distend, apply a blood pressure cuff and inflate it to a few points below his diastolic pressure. (See *I.V. therapy: veins; I.V. therapy: vein selection.*) Or tap his vein gently, and have him open and close his fist or hang his arm over the side of the bed.

4. If these techniques fail to distend the veins, have him hold a warm, dry compress, such as an instant hot pack, in his hand. When the veins are adequately distended, choose one of the most distal sites for the insertion.

5. Clean the site with alcohol sponges. Start at the center of the site and wipe outward in a circular motion. Use as many sponges as necessary until the last one comes away clean. (See also *I.V. therapy: skin preparation.*)

6. Repeat this procedure using povidone-iodine solution. (If the patient is allergic to iodine, skip this step. Just scrub the site with an alcohol sponge for 1 minute.) Use a gauze pad to wipe off the excess.

7. Hold the skin and selected vein taut below the site to stabilize the vein.

8. Insert the catheter by the indirect or direct method. To use the indirect method (preferred for small veins), first pierce the skin with the catheter's bevel up and at a 15 to 20-degree angle. To use the direct method (preferred for large veins), thrust the catheter through the skin and into the vein with one quick motion.

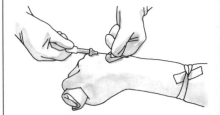

9. Lessen the catheter's angle and gently advance the catheter. You should feel resistance when it reaches the vein wall. As you advance the catheter into the vein, you should feel a "popping" or "giving way" sensation. Watch for a blood return in the flashback chamber.

10. Once you see a blood return or feel the vein wall give way, advance the catheter about ¼" (.5 cm) farther to ensure that the catheter itself (not just the introducer needle) has entered the vein. Then remove the tourniquet.

11. Withdraw the needle. Advance the catheter up to the hub or until you meet resistance.

12. Attach the I.V. tubing to the hub.

13. Begin the infusion slowly, checking line patency.

14. Check the skin above the insertion site for signs of infiltration or hematoma formation, such as swelling and discoloration.

I.V. therapy: intermittent devices

Guidelines for insertion

Gather the following supplies: an I.V. start pack containing a tourniquet, alcohol sponges, povidone-iodine ampulet and ointments, two 2″ x 2″ gauze pads, tape, adhesive bandage strip or transparent occlusive dressing, and insertion site label; a plastic catheter; an injection cap; an extension set; a cartridge containing 100 units/ml heparin flush solution; and a cartridge syringe.

1. Check the patient's identification bracelet against the name on the order, then explain the procedure to him. Wash your hands and put on gloves. Attach the injection cap to the distal end of the extension set and prime it with heparin. Clean the site and insert the catheter.

2. Attach the primed injection cap and extension set to the catheter hub.

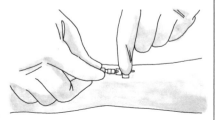

3. Swab the injection cap port with the alcohol sponge. Insert the syringe containing the heparin flush solution and aspirate, checking for blood return. Then slowly inject 1 ml of heparin. Check the site for signs of infiltration. If the I.V. is patent, tape the catheter securely in place.

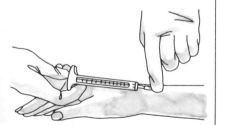

4. Apply a small amount of povidone-iodine ointment to the site (unless the patient is allergic to iodine).

5. Cover the site with either an adhesive bandage strip or a transparent occlusive dressing. Loop the extension set tubing and tape the device in place.

Record the date, time, your name, and type and size of catheter on the dressing or insertion site label.

6. Cover the site with stockinette to protect it. Then record the procedure in your nurses' notes and the patient's medication administration record.

To keep the device patent when no medication is being given, flush it every 8 hours with 1 ml of 100 units/ml heparin flush. (See also *I.V. therapy: devices; I.V. therapy: dressings; I.V. therapy: heparin locks.*)

I.V. therapy: I.V. solutions

Choosing the right one for your patient

An I.V. solution's effect on body fluid movement depends in part on its osmolarity, or concentration. A solution is isotonic if its omsolarity falls within (or near) the normal range for blood serum—from 275 to 295 mOsm. A hypotonic solution has lower osmolarity; a hypertonic solution has higher osmolarity.

Here are some common examples:

Isotonic solutions
• Lactated Ringer's (275 mOsm)
• Ringer's injection (275 mOsm)
• Normal (0.9%) saline (308 mOsm)
• D_5W (260 mOsm)
These solutions expand the intravascular compartment, so closely monitor the patient for signs of fluid overload—especially if he has hypertension or CHF.

The liver converts lactate to bicarbonate, so don't give lactated Ringer's solution if the patient's serum blood pH is above 7.50.

Don't give lactated Ringer's solution if the patient has liver disease, because he won't be able to metabolize lactate.

Avoid giving D_5W to a patient at risk for increased ICP, because it acts like a hypotonic solution in the body.

Hypotonic solutions
• 0.45% saline (154 mOsm)
• 0.33% saline (103 mOsm)
• 2.5% dextrose (126 mOsm)
Administer cautiously: These solutions can cause a sudden fluid shift from blood vessels into cells. This may lead to cardiovascular collapse from intravascular fluid depletion and increased ICP from fluid shift into brain cells.

Don't give hypotonic solutions to patients at risk for increased ICP from cerebrovascular accident, head trauma, or neurosurgery.

Don't give hypotonic solutions to patients at risk for third-space fluid shifts (abnormal fluid shifts into the interstitial compartment or a body cavity)—for example, patients suffering from burns, trauma, or low serum protein levels from malnutrition or liver disease.

Hypertonic solutions
• 5% dextrose in 0.45% saline (406 mOsm)
• 5% dextrose in normal saline (560 mOsm)
• 5% dextrose in lactated Ringer's (575 mOsm)
Because these solutions greatly expand the intravascular compartment, closely monitor the patient for circulatory overload.

Hypertonic solutions pull fluid from the intracellular compartment, so don't give them to a patient with a condition causing cellular dehydration—for example, diabetic ketoacidosis.

Don't give hypertonic solutions to a patient with impaired heart or kidney function—his system can't handle the extra fluid.

I.V. therapy: needle placement

Ensuring good placement

One way to tell whether or not you've correctly entered the vein is by checking for blood backflow. Lower the I.V. container below the venipuncture site. Then, bend the tubing at a point several inches away from the needle or catheter and release it. If the needle's properly placed in the vein, gravity should pull blood into the tubing.

But backflow's not a foolproof indication of correct placement. You could get backflow when the needle's only partially in the vein. In this case, the flow rate may be sluggish when you begin the infusion. If this happens, slightly advance the needle or catheter and check the flow rate again.

You may also get some backflow if the needle pierces the vein's opposite wall. Backflow will be minimal and short lived; however, the absence of backflow doesn't necessarily mean the needle or catheter's improperly placed. A tourniquet that's too tight could be at fault. Loosen it and see what happens. You may also fail to get backflow when the vein's small or when the patient's elderly or has low blood pressure. In such cases, try drawing blood with a needle and syringe from the tubing port. (Remember to pinch off the I.V. tubing first, so you don't aspirate I.V. fluid instead of blood.) (See *I.V. therapy: aspiration-irrigation.*)

Or maybe you can't get backflow because the needle or catheter tip's pressed against the vein wall. If you're using a steel winged-tip needle, try pulling the needle back slightly. If you're using an over-the-needle catheter, withdraw the inner needle first. Then, pull the catheter back slightly.

After beginning the infusion, you can make sure the needle or catheter's placed properly by tightly applying a tourniquet just above the insertion site. If the infusion continues to flow, fluid may be infiltrating surrounding tissue. Stop the infusion immediately and remove the I.V. device. (See also *I.V. therapy: complications.*)

I.V. therapy: needle safety

Protecting yourself

Most accidental needle punctures stem from carelessness: from hasty recapping or inappropriate disposal. Here's how to avoid such accidents:
• Always have someone help you when giving an injection to a restless or agitated patient.
• Never try to force a needle into a full needle disposal receptacle.

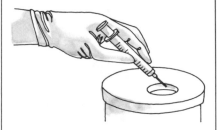

• Change the receptacles regularly. (If possible, assign someone to be responsible for this task each day.)
• If a receptacle is full, tape it securely, then put it in a bag before asking someone from the maintenance department to dispose of it.
• Never return a tray containing used or exposed needles to the central supply department. (See also *Syringe disposal.*)

I.V. therapy: patient teaching

What to do first

Ask your patient if he's had an I.V. before, and try to dispel any fears or misconceptions he has about it.

Tell him why he needs I.V. therapy; how the venipuncture is done; how much discomfort he'll feel.

Do your best to appear self-confident. If the patient senses that you're anxious, he'll feel the same way. Anxiety can trigger vasoconstriction, making venipuncture more difficult for you and more painful for him.

I.V. therapy: pediatrics

Special considerations

Children and I.V.s don't always mix well. For instance, even if a child resists the urge to pluck the I.V. out of his arm, he may bend his arm and inadvertently dislodge the I.V. Normally an armboard should be used to stabilize the I.V. But when one's not available, follow these tips.
Making a splint
Make a splint for the child's arm using tongue depressors. Place some tongue depressors—enough to encircle the child's arm—side by side. Tape them together to make the splint. Cover it with a washcloth, and wrap it around the child's arm and the I.V. site. Tape the ends of the splint together, and it'll keep the child from bending his arm and dislodging his I.V. The splint's lightweight and easy to remove, too.

Another idea is to tape a 1- to 5-lb (0.45- to 2.2-kg) sandbag to the child's arm or leg. The bag's weight will limit movement of the extremity just as well as an armboard and will stabilize the I.V. (See also *I.V. therapy: armboards.*)

I.V. therapy: restraints

Deciding if your patient needs them

A patient who's restless or confused may accidentally dislodge his I.V.

needle or catheter—causing complications such as infiltration and phlebitis. You can usually prevent this and protect the I.V. site by applying a 2″ (5 cm) net stockinette over his hand or arm (cut a hole for the patient's thumb). Or you can apply an elastic, self-adhesive bandage (such as Kling or Coban wrap) over the I.V. dressing; you can remove it easily for dressing and tubing changes. But if these measures aren't adequate, consider asking the doctor to order restraints. (See *Legal risks: restraints; Restraints: precautions.*)

Before applying a restraint, make sure the patient understands why it's necessary. Be tactful—he'll probably resent being restrained.

If his I.V. site is below the antecubital fossa, don't apply the restraint directly to his arm. If he struggles, the restraint could impede circulation and cause the catheter to become clotted or dislodged. Instead, wrap a folded washcloth around his arm and loop the restraint over the washcloth. Tie the restraint snugly. The padding will prevent skin edema and protect the I.V. device from accidental dislodgment.

If you use an armboard, loop a gauze strip around the armboard and tie the strip to the bed frame. (See *I.V. therapy: armboards.*)

I.V. therapy: skin preparation

Proper method

You'll generally start by cleansing the insertion site with a povidone-iodine preparation. But if the site is hairy, you may want to first remove the tourniquet and shave the site, including the area where you'll apply tape. This will help you see the vein more clearly and makes subsequent tape removal more comfortable for the patient. Shaving is controversial, however, so check

your hospital's policy; it may mandate clipping instead.

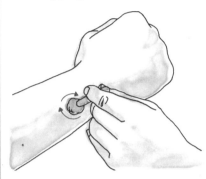

If you shave the site, use a disposable razor and hold the skin taut as you work. Then, reapply the tourniquet and prepare to cleanse the insertion site. (See *I.V. therapy: insertion.*)

I.V. therapy: taping

Securing the line

When you're certain the I.V. line is patent, tape the catheter in place. To use the chevron method of taping, first place a ¼-inch-wide (.5 cm) strip of tape, sticky side up, under the catheter hub. Next crisscross the tape over the hub, toward the fingers. Then place another strip of tape over the hub. Then:

1. Apply a small amount of povidone-iodine ointment to the site (unless the patient is allergic to iodine).

2. Cover the insertion site with a sterile adhesive bandage strip.

3. Loop and tape the tubing so it won't catch on the patient's clothing or bedclothes, which could injure the vein or disconnect the tubing from the catheter.

4. Record the following information on the insertion site label: date, time, your name, and type and size of catheter. Attach the label to the site.

5. If the insertion site is over an area of flexion, use an armboard to

immobilize the site. (See *I.V. therapy: armboards.*)

6. Cover the site with stockinette to protect it and prevent pulling on the I.V. tubing.

7. In your nurses' notes, record the date and time of insertion, the type and size of catheter, the location of the insertion site, and your name.

Remember that the site should be changed every 48 to 72 hours to reduce the risk of complications.

I.V. therapy: veins

When your patient has poor ones

If your patient has poor veins, make it easier on yourself and him by using a blood pressure cuff. Put the cuff on his arm and inflate it to about 100 to 120 mm Hg. This is low enough to avoid rupturing the vein but high enough to dilate it so you can easily insert the needle.

Immediately after you see a backflow of blood, thread the catheter about half-way, deflate the cuff, complete the threading, and securely tape the catheter to the patient's arm.

Another suggestion for a patient with poor veins who needs frequent I.V. therapy is a simple exercise program to build up his veins.

Have him squeeze a small rubber ball in each hand as often as possible every day. In a few weeks, veins should protrude above the dorsal surface of his hands and lower arms, making the I.V. insertion much easier and less painful. (See also *Blood specimen: elderly patients; I.V. therapy: vein selection.*)

I.V. therapy: vein selection

Choosing a good vein

In general, the best sites for I.V. therapy are the hand and lower arm.

Any vein there can accommodate most I.V. fluids; even finger veins can accept an infusion for days. If the patient's obese or has extremely deep veins, a hand vein may be your only choice. When you anticipate that the patient will need long-term I.V. therapy, start low in the hand

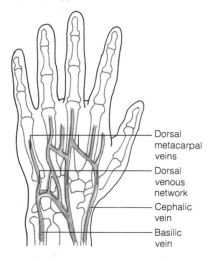

Dorsal metacarpal veins

Dorsal venous network

Cephalic vein

Basilic vein

and advance upward with each successive venipuncture.

Use a larger vein on the lower arm if you're giving a viscous or irritating drug or solution (for example, high doses of potassium chloride, antibiotics, amino acids, or lipid solutions). Because of its greater volume of blood flow, a larger vein is less likely to become irritated.

Try to avoid using these veins:
• the weaker, thin-walled inner-arm veins branching off the tough-walled cephalic and basilic veins.
• the median antebrachial vein on the wrist's inner aspect, sometimes called the "desperation vein." This site's very uncomfortable for the patient; use it only as a last resort.
• a leg vein, because thrombophlebitis or an embolism is likely to develop. This site should also be used as a last resort and may require a doctor's order (check your hospital's policy). If you have no alternative, choose a leg vein that's soft, full, unobstructed, and free of scarring or inflammation.

A site over a joint (for example, the antecubital fossa) is another poor choice for long-term I.V. therapy. To stabilize the site, you'll have to apply an armboard, limiting the patient's mobility and increasing his discomfort. If you choose an insertion site near a joint, make sure the catheter won't rest over the joint after insertion. (See also *I.V. therapy: veins.*)

I.V. therapy: volume-control set

Proper technique for filling one

A volume-control set works well with an intermittent I.V. device. (See *I.V. therapy: intermittent device.*) It delivers a measured amount of medication, then seals itself (using an air-lock mechanism to prevent air from entering the I.V. line). Because it's an alternative to more expensive minibags, it cuts costs.

Gather the following supplies: two 22- or 23-gauge needles, alcohol sponges, adhesive tape, a cartridge containing 100 units/ml heparin flush solution, and a cartridge syringe. Obtain the volume-control set, the I.V. solution (the diluent), and the ordered medication. Be sure you know whether the set has a membrane filter, hinged latex valve, or floating latex diaphragm. Each of these sets has specific considerations. A membrane filter set can't be used to infuse suspensions, emulsions, blood or blood components. Check the order against the I.V. solution label, then check the patient's identification bracelet and explain the procedure to him. Wash your hands with povidone-iodine soap.

1. Close the upper clamp on the volume-control set.

2. Position the lower clamp directly under the drip chamber, then close the clamp.

3. Hang the I.V. solution container. Remove the protector from the spike on the volume-control set

and insert the spike into the I.V. port on the solution container.

4. Open the upper clamp and let 30 ml of solution flow into the metered chamber. Then close the clamp.

5. Squeeze the drip chamber until it's half full. Attach a 22- or 23-gauge needle to the set's tubing, then open the lower clamp to prime the tubing and needle. Close the clamp.

Squeezing the drip chamber

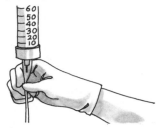

6. Check the medication syringe label against the order. Swab the medication port on the metered chamber with the alcohol sponge. Inject the medication into the metered chamber. Remove the label from the syringe and attach it to the chamber.

Injecting medication into fluid chamber

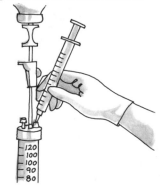

7. Open the upper clamp and fill the metered chamber up to 50 ml (or as ordered). Then close the clamp and rotate the chamber to mix the medication and solution. Check the patient's I.V. site for swelling, redness, coolness, warmth, or signs of discomfort. If the I.V. is patent, clean the port on the injection cap with alcohol. (See *I.V. therapy: drugs.*)

8. Insert the volume-control set needle into the injection cap port. Tape the needle and tubing in place, and open the lower clamp to start the solution flowing. Check to see that the equipment is functioning properly, and adjust the flow rate as needed. When the metered chamber is empty, flush the set. First remove the label. Then open the upper clamp and let about 20 ml of solution flow through the set. Close the upper and lower clamps, and disconnect the tubing and needle from the injection cap port. Then attach a new sterile needle to the set's tubing and hang the tubing over the I.V. pole. With a hinged latex valve set, the diaphragm may stick after repeated use. If it does, close the air bent and upper clamp, invert the drip chamber, and squeeze it. If the diaphragm opens, reopen the clamp and continue to use the set. If the drip chamber overfills in a set with a hinged latex valve or floating latex diaphragm, immediately close the upper clamp and air vent, invert the chamber, and squeeze the excess fluid back into the metered chamber.

9. Flush the intermittent I.V. device with 1 ml of 100 units/ml heparin flush.

10. Record the procedure on the patient's medication administration record and the volume of fluid given on the intake and output sheet.

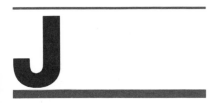

Jaw-jerk test
Checking for trismus

If your patient reports difficulty in opening his mouth, perform the jaw-jerk test because even slight trismus may indicate an otherwise asymptomatic mild localized tetanus. Here's how to elicit and interpret this important reflex: Ask the patient to relax his jaw then slightly open his mouth. Then place your index finger over the middle of his chin and firmly tap it with a reflex hammer.

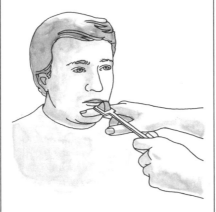

Normally, this tap produces sudden jaw closing. Then an inhibitory mechanism abruptly halts motor nerve activity, and the mouth remains closed. In trismus, however, this inhibitory mechanism fails and motor nerve activity increases, causing immediate spasm of the jaw muscles.

Jaws, wired
Airway maintenance and mouth care

Routine airway maintenance includes keeping the head of the bed elevated 30 degrees or more and observing the patient for increased neck swelling and diminished respirations. For the first 3 postoperative days, have the patient use nasal decongestant spray three times daily. He should wait 4 hours between each instillation to prevent tissue rebound in the nares caused by the drug.

Keep a pair of wire cutters taped to the head of his bed in case of emergency. If he starts to vomit, turn him on his side and suction the vomitus from inside his cheek. If you can't clean his airway and he looks as though he's going to aspirate the vomitus, cut the wires at the middle of his mouth along the bottom teeth. As soon as possible after cutting them, notify the patient's doctor.

Begin mouth care on the first postoperative day by having the patient rinse with saline solution after meals and before bedtime. Tell him to apply dental wax to areas of the mouth and gums that might be cut by the wires. (He must remove this wax before he rinses with the saline solution.)

On the second postoperative day, have him start brushing his teeth. This will toughen his gums, which will be tender from surgery, and keep debris off the wires. He may use mouthwash to eliminate odor.

Finally, before he's discharged, tell him how to make his own saline solution at home by mixing a tablespoon of salt with with a quart of water. If he has a Water-Pik at home, tell him to use it three times a day.

Jaw-thrust maneuver
Doing it properly

If you suspect cervical spine injury, use the jaw-thrust without head-tilt maneuver. Begin by resting your elbows on the surface supporting the victim's head, and place a hand on each side of his lower jaw, at its angles. Lift with both hands to displace the mandible forward. Support his head so that it doesn't tilt backward or turn to the side. If his

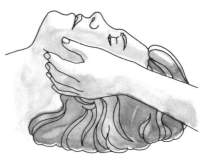

lips close, retract them with your thumb. After opening the victim's airway, check to see if his breathing has been restored.

Job assignments

Coping with the stress of floating

Adjusting to a new group and being separated from your usual team is trying. Here's how to cope:

Act professionally

First, introduce yourself to the charge nurse and tell her your usual clinical responsibilities. Be cooperative and respectful; use a self-assured voice and maintain eye contact. Show your willingness to work. The charge nurse will realize that you're assertive and able to handle yourself.

As introductions are made and assignments are given, assess the charge nurse as a leader and as a resource person. If she has a laissez-faire approach or isn't available as a resource, ask her to designate a specific nurse to help you. You have a right to request this, for the well-being of your patients.

If the charge nurse is autocratic or overly directive about responsibilities you're uncomfortable fulfilling, gently but firmly define your capabilities. Reassure her that you plan to stay in touch with her to offer periodic reports about your work. But don't take her need for information personally. After all, you have the authority to care for patients, but ultimately she's accountable for what happens on the unit.

Clarify your assignment and communicate your limits

Find out as much as you can about what's expected of you on the unit and what the usual routine is. When are meals served? Who takes patients to other departments? What are the visiting hours?

Get a report on the patients assigned to you and be sure that the assignments are appropriate; never accept any you're not qualified to handle.

If you have any reservations about your assignment, tell the charge nurse and suggest an alternative plan. Remember, making safety your first priority protects both you and your patients.

Get the job done

After you've accepted the assignment, make the best of the situation. Approach co-workers in a spirit of cooperation. For example, ask someone to familiarize you with the unit layout and procedures. If you have extra time, offer to help with other patients. Be flexible; integrate your style of doing things with the way the staff does things on the unit. Use your floating experience to learn new things, to share information, and to test your interpersonal and professional skills.

Evaluate how well you did under the circumstances

At the end of the shift, you'll have many thoughts and feelings about the experience. To determine how well you did, consider the dynamics of the situation: What was the atmosphere on the unit? How could you have been better accepted into the work group? What did you need that you didn't get? What was the quality of your patient care?

Job change: planning

Effective strategies

Here are some guidelines for making a job change truly worth your time and effort:

1. *Set goals.* A job change should be part of your overall career plan. (See *Career strategies.*)
• Think about where you are, where you're going, and your short- and long-term goals—both personally and professionally.
• Read career-planning guides, attend a career-planning workshop, or discuss your ideas with a career counselor.

2. *Take stock of yourself.* Match your goals with realistic self-analysis. Ask yourself the following questions.
• What are your strengths, weaknesses, limitations, and interests? List them.

• What kinds of activities do you do best, and why? Independent activities, such as patient teaching or direct patient care? Or highly structured activities, such as intensive care, supervisory activities, and peer education?

3. *Review your present job.*
• Does it offer career mobility?
• Is it challenging?
• Do you get recognition for a job well done?
• Is the job compatible with your life-style?
• Does it offer you support and friendships?
• Are you paid in proportion to your responsibilities?
• Do you like where you live and work?

4. *List what you don't like about your present job—worst things first.* Decide if you can change the things you don't like.

```
GOAL:
TO BECOME HEAD NURSE.

STRENGTHS:
ORGANIZED; ASSERTIVE.

WEAKNESSES:
DELEGATING; CONFRONTING.

PRESENT JOB:
LITTLE CAREER MOBILITY;
AVERAGE SALARY;
CHALLENGING.
```

After following these steps, consider what you'd be most happy with and start achieving that goal.

Job change: relocation

Moving to a different city

How do you line up a nursing job before you relocate to another city? Start by researching the new area.

1. Check a copy of *The American Hospital Association Guide to the Health Care Field* (available in most libraries) to find hospitals in your new location. Then write to all of them about job openings.

2. Read newspapers from your new location to find out which institutions need nurses and which are adding new departments, expanding, or building new facilities. (You can subscribe to most local newspapers or possibly look through them at your public or university library.)

3. Ask the new city's local chamber of commerce for information about the area, including housing, schools, government, businesses, industries, and so on. Some businesses and industries might have nursing positions open. Ask the chamber of commerce for the names of people to contact at those firms.

4. Write to state and local nursing organizations for up-to-date information. Ask if they can put you in touch with a nurse who works in a position similar to the one you're seeking.

5. Write to the state board of nursing for licensing information. In some states, getting your license may take several months. But most states will issue a temporary license if your current one is still valid.

6. Contact employment agencies that have branch offices nationwide. They may be able to provide some of this information free. (See also *Career strategies; Job change: planning; Job-hunting.*)

Job change: resignation

Smoothing your departure

Here are some tips to follow if you're quitting your job:
• Make sure you give enough notice. If you're a manager, you may need

to give at least 1 month's notice. For other positions, 2 weeks is generally acceptable.
• Tell your supervisor before you tell anyone else. She shouldn't find out through the grapevine that you're leaving. You may need her as a reference in the future, so you'll want to leave on good terms.
• Train the person replacing you. Review important policies and procedures to make sure she understands her responsibilities. Show her where to get equipment or supplies she might need. Introduce her to people in other departments she may be working with.
• Don't dwell on the negative aspects of your job change. Let everyone know you're leaving for positive reasons—for example, to move into management or to start your own business. That way, their last impressions of you will be positive ones.

Job change: unit transfer

Transferring to another unit to alleviate stress

Sometimes the only way to relieve the relentless stress of a particular job is by transferring to another unit. But transferring may not be all that easy to do unless you go about it professionally. Here's how to do it properly:
• Put your request in writing, specifying the unit and shift you want. Then briefly list your reasons, keeping the tone positive. Make two copies and keep one for yourself.
• Tell your current supervisor about your request and give her a copy. Maintain rapport with her, even though you hope to leave.
• Make an appointment with the person responsible for transfers in your hospital, and give her your request personally. Explain why you want to transfer—for example, for new or different challenges.

• Follow up on your request in a few weeks to show the supervisor in charge of transfers that you're serious about your decision.
• Be patient; don't expect the transfer immediately. Administration will need time to consider your request, and, of course, you may have to wait for an opening. Even after your request is approved, you may still have to wait for management to find a replacement for you.

Job-hunting

Using a "headhunter"

If you're a manager who wants to change positions, consider hiring an agent or "headhunter" to help you. Follow these steps:
• Commission only one headhunter at a time. Having an "exclusive" will make her work harder to place you. If you're dissatisfied with the results, make a switch.
• Instruct her not to distribute your resume to any prospective employer without your authorization.
• Be honest. If you want to relocate, tell the headhunter why, even if it's because of a "romantic interest." And if you've been fired, say so, and give the reason. A responsible headhunter will treat sensitive information confidentially.
• Ask for advice about your most marketable skills. Remember, your headhunter knows more about the market than you do.
• Don't quit your present position until you have another. Potential employers might question why you're unemployed.
• Give only 1 month's notice to your present employer. This is standard procedure for administration and management positions in nursing. If you feel obligated to stay on longer, a potential employer may hire someone more readily available.
• Be patient. Expect that finding the position you want will take time. (See *Career strategies; Job change: planning; Job interviews.*)

Job interviews

Responding to a recruiter's questions

Here are some suggestions for making your answers match what the recruiter wants to hear.

1. *"What position interests you most?"* Titles vary from one hospital to the next, so don't answer by saying "staff nurse" or "clinical coordinator." Instead, describe the work that interests you.

2. *"What's your work history?"* Start with your most recent job. Or if you're a recent graduate, describe your clinical experience and what you enjoyed most. If you left a position on unfavorable terms, don't criticize your former employer. Tell your side and the employer's side calmly and objectively.

3. *"Why do you want to work here?"* Rather than tell the recruiter how wonderful the hospital is, concentrate on specifics. For example, focus on how you share similar values with those the hospital's reputed for.

4. *"What's your salary requirement?"* The salary for new graduates is usually set. But an experienced nurse has room to negotiate. Ask the recruiter the salary range for the position, and discuss your previous salary only if asked. Also remember that money isn't everything: Ask about benefits and working conditions, too.

5. *"Do you want full-time or part-time work?"* If you're looking for full-time employment and the recruiter has only part-time positions available, find out if you can accept one until another position opens up. If you're applying for a specific position, such as working nights on the intensive care unit, tell the recruiter.

6. *"What are your strengths and weaknesses?"* Be honest. Play up your strengths and play down your weaknesses. After all, the recruiter wants to put you in a position best suited to your ability.

7. *"What can you contribute to this hospital?"* Tell about your special qualities or experiences that you haven't yet discussed. Are you especially skilled at starting intravenous lines, for instance? Explain what you have to offer.

8. *"What would you do if...?"* When the recruiter asks how you'd handle a hypothetical situation, show your decision-making skills. If he asks how you'd manage your work if you were short-staffed, say that you'd quickly assess your responsibilities, decide which were priorities, which would wait, and which you would delegate.

9. *"What are your long-range plans?"* Have a goal—especially one this job can help you reach. You might tell the recruiter "I'd like to spend a few years expanding my experience in medical-surgical nursing. Eventually, I'd like to move into a position in nursing management." This will let her know you want to grow in your work and that you can do so at this hospital.

10. *"Do you have any questions?"* That's the big question. Has the recruiter covered all important details? Are you unsure of any information you've received? When you ask questions, be sincere and enthusiastic. If you don't have questions, tell the recruiter they were covered earlier.

Practice your answers so you can respond confidently. (See also *Interviewing technique.*)

Job negotiation

Techniques for getting the job you want

Use the following tips and techniques to maintain a position of negotiating strength:

• Recognize that, in every negotiation, both the other party and you want something. Therefore, you're as potentially important to the other person as he is to you. If you've done your homework, you'll know what you want. Find out what

the other party wants. Get specifics. The institution is expecting to fill its needs, and you'll negotiate more effectively if you identify what those specific needs are.

• Be positive about what you have to offer — you're very good at what you do and you have the credentials to prove it. Don't be afraid to tell the interviewer what you do well.

• Learn about any "challenges" (problems) the institution is encountering in its delivery of care. Decide how you could best help the institution meet those challenges, and share your ideas with your interviewer. What skill, experience, and enthusiasm do you have that would indicate you're fit for the job? Your prospective employer will be more amenable to negotiating salary, benefits, and working conditions with you if you show the negotiator that you can help the institution in specific areas.

• Avoid dead-end situations. Don't get side-tracked by differences of opinion or feeling. To establish a battleground over a difference of opinion is to lose the negotiation.

• Avoid making the other person feel he's wrong. Your aim is to promote agreement, not argument. Phrases that can help you get past areas of disagreement include: "That's a good point." "It's interesting that you bring that up." "I can see why it would be important for you to do it this way." If you're asked a direct question about a specific subject, say how you feel, but if you don't agree and you're not asked to comment, allow the discussion to move on.

• Ask questions and *listen* to the answers. Write down your questions beforehand, so you won't have to worry about forgetting what you want to ask. Concentrate on what's being said. If something doesn't sound right to you, ask for clarification.

If you anticipate feeling uncomfortable about asking key questions, practice beforehand with a friend. Say out loud what you want to say to the interviewer. If you practice, you'll be more comfortable, and you'll project confidence. And if you're confident when you're negotiating, you'll get better results.

• Don't let a negotiation become a confessional. When you can, help the interviewer consider your weakness in a positive light. You might say, "I'm a terrible workaholic. I tend to get so caught up in following a patient that I forget to go to lunch." Stay away from any form of negative admission. However, if there are specific negatives — in your references, for example — discuss them honestly.

• Don't fall into the trap of thinking of yourself as unequal, or of thinking the doctors and administrators are in control. Temerity in negotiating only perpetuates these feelings of inferiority. So negotiate for your own good. You're worth it! Know what you do well. Know why you're special. Figure out how you'll be an asset to the organization, and communicate it.

A last word of advice: Don't go into a negotiation acting as if your life depended on it or as if the outcome was cast in stone. One bad interview or one bad job selection doesn't have to blight your entire career.

As the negotiating session comes to a close, be sure to recap the important points you covered, such as salary range, working hours, shift, and benefits.

Job termination

When you're wrongfully discharged

Unless you're protected by an individual or collective contract, your employer has the power to fire you without cause at any time. This action is based on the common-law principle of "terminable at will." On the other hand, the legal principle of retaliatory or wrongful discharge has evolved rapidly in the last few years. Courts have awarded damages to employees who were discharged for refusing to commit an unlawful act, for exercising or seeking to exercise a legal right or privilege, and for whistle-blowing on improper conduct.

In short, if you're ever fired for taking a stand, talk to a lawyer about the legal principles that protect your professional principles. A person of honor shouldn't be easy to dismiss. (See also *Legal risks: wrongful discharge.*)

Jugular venous pressure

Identifying jugular pulsations

Remember that patient positioning affects jugular pulsations, but not carotid pulsations, as follows:

• If the patient is supine, his jugular veins will be visible (or "distended") up to the angle of the jaw.

• If the patient's upper body is raised 45 degrees, the blood column should extend about halfway up the jugular vein. In other words, the top of the blood column, where you'll see the pulsations, is usually visible ¾" to 1" (2 to 3 cm) above the sternal angle. With the patient in this position, the upper normal limit for jugular venous pulsations has been estimated at 1¾" (4.5 cm) above the sternal angle.

• If the patient is standing or sitting with his upper body erect, you won't normally be able to see the top of the blood column in the jugular vein. If the top of the column is visible, it indicates increased right atrial pressure.

To measure jugular venous distention (JVD), you'll need a penlight and two rulers. Raise the head of the bed 45 degrees. Shine the penlight tangentially across the side of the patient's neck to get the best possible view of the jugular vein. Line up the bottom edge of the second ruler with the top of the nickel-sized area of pulsations in the jugular vein.

Next, take the centimeter ruler and place it alongside the second ruler, perpendicular to it, at the level of the sternal angle. The distance between the second ruler and the sternal angle, as measured on the centimeter ruler, is the degree of JVD.

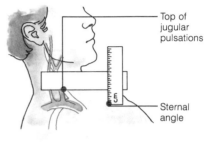

Top of jugular pulsations

Sternal angle

As an example, you might chart "internal jugular measures 1½" (4 cm) above sternal angle with patient at 45 degrees."

Since the distance between the sternal angle and right atrium in most patients averages about 2" (5 cm), you can use your JVD measurement to obtain a rough approximation of central venous pressure by adding 2" to it. Central venous pressure, remember, is the pressure within the right atrium, which can be measured directly through catheterization. Normally, it's 4 to 12 cm H_2O.

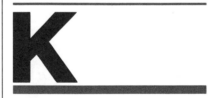

Kidnapping

Safeguarding pediatric patients

Here are some tips you can pass along to parents. Tell them to:

• have their child fingerprinted by local police

• take frequent photographs of their child for up-to-date identification

• avoid putting their child's name on toys and clothing (If a stranger calls a child by his first name, the child may think that person knows him.)

• never leave their child unattended in a car

• put tags inside their child's shoes with his name, address, and telephone number

• give their child a card with a quarter taped to it and the emergency number 911. (The child should carry this card with him at all times.)

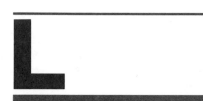

Lacerations: emergency care

Dealing with glass cuts

When accident victims come to the emergency department covered with small glass particles, remove the glass with a wall suction unit. Turn the unit on to medium or low and gently pass the suction tubing over the glass-covered area. Afterward, throw away the tubing and carefully clean out the suction bottle.

Another way to remove small glass fragments is to gently brush them with a towel. If that doesn't remove all of them, wrap a piece of adhesive tape—with the sticky side out—around the fingers of one hand. Then lightly touch the tape to the patient's skin. The glass will lift right off and won't fall onto the stretcher or floor.

Lacerations: tendon damage

Testing for it

When your patient's had a major laceration of his hand or arm, be sure to check for hidden tendon damage. Why? Because untreated tendon damage can lead to per-

manent deformity.

You should always test a lacerated hand for deep and superficial tendon damage. Begin by asking your patient to spread his fingers apart; then ask him to make a fist. This test assesses *general tendon function*.

Next test *deep tendon damage* by immobilizing the proximal interphalangeal joint of your patient's

Testing for deep tendon damage

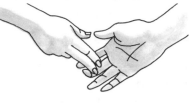

lacerated finger. Then ask him to flex the finger. If he can't, he may have deep tendon damage.

Now, test for *superficial tendon damage* by immobilizing the two fingers on either side of the patient's

Testing for superficial tendon damage

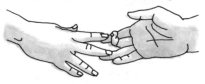

middle finger. Then ask him to wiggle the middle finger. If he can't, he may have damage.

Laminectomy, lumbar

Preoperative patient teaching

Expect the patient hospitalized for a lumbar laminectomy to have mixed emotions. Support his hopes while you help relieve his fears and anxiety with thorough teaching.

Start by explaining what the surgery will accomplish. Using a model of a herniated disk, show him how the extruded material presses on the spinal nerves, causing back pain and sometimes pain and tingling down the legs. Explain that the surgeon will make an incision, remove a small piece of bone from

the vertebra to expose the disk, then open the disk's capsule and remove the herniated material along with any bone fragments. He'll finish by closing the incision and applying a dressing.

Herniated disk

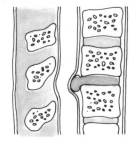

After answering the patient's questions, teach him what he'll need to do after surgery. First, explain that he'll have to deep-breathe and cough about every 2 hours after surgery.

Next, teach him how to turn in bed. Explain that turning is necessary to lessen pain and prevent pneumonia, and reassure him that, done correctly, it won't injure his back. Tell him to make sure the bed is flat. He should turn his body as a unit, keeping his shoulders and hips aligned. After he turns, he should place a pillow between his knees—he'll be more comfortable that way. Explain that you'll help him turn the first few times after surgery.

Give him the following instructions on how to get out of bed after surgery (explain that two nurses will help him the first time):

• "Lying on your back, move as close to the edge of the bed as possible. Then turn on your side, facing the edge.

• "Use the hand control to raise the head of the bed as far as you can without discomfort.

• "Use the arm you're lying on to push yourself away from the head of the bed while you swing your legs over the side.

• "Keep your back straight and push down on the bed with your hands and arms to steady yourself. Then use your thigh muscles to stand up."

Watch the patient practice turning and getting out of bed.

When your patient's discharged, make sure he understands how to practice proper body mechanics. Finally, reassure him that his recovery should be steady: Each day, he should feel stronger and have less discomfort.

Laryngectomy patients

Valuable communication techniques

The best approach is to start early and go slowly. For example, before surgery, tell the patient that he'll be communicating by writing or drawing. Then, immediately after surgery, have him use a pen and paper or a Magic Slate (See *Communication: respirator patients.*) If he can't write English, ask him to draw pictures so you'll have some idea what he's trying to tell you.

When he's able to speak again, you'll probably have trouble understanding his esophageal speech. It'll be quieter than normal speech and, at first, far less intelligible. But here are some tips that will help you understand him better:
• Close the door to the room to make sure the environment is as quiet as possible before you attempt to communicate with him.
• Watch his lips carefully as he speaks. Because a laryngectomy does not affect articulation, his lip movements will provide clues to what he's saying.
• If you don't understand him, repeat what you think he's saying and ask if you're right. If you're not, ask him to repeat the message.
• Don't talk to him as though he's a child. Remember, he can still understand you as well as he could before his surgery.

To make communication easier, the same nurse should work with the patient every day. (See also *Emergency tapes.*)

Laryngospasm

Emergency intervention

If your patient's larynx goes into spasm while you're performing tracheal suctioning, what should you do? Leave the suction catheter in place. Small as it is, it's the patient's only airway.

Then call for help, and tell whoever responds to page the anesthesiologist and the patient's surgeon. Keep the head of his bed raised (as long as vital signs allow). Stay with him and try to calm him. Anxiety and movement will increase oxygen demand.

Administer oxygen, but don't attach oxygen tubing to the suction catheter, because then the patient won't be able to exhale. Place an oxygen mask over his face so that the end of the catheter is within the mask.

While you check his vital signs, ask someone else to get supplies for endotracheal intubation and tracheotomy—either procedure may be required. You'll need endotracheal tubes of various sizes (including a pediatric tube, because the constricted airway may not allow passage of an adult-size tube), a laryngoscope, tape to secure the tube, and a tracheotomy tray. See that suction apparatus and catheters are also at hand.

When the doctors arrive, they'll assess the patient's condition to determine what action to take. If the spasm has subsided, the anesthesiologist will remove the suction catheter while the surgeon stands by, ready to perform an emergency tracheotomy in case laryngospasm recurs.

Once the catheter is removed, an endotracheal tube will be inserted to provide a larger and more stable airway—if the larynx doesn't go into spasm again. If laryngospasm occurs when the catheter is removed, or if the patient goes into respiratory arrest, an emergency

tracheotomy will have to be performed at the patient's bedside.

Even if an endotracheal tube is succcessfully inserted, the patient will have to have a tracheotomy, but it can be done later in the operating room. The procedure is necessary because the endotracheal tube would further irritate the larynx, and the patient could again develop laryngospasm when he's extubated. The tracheostomy will ensure an airway if this occurs. It will also give the vocal cords a rest while providing access for removal of secretions. (See also *Endotracheal tubes: insertion.*)

Lavage, gastric

Ensuring good technique

First you'll need:
• a lavage setup (two calibrated containers or bottles, three pieces of large-lumen rubber tubing, a Y connector, and a hemostat)
• a container of irrigating solution
• an I.V. pole
• water soluble lubricant or anesthetic ointment
• an Ewald tube (#28 to #36 French) for poisoning or drug overdose, or a Salem pump or Levin tube (#18 French) for gastric or esophageal bleeding
• a stethoscope
• ½" (1 cm) hypoallergenic tape
• optional: two bath basins or graduated containers filled with ice (for gastric or esophageal bleeding), and a 50-ml bulb or catheter-tip syringe.

1. Prepare the lavage setup by connecting one piece of large-lumen rubber tubing to the container of irrigating solution. Attach the other end of tubing to the Y connector, which should be upside down. Then attach the remaining two pieces of rubber tubing to the other ends of the connector.

2. Place the lower end of one of the two pieces of tubing into one of the calibrated containers or bottles.

(Later, you'll connect the other piece of tubing to the patient's nasogastric (NG) tube.) Attach the hemostat to the tube that's connected to the solution container.

3. Suspend the entire setup from the I.V. pole, hanging the solution container at the highest level. To prevent a drop in the patient's body temperature, warm the irrigating solution before filling the bottle. Lubricate the end of the NG tube with the water-soluble lubricant or anesthetic ointment.

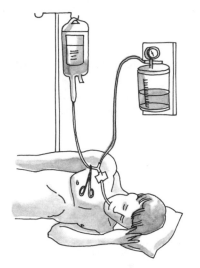

4. Explain the procedure to the patient, provide privacy, and wash your hands.

5. Insert the NG tube, and check its position by injecting about 30 cc of air and auscultating the patient's stomach with the stethoscope. If the tube's in place, you'll hear air being injected into the stomach.

6. After making sure the inflow tube is clamped, connect the remaining piece of tubing to the NG tube. Allow stomach contents to empty into the drainage bottle before instilling any irrigating solution. This will help confirm proper tube placement. It'll also decrease the risk of overfilling the stomach with irrigating solution and inducing vomiting. If you're using a disposable irrigation set, aspirate stomach contents with a 50-ml bulb or catheter-tip syringe before instilling the irrigation solution.

7. After confirming proper tube placement, remove the hemostat from the inflow tube and clamp it on the outflow tube.

8. Begin gastric lavage by instilling 250 ml of irrigating solution to evaluate the patient's tolerance and to prevent vomiting.

9. Remove the hemostat from the outflow tube and clamp the inflow tube. This will allow the irrigating solution to flow out. If you're using the disposable irrigation set, aspirate the irrigating solution with the syringe and empty it into a graduated container. Record the amount of outflow to make sure it at least equals the amount of irrigating solution you instilled. This will prevent accidental stomach distention and vomiting. If the amount drained is significantly less than the amount instilled, reposition the patient or the tube until sufficient solution flows out.

10. Repeat the procedure, increasing the amount of irrigating solution to 500 ml.

11. Repeat this inflow-outflow cycle until the returning solution becomes clear. This will mean the stomach's been emptied of all harmful substances or bleeding has stopped.

• If ordered, remove the NG tube.

Lawsuits: torts

What you need to know

Most lawsuits against nurses fall into the tort category. If you're ever a defendant in a lawsuit, you'll find that the various distinctions within this broad legal category can make a big difference to you.

The general legal definition of a tort is a "civil wrong." But a more comprehensive definition is "any action or omission that harms somebody." You've probably heard the term "malpractice" more often: It refers to a "tort committed by a professional acting in his or her professional capacity."

Nursing errors are characterized as ordinary torts in some jurisdictions and as malpractice in others. If an error is characterized as malpractice, the plaintiff will usually have to get one or more experts to testify on his behalf about the "professional" duty you (as the defendant) owed him. If the error is considered an ordinary tort, the plaintiff may not have to locate and pay for any experts to testify. The testimony of ordinary (that is, nonexpert) witnesses like the patient himself may be sufficient to prove his case. (See *Testifying: expert witness; Testifying: preparation.*)

You also need to know about two other distinctions within the tort category: *negligent* versus *intentional.* Most malpractice cases involve *negligent* torts—accidental omissions or incorrect actions. Practically speaking, what that means is that if someone sues you for negligence, he as the plaintiff must prove four things in order to win:

1. That you owed him a specific duty. In nursing malpractice cases, this duty is equivalent to the local or specialty standard of care.

2. That you breached this duty.

3. That the plaintiff was harmed. The harm can be physical, mental, emotional, or financial. It also must be given a financial value, called "money damages." The nature and the amount of the damages must be proved to the jury.

4. That your breach of duty caused the harm.

Occasionally, a malpractice case involves an *intentional tort.* In this kind of case, the plaintiff doesn't need to prove that you owed him a duty. The duty at issue (for example, not to touch people without their permission) is defined by law, and you're presumed to fulfill this duty. The plaintiff must still prove that you breached this duty, however, and that the breach caused him harm.

The most common intentional tort alleged against hospital staff is battery (unpermitted touching). These cases usually stem from operating room errors, such as performing nonemergency surgery without the consent of the patient (or his responsible adult relative or guardian).

Note that when lawyers use the word "intentional" in a noncriminal case they don't mean that the defendant meant to do harm. "Intentional" here indicates that you "meant to perform the complained-of action," whether or not you also meant to hurt the patient.

At times an action that is considered an intentional tort in some jurisdictions will be considered negligence in others.

Again, what difference does it make?

No difference, when a jury is calculating compensatory money damages. But the characterization of the action can determine whether the plaintiff can get punitive or exemplary damages. These kinds of damages are awarded for intentional torts and "willful" or "gross" negligence but not for simple negligence. (See also *Legal help; Malpractice settlement.*)

Leadership skills

Sharpening them

Being a nurse means being a leader, regardless of your title, salary, or educational background. Even if you don't consider yourself a natural leader, you can learn to lead more confidently. Follow these steps:
1. *Get reacquainted with yourself.* List your strengths. Are you honest? Assertive? Experienced? Now list your weaknesses. Do you talk too fast? Avoid delegating responsibility? Rarely listen to what others say?

Take time to appreciate your strengths, to assess how much you've grown. Then, choose one or two weaknesses to work on and set realistic goals for improvement.

2. *Believe in others.*
Nurses often seem to doubt each other's abilities. And such doubts have a way of reinforcing themselves: The more we doubt, the more we find to doubt. Luckily, this process can work the other way too: The more we believe in each other, the higher expectations we have of each other. This tends to boost everyone's performance.
3. *Listen actively.*
A good leader must be flexible and open-minded enough to listen to suggestions without feeling threatened. Make sure you concentrate fully on what the other person is saying, *not* on how you're going to answer. Watch expressions and body language too—they might contain a hidden message that needs a response. Good listening will gain you more respect as a leader. (See *Listening to co-workers.*)
4. *Set common goals.*
You and your co-workers should agree on the basic goal of your work. No matter what your staff position, accept your responsibility to help define that goal. And don't give up if everyone seems to want something different. You may discover that you can uncover a single common goal among many different ones.
5. *Capitalize on people's strengths.*
A good leader lets others work independently and be responsible for their actions. To decide whether a staff member is competent to handle certain specific tasks, look at the results of what she's done. For example, if you assign a staff member to insert a Foley catheter, evaluate her skill at performing the task. Were her actions confident, smooth, and successful? How much supervision did she need? If your evaluation is positive, you can feel confident giving her this task in the future.
6. *Set priorities efficiently.*
Every day, you're faced with multiple—and sometimes conflicting—demands for your time and skills. So, planning and setting priorities can help you meet those

demands. List all the day's tasks, then rank them in order of importance or priority. For example, you might rate a dying patient's need for companionship higher than the need to have fresh water for other patients at 2 p.m.
7. *Keep a positive attitude.*
Whatever your position, the environment you help create can affect your co-workers' performance. Show them you're eager to do a good job no matter what's happening in your personal life. Your enthusiasm—especially in the face of adversity—will inspire and support them. And *that's* leadership.

Being a leader isn't always easy or obvious. But if you keep these steps in mind, you'll not only feel better about yourself, you'll set an example that others will *want* to follow. (See also *Leadership strategies.*)

Leadership strategies

Dealing with objections

When you're trying to get people to see your point of view, you're bound to meet some resistance. But you can learn how to overcome it and sell your ideas by knowing how to respond to your challenger. Follow these steps to keep control of the discussion:
1. *Relax.* If you're sitting down, sit back in your chair. Avoid frowning or looking displeased. A relaxed posture and expression will make you appear confident and open to the other person's point of view.
2. *Listen.* This is the hardest advice to follow when someone's giving you a hard time. But listening serves two important purposes: It's a courtesy that compliments the other person, making him more likely to want to give in. And it's the only way you'll find out whether you've analyzed the other person's resistance correctly. (See *Listening to co-workers.*)
3. *Agree.* Not with the other person's reasons for rejecting your idea,

of course, but with his feelings. Remember, you have to deal with his anxiety before he can deal with your suggestion. "Yes, I can understand that it's a problem...."I can see why you feel that way...."

One result of your supportive response may be that, as he elaborates on his feelings, he'll realize that they are feelings, not logical objections to your suggestions.

4. *Stay with your main idea.* You've probably had the experience of losing your way during an exchange of views with a colleague. Suddenly, you're talking about something else. What happened? You shifted from stressing your main idea to answering the other person's objections: You stopped "selling" what you wanted and started "buying" the other person's reason for not doing it.

Next time someone interrupts your presentation with an objection, nod slightly to show that you've heard it, then move on to your next point. Besides ensuring that you get to complete your presentation, moving on may divert the other person so he never brings up his objection again.

5. *Make the other person's objection work for you.* After completing your presentation, listen to each objection, dealing first with the person's feelings, then with the objection itself. Then try to ensure that even if you can't satisfy all objections, you still have a chance to get what you want: "If I can get everyone else to agree, how would you feel about going ahead with my suggestion?"

Some people promise to consider your idea, but never seem to get around it. Other people quickly agree with your idea, but every time you check back with them, they come up with a new objection. If you can't get an immediate decision, get a firm date when it will be made. Don't settle for "I'll let you know." If you don't get an answer by the date promised, follow up. Even a "no" is better than nothing. At least then you can pick yourself up and

start over. (See also *Staff management: group dynamics; Staff management: problem solving.*)

Legal help

Finding a good attorney

Suppose a patient sues you, and you don't have an attorney. If you work for a hospital and the patient sues the hospital too, the hospital's insurance company will handle the case, supplying an attorney to defend you as the hospital's employee.

But what if the patient sues you alone? First, contact your professional liability insurance agent; your insurance company will probably appoint an attorney to defend you. But if you don't have insurance or you're not satisfied with the attorney the insurance company provides, or if the company doesn't cover you, here's how to find an attorney experienced in nursing malpractice cases.

1. If you work in a hospital with a legal services department, find out if the hospital will provide you with an attorney or refer you to one.

2. If you have a relative or friend who is an attorney or a judge, ask him for a referral.

3. If you belong to a professional association, ask if it can refer you to an attorney.

4. If none of these situations apply to you, contact your local bar association, listed in your phone book, for a referral. Ask for an attorney who's experienced in medical malpractice cases.

Legal risks: advice

When neighbors ask your opinion

When you respond to a neighbor's or friend's request for your professional advice, you may be setting up a nurse-patient relationship. This happens when you know (or ought to know) that the person will

act on your advice or be affected by your assistance.

Once your assistance or advice has created this relationship, you've assumed a legal duty to the neighbor-patient, and he may successfully sue you if you don't live up to it.

Your legal duty can be summed up this way: *You must help your neighbor in the same manner as would the average, reasonable, and prudent nurse in the same or similar circumstances.* If you fail to meet these standards and—as a reasonable foreseeable result—your neighbor is injured, it's considered negligence.

How can you minimize your risks? Because you can be held responsible for nursing negligence when you help people away from your job, you ought to find out whether your employer's malpractice insurance covers you off duty.

Even if you carry your own malpractice insurance, don't assume that your policy provides off-duty coverage. If your policy doesn't cover you off duty, you'll have to decide whether you want additional insurance. (See *Liability insurance.*) To minimize your off-duty risks, take these precautions:

• Don't express an opinion or offer assistance unless you're experienced and up-to-date in that field of nursing.

• Don't give medical advice when serious or permanent injury could result if your advice is wrong. Anytime there's danger of permanent injury, encourage your neighbor to call a doctor.

• Don't encourage anyone to contravene his doctor's orders. If you or your neighbor-patient is unhappy about his medical care, encourage him to talk with his doctor or seek a second opinion.

• Don't guess. If you're uncertain, encourage your neighbor to see a doctor.

• Don't allow your neighbor to rely on you for more than first aid or traditional nursing care and certainly not for regular medical care. (see *Good Samaritan acts.*)

Legal risks: dispensing

Protecting yourself from practicing phamacy

How can you avoid dispensing drugs—and avoid a charge of practicing pharmacy without a license? Follow these guidelines:
• Never take a container of medication from the pharmacy after hours for use on a unit.
• Never refill empty containers.
• If you work in an institution that allows patients to go on weekend and day trips, don't ever place medication in a container you've labeled so the patient can take it while he's away. (Even though this is common practice in many hospitals, you're on shaky legal ground if you do it.) Instead, plan ahead so the *pharmacist* can fill the medication order before the patient leaves.
• To avoid having to refill stock medication containers, make sure you order adequate supplies during pharmacy hours.
• If you find that you or your supervisor must frequently enter the pharmacy after hours to fill new drug orders or refill stock orders, discuss your concerns with your director of nursing. (She may not know about the situation.) Then, ask her to meet with the hospital's pharmacy director to try to improve pharmacy staffing—or at least to arrange to have a pharmacist on call for emergency drug orders.

Legal risks: doctors' orders

Five orders you should question

Are you sure you're legally safe when you follow direct orders of an attending doctor? Protect yourself by questioning these orders:
1. Ambiguous orders. Follow your hospital's procedure for clarifying ambiguous orders or questioning orders that seem inappropriate, and document your actions. If your hospital doesn't have a step-by-step procedure, ask for one that clearly defines correct nursing action in such situations.
2. Orders that a patient questions. If your patient protests that his medication order has been changed, be sure to check with his doctor.
3. Orders if the patient's condition has changed. Nurses have a duty to report any significant changes in a patient's condition—whether the doctor requests that information or not. So, you should also discontinue treatment that's affecting the patient adversely until the situation's clarified.
4. Standing orders if you're inexperienced. If you know you don't have enough experience to exercise proper judgment, contact the prescribing doctor for guidance in deciding when to follow the order; she can then delegate the responsibility to a more experienced nurse.
5. Verbal orders. To minimize your risks in taking telephone orders, see *Telephone orders*. (See also *Doctors' orders; Medication orders by nonphysicians.*)

Legal risks: ED

Important guidelines

In the emergency department (ED) you're expected to meet the same standard of care any reasonable and prudent nurse with similar education and experience acting in a similar circumstance. So if an injured patient died, and a lawsuit alleged you were negligent, the court would have to decide whether you provided him with appropriate care under the circumstances.

A common error is failure to record unstable vital signs. If other patients need your attention, and you fail to stay with an unstable patient constantly, you probably won't be found negligent. But you could be found negligent—and liable—if you failed to record an unstable patient's vital signs and he later developed a serious complication.

ED flowsheet

Time	B.P.	Temp.	Pulse	Resp.
0900	140/80	98	90	24
0915	100/60	—	100	26
0930	90/60	—	120	28
1000	80/60	—	140	30

Verbal orders are legally acceptable in *any* situation as long as they're written on the patient's chart as soon as possible. But getting some doctors to document their verbal orders can be an uphill battle. To protect your patients from harm and yourself from liability, ask your manager, the ED's medical director, or the hospital administrator to inform doctors that ED nurses won't carry out verbal orders except in emergencies. Explain to the doctors the shaky legal position verbal orders put *you* in.

As you're aware, emergency *and* nonemergency verbal orders are fraught with danger to both you and your patient. So when any doctor gives you a verbal order, take the following precautions:
• Repeat the order aloud so the doctor can confirm it.
• As soon as possible, write the order in the patient's chart, noting both the doctor's name and the fact that the order was given verbally. Sign your name to the order.
• Ask a colleague who also heard the order to co-sign your entry on the chart.

Patient care in the ED, of course, is ultimately the ED doctor's responsibility. But if you're a triage or charge nurse (rather than a staff nurse), you can be held liable for a

L

patient's injury that results from incorrect triage.

The *best* plan is to always use a nurse for triage. If that isn't possible, the hospital should educate the admissions clerk to perform initial assessments and recognize emergency conditions.

If you have reason to believe that patients in your ED aren't receiving treatment quickly enough from appropriate medical personnel, document your concerns by writing a memo. Then give copies to your manager, the medical director of the ED, and the hospital administrator.

Legal risks: equipment

Coping with malfunctions

Sophisticated equipment can be a lifesaver for the patient—or a source of liability for you. Although most hospitals do routine safety checks, equipment can still fail at the worst possible moment, leaving you and the hospital at risk for a lawsuit.

The general rule is: If you know a piece of equipment isn't functioning properly, you're legally obligated to take steps to resolve the problem, then document what you did. Most often, this means calling the maintenance department and asking them to replace or repair malfunctioning equipment.

But suppose the defect isn't readily apparent? Are you still liable if something goes wrong? No—as long as adequate checks were made. Unless the equipment's obviously defective and you use it anyway, neither you nor the hospital is liable for the patient injury it may cause. Who *is* liable in such a situation? Usually, the manufacturer.

You can reduce your risk of being held liable for patient injury from equipment failure by following these guidelines:
• Follow the manufacturers' instructions for operation and maintenance of all equipment.

• Know your hospital's policy on equipment checks and maintenance. Nurses routinely check some equipment (for example, intubation equipment, monitors, and defibrillators); the maintenance department or a biomedical specialist checks the rest. Be sure you know what equipment you're responsible for checking and whom to call if you find a malfunction or if the equipment needs to be serviced.
• Fix or report any defective equipment immediately. And ask that it be removed from the unit before someone else tries to use it.

Common equipment malfunctions

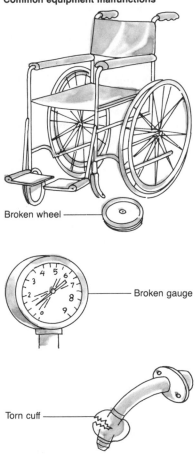

Broken wheel

Broken gauge

Torn cuff

• When equipment fails while you're using it, document the incident, including the actions you took, and advise your hospital's risk manager.
• Urge your hospital to hold continuing education classes (if it's not already doing so) to review proper

use of new equipment and equipment already in use.

Legal risks: OR

Precautions to take

Working in the operating room (OR) or recovery room (RR) presents its own special legal risks. Here are the most common causes of malpractice suits arising from these areas and the best ways to protect yourself.

Failing to perform procedures correctly
Malpractice lawsuits can arise from:
• *failure to check the chart* for a consent form; preoperative laboratory, electrocardiogram, or X-ray results; or allergy warnings.
• *failure to perform a sponge and instrument count* or *performing it incorrectly.*

Sponge count

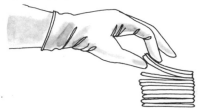

• *inadequate postoperative observation* of the patient in the OR or RR, in transit between these two places (where most malpractice lawsuits arise), or in transit to the medical-surgical unit.

Ideally, *all* postoperative patients should be accompanied to the medical-surgical unit by an RR nurse. But if that's impossible because of tight staffing, an RR nurse should at least accompany *high-risk patients*—those with chest tubes, for example.
• *anesthesia errors by nurse anesthetists.* In most states, if you're responsible for anesthetizing patients, the medical standards for anesthesiology apply to your performance. If you don't meet them and you harm a patient, you're liable.

Following incorrect or inappropriate orders

You have to evaluate every order for its safety and appropriateness. As an independent professional, you're held accountable for every order you carry out.

Taking other precautions

Here's some more advice for avoiding legal errors in the OR and RR:

• Familiarize yourself with your state's nurse practice act, the nurse practice standards of the Association of Operating Room Nurses, and your hospital's written policy on OR emergencies.

• Document carefully. Documentation may not help you avoid legal problems completely, especially if an incident has already happened, but it can *reduce* your legal risk. (See *Documentation.*)

• Carry adequate malpractice insurance before setting foot in an OR. Generally, a hospital's malpractice insurance policy covers both OR and RR nurses. But in the rare case that your hospital's policy is inadequate, you may need your own professional liability insurance. Check with the personnel department or hospital administration for information on the extent of their coverage.

• Don't let yourself be intimidated. If a doctor gives you an inappropriate order, *don't* follow it. The law requires you to consider the patient's safety first. In fact, by putting your patient's best interests first and standing your ground when you know you're right, you can avoid most legal risks in the OR. (See *Postanesthesia recovery.*)

Legal risks: patient falls

Protecting yourself and your patient

Patient falls are responsible for more lawsuits alleging negligence

by hospitals and nurses than any other kind of injury.

Patients who are elderly, infirm, sedated, or mentally incapacitated are most apt to fall, although any patient can fall when the circumstances are right.

Nurses and doctors aren't *automatically* liable for patient falls. The courts expect you to continually evaluate your patients' needs and take proper precautions, so you may be held liable if a patient falls because you neglected to do this. But if he falls despite your having taken all proper precautions to protect him—and you can produce documented evidence of the quality of your care—your risk of liability is much less.

How can you protect your patients from falls—and yourself and your hospital from lawsuits? Assess *every* patient carefully to determine his risk of falling; if he's at high risk, follow these guidelines:

• Write your nursing diagnoses and care plan to reflect his risk of falling.

• Monitor him regularly, following your hospital's policy.

• Keep his bed rails raised, as indicated.

• As always, provide adequate lighting and a clean, uncluttered environment.

• Help him when he gets out of bed, and make sure he wears proper shoes when walking.

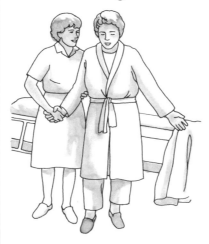

• Have adequate staff available if he needs help getting in or out of bed.

• Take special precautions with an elderly or medicated patient, especially if the doctor's orders include having him sit in a chair several times a day. If you can't supervise him, assign someone else.

• Keep the patient oriented to time and place, especially if he's elderly or confused. (See *Patient falls.*)

Legal risks: patient teaching

Reducing your risk of liability

For more than 40 years, courts have recognized patient teaching as a nursing function. But the more you get involved in teaching, the greater your risk of being found liable for giving incorrect or incomplete discharge instructions. And now, with Diagnosis-Related Groups shortening hospital stays, reducing the time available for patient teaching, your chances of making an error increase even more.

To reduce your risk of liability, follow these guidelines:

• Encourage the patient and his family to ask questions about his postdischarge care.

• Make sure the patient signs the patient record, indicating that he's received discharge instructions, after you've explained them.

• Take special care when teaching geriatric or pediatric patients (you might have to teach a family member, too) or patients with visual or hearing impairments or language problems.

• Suggest that the patient tape-record your discharge instructions if the information's very detailed. Then he can bring a cassette to follow-up visits and record any new instructions. (See also *Elderly patients: discharge planning; Patient-teaching errors; Patient-teaching techniques.*)

L

Legal risks: pediatrics

Strategies to use

Besides documenting patient care accurately, pay close attention to the physical safety of your young patients. When children are injured in pediatric units, nursing negligence is *commonly* the cause. So be sure to follow your hospital's policy regarding the appropriate patient ages for cribs and youth beds. And check that each bed works properly.

Also, make sure each room is child-proofed. Unused electrical outlets should have child-proof protectors on them, and all medications, disinfectants, and equipment should be securely locked away.

Finally, supervise all hospitalized children when they're playing together: You can be held liable if one child hurts another while they're under your care.

Follow these guidelines for reducing your legal risks:
• Establish rapport with both the child and his family. Because a child's illness is stressful to everyone in the family, make effective communication the keystone of your care plan. By helping to build trust between you, the child, and his family, you may also be preventing a future lawsuit.
• Keep up to date with the latest developments in pediatrics. Even if your state doesn't require you to take continuing education courses, keep up to date by reading professional literature and by attending seminars.
• Become thoroughly familiar with your hospital's policies and procedures, and follow them carefully—remember, they help set the standard of care. If any procedures seem out of date, notify your manager.
• If a patient, a member of his family, or his lawyer contacts you with questions about the care you gave him, don't discuss anything before talking to your own or your hospital's lawyer.
• Get your own professional liability insurance. (See *Liability insurance.*) Remember, even if a court orders the hospital to pay all damages in a lawsuit because your care was negligent, the hospital can sue you, in turn, for the amount of the damages. Although most hospitals don't sue their employees, you'll be sure of protecting yourself if you have your own professional liability insurance.

If you do become involved in a lawsuit, make sure your lawyer prepares you for giving pretrial evidence (the deposition) and, if the case goes that far, for testifying at the trial. (See *Deposition.*)

Legal risks: restraints

Using them without a doctor's order

If the doctor orders restraints, follow his order. If you don't, you're risking liability if the patient falls and injures himself. But think twice about restraining a patient *without* a doctor's order. Unless you can show that the patient posed a threat to himself or others, you could be held liable for false imprisonment.

These guidelines will help:
• Use restraints only as a last resort or as ordered; use minimal restraints when possible.
• Check your hospital's written protocol. Besides reflecting state laws, it should specify when you can use restraints and who may order their use. A doctor's order may be required.
• In an emergency—such as when you believe a patient's condition will lead to violent behavior—you may need to apply restraints without an order, but be sure to get a written order afterward.

• Assess and document the reason for restraining the patient, and record what type of restraints you use, how you supervise their use, and what time you apply or remove them.
• Once you've applied restraints, you may be liable for any injuries they cause. Check at least every half hour to make sure that the patient doesn't work his way out of them (or strangle himself) and that they're still properly placed.

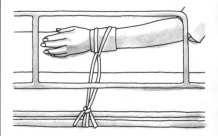

• Reassess him frequently for signs of impaired circulation and skin irritation. Loosen the restraints every 2 hours; if he's awake, be sure to take proper precautions.
• Place him in an upright position for eating to help keep him from aspirating food or choking.
• Don't use restraints as punishment or as a substitute for treatment. (See *Restraints: padding; Restraints: precautions*)

Legal risks: SPU

Identifying major risks

Here are the major risks for each aspect of your nursing care done in the short procedure unit (SPU), beginning with preprocedure assessments. Before the procedure, the legal risk you're most likely to encounter occurs when you first assess a newly admitted patient and check his informed consent.
• *Assessment.* Despite the thoroughness of early screening tests, you should still perform your *own* nursing assessment when the patient's admitted. You must determine whether he really is ready for surgery that day.

Some of the questions you should answer: If his doctor instructed him to go without food after midnight the previous evening, did he follow those instructions? Does he have any cold symptoms, a fever, a suspicious rash, or any other signs or symptoms that might affect his reaction to anesthesia and surgery? If he regularly takes morning medications, did he take them today?

• *Informed consent.* As you know, obtaining informed consent is the *doctor's* responsibility. But many hospitals make sure the patient understands what the doctor told him. So, if a patient's confused about the procedure he consented to, you can give him more information; if he remains confused, or if you don't feel qualified to give him the information he needs, document your observations on his chart and make sure the doctor answers his questions. Whatever the outcome, document the entire conversation.

• *Never prepare a patient for surgery unless you have his signed consent form in hand.* To avoid legal problems arising from consent forms that are missing or that consistently arrive late, encourage your hospital administration to implement this policy: Every patient's consent form must be attached to his chart 24 hours before surgery—or his surgery will be rescheduled.

• *Observing and reporting.* Many short procedures are performed under general anesthesia, so they present the same risks as *any* surgery performed under anesthesia. You must report all adverse reactions to the anesthesiologist and surgeon.

• *Discharge assessment.* SPU patients are typically scheduled to be discharged the same day they're admitted. So be especially alert when assessing patients for postoperative problems.

Depending on your hospital's policy, you may have to arrange for someone to accompany your patient home after surgery. Suppose he's still under the effects of sedation. As you're wheeling him to the door, you find out that he plans to take public transportation or to drive his own car home. Try to persuade him to have somone pick him up—or call a taxi for him. If he were to injure himself or someone else on his way home because of his impaired faculties, you could be held liable.

• *Patient teaching.* In the SPU, patient teaching is mostly discharge teaching. The patient's doctor should give him discharge instructions before surgery, but don't assume he's done so or that he understands the instructions his doctor gave him. Take the following steps:

1. If your hospital doesn't have a policy on discharge teaching, try to establish one. It should require that patients receive discharge instructions *before* admission.

2. Make sure your SPU has preprinted discharge teaching instructions, especially for the most frequently performed procedures. Individualize your teaching with specific written instructions whenever necessary. If preprinted instructions aren't available, write them yourself.

3. Have your patient repeat your instructions to you to make sure he understands them.

4. Make sure he's capable of following the instructions; if he isn't, contact the appropriate support services. (See *Legal risks: patient teaching.*)

5. Document *painstakingly* what you taught the patient; what written instructions you gave him, if any; how he responded to those instructions; and what other actions you took, such as contacting a support person or agency.

Legal risks: telephone advice

Protecting yourself

First, devise a protocol for handling "routine" problems, such as diarrhea or sore throat (get the supervising doctor's approval first). That way, you'll be giving uniform advice and you'll have some legal protection if your advice is questioned.

Be meticulous about documentation. Include the patient's name, his problem, the date and time of the call, your name, and a brief summary of any advice you give.

Refer unusual calls to a doctor, and document his involvement in the logbook.

Conclude all phone conversations by advising the patient to seek medical treatment immediately if his condition doesn't improve or if any other signs or symptoms occur.

To be sure your advice meets legal standards, write protocols using the above guidelines, getting input from the ED doctors, hospital administrators, and the hospital lawyer. (See *Legal risks: ED.*)

Legal risks: understaffed unit

Preventing lawsuit

Understaffing can lead to substandard patient care, increased errors, and careless documentation. But most lawsuits related to understaffing involve nurses who fail to continually monitor patients or to report significant changes in the patient's condition to the doctor.

The courts generally hold hospitals primarily responsible in lawsuits where understaffing is the key issue. But they may find charge nurses liable as well, because charge nurses are responsible for making work assignments.

One way hospitals remedy staffing problems is by floating nurses from well-staffed units to understaffed units. But floating can also increase nurses' legal risks, especially for nurses who float to unfamiliar areas. (See *Job assignments.*)

L

Here's how to reduce your legal risk of legal problems stemming from understaffing:

• Be sure you're familiar with your state's nurse practice act so you know what extra responsibilities you can legally take on when you float to other units.

• Inform your supervisor and request more help if you notice a staffing problem that could seriously compromise patient care.

What if help isn't available? No matter how concerned you are about your legal risks, do the best you can. If you feel patient care is being compromised, file a documented report after your shift's over and send it up the chain of command or to your risk manager. This won't necessarily protect you if a patient's injured while in your care, but it'll show that you made a sincere attempt to protect your patients.

• If you're a director of nursing or a charge nurse: Assign your staff properly, make sure they're competent to perform the tasks you assign them, and supervise their actions continually.

• Know your hospital's policies concerning floating. For example, if your employment contract says you aren't required to float, you can refuse; otherwise, you can't. If you feel uncomfortable with a floating assignment, however, voice your concerns to your supervisor and document them.

• Push for continuing education programs if you work in a small hospital where staff is floated freely. These programs will help you maintain and broaden your clinical skills.

Legal risks: wrongful discharge

Avoiding being named in a lawsuit

To avoid being named in a wrongful discharge suit, follow these guidelines.

Make sure your performance appraisals are factual, up-to-date, and accurate. Many nurse-managers have lived to regret firing a nurse who had been causing problems for a long time but, because no one wanted to rock the boat, had still been getting excellent appraisals. (See *Appraisals: records.*)

Have a legitimate reason—whether disciplinary or economic—for the discharge. Ask yourself, "Am I discharging this employee for a reason I can defend in open court?" If you can't answer yes to this question with confidence, discuss the matter with your hospital's lawyer.

If institutional policy calls for a progressive course of disciplinary actions, don't sidestep it. Follow it consistently with all staff members. If you "walk the extra mile" with your employees and act in a reasonable, fair, and consistent manner, you'll protect yourself from being charged with outrageous conduct. Even if your institution doesn't have such a policy, document all previous disciplinary actions you've taken, such as giving fair warnings.

Finally, when discharging an employee, remember to show the same sensitivity you'd show to a patient who had just received crushing news. A staff member who is being dismissed will most likely be upset and angry. Explain the reasons for the dismissal as objectively as possible. If you've followed the legal guidelines above, you'll be protected and so will your institution. And, most important, you'll know that you've carried out an unpleasant but necessary duty as fairly and evenhandedly as possible. (See also *Job termination.*)

Legislation

Effecting a change

When writing to legislators, remember these important points:

1. Use your own stationery, not hospital or agency stationery. A letter is better than a postcard or telegram. Use your own words—form letters are not as effective as original ones.

2. Identify your subject clearly. State the name of the legislation you're writing about. And give the House or Senate bill number, if you know it.

3. Be brief when giving the reasons why you are for or against the legislation. Explain how the issue would affect you, your business or profession, or what effect it could have on your state or community.

4. Know what committees your legislators serve on and indicate in the letter if the bill is being taken before any of those committees.

5. Sign your name with "RN" after it. Be sure your correct address is on the letter as well as on the envelope because envelopes sometimes get thrown away before the letter is answered.

6. Be courteous. A rude letter neither makes friends nor influences legislators. Be sure to express your appreciation for work well-done, a good speech, favorable vote, or fine leadership.

7. Try to write about a bill while it's still before the committee. Your senators and representatives will usually be more responsive to your appeal at that time rather than later on, when the bill has already been approved by a committee.

8. Limit your letter to one issue and don't write more than once or twice on the same subject.

9. Keep a copy of all correspondence for your files.

10. Address written correspondence as follows:

• To a U.S. Senator:
Honorable Jane Doe
United States Senate
Washington, DC 20510

Dear Senator Doe:
• To a U.S. Representative:
Honorable Jane Doe
House of Representatives
Washington, DC 20515

Dear Representative Doe:

The same format applies to state and local officials.

Liability insurance

Why you need your own

Should you get your own professional liability insurance? That's a personal decision, but more and more nurses are deciding that they should.

For one thing, times have changed: More nurses are now being named as defendants in lawsuits and are being held personally responsible for their nursing acts.

For another: The coverage your hospital provides probably doesn't extend to any activities outside your employment. If you moonlight, volunteer your professional services, or help friends on a continual basis—giving insulin shots, for example—you probably need a personal policy to ensure coverage for these activities.

If you're covered under the same liability policy your employer has, the insurance company wouldn't be likely to sue you. If you're covered by a policy other than your hospital's, the likelihood of a suit increases slightly. And, of course, if you're covered by a different insurer, the chance increases still more that the hospital's insurer will sue yours.

Ask your employer for a written description of the coverage it provides—the amount of coverage and the activities covered. Talk to an insurance advisor about individual policies available—and the cost and coverage. Then decide.

Limb measurements

Getting consistent readings

To ensure accurate and consistent limb circumference measurements, use the same reference point each

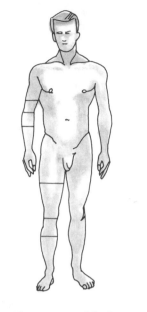

time and measure with the arm or leg in full extension.

Listening to co-workers

Improving your skills

Fortunately you have the power to do something about misunderstandings—by developing the skills you need to be a good listener. Here's how:

1. *Show* the person talking to you that you'll give him time to express his ideas fully. Set aside the chart you're writing in, and look him in the eye. Nod your head to show your understanding. And ask questions.

2. *Learn* to concentrate. One of the most helpful techniques is to adapt your thinking speed. Keep analyzing what the speaker's saying as he talks: What's his point? How well has he looked at all sides of the question?

3. *Do not interrupt or finish people's sentences for them,* which would break down communication. Apologize every time you interrupt. After a few apologies, you'll think

twice before jumping in while someone's speaking.

4. *Avoid* getting wrapped up in someone's speech style: you'll lose track of his message. Instead of marveling that anyone could speak so slowly, have such an accent, cope with such a speech impediment, or get through life with such disorganized thoughts, force yourself back to the message. Ask yourself: "What's he saying that I need to know? What can he add to my knowledge and experience?"

After you recognize that you have something to gain by listening, you'll be willing to overcome any delivery problems by putting the message in your own words.

5. *Learn* to listen to ideas you don't want to hear—this may be difficult because you've trained yourself to hear some things and shut out others: you hear what you want to hear or what you're listening for.

You may unconsciously tune out ideas that don't match your own because you perceive them as threatening. If you'll start taking the risk—and listening to ideas you think you disagree with—you'll find it more of a challenge than a threat. You'll understand your own reasoning better by hearing what others think. And you may change your mind.

6. *Look* between the lines when other people's messages seem garbled or repetitious. Ask yourself what the facts mean, how they relate to one another, and what key idea binds them together. You'll get a clearer picture when you match facts with ideas.

7. *Pay attention* to slumping shoulders, a downward gaze, and crossed arms—they may indicate a conflict between feelings and words. Few people put their entire message into their words. They also communicate with their voice tone, volume, facial expressions, gestures, and body movements. (See also *Communication, nonverbal; Staff management: communication.*)

Listening to patients

Tuning in for better care

Many patients hesitate to tell anyone how worried they are. They don't want to upset their families. And they don't want to interrupt their doctors' busy schedules. But many of these patients send out feelers or hints, hoping someone will realize they're afraid. You may be in the best position to help them—if you can pick up their hidden messages. Try these listening techniques.

1. *Let your patient direct the conversation.* Most of us concentrate on what we're going to say next instead of actually listening to what the other person's saying. But that won't help a patient who can't express his fears without a great deal of subtle urging. He doesn't need to know what *you* think. He needs help exploring his own thoughts.

2. *Define your patient's feelings.* One good way of letting your patient know you're listening is to reword or paraphrase what he's just said to you. Just reflecting back the thought or feeling your patient communicated to you lets him know he's been heard. But be careful to not repeat what he's said over and over because you'll start to sound like a parrot, which can be very irritating. Another technique that'll help you draw a patient out is to let him know what mood or emotion you think he's experiencing. If you're right, the patient will be relieved that you understand. And you'll have helped him come to grips with an emotion he may not have had the courage to face alone.

3. *Give an opinion; don't ask a question.* Tell the patient what you think he feels, don't ask him what he feels. The distinction is important when you're trying to reassure a patient that he can safely tell you his fears.

An insecure or frightened patient may think your question implies that his feelings are inappropriate. In that case, he'll quickly deny them, and true communication will end.

4. *Look interested.* If you've ever tried to talk to someone who was filing her nails or staring out a window, you know how unimportant such behavior made you feel. That person could have said all the right things, but it wouldn't have mattered because body language spoke louder than words.

Remember that when you're talking to a patient *show* him you're interested. You can do this by positioning yourself appropriately (sitting instead of standing), with eye contact, and attentive behavior. (See also *Communication, nonverbal.*)

Liver assessment: percussion

Percussing your patient's liver

Use percussion to judge the liver's size. Position your patient comfortably on his back with his abdomen exposed. Start by percussing directly beneath the clavicle; listen for the resonant note of the lung. Percuss downward along the midclavicular line, placing your fingers between the ribs; otherwise, you may hear dull percussion notes caused by bone rather than the liver. From the fourth to the seventh intercostal spaces, you should hear dull, distinctive percussion notes, which identify the liver's upper border. Mark the upper border using a nontoxic pen.

To locate the lower border (the edge), percuss upward along the midclavicular line, starting in the abdomen's lower right quadrant. The first notes should sound hollow as you percuss the hepatic flexure of the large bowel. When you hear the first dull note, percuss several spaces further up until you find the dullest sound, which is produced by the liver. Then mark the edge.

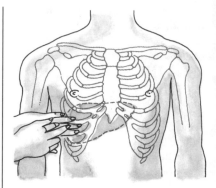

Measure the distance between the two marks. The normal liver span along the midclavicular line varies from 2.4″ to 4.8″ (6 to 12 cm) in an adult. (See also *Abdominal exam: palpation.*)

Lumbar puncture

Explaining it to your patient

Prepare your patient by giving him the following instructions:

"If you're having the lumbar puncture done as an outpatient, you must arrange for someone to drive you home. For the test, you'll lie down on your side with your knees bent and your neck flexed. This position allows the doctor to see the bony structures of your spine. Then your lower back area will be cleansed with two solutions that feel cool.

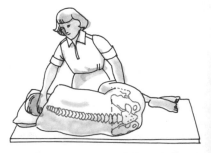

"Next, the doctor will inject a local anesthetic with a needle. You'll feel pinching for a second or two; the anesthetic will take effect in a few minutes. After this, a long, hollow needle will be inserted to collect the spinal fluid.

"You may feel a sensation—something like pressure—as the doctor inserts the needle. While he positions it, your legs may tingle or twitch. During the test, be sure to describe to him everything you feel.

"After the procedure is over, you'll have to lie flat, but you can use a pillow under your head. For 24 hours, your activity will be restricted to going to the bathroom and sitting up for meals. You'll need to drink plenty of fluids to build up your spinal fluid level again. If you get a headache, it will go away when you lie down. It will stop when your spinal fluid reaches the normal level, probably in a day or two."

Lung volumes

Measuring them

Use a Wright respirometer to measure tidal volume (the amount of air inspired with each breath) and minute volume (the volume of air inspired in a minute—or tidal volume multiplied by respiratory rate). You can connect the respirometer to an intubated patient's airway via an endotracheal tube or a trache-

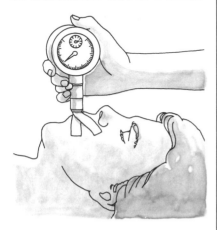

ostomy tube. If the patient isn't intubated, connect the respirometer to a face mask, making sure the seal over his mouth and nose is airtight.

Lymphadenopathy

What to ask and do

Ask the patient when he first noticed nodal swelling and if it's on one side of his body or both. Are the swollen areas sore, hard, or red? Ask if he's recently had a cold or virus, or any other health problems. Also ask if a biopsy has ever been done on any nodes, for this may indicate a previously diagnosed cancer. Find out if his family has a history of cancer.

Palpate the entire lymph node system to determine the extent of lymphadenopathy and detect any other areas of local enlargement.

Head and neck lymph nodes

Use the pads of your index and middle fingers to move the skin over underlying tissues at the nodal area.

Axillary lymph nodes

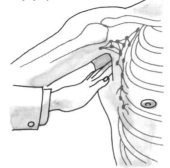

If you detect enlarged nodes, note their size in centimeters and whether they're fixed or mobile, ten-

der or nontender. Also note its texture: Is the node discrete or does the area feel matted? If you detect tender, erythematous lymphadenopathy, check the area drained by that part of the lymph system for signs of infection, such as erythema and swelling. (See also *Palpation.*)

M

Malpractice

What to do if you get sued

Here's what to avoid doing if you are summoned:
• Don't discuss the case at your hospital with anyone other than the risk manager.
• Don't discuss the case with the plaintiff or the plaintiff's lawyer.
• Don't discuss the case with anyone testifying for the plaintiff.
• Don't discuss the case with reporters.
• Don't alter the patient's records.
• Don't hide any information from your lawyer.
• Don't go on the witness stand unprepared.
• Don't be discourteous on the witness stand.
• Don't volunteer any information. (See also *Legal help; Malpractice settlement.*)

Malpractice prevention

Tips to keep you out of court

Here are the best ways to keep yourself out of court:
1. *Recognize that your first duty is to defend your patient, not his doc-*

tor. If your judgment tells you to call the doctor because of a change in your patient's condition or to clarify orders, don't hesitate.

If your hospital doesn't already have a policy covering nurse-doctor communications, ask for one and keep asking until you get one. Meanwhile, record all communications with doctors.

2. *Keep your nursing skills up-to-date.* Read nursing journals, attend staff-development programs, and seek advice from nurse specialists. If your hospital doesn't offer needed staff-development programs, ask for them.

Remember, if you're ever sued for malpractice, your care will be judged by current standards.

3. *Include all parts of the nursing process in your patient care.* Taking shortcuts endangers your patient's well-being and your own.

4. *Document every step of the nursing process for every patient.* Chart your observations immediately, while facts are fresh in your mind. (See *Documentation; Documentation, computerized.*)

5. *Audit your nursing records consistently and comprehensively, using specific criteria to evaluate the effectiveness of patient care.* Ask for a charting class—or start one yourself—to encourage staff nurses to chart patient care correctly and legibly. Use problem-oriented charting (to be sure you're documenting all parts of the nursing process) and flow sheets (to record large volumes of data).

6. *Use your nursing knowledge to make nursing diagnoses and give clinical opinions.* You have a legal duty to your patient not only to make a nursing diagnosis but also to take appropriate action to meet his nursing needs. Doing so will help protect your patient from harm and you from malpractice charges.

7. *Delegate patient care wisely.* Know the legal practice limits of the people you supervise. If your del-

egation of skilled tasks to an unskilled person harms a patient, you could be held liable.

8. *Know your nursing service policies.* Review the policies at least yearly. Ask for new policies, if needed.

9. *Treat patients and their families with kindness and respect.* When you help relatives cope with the stress of your patient's illness and teach them the basics of home care, they are more likely to remember you with a thank-you card than with a legal summons. (See *Malpractice; Malpractice settlement.*)

Malpractice settlement

Settling out of court

About 10% of malpractice cases end up in court—and of those, only about 10% end with a final judgment. The rest are settled out of court.

If you're involved in a malpractice case, remember these two points:

1. If you're covered by professional liability insurance, your policy will state if you and your lawyer, or the insurance company, can control an out-of-court settlement. Most policies don't permit the nurse to settle without the insurance company's consent. In fact, many policies let the insurance company settle without the *nurse's* consent. Review your policy to learn your settlement rights.

2. Tell your insurance company's representative and your lawyer all you know about the case. Then they can evaluate your liabilities and the plaintiff's liabilities to figure the best settlement with the plaintiff. As the attending nurse, you'll be able to give observations about the patient's state of mind—the basis of many successful settlements. (See *Liability insurance; Malpractice; Malpractice prevention.*)

Mastectomy, bilateral

Helping a patient get out of bed

One of the most painful tasks for a patient with bilateral mastectomy is raising herself to get out of bed. Here's a way you can make getting up easier and less painful.

When making the patient's bed, lay a drawsheet over the top half of her bed. When she wants to get out of bed, ask her to fold her arms under her chest area for comfort, then raise the head of her bed as far as it will go. Grab the top of the drawsheet on both sides of her and pull it towards you. As she rises, she should swivel sideways and put her legs over the side of the bed. After she rests there a minute or so, *again* pull the drawsheet towards you to help her to put her feet on the floor.

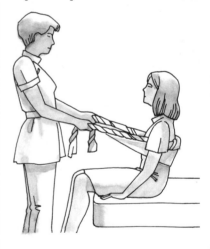

The sheet gives her the boost she needs without any painful tugging or pulling.

Mastectomy: flap necrosis

Odor control

If a patient who's had a mastectomy develops some flap necrosis, you'll need to teach her how to cleanse the wound, recognize the need for debridement, reduce the bacteria, and dress the wound. Here's a tip on odor control. Soak some pieces of gauze in oil of wintergreen and pin them near the neckline of her pajamas.

The patient will love her fragrant "sachets" and the clean, fresh feeling they give her. (See *Wound care dressings: taping.*)

Mastectomy: incisions

Proper care

The doctor may order a sterile towel to be draped over the patient's incision after the original dressing and drains are removed. But by this time, the patient is moving and exercising, so the towel just won't stay taped in place.

To solve this problem, hold the towel in place over the patient's incision and pin a strip of ½″ (1 cm) gauze to one of the top corners. Bring the gauze over her shoulder and the opposite corner of the towel around to her back. Pin the gauze to this corner. Then pin some gauze to the bottom corner of the towel in front, bring the gauze around to the back of the patient's waist, and pin that end of the gauze to the bottom corner of the towel in back.

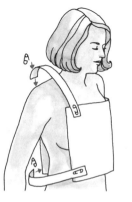

Now the towel will stay in place while the patient has enough freedom to move and exercise comfortably. (See also *Mastectomy, radical.*)

Mastectomy: phantom sensations

Patient-teaching strategies

Women who've had a mastectomy may feel phantom sensations (pseudesthesia) in the operative area of the inner part of the arm—as though they still have the breast. This phenomenon may result from feelings of grief or loss, and from difficulties in adjusting to a radically altered body image.

If your patient has them postoperatively, reassure her that they're common among women who've had mastectomies. If indicated, arrange consultations with a psychiatric nurse clinician, psychologist, psychiatrist, social worker, or clergyman.

Mastectomy, radical

Keeping fabric away from grafted areas

After a radical mastectomy with extensive muscle and skin autografting, a patient may be told to keep any fabric (even a hospital gown) from touching the grafted areas, but to get out of bed and walk. To help compliance and permit some modesty, use a plastic laundry basket. Cut a hole large enough for her head in the bottom of the basket, tape gauze around the edge of the hole, and pin sheets to the gauze. Then put the basket over her head so it rests on her shoulders. The sheets will cover her, yet the basket will hold them away from her body. (See also *Mastectomy: incisions.*)

MAST suit

Correct use

Your hospital may use medical antishock trousers (MAST suit) for trauma patients. Use the following guidelines for inflating or deflating them.

Inflation

Position the suit on the patient so that the abdominal chamber's top just touches his lower rib margin. Then, strap on the suit and begin inflating it with the foot pump. Inflate the leg chambers first, then the abdominal chamber. As the suit inflates, check the patient's blood pressure every 15 seconds. Use this as your guide: if blood pressure starts rising after you've inflated one or both leg chambers, you may not need to inflate the abdominal chamber.

If the patient's conscious during inflation, he may complain of respiratory discomfort. As pressure in the suit builds, he may even vomit or defecate. Reassure him that the MAST suit normally causes a feeling of extreme pressure on the legs and abdomen.

After inflation, monitor the patient's vital signs closely and check his blood pressure every minute. Also check his apical heart rate, lung sounds, skin color and temperature, and peripheral pulses for signs of fluid overload or constricted peripheral circulation. Therapy duration depends on the patient's condition and response to treatment.

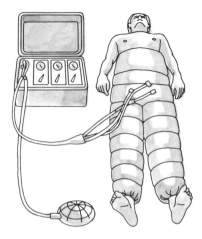

Deflation

Never cut a MAST suit off a patient. And don't deflate it until his circulating volume has been restored,

M

he's stabilized, or he's ready to undergo surgery. Suit inflation compresses his lower venous system, inducing lactic acidosis in his legs. This produces carbon dioxide, a potent vasodilator. Rapid deflation would cause carbon dioxide to dilate leg veins and increase the vascular bed enough to cause severe hypotension.

Deflate the MAST suit *gradually* before removing it. Start with the abdominal chamber and continue with the leg chambers one at a time. Monitor the patient's blood pressure after each release of air. If it drops by 5 mm Hg or more, reinflate the chamber and administer I.V. solutions as ordered to increase circulating volume. Continue gradual deflation only when his blood pressure's stable. Deflate a MAST suit rapidly *only* if the patient suffers an abdominal trauma and needs immediate surgery.

McBurney's sign

Patient positioning and palpation

Before McBurney's sign is elicited, inspect the abdomen for distention and auscultate it for hypoactive or absent bowel sounds.

To elicit McBurney's sign, position the patient supine with his knees slightly flexed and his abdominal muscles relaxed. Then, palpate deeply and slowly in the right lower quadrant over McBurney's point—located one-third of the distance from the anterior superior iliac spine to the umbilicus. Point tenderness, a positive McBurney's sign, indicates appendicitis. (See *Appendicitis.*)

McMurray's sign

Eliciting it

McMurray's sign is used to confirm a torn meniscus. Checking for McMurray's sign requires gentle manipulation of the patient's leg to avoid extending a meniscal tear or locking the knee. If you've been trained to elicit McMurray's sign, place the patient in a supine position and flex his affected knee until his heel nearly touches his buttocks. Place your thumb and index

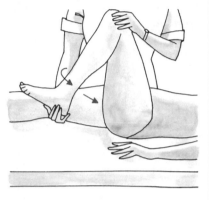

finger on either side of the knee joint space and grasp his heel with your other hand. Then rotate his foot and lower his leg laterally to test the

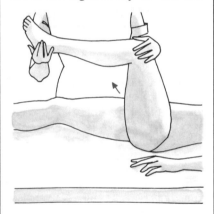

posterior meniscus. Keeping his foot in a lateral position, extend his knee to a 90-degree angle to test the anterior meniscus. A palpable or audible click—a positive McMurray's sign—indicates a meniscal tear.

Medication

Breaking a scored pill

Here's a way to break a scored pill in half. Just insert a sterile needle

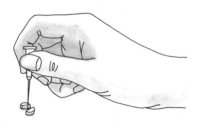

into the groove. The pill will break apart cleanly.

Medication, antituberculosis

Nursing implications

When caring for a patient on isoniazid (INH):
• Tell him to report signs and symptoms of neuritis (numbness and tingling in hands and feet) and hepatitis (anorexia, nausea, vomiting, jaundice, malaise, or dark urine.) Give Vitamin B_6 if he develops neuritis.
• Lower the dosage if isoniazid interferes with phenytoin (Dilantin) metabolism. Tell him to take INH on an empty stomach and to avoid alcohol. Monitor liver enzymes in elderly or symptomatic patients.

If your patient's taking ethambutol (Myambutol):
• Tell him to notify his doctor if his vision blurs or if he can't see red or green.
• Use the drug with caution in patients with renal impairment or those who can't undergo a visual exam.

If the patient you're caring for is on rifampin (Rifadin, Rimactane):
• Tell him to expect orange-tinged body fluids.
• Don't administer the drug at mealtime since food decreases absorption.
• Tell him to report anorexia, nausea, vomiting, jaundice, malaise, or dark urine.
• Use the drug with caution in patients with liver disease.
• Check his other medications; rifampin decreases the effectiveness

of anticoagulants, oral contraceptives, methadone, oral hypoglycemics, digitalis, and quinidine.

Be sure to do the following when caring for a patient on streptomycin:
• Obtain baseline renal and audiology studies before therapy.
• Tell the patient to report any dizziness, vertigo, tinnitus or ringing, roaring, or fullness in his ears.
• Help coordinate outpatient arrangements for I.M. injections, as needed.

When you have a patient on pyrazinamide:
• Monitor uric acid and liver enzymes after obtaining baseline measurement.
• Instruct the patient to report any signs and symptoms of gout (painful swelling in joints, chills, and fever); hepatitis (anorexia, nausea, vomiting, jaundice, malaise, and dark urine); or hepatotoxicity (jaundice).
• Use with caution in patients with liver disease, gout, or renal impairment.

Medication, endotracheal

Using an endotracheal tube as an alternative

An endotracheal tube can be a lifesaver. When you use it to give a first-line emergency drug, the drug enters the lungs, passing quickly through the alveoli into the circulation. Take these steps:

1. Prepare the medication. If a prefilled syringe isn't available, use a standard 5-ml or 10-ml syringe with a needle or catheter securely attached. (Use the longest needle or catheter available so you can inject the drug deeply.)

With your stethoscope, check placement of the endotracheal tube. Make sure the patient is supine and his head is level with or slightly higher than his trunk.

2. Quickly compress a positive-pressure oxygen-delivery device (such as an Ambu bag) three to

five times, then remove the device.

3. Inject the drug deep into the tube.

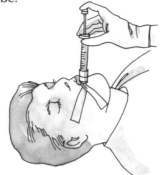

4. To prevent medication reflux, briefly place your thumb over the tube opening. Then reattach the Ambu bag and quickly compress it five times to distribute the medication and oxygenate the patient.

Monitor the patient's response. And be prepared: The onset of action may be quicker than it would be following I.V. administration. If he doesn't respond quickly, the doctor may order a repeat dose.

Medication, nasogastric

Administration of tablets and capsules

If you have to administer tablets or capsules through a nasogastric tube because no liquid replacements are available, remember that the medication will dissolve more rapidly and completely in warm water. And since less warm water is needed to dissolve the medication, a patient on fluid restriction won't get too much liquid.

Medication: nausea

Keeping your patient nourished

Besides causing nausea, vomiting, and anorexia, some of the medications your patient will be taking may

leave an unappetizing taste in his mouth. So, one of your most important nursing goals—keeping the patient nourished and hydrated—will become that much harder to reach. To encourage him to eat and drink, follow these guidelines:
• Avoid giving the drug at mealtime, if possible.
• Provide antinauseants or antiemetics as needed.
• Encourage his family and friends to bring his favorite foods.
• Keep bedside commodes clean, and remove emesis basins promptly after use.
• Offer a toothbrush and toothpaste after episodes of vomiting.
• Keep in mind that even normally pleasant smells, such as the scent of perfume or cologne and strong food odors, can nauseate a patient.

Medication, pediatric

Teaching parents how to give it

When teaching parents how to give medication to their school-age child, tell the parent to keep these pointers in mind:
• "Find out if the medication is available in syrup or chewable tablet form. Although the child may be able to swallow a tablet or capsule safely, he may be more willing to take a sweet-tasting syrup or chewable tablet.
• "If the child needs an elixir, dilute it first with a small amount of water. This will decrease the alcohol flavor in the elixir.
• "Act as though you expect the child to cooperate. However, if he balks, don't threaten or embarass him. And never insist that he swallow the medication because he may aspirate it.
• "Avoid mixing medication with food. If the child detects a strange taste, he may refuse that particular food in the future.
• "When you know medication won't taste good, tell him. Don't try

M

to trick the child. Doing so will make him less cooperative next time. Never tell a child that medication's candy. He may look for an opportunity to eat or drink the entire contents of the bottle.

• "Praise him if he cooperates." (See *Medication: taste.*)

Don't just worry about whether parents are giving their children's antibiotics properly. Instead, create a visual aid for parents—a cross-off-the-pill chart. Each chart should have 10 boxes (one for each day of the antibiotic course). Inside each box, write, "1, 2, 3, 4" to designate the number of pills to be taken each day. Have the patient cross off a number after each pill he takes. On the flip side of the chart, list general instructions for taking antibiotics.

Patients can hang their charts in a prominent place, remind their parents when they need a pill, and cross off the numbers themselves.

Medication: taste

When your patient dislikes the taste

If your patient dislikes the taste of his medicine, tell him to suck on some ice for a few moments before you administer the medicine. The ice will numb his taste buds so the medicine will go down easier.

Medication, topical

Applying it properly

If the patient's skin is red, irritated, sore, and oozing, the doctor will probably order a lotion or spray. If the skin is red and wet but not painful to the touch, he may order a cream or gel. These are also ordered for chronic, scaly skin conditions such as seborrheic dermatitis. Ointments are used to treat the thick, hyperkeratotic skin found with psoriasis.

To apply a topical medication, begin by reviewing the doctor's order and noting how often you should apply the medication. Assemble the medication and the supplies you'll need, such as drapes, gloves, tongue depressors, paintbrushes, or gauze pads.

Ensure the patient's privacy and drape him properly. Make sure the skin site is clean and dry. If topical medication previously applied is caked, remove it before applying more medication. To remove cream, use a water-soaked gauze pad or, if possible, gently wash the area with tap water. To remove an ointment or paste, use a gauze pad dampened with cottonseed or mineral oil.

To apply cream, ointment, or paste, squeeze a small amount (about a ½″ [1 cm] ribbon) onto your gloved hand. Then with long, downward strokes, apply it to the affected area. Don't rub up and down; you might cause folliculitis.

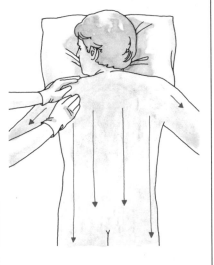

Systematically cover the entire site. When you're finished, the area should be lubricated but not greasy. A very thin coating is adequate. Excess medication would rub off on clothing or bedclothes and increase the chance of adverse reactions.

To apply a lotion or solution, shake the container well, then pour a small amount into your gloved hands. If the lotion has a water or alcohol base, apply it directly to the patient's skin. Use a brush or gauze

only if the lotion's too thin to control. Don't use cotton because it can filter out the suspended medication and can stick to the patient's skin, causing inflammation.

To apply a spray or aerosol, shake the container well. Direct the spray toward the affected area from the distance recommended in the package insert (usually 6″ to 12″ [15 to 30 cm]). Spray in short bursts.

To apply a powder, again make sure the area is dry to minimize caking. Gently "dust" or shake the powder on to apply a thin layer. If you have difficulty reaching the area, use gauze or a powder puff.

If the doctor orders a lotion or spray for the patient's scalp, use the applicator supplied. Part the patient's hair at ¼″ (.5 cm) intervals and direct the applicator along the parts until you systematically cover the scalp.

After you've applied the topical medication, remove your gloves and wash your hands. Then note the following information on the patient's chart:
• how the area looked before the treatment
• any adverse reactions, such as irritation, thinning of the patient's hair, or atrophy
• how the patient accepted the treatment.

Sometimes the patient's skin condition will worsen, despite adequate topical therapy. If that happens, suspect allergic contact dermatitis. The patient may be allergic to the medicaton's active ingredients (such as neomycin), to its vehicle components (such as propylene glycol), or its preservatives (such as paraben compounds).

Medication administration

Methods for hospitalized infants

Sometimes administering medication to an infant can be difficult—even with the aid of special spoons and syringes. Here's an easier way:

Put the medication in the infant's bottle and add water to make 1 ounce. (Check first to see if the medication can be diluted in water.) Use a regular nipple for clear medications such as cough medicines and acetaminophen drops; use a crosscut nipple with larger holes for opaque medications that are more viscous.

You can add more water to any medication left in the bottle, and make sure the infant drinks it all. Don't mix medication with formula, milk, or juice because of the risk of drug incompatibility. (See also, *Medication, pediatric.*)

Medication compliance

A good way to ensure it

To ensure compliance with drug therapy, your patient teaching must go beyond merely accurate information. You must motivate him to participate in his own treatment and to see himself as the most important member of the health care team.

Start by trying to anticipate any problems the patient might have in following your instructions. If he has poor vision or poor muscle control, find a pharmacy that carries preloaded syringes or syringes with a spring release. Or teach a family member, friend, or neighbor how to give an injection. Remember, too, that a patient who has poor vision may not be able to read the label on his medication. Suggest that he use a magnifying glass or ask the pharmacist to use larger print. (See *Blind patients.*)

For a patient who can't open a pill bottle because of arthritis, make sure the pharmacist uses a flip-top cap instead of a childproof one. The doctor can specify this on the prescription, too.

If your patient's worried because the prescribed drug is too costly, discuss the problem with his doctor and pharmacist. A generic version may be available. If it is, make sure the doctor specifies on the prescription that a generic substitute can be used. If one isn't available, find out if a different, less expensive drug can be used instead.

If your patient's annoyed about having to take too many pills, too many times a day, check with his doctor. The drug may be available in higher doses or in an extended-release form that would simplify things and ensure cooperation.

When your patient's not complying with his drug regimen, ask him if he has difficulty swallowing his pills. If he does, find out whether the drug also comes in liquid form. Or maybe the problem is that he doesn't speak or understand English very well. Then make sure all labels and instructions are printed in his native language. Or perhaps he's confused by all the different pills he has to take. You may be able to solve that problem by asking the pharmacist to use color-coded caps on each pill bottle.

Medication errors

Safeguards against giving the wrong drug

Follow these guidelines:
• Pay attention at all times, even during routine procedures you think you could perform blindfolded.
• Check and double-check the label before using a medication.
• Make sure your hospital storage procedure separates look-alike medications, and separates medications from toxic chemicals.
• Discard out-of-date drugs.
• Use accepted injection sites. Heparin, for example, should be injected into the buttocks or the lateral aspect of the thigh.
• Aspirate before giving an I.M. injection. Pull back on the syringe

slightly. If a backflow of blood appears, you've punctured a blood vessel.
• Use the right length needle. Standard needles will rarely deliver an I.M. injection in patients weighing more than 250 lb (112.5 kg). Many nurses use spinal needles for I.M. injections in obese patients. You could ask the prescribing doctor to specify in the order "a 3- to 3½-inch needle for thigh or hip."
• Listen to the patient and record the information he gives you. Don't ignore a patient's saying he's allergic to a certain medication.
• Maintain good records and read them.
• Know the peculiarites—and particular dangers—for every drug you give.
• Read—and follow—drug labels. Never ignore a manufacturer's warning.
• Before administering the first dose of a newly ordered medication, check the transcribed order against the doctor's order sheet.
• If you're unfamiliar with a drug, verify its dosage in a drug reference before giving it.
• Before giving any drug, ask yourself if the drug corresponds with the patient's diagnosis.

Hospital administration can help prevent errors by establishing and enforcing a policy that the hospital pharmacy be contacted before any medication is obtained from a source other than the hospital pharmacy. (See also *Legal risks: dispensing.*)

Medication orders by nonphysicians

If NPs or PAs write them

What should you do if a nurse practitioner (NP) or physicians' assistant (PA) writes treatment or medication orders in the hospital where you work?
• Get a copy of your nurse practice act from your state nurses' asso-

ciation, and read it to find out whose orders you can follow.

• Check your hospital policy. If it says you can't take orders directly from NPs or PAs, refuse to follow any such order until the attending doctor countersigns it. If the situation is life-threatening, you shouldn't wait for his signature. (But even then, you could be liable for practicing outside the scope of your nurse practice act or for violating hospital policy.)

• Discuss any concerns you have with your nurse-manager, director of nursing, or hospital administrator.

• Ask for assignment to your hospital's policy and procedure committee. Then help make sure hospital policy conforms with your state's nurse practice act—and work to change the policy if it doesn't.

• Become involved in your state nursing association so you can have some say about whose orders you should follow. (See *Doctors' orders; Legal risks: doctors' orders.*)

Medication schedules

Helping home care patients

To help home care patients keep track of their medication schedules, use cardboard "sliding pill boxes." (They look like matchstick boxes with an inside compartment that slides in and out. Some pharmacies stock them for patients.)

Stack four boxes on top of one another and tape them together. Then set seven of these taped stacks side by side and tape the seven

stacks together. Label the top of each stack with a day of the week. Label the four boxes in each stack "breakfast," "lunch," "dinner," and "bedtime."

When you visit the patient each week, fill the boxes with medications for the upcoming week. At the next visit, you can tell by checking the boxes whether he's missed any medications.

Medication teaching

Discharge instructions

• First, ask your patient if and when he'll take his medication, to make sure he understands and remembers your instructions. By doing this, you'll identify if he's been noncompliant in the past or has memory problems. Then you can take appropriate steps, such as home health care referrals and more suitable discharge orders.

• Make sure he reads the labels of his medications aloud, to find out if he has problems seeing the print. Elderly patients who can't read the labels usually make more errors.

• Find out if he has any of the discharge medications at home. If he doesn't know the doses, double-check his admitting history.

• Be careful about overemphasizing the adverse effects of his medications. Use your judgment about how much to write down. Consider what he needs to know to be safe. Elderly patients are often readmitted because they've experienced an adverse reaction to their medications.

• Make sure a person who frequently sees the patient (a family member, friend, or neighbor) also hears your discharge instructions. That person will serve as a backup if the patient forgets something.

• Don't wait until you get discharge medication lists to do your medication teaching. You'll overwhelm your patient. Weave the information into his hospital stay by telling him what he's taking when you give him medication.

• Don't assume he remembers what he's taking just because you've explained the medications three times. The best way to find out how much he's understood is to ask. Be discreet. Say something like, "Here's the pill you took at home. Do you remember what it's for?" Repetition is important. Make sure you use the same words each time. (See *Medication compliance; Medication schedules.*)

Meetings: efficiency

Keeping them from breaking down your unit

Too many meetings infect everyone with the feeling that they need more meetings. They prompt some people to make speeches and inflame other people's desire to work. To keep meetings from breaking down your unit's organization:

1. Have a definite reason for any meeting you call.

2. Cancel a regular meeting occasionally to test the need for it.

3. Question the need for each item on the agenda before the meeting.

4. Schedule the meeting right before lunch or before the end of the shift.

5. Begin on time.

6. Limit attendance to those people whose concerns are on the agenda.

7. Set a time limit for each item on the agenda and stick to it. (See also *Meetings: goal setting.*)

Meetings: goal setting

Increasing productivity

Here's a checklist that will help you plan your meetings more effectively:

1. Set clear goals. Knowing where you're headed will help you organize the meeting and increase your

satisfaction when you get there. But make sure your goals are realistic—why set yourself up for failure?

2. Develop an agenda. Circulate a list of topics well before the meeting, asking the participants to select their favorite five or six topics for discussion. That way, they'll know you value their input—and they'll be better prepared for the meeting.

3. Analyze potential personality problems. Consider the participants' needs, concerns, talents, and weaknesses. Will any "hidden agendas" be present? How will you encourage the shy person to contribute or the aggressive person to listen?

4. Match your leadership style to the meeting's objectives. If participants are unfamiliar with the topic, they might welcome a more direct leadership style from you.

On the other hand, if you need everyone's cooperation and good will to carry out the meeting's objectives, use a more democratic style.

5. Explore different problem-solving techniques. What will serve the meeting's purpose better—brainstorming, small-group discussions, or parliamentary procedures?

Whichever technique you choose, don't get locked into it. Using a new technique during a routine meeting can increase involvement and spark creativity. (See also *Meetings: efficiency; Staff management: group dynamics; Staff management: leadership.*)

Melanoma, malignant

Prevention and detection

Melanoma are malignant tumors made up of melanin-pigmented cells. They're most frequently caused by exposure to sunlight. Give your patient these guidelines:
• When he's out in the sun, he should use a sunscreen with a pro-

tection factor of a least 15. Tell him to reapply the sunscreen after swimming or perspiring heavily. His children should also use a sunscreen.

During the summer, he should stay out of the sun as much as possible between 10 a.m. and 2 p.m. If he's out in the sun during these hours, he should wear protective clothing, including a hat.
• Certain medications (such as birth control pills and antibiotics) can make your patient's skin more sensitive to the sun. Tell patients who are taking such medications to limit their time in the sun. When they are out in the sun, they should use a sunscreen.
• Caution your patient not to use a sunlamp. It can be as damaging to the skin as sunlight.
• If your patient has dysplastic nevi or a personal history or family history of melanoma, explain that he'll need regular examinations. Typically, a dermatologist will schedule them at intervals of 3 to 12 months. Teach this patient how to do self-examinations, too. After a bath or shower, he should use a mirror to check his entire body (including his scalp, palms, and soles), looking for changes on his skin. He should perform these examinations once a month.

Explain to the patient that if a mole itches, bleeds, or changes color, size, or shape, or if one mole just looks differently from the others, he should report it immediately.
• Teach him the "ABCDs" of identifying melanoma:
—Asymmetry (one side of the lesion doesn't match the other)
—Border irregularity (the edges of the lesion may be ragged,

Lentigo maligna melanoma

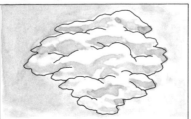

notched, or blurred; scaling or nodules may be present)
—Color (the lesion has a mottled appearance; colors may include tan, brown, black, red, blue, and white)
—Diameter greater than 6 mm (an increase in size usually indicates pathology).

Make sure he understands that the earlier melanoma is detected, the better the chance of curing it.

Melena

Assessing your patient

If your patient is experiencing severe melena, quickly take orthostatic vital signs to detect hypovolemic shock, while another nurse immediately notifies the doctor. (See *Blood pressure, orthostatic.*) Quickly look for other signs of shock, such as tachycardia, tachypnea, and cool, clammy skin. Insert a large-bore I.V. to administer replacement fluids and a blood transfusion, if needed. Place the patient flat with his head turned to the side and his feet elevated. Administer supplemental oxygen if your patient is dyspneic or has cyanosis.

Next, inspect his mouth and nasopharynx for evidence of bleeding. Take a complete history. Then perform an abdominal examination that includes auscultation, palpation, and percussion. (See *Abdominal exam: auscultation, Abdominal exam: palpation,* and *Abdominal exam: percussion).*

MI: anxiety

Helping your patient deal with anxiety and denial

The more you can replace your patient's anxiety with trust, the more likely he'll cooperate with treatment that will improve his chances of recovering from a myocardial infarction (MI). Do your best to instill

M

trust by including these components in all your discussions:
• *Information*. Explain the purpose of the equipment that's near your patient and the treatments he may need. Give him details of the routine he'll be following in the hospital.
• *Listening*. Encourage him to tell you how he's feeling. He needs to know someone's listening to him, and you need to know his fears. (See *Listening to patients*.)
• *Acknowledgment*. Let him know— by the way you respond to his words and behavior—that his feelings are reasonable and understandable.

MI: denial

How it can help your patient

If your patient completely denies that he's had a heart attack, he may ignore or defy the treatment regimen his doctor sets up for him. Such behavior invites another MI. But denial in its milder form—selective inattention—can actually enhance his recovery.

Concentrating on the positive rather than negative aspects of any situation makes it possible to tolerate some element of risk or unpleasantness. In the aftermath of an acute MI, studies show that patients who focus on the positive aspects of the care they're receiving have not only a higher-than-average survival rate while in the hospital, but also a shorter-than-average delay before returning to normal activities.

You can help your patient join this high survival rate group. Talk with him about his current treatment program, including any rehabilitation program he may begin in the hospital and continue after discharge. By doing so, you'll encourage him to replace his vague fears about the future with positive planning. And you'll help him focus on the contributions he can make to his own recovery effort, rather than on the seriousness of his condition. (See *MI: psychological problems*.)

MI: emergency intervention

Quick emergency techniques

If you suspect your patient's had a myocardial infarction (MI), take the following steps at once:
• Notify the doctor immediately.
• Adminster oxygen, as ordered.
• Establish an I.V. line, as ordered.
• Run a 12-lead ECG.
• Be prepared to administer nitroglycerin and an analgesic, such as morphine, as ordered.
• Gather emergency equipment.
• Reassure the patient.

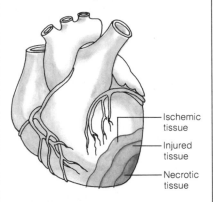

Ischemic tissue
Injured tissue
Necrotic tissue

Concentrating on the positive rather than negative aspects of any situation makes it possible to tolerate some risk or unpleasantness. Besides an ECG, the doctor may also order cardiac enzyme tests, arterial blood gas levels, complete blood count, and serum electrolyte tests to determine the location and extent of MI damage.

MI: family problems

Helping the patient's family

As anxious and helpless as your patient may feel after an MI, his family may feel even worse. By identifying their needs and making an effort to help them, you may win the family members' gratitude—and enlist their cooperation.

Although each family has special needs, all family members need to feel that hospital personnel care about the patient and about them. Seeing the way you and other health care members touch and talk to the patient can reassure them about the quality of care he's receiving. And they need to know the facts of the patient's condition and treatment. Even a prognosis that's not so bright is better than uncertainty. Be sure the doctor talks with them, and follow up on what he says. If a family member asks a question you can't answer, promise to get back to him.

Make sure they know they can see the patient as much as possible. Obviously, you must make them understand that the patient shouldn't be overtaxed, but never make them feel shut out. If visiting hours present a problem, get permission for special arrangements.

Reassure them that they'll be notified promptly of any changes in the patient's condition. Find out how to reach his spouse or another close family member at work and at home, and assure them that someone will call immediately if changes occur. Then, keep your word. Let the family know how to reach your nurses' station if they have questions, too.

As the family members struggle to come to terms with the patient's heart attack, they may feel shock, disbelief, and helplessness. Encourage them to talk about their feelings. An understanding listener— you, the hospital chaplain, or a member of the social services staff—can help them find effective ways to adapt and cope. (See also *Communication: family*.)

MI: psychological problems

Overcoming barriers to your patient's recovery

Typically, an acute myocardial infarction (MI) patient experiences three major emotional states:

• *Anxiety*. This is usually his first response to an acute MI—for good reason. He faces the threat of sudden death. Other fears may also weigh heavily on his mind: Will he be able to keep his job, to function physically (particularly, sexually), or to resume his role as a responsible family member?

Anxiety usually is most obvious early in an acute MI. In some cases, the patient may be anxious only during his first day in the hospital. After that, the combination of pain medication, tranquilizers, and the skilled nursing care helps diminish his fears. Later, however, these fears can return—when he's transferred out of the coronary care unit and when he's discharged.

• *Denial*. Depending on your patient's personality, he may use denial (and possibly anger) as the principal means of dealing with acute MI. Denial commonly occurs in the first 24 to 48 hours after the pain begins. But some patients persist in denying their condition well into convalescence.

• *Depression*. Most patients experience some depression after an acute MI. This feeling commonly surfaces the third day after infarct but may not appear until after the patient's discharged.

Many patients attempt to conceal their depression or to minimize it. However, by using careful, open-ended questions, you can help your patient talk about his feelings more freely and work them through. (See *MI: anxiety.*)

Mouth care: plaque removal

Using a gauze pad and soda

A patient on a ventilator can easily get a hard white caking on his tongue. To remove this caking, gently scrub the patient's tongue with a gauze pad moistened with soda water. This will keep his tongue pink and moist, and won't leave any unpleasant aftertaste. (See also *Mouth care: stomatitis.*)

Mouth care: stomatitis

Advising your patient

Have your patient rinse his mouth out with water, normal saline solution, a solution of normal saline and sodium bicarbonate, or a 1:6 solution of hydrogen peroxide and water. Advise him not to use commercial mouthwashes; they contain alcohol that can irritate and dry out his mouth.

For a serious case of stomatitis, your patient can use a Toothette. This specially designed toothbrush has a soft sponge instead of bristles. The sponge is impregnated with a mild dentifrice that won't irritate the inflamed mucosa. (See also *Mouth care: plaque removal.*)

MRI

Preparing your patient

Instead of using radiation, like a CT scan, magnetic resonance imaging (MRI) uses magnetism. Before the test, find out if your patient's preg-

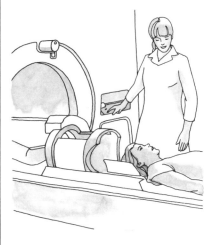

nant, claustrophobic, or has a cardiac pacemaker, a metal prosthesis, or aneurysm clips. Notify the laboratory if any of these conditions are present.

Then tell the patient he can take his usual medications and eat or drink what he wants unless he's having an abdominal or pelvic scan. In that case, tell him he can't have anything by mouth for 4 to 6 hours before the scan. Advise him to use the bathroom before the test begins because it can take up to 1½ hours.

Tell him to remove any metallic items, including hair clips, bobby pins, jewelry, watches, eyeglasses, hearing aids, and dentures. He should also remove clothing that has metal zippers, buckles, or buttons, and any credit, bank, and parking cards bearing metallic strips, because the scan will erase their magnetic codes.

To allay his anxiety, explain the procedure thoroughly, and tell him it's not painful in any way. If you find he's especially anxious, see about getting an order for a mild sedative. Otherwise, demonstrate simple techniques, such as visual imagery, that will help him relax. (See *Diagnostic studies.*)

MUGA scan

Preparing your patient

Your patient won't need to go through any special preparations for the MUGA scan. And he won't have to do anything except lie under the camera. Still, he'll be anxious, and he'll depend on you to teach him about the scan.

The camera can look ominous, so start by showing him picture of it (your radiology department should have pamphlets). Explain that he'll have ECG electrodes on his chest and that he'll receive two injections—a nonradioactive substance first, then the radioactive isotope. Reassure him that the isotope isn't

M

harmful, and that it weakens and loses most of its radioactivity in a few hours.

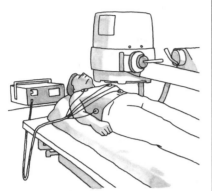

Tell him the injections may cause some discomfort; otherwise, the procedure is painless. Explain that he may be asked to change his position to help the camera scan different areas of his heart, and that the study takes about an hour. (See *Diagnostic studies.*)

Mumps

Reducing complications

Mumps, infectious or epidemic parotitis, is an acute viral disease caused by a paramyxovirus. It is most prevalent in children ages 5 to 15. Prognosis for complete recovery is good, although mumps sometimes causes complications. You can reduce the risk of complications by providing good care.

Stress the need for bed rest until the swelling subsides. Give analgesics as prescribed and apply warm or cool compresses to the neck to relieve pain. Give antipyretics and tepid sponge baths for fever. To prevent dehydration, encourage the patient to drink fluids; to minimize pain and anorexia, advise him to avoid spicy, irritating foods and those that require a lot of chewing. During the acute phase, observe the patient closely for signs of central nervous system involvement, such as an altered level of consciousness and nuchal rigidity.

Because the mumps virus is present in the saliva throughout the course of the disease, respiratory isolation is recommended until symptoms subside.

Emphasize the importance of routine immunization with live attentuated mumps virus (paramyxovirus) at age 15 months and for susceptible patients (especially males) who are approaching or are past puberty. Remember, immunization withing 24 hours of exposure may prevent or attentuate the actual disease. Immunity lasts at least 9½ years.

Report all cases to the local public health authorities.

Myelogram

Explaining one

A myelogram is done to rule out a space-occupying lesion in the spinal cord (a tumor, for example) or orthopedic problems, such as a herniated disk. Spinal fluid can be taken during a myelogram.

Here's how to describe a myelogram:

"Dye will be injected through a needle that's been inserted into your lower back. (See *Lumbar puncture.*) We'll have to find out if you

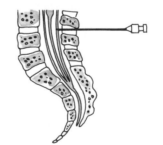

have any allergies or have had reactions to dyes in the past. Also, you won't be permitted to eat or drink anything for at least 3 to 4 hours before the test. You'll lie on a table that will tilt slowly—head down first, then up to a standing position. This will let the dye flow evenly throughout your spinal

canal. You may feel a burning or flushing sensation as the dye is injected or immediately afterward.

"To make sure you don't slip off the table, you'll be secured to it with straps. Your chin will rest on soft padding, and your shoulders will shoulders will rest snugly against metal supports. After the dye is injected, X-rays of your spine will be taken." (See *Contrast dyes; Myelography: patient positioning.*)

Myelography: patient positioning

Post-procedure guidelines

Patient positioning after myelography depends on which dye is used. Pantopaque, an iodine compound with an oil base, is not very soluble and takes a long time to clear from cerebrospinal fluid (CSF). After the procedure, Pantopaque is aspirated to prevent irritation of neural tissue. Inevitably, some CSF is withdrawn with the dye.

If your patient had a myelogram using Pantopaque, keep the head of his bed flat for 6 to 24 hours. This will help prevent the most common problem after the procedure—headache. As you know, CSF normally cushions the brain. When CSF is removed, the weight of the brain stretches dural surfaces, producing intense pain. Lying flat will maintain uniform pressure and help prevent this pain.

Encourage the patient to drink fluids, which will aid CSF formation. Gradually, over the next several hours, his body will replace the CSF he lost. But in the meantime, he must lie flat.

Unlike Pantopaque, both Amipaque and Omnipaque mix well with CSF. They're absorbed rapidly from the subarachnoid space, and then excreted relatively quickly.

For 6 to 8 hours after a patient undergoes myelography with either Amipaque or Omnipaque, position the head of the bed at 30 to 45 degrees to reduce the amount of dye reaching the higher cervical region and intracranial vault. This will minimize irritation of cerebral tissue, which could lead to headache, nausea, vomiting, seizures, and other transient neurologic disturbances such as confusion and language dysfunction. Typically, patients who receive Omnipaque will experience significantly fewer and less severe adverse reactions than patients who receive Amipaque.

Changes in position will cause the dye to move toward the brain. Caution the patient not to lean over or place his head lower than his waist. Such positioning would exacerbate the adverse effects of the dye. Also, encourage him to drink plenty of fluids after the procedure to speed elimination of the dye. After 6 to 8 hours, you should be able to place the patient in a horizontal position for the next 12 to 18 hours. (See *Contrast dyes; Myelogram.*)

Myocardial contusion

Swift intervention

A patient with myocardial contusion will show the following signs and symptoms: ecchymotic area on chest, dyspnea, pericardial friction rub, increased heart rate, decreased blood pressure, chest pain, cardiac dysrhythmias, and ECG changes. Here's how to manage your patient:

1. Assess the patient's airway, breathing, and circulation, and intervene as necessary.
2. Place him on a cardiac monitor, and observe for dysrhythmias.
3. Start I.V. fluids, and administer oxygen at a high flow rate.
4. Manage dysrhythmias as needed.
5. Place him in semi-Fowler's position.
6. Draw samples for blood tests, including arterial blood gas and cardiac enzyme studies.

7. Run a 12-lead ECG.
8. Administer pain medication, as ordered.

Myotherapy

Relieving your patient's muscle pain

When you do a back massage, feel for trigger points.

These tiny, tender spots can be activated when a muscle is injured—whether from a fall, blow, knock, or strain. Trigger points are usually concentrated along the muscles of the neck, shoulders, back, or legs, just under the skin. But they're also in the face, fingers, and feet—anywhere there's a muscle. When you massage a patient's back, for instance, you're probably going over scores of them.

Trigger points can lie dormant in muscles for years. Suddenly—especially during physical or emotional stress—they "fire." Then, the muscle goes into spasm. To stop it, you can locate the release trigger points. While you're massaging your patient's neck, you have to apply only slight pressure with the tips of your fingers to feel a highly sensitive spot. Your patient will let you know if you've found a trigger point. He'll grimace, groan, twist, or twitch. After finding the first one, search for others by moving along the muscle an inch at a time, applying slight pressure with your finger each time.

Trigger points can be located just about anywhere on a muscle. When you find one, simply apply the same, slight pressure with your finger or elbow for 7 seconds. Your patient may complain as he did when you located the trigger point. Just explain to him exactly what you're doing. And tell him the pain will stop shortly.

By releasing each trigger point, you'll ease some of his pain, helping him to relax. If you use the tech-

nique near bedtime, he'll get a better night's sleep, and he'll feel better in the morning.

This technique is called "myotherapy" (muscle therapy). To use it you'll need the cooperation and approval of the patient's doctor. Of course, you can use it for short periods just to relax your patient and relieve his muscle aches—such as when you're massaging his back.

Nasogastric tube: children

Getting an accurate drainage measurement

As you know, a young child on intermittent nasogastric suctioning usually has only minimal drainage. So getting an accurate measurement of the amount can be a problem.

To solve this, channel the drainage into a plastic container for a 35-ml syringe. The container should be taped to the inside stopper of the patient's suction bottle. By using only one thickness of tape to secure the container, you can easily fit the bottle stopper in place.

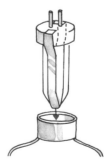

After each suctioning, simply remove the bottle stopper and empty the drainage into a small measuring device. Then take the reading and chart the amount accordingly.

Nasogastric tube: clamps

A time-saving method

If you need to briefly clamp a nasogastric tube (for example, to ambulate a patient or between feedings), use the tube itself as the clamp. Just fold the tubing 6" (15 cm) from the end and insert the folded section into the opening. This

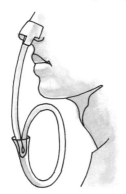

time-saving method doesn't strain the tubing with the added weight of a clamp.

Nasogastric tube: fastening

Proper procedure

Instead of using tape to hold a nasogastric tube in place, use tincture of benzoin and Steri-Strips. Apply a small amount of benzoin across the bridge of the patient's nose. When it's dry, wrap the Steri-Strip around the tube and place it over the patient's nose.

The strips not only adhere to the tube securely, but also look better than tape, so the patient appreciates them, too.

Here's another tactic: Before taping a nasogastric tube to a patient's face, wipe the area with a Skin-Prep pad. This will remove oil from the skin, so the tape will stick better.

Let the invisible residue dry for 30 to 45 seconds before applying tape. (The unpleasant odor will subside when the area is dry.)

Nasogastric tube: patient care

Recognizing patients' needs

The doctor will choose a nasogastric (NG) tube that suits the patient's needs: lavage, aspiration, enteral therapy, or stomach decompression (when the tube's connected to suction). The patient's needs will also dictate tube diameter—measured by the French scale in which each unit equals roughly 0.33 mm. For example, a #16 French tube measures 5.28 mm in diameter; a #42 French tube, 13.86 mm.

Keep these important points in mind when caring for a patient with an NG tube:
• Before instilling anything through the tube, always verify its placement by aspirating gastric contents or auscultating the patient's stomach while injecting 50 cc of air into the tube. (If you hear gurgling, the tube's in place.)
• Follow hospital policy and doctor's orders regarding tube irrigation.
• Monitor the patient for dehydration and electrolyte imbalance, as aspiration of gastric contents can cause fluid and electrolyte loss.
• Check for signs of a tube-induced stress ulcer.
• Make sure the tube doesn't interfere with the patient's breathing. (See also *Feeding tube: complications.*)

Nasogastric tube: suctioning

Problem-solving strategies

Assume that your patient has had a partial gastrectomy, and a nasogastric (NG) tube is in place.

Suppose you see nonfluctuating fluid in the tube. Is it clogged? Has drainage stopped? Has the machine malfunctioned? You must take a few steps to test your assumption of a problem in the tubing.

First, determine what type of tube is being used. You're probably familiar with the standard Levin tube; perhaps less so with the Salem sump tube. Although the low-suction machines can help drainage, both these tubes can also work by gravity alone to drain fluid from the stomach. Unlike the Levin, the Salem tube has two lumens instead of one.

The Salem tube's second lumen appears externally as the pigtail port at the tube's distal end. Through this external opening, enough atmospheric air enters the stomach to let the tube float freely within the stomach. This keeps the tube's drainage ports from adhering to and damaging the fragile gastric mucosa.

You've checked the suction machine's light or gauge; now ask yourself, is the right amount of suction being given? With either suction machine model, disconnecting the tube at the junction of the NG tube and drainage tube will cause a "whoosh" sound if the suction force is on. This "whoosh" further validates that the suction machine is working: Thus, the problem *must* lie between the patient's body and the external NG tube/drainage tube junction.

Ask yourself some more questions: What do you see? Is the tubing so far outside the patient's nostril that the drainage ports can't be in position with the stomach?

Has the drainage itself become too viscid for passage? Are particles clogging the exit ports? Maybe irrigation would help; but of course, as you remember, you'd never instill any irrigating solution until you're certain of the tube's placement.

Using an irrigating syringe, aspirate gently. The return of gastric contents tells you that you're indeed in the stomach and one vari-

N

able—either thickening, positioning, or clogging—has blocked the tube's exit ports. At this point you may—with a doctor's order, if needed—irrigate the tube gently to correct any of these conditions (see *Salem sump tubes*).

You can aid continuous outflow of contents by positioning the tubes properly. For instance, place the drainage end of the Levin tube downward toward the patient's chest to improve the flow.

With the Salem, drape the tube in a U-shape so the pigtail points up. Thus air can enter and permit the tube to float freely. Also, this position prevents the pigtail port from becoming a siphon that would dump gastric drainage all over the patient and the bed linens.

Nasotracheal tube: suctioning

Proper technique

Here's what to do:

1. Collect all of your equipment and wash your hands. You'll need a suction kit containing a suction catheter (usually #12 or #14 French), a receptacle for saline solution, and a sterile glove; sterile normal saline solution; water-soluble lubricant; a nasopharyngeal airway (usually #28 French); and an oxygen-delivery device.

At the patient's bedside, you should have an oxygen flowmeter, suction equipment, connecting tubing, a collection bottle, and a plastic bag for your used supplies.

2. Unless contraindicated, elevate the head of his bed about 45 degrees. This will allow maximum movement of his diaphragm, promoting deep breathing and effective coughing.

3. Be sure the connecting tubing is accessible and maneuvers comfortably once the catheter is attached. Whenever you're not sure, add extension tubing. Hook up your oxygen-delivery device.

4. Open the suction kit. Be sure to maintain sterile technique.

5. Place the glove from the kit on your dominant hand. (Hospital policies and procedures may require you to wear a glove on each hand.)

6. Set up your cup for the saline solution to rinse the catheter and check its patency.

7. Using your ungloved hand, pour the solution into the cup.

8. Squeeze some water-soluble lubricant onto the paper that contained your glove. (Because you will introduce this lubricant into the airway, it must be water-soluble. Oil-based lubricants can cause aspiration pneumonitis.)

9. Generously lubricate the airway. (If you think that the patient will be more comfortable with his nasal mucosa anesthetized, ask the doctor to order lidocaine [lignocaine] for the lubricant.)

10. Now attach the suction catheter to the connecting tubing. Turn on the suction.

11. Occlude the lumen of the catheter by pinching it between your fingers. Place your thumb over the suction port to apply suction, then look at the gauge on the suction apparatus. It should read between 80 and 120 mm Hg. Adjust the suction pressure accordingly, but be sure to release and reapply suction between test adjustments.

12. Check for catheter patency: Apply suction and draw up saline solution through the catheter and connecting tubing until you see it in the collection bottle. Then, disconnect the catheter from the connecting tubing, and wrap it around your glove to maintain sterility.

13. Generously lubricate the catheter and lay it on the paper.

14. Place the oxygen-delivery device over the patient's mouth, leaving his nose free. Take care in using oxygen if the patient has chronic lung disease and is breathing on the hypoxic drive. Don't avoid using oxygen, however, or he'll become hypoxic during the procedure. Just monitor him closely for any indica-

tion of respiratory depression, lethargy, and other signs of CO_2 narcosis.

15. Leave his pillow behind his head, but slide it down closer to his shoulder blades. This way, his head will rest on the bed, not the pillow. This will help stabilize the patient's head, giving you better control during the insertion. Encourage him to breathe through his mouth and try to relax.

16. Using steady, gentle pressure, insert the airway into his nostril until the flanged end is at the nostril's opening. Expect some resistance, but if you encounter too much, use the other nostril.

Inserting the airway

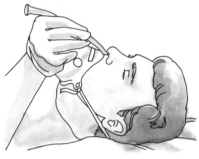

17. Have him stick out his tongue as far as he can while you insert the catheter into the airway. This will help keep him from swallowing the catheter. Throughout the insertion, remind him to keep his tongue out. Watch his breathing, and advance the catheter during inspiration.

18. When you've advanced the catheter past the tip of the airway, bring your ear down to the catheter opening as you continue inserting it. You should be able to hear the air moving in and out with each respiration, indicating the catheter's still in the airway. If the sound of air movement stops, you have accidentally passed the catheter into the esophagus.

19. As you enter the trachea, past the epiglottis, the patient will probably cough violently. Continue to advance the catheter slowly, as tolerated, until you meet resistance. Then pull it back ½″ (1 cm).

N

20. Attach the connecting tubing to the catheter.

21. To apply suction, slide your thumb over the suction port and ask him to cough as hard as he can. Rotate and slightly withdraw the catheter as you apply suction. Try not to withdraw the catheter all the way out of the trachea. Don't suction for more than 10 to 15 seconds.

Inserting the catheter

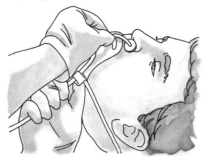

Ideally, you'll want to introduce the catheter into the trachea only once. But if you don't see secretions moving in the connecting tubing, thick mucus may have plugged the catheter's tip. Then, if you can't suction, you'll have to withdraw the catheter completely, rinse it with saline solution, and begin again.

22. When you've finished suctioning, remove the catheter. If the patient will need to be suctioned again soon, leave the airway in place, but not for more than 8 hours.

Wrap the catheter around your gloved fingers.

23. As you pull the glove off your hand, turn it inside out so the catheter is inside it. Discard the catheter and glove into the plastic bag.

24. Encourage the patient to relax and breathe deeply. Place the oxygen mask over his nose and mouth and ask whether he's having any trouble breathing.

25. Auscultate his breath sounds again to determine whether the suctioning was effective. Also, listen to his heart sounds and check his pulse for any changes. Make him comfortable and then turn the oxygen-delivery device back to the prescribed setting.

Near-death experiences

Ways you can help your patient

A near-death experience (NDE) is a phenomenon in which a person comes very close to death and has an experience with certain universal characteristics.

By alleviating your patient's fears and providing a trusting, caring environment, you can help him come to terms with the experience. In a sense, your acceptance can help "welcome" him back. Here are some guidelines to follow:
• Be alert to signs of an NDE. A patient who's afraid to come right out and tell you of his experience might say something such as, "I had the funniest dream" (or the "funniest experience"), although he doesn't look on it as a dream or as funny.

Many don't say even that. But look for certain clues in patients who've pulled through a life-threatening crisis: They might seem angry on awakening, become withdrawn or suddenly calm or silent, or display some other change in behavior.

The best way to get a patient to talk about an NDE is to approach him subtly. You might begin by saying something such as, "People who've gone through a crisis like yours have many different experiences. Is there anything you'd like to talk about?"
• Explore your own attitude toward NDEs.
• Avoid judgment about the NDE.
• Allow the patient to express his emotions.
• Work toward mutual trust.
• Avoid labeling the NDE or the patient.
• Don't give the impression of abandoning the patient.
• Provide human contact during and after unconsciousness.
• Give the patient information about NDEs. Above all, you want to reassure the patient that he's not the only person to ever have this experience. If he wants more information than you're able to give, recommend that he read books and articles about NDEs written for the general public.
• Most patients don't need to be referred to anyone. But if you see that the patient is still upset about his NDE, or is having trouble integrating it into his life, refer him. Just be sure to refer him to someone who understands the phenomenon. Not every professional is familiar with NDEs.

Near-drowning

Assessment and care

Treatment begins immediately with CPR and administration of 100% oxygen. When the patient arrives at the hospital, assess him for a patent airway. Establish one, if necessary. Continue CPR, intubate him, and provide respiratory assistance, if needed. Then do the following:
• Assess arterial blood gas levels.
• If the patient's abdomen is distended, insert a nasogastric tube.
• Insert a Foley catheter; start intravenous lines.
• Give medications, as ordered. Much controversy exists about the benefits of drug treatment for near-drowning victims. However, such treatment may include sodium bicarbonate for acidosis, corticosteroids for cerebral edema, antibiotics to prevent infections, and bronchodilators to ease bronchospasms.
• Remember, all near-drowning victims should be admitted for an observation period of 24 to 48 hours because of the possibility of delayed drowning.
• Observe for pulmonary complications and signs of delayed drowning (confusion, substernal pain, and adventitious breath sounds). Suction as necessary. Pulmonary artery catheters may be useful in assessing cardiopulmonary status. Monitor vital signs, intake and out-

put, and peripheral pulses. Check for skin perfusion. Watch for signs of infection.
• To facilitate breathing, raise the head of the patient's bed slightly.

Neonatal assessment

Using the Apgar test

The Apgar neonatal assessment system indicates a newborn infant's overall health by assigning him a score based on his heart rate, respirations, muscle tone, reflex irritability, and color. Normally, Apgar scoring reflects the infant's status 1 minute and 5 minutes after his complete birth (with reassessment every 5 minutes following a 5-minute score below 7). If indicated, however, begin resuscitation efforts immediately without waiting for even a 1-minute score.

Heart rate, respiration, and color are the best indicators of neonatal distress. Assess heart rate by listening to the apical heartbeat with a stethoscope, feeling the pulse at the umbilical cord's base, or monitoring with a cardiotachometer.

Administer neonatal resuscitation in four steps:
• Position, suction, and stimulate. (See *Neonatal resuscitation*.)
• Ventilate with bag, mask, and endotracheal tube (if necessary).
• Perform chest compressions.
• Give drugs and fluids.

Most infants respond to the first two steps; only a few need chest compressions and drugs. Nevertheless, every delivery room team should be prepared to handle a crisis. At least one person who's skilled at neonatal resuscitation should be present at each delivery. Another skilled professional should be readily available because life support for a severely depressed and asphyxiated infant requires intubation and closely coordinated ventilations and chest compressions. During prolonged resuscitation efforts, a third person should be ready

to insert I.V. catheters and administer drugs.

Hypothermia, a particular danger to asphyxiated infants, can delay recovery from acidosis. Prevent heat loss by keeping the delivery room warm, placing the infant under a warmer immediately after birth, and drying him quickly. (See also *Airway obstruction: infants.*)

Neonatal care

Preventing diaper rash

Have you ever been told to expose the red, sore buttocks of a premature infant to room air? To do it without risking temperature loss, put another undershirt on him—a bit differently, though. Put the in-

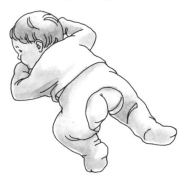

fant's legs through the arms of this undershirt and leave his buttocks exposed through the neck opening.

Neonatal resuscitation

Positioning, suctioning, and stimulation

Here's how to properly resuscitate an infant:
1. Position the infant on his back or left side in a slight Trendelenburg position, with his neck in a neutral position. (Overextension or underextension may obstruct his airway.) Place a 1″ (3 cm) thick blanket or towel under his shoulders to help maintain head position.

2. Suction with a bulb syringe, DeLee trap, or mechanical suction device attached to a suction catheter. Avoid pressures exceeding 100 mm Hg (−136 cm of water). Limit suctioning to less than 10 seconds at a time, and monitor for bradycardia and apnea (possible consequences of deep suctioning, which may produce a vagal response).

Suctioning with bulb syringe

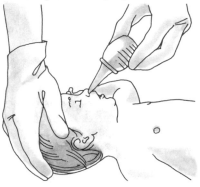

3. Between suctionings, give the infant time to breathe spontaneously, or provide ventilatory assistance with 100% oxygen. (To guard against meconium aspiration, the doctor suctions as soon as crowning occurs, if possible.)
4. If suctioning doesn't stimulate effective respirations, try slapping or flicking the soles of the infant's

Stimulation

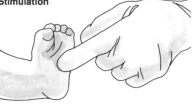

feet, or rub his back. Avoid more vigorous methods. (See also *Airway obstruction: infants; Neonatal assessment.*)

Neonatal ventilation

Proper procedure

Most infants needing ventilatory support respond to assistance from positive-pressure ventilation. Initial

N

lung inflation may require pressure between 30 and 40 cm of water; subsequent inflations should require less pressure. While providing a ventilatory rate of 40 breaths/minute, watch for bilateral lung expansion and auscultate for breath sounds. A distended stomach may require periodic decompression.

If you can't inflate the lungs adequately, first suction, then reposition the head and face mask. If the problem persists, the doctor will perform a laryngoscopic examination of the upper airway and intubate the trachea. Other indications for intubation include apnea, a heart rate below 100 beats/minute and persistent central cyanosis despite administration of 100% oxygen.

After you've established adequate ventilation for 15 to 30 seconds, your next step depends on the heart rate. Follow these guidelines:

• *Heart rate greater than 100 beats/minute; spontaneous respiration:* Discontinue positive-pressure ventilation. Maintain spontaneous respiration with gentle tactile stimulation. If spontaneous respiration ceases, resume positive-pressure ventilation.

• *Heart rate below 60 beats/minute:* Continue positive-pressure ventilation and begin chest compressions.

• *Heart rate 60 to 100 beats/minute and rising:* Continue assisted ventilation; stop chest compressions.

• *Heart rate 60 to 100 beats/minute and not rising:* Make sure you're providing adequate ventilation. If the heart rate remains below 80 beats/minute, begin chest compressions. (See *Neonatal assessment; Neonatal resuscitation.*)

Nephrostomy, percutaneous

Changing the dressing

First, have the patient lie on his stomach or on the side opposite the dressing site. Wash your hands and put on sterile gloves before removing the old dressing. When removing the dressing, be careful not to dislodge the nephrostomy catheter. Use adhesive remover to clean off the residue from the old bandage.

Check the catheter site for signs of infection or tube displacement. Notify the doctor if there's any bleeding or if the patient complains of pain at the site. Normally, he shouldn't have pain or bleeding by the second or third day after the nephrostomy.

Change to another pair of sterile gloves. Then, beginning at the catheter insertion site, clean the area with an outward circular motion, using povidone-iodine (Betadine) or another antiseptic solution. Remove the Betadine with alcohol and allow the area to dry. Next, apply an antibacterial ointment to the site. You'll probably do this during every other dressing change, but more often if the site becomes red or irritated.

If a Molnar disc is used to stabilize the catheter, tape it to the skin. Place precut dressing pads around the catheter site. (If you cut your own pads, use sterile dressing scissors.) Put pads under the tubing to protect the patient's skin at pressure points. Apply extra padding as needed for comfort and to keep the catheter from kinking or bending.

Cover the extra padding with 2″ (5 cm) cloth or paper tape. Tincture of benzoin will help the padding adhere longer. Label the dressings with your initials and the date you changed it.

At certain times you may have to change the extension tubing and the drainage bag. When disconnecting the tubing, ask the patient to take a deep breath. This should cause urine to flow from the catheter, indicating the system is patent. Tape any excess tubing to the patient's hip or thigh to prevent unnecessary tension. Make sure you protect his skin from the plastic extension connectors that are used to attach the nephrostomy catheter to the drainage bag.

Document the dressing change and your assessment. Generally, after the first week, you'll probably change the dressing every fourth day, provided the site appears healthy and the dressing stays dry and intact. (See *Wound care dressings: changes.*)

Nephrostomy tubes

Nursing management

Genitourinary trauma, disease, or surgery can obstruct your patient's normal urine flow or necessitate diverting it. In either case, the doctor will insert a drain, catheter, or tube into the patient's urinary tract to keep his urine flowing. When caring

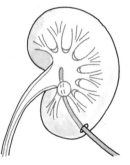

for this type of patient, give special attention to his nephrostomy tube, according to the guidelines below:

• Check tube patency frequently to prevent urine flow obstruction and possible kidney damage.

• Tape the tube to the patient's skin to prevent displacement. If it becomes dislodged, call the doctor immediately.

• Clean the tube site twice daily. (See *Nephrostomy, percutaneous.*)

• Watch for bleeding or urine leaks at the nephrostomy site. Expect hematuria for 24 to 48 hours after percutaneous tube placement.

• Maintain a closed drainage system to prevent kidney infection.

• Make sure the tube doesn't kink when the patient lies on his side. Never clamp the tube.

N

• Keep separate output records for each kidney, if both have tubes.
• Never irrigate the nephrostomy tube unless ordered. Never use more than 5 ml of warm sterile saline solution.

Nerve damage, peripheral

Assessing your patient after a fracture or dislocation

When you're assessing a patient's fracture or dislocation, always check for peripheral nerve damage. Here are the most commonly used tests of sensory and motor function. Decreased sensation or inability to perform range-of-motion tests indicates possible nerve damage.

Upper extremities

• *Median nerve*

—*Sensory:* Test sensation over the palmar side of the patient's thumb, index and long fingers, and half of the ring finger.

Median nerve: sensory function

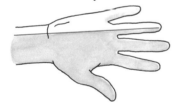

—*Motor:* Ask the patient to rotate his thumb to a grasp position.

—*Motor:* Ask the patient to oppose his thumb to his little finger.

• *Radial nerve*

—*Sensory:* Test sensation over the dorsum of the patient's thumb, index and long fingers, and half of the ring finger.

Radial nerve: sensory function

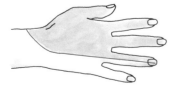

—*Motor:* Ask the patient to extend his wrist and fingers at the metacarpophalangeal joint and his thumb at all joints.

• *Ulnar nerve*

—*Sensory:* Test sensation of the patient's dorsal and palmar side over his little finger and the ulnar half of his ring finger.

Ulnar nerve: sensory function

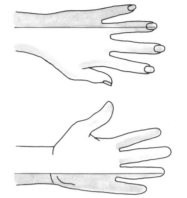

—*Motor:* Ask the patient to spread and close his fingers or to flex his metacarpophalangeal joints without interphalangeal flexion.

• *Axillary nerve*

—*Sensory:* Test sensation over the lateral aspect of the patient's upper arm and shoulder (military patch area).

Axillary nerve: sensory function

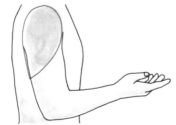

—*Motor:* Ask the patient to abduct his arm at the shoulder joint.

Lower extremities

• *Peroneal nerve*

—*Sensory:* Test sensation over the dorsum of the patient's foot in

Peroneal nerve: sensory function

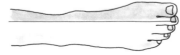

the area adjacent to his great and second toes.

—*Motor:* Ask the patient to dorsiflex his foot or to extend his toes.

• *Tibial nerve*

—*Sensory:* Test sensation over the lateral part of the patient's foot.

Tibial nerve: sensory function

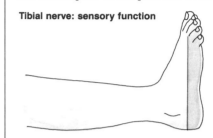

—*Motor:* Ask the patient to plantar flex his ankle and toes. (See also *Dislocation, leg; Fracture assessment; Fracture care.*)

Networking

Polishing your skills

If you don't already belong, join one or more professional organizations. Attend meetings, conferences, and conventions so others will start to recognize you. Get out and meet the "movers and shakers" in nursing.

While at these gatherings, act like a hostess, not a guest. (A hostess introduces herself first; a guest waits to be introduced.) Take the initiative and ask people to lunch. Others will be networking, too, and they'll be glad to meet you.

Enjoy these lunches; don't cross the fine line between assertive and aggressive behavior by doing business while networking. If you want to ask about job leads, get to know people first. Then set up a separate meeting time for business.

Follow up with those you meet. When you tell someone you'll call, do it as soon as possible so she'll remember meeting you. And keep in touch. You might schedule a monthly or quarterly contact with the people you meet, whether by phone, letter, or in person.

N

Once you've made contacts, you'll want to keep them, so set up a file to store names and addresses. For example, sort business cards alphabetically or geographically in a card file. To help you remember each person, jot down a key phrase on the back of the business card. Or note where you met the person so you can match the face with the name.

You can't network alone; successful networking means sharing your sources and ideas with others. But don't abuse your contacts by referring more people to them than they can handle. Treat your sources as you'd like to be treated: Rely on them for quality information, but don't take up too much of their time. And try to help those who have helped you.

Be a good listener; learn to actively listen and pay attention to what people say as well as how they say it. Ask open-ended questions that draw diverse answers.

You'll gain more from your contacts if you don't make assumptions. Stay open to their perspectives and new ideas. You'll be surprised how often one thing leads to another.

The people you meet outside of nursing may also prove helpful, and you never know when you'll make a valuable contact. So carry business cards with you—yes, to the supermarket, the health club, and wherever else. And, even in casual situations, dress neatly to make a good impression.

You can network to improve your current job or to help find a new job. If you're looking for a new job, call or write to your contacts and let them know you're looking. Ask them to keep you in mind if they hear of an appropriate opening. Another networking avenue is your specialty organization; call your contacts there, too.

Be practical about networking; accept the limits of what you can accomplish with it. Remember, networking is volunteer work, so don't let it wear you down. (See also *Career strategies; Job change: planning.*)

Neurologic exam: assessment

Assessing your patient quickly

How can you assess your patient's neurologic status accurately yet quickly? After taking his health history and performing a complete physical examination, follow these guidelines for neurologic screening:
• Evaluate mental status and speech (cerebral function).
• Test cranial nerves II, III, IV, V, VI, and VII for function. (The other cranial nerves will be tested later during the complete physical exam.)
• Assess balance and gait (cerebellar function).
• Test wrist and arm extension, foot dorsiflexion, and knee flexion (motor function).
• Check sensation in both arms and legs (sensory function).
• Test biceps, triceps, patellar, and Achilles reflexes.

Neurologic exam: coordination

Checking coordination and balance

After testing your patient's muscle strength (see *Neurologic exam: muscle strength*), evaluate his coordination and balance. Begin by having him perform rapid alternating movements.

First, tell him to pat his upper thigh with his dominant hand, alternately using the palm and the back of the hand as quickly as pos-sible. Have him repeat this exercise using his other hand.

Rapid alternating movements

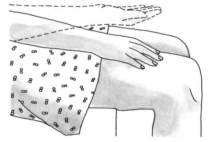

Next, tell him to touch the thumb of his dominant hand with each finger of that hand as quickly as possible then tell him to do the same with his other hand.

Point-to-point tests will help you evaluate coordination and detect intention tremors. Tell the patient to use his forefinger to touch first your forefinger, then his nose. Instruct

Point-to-point localization

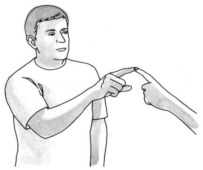

him to move back and forth as fast as he can. Test both hands. Observe for accuracy; note any tremors.

Now, check leg coordination. Ask the patient to touch your hand with the sole of his foot as fast as he can.

Leg coordination

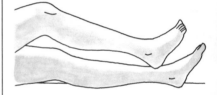

Then have him run his right heel down his left shin, then his left heel down his right shin, as you observe for equal coordinated movement. If your patient has difficulty performing any of these coordination exercises, he may need to be evaluated further for cerebellar disease.

If your patient is confined to bed, you won't be able to test his balance. But if he can stand beside the bed, you can perform the *Romberg* test. He should stand with his feet together, arms at his sides. Have him maintain this position for about 30 seconds with his eyes open, then another 30 seconds with his eyes closed. Stay close to him in case he starts to fall.

Neurologic exam: mental status

Guidelines

When you perform a mental status examination, you're really assessing the patient's cerebral function.

The health history interview provides you with an excellent opportunity to assess your patient's mental status. As you talk to him during the interview, you can evaluate his orientation, judgment, memory, affect, speech, and language. If you suspect a problem in one of those areas, investigate further.

Evaluate the patient's judgment by noting whether his ideas and thoughts make sense. Does he draw logical conclusions?

You can assess short-term memory by asking the patient about events that occurred during or just before his hospitalization. To evaluate long-term memory, you can ask about past hospitalizations, surgeries, and the like. If you suspect a memory deficit, check his responses against his health records or family members' recollections.

Note if the patient's emotional state seems appropriate. For example, how does he react to being hospitalized? Also, observe his posture, grooming, and behavior.

When you document the patient's level of consciousness, avoid vague terms, such as lethargic, obtunded, or stuporous. Be as specific as possible about how the patient responds to verbal or tactile stimulation. If you must assess a patient's level of consciousness frequently, say every 2 hours, use the Glasgow Coma Scale. That should help make your assessments more objective and consistent. (See *Glasgow Coma Scale.*)

As you talk to the patient, evaluate his speech and language. Normally, a patient's speech should be clear, well-paced, and coherent. His language should be appropriate for his educational and socioeconomic levels. Aphasia or altered speech patterns would alert you to the possibility of neurologic problems.

Neurologic exam: muscle strength

Assessing your patient's motor system

Start by inspecting the patient's arm and leg muscles, look for atrophy and abnormal movements, such as tremors or fasciculations. For a quick check of muscle tone, use passive range-of-motion exercises and note any resistance. (See also *Orthopedics: inspection.*)

Now, assess the strength of specific muscle groups against resis-

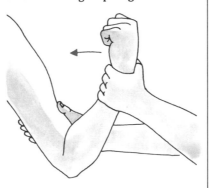

tance. For instance, to test the biceps, hold your patient's wrist and instruct him to flex his arm as you

pull on the wrist. Then test the triceps by having him extend his arm while you push against his wrist. If you suspect distal muscle weakness, test wrist flexion and extension as well as hand grasps.

To assess leg muscle strength in a patient who must remain in bed, have him flex his hip and knee so that his knee is about 8 inches off the bed. Then tell him to maintain this position while you push down against his thigh.

Next, test knee flexion and extension. Have the patient flex his knee and place his foot flat on the bed. As with the previous test, tell him to maintain this position as you first push down on his lower leg, then pull up.

To test plantar flexion and dorsiflexion at the ankle, have the patient push his foot down against your hand, then have him pull it up against your hand.

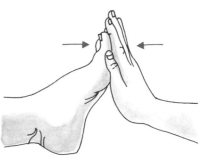

For all these tests, note whether you find weakness on one or both sides. If your patient can't perform these resistive tests, note whether he can simply raise his arms and legs. If not, can he slide them back and forth on the bed?

Now assess for mild hemiparesis of the arms. While the patient is sitting up, tell him to close his eyes and hold his arms out in front of him with his palms up. Have him hold the position for 30 seconds as you observe for drifting and pronation.

Grade muscle strength from 0 (no contractions) to 5 (normal muscular contractions).

N

Neurologic exam: sensory system

Assessing it properly

Keep these points in mind:
• The patient's eyes should be closed during all the tests.
• Compare one side with the other, noting whether sensory perception is bilateral.
• When testing position and vibration, assess the distal aspects of the arms and legs. When testing temperature, touch, and pain, assess both the distal and proximal aspects of the arms and legs.
• If you detect an area of increased or decreased sensation, mark it with a water-soluble marker and note which peripheral nerves carry sensation to that area.

Begin your examination by assessing the spinothalamic tract, testing pain sensation first. If that's intact, you usually won't have to test for temperature and touch. To test for pain, you'll need a sterile needle. Have the patient close his eyes and tell him to let you know when he feels the needle on his skin. Then lightly touch the proximal and distal aspects of his arms and legs with the sterile needle.

Pain sensation

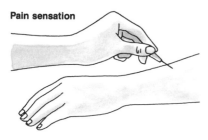

Next, assess the posterior column by testing your patient's perception of light touch, vibration, and position. With a wisp of cotton, lightly stroke the proximal and distal aspects of his arms and legs. Have the patient tell you when he feels each stroke.

To test vibratory sensation, place a vibrating tuning fork on the distal joint of one finger of each hand and on the great toes. When you position the tuning fork, ask the patient what he feels. If he doesn't feel the vibration at the distal joint, move the tuning fork proximally to the next joint.

Vibratory sensation

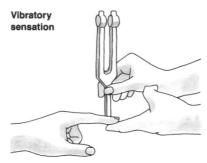

To test position sense, grasp your patient's great toes. As you move the toe up and down, ask your patient which way it's pointing. Using the same technique, check all his

Position sense

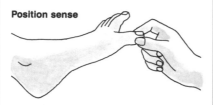

fingers. If the patient's position sense isn't intact, move proximally to the next joint and repeat the test.

The ability to distinguish fine sensations is controlled by the posterior column and the sensory cortex. To test this function, check for *stereognosis* (the ability to distinguish objects by touch). Place a common object such as a coin, key, or safety pin in your patient's hand and ask him to identify it. Test the other hand using different objects.

If he can't identify the objects (or if he simply can't perform the fine motor movements necessary to identify small objects), evaluate *graphesthesia*. Have your patient open his hand, then draw a number on his palm, using a dull pointed object (the eraser of a pencil will do nicely). Make the number as big as possible. Then ask the patient to identify the number. (See also *Nerve damage, peripheral.*)

Nitroglycerin: aerosol

Helping your patient relieve angina

Angina sufferers have a new alternative to standard nitroglycerin tablets. Nitrolingual aerosol comes in a spray canister and contains 200 0.4-mg metered doses of nitroglycerin—the same dose as in most sublingual tablets. Most tablets need a short time to dissolve, but the spray gets rapidly absorbed

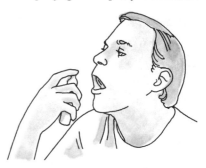

through the oral mucosa, providing almost instant pain relief.

For angina, instruct your patient to spray one dose on or under his tongue, then to close his mouth. Warn him not to inhale the spray or swallow immediately. If he needs another dose, he can repeat the application in 3 to 5 minutes, but he shouldn't exceed three doses in a 15-minute period. To prevent angina, tell him to use the spray 5 to 10 minutes before engaging in strenuous activities. Advise him to sit down when he applies the spray, to prevent postural hypotension.

Nitroglycerin: I.V.

Giving it properly

When giving nitroglycerin by the I.V. route:
• Never give it in a bolus. Dilute the concentrated drug with either 5% dextrose in water injection or nor-

mal saline injection. Follow the manufacturer's preparation procedures.

• Use only a glass bottle and the manufacturer-supplied tubing. Up to 80% of the drug can be absorbed by plastics, including the bottles, tubing, and filters you'd normally use for infusions.

• Don't mix I.V. nitroglycerin with other drugs because of the danger of incompatibility.

• Use an infusion pump to administer the drug.

• Monitor the patient's blood pressure and heart rate when titrating the drug to achieve the appropriate dosage for his condition. Intravenous nitroglycerin has no optimum dose.

• Monitor for the same adverse reactions caused by nitroglycerin tablets and ointment. (See *Nitroglycerin precautions*.)

• Watch for overdose, as evidenced by hypotension and tachycardia. If they occur, stop the drug and notify the doctor. He may order an I.V. alpha-adrenergic stimulant (for example, phenylephrine).

Nitroglycerin: ointment

Teaching your patient

When giving the following instructions to your patient, tailor your teaching to suit his needs. Tell him:

• "First, choose your application site: a hairless area of skin on your chest, thigh, or abdomen. Remove

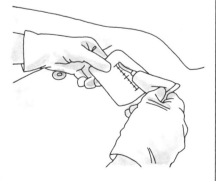

any traces of ointment left from a previous application.

• "Next, use the ruled applicator paper that comes with the ointment to measure your dose accurately.

• "Then, use the applicator paper to apply the ointment in a thin, uniform layer over an area of about 3″ to 6″ (7.5 to 15 cm).

• "Now, cover the area with plastic wrap and secure it with tape. This will protect your clothing and ensure maximum absorption.

• "Call your doctor if you experience headache, feel dizzy or faint, or notice any redness or irritation at the application site. He may want to adjust your dosage or check the site.

• "The ointment prevents angina from occurring rather than treats it. If you experience acute angina, take a sublingual tablet." (See also *Medication, topical.*)

Nitroglycerin: tablets

Patient teaching

Incorrect use of the *forms* of nitroglycerin can seriously affect how well the drug works, so you must be especially diligent with patient teaching. For sublingual tablets, give your patient these instructions:

• "When you experience angina, sit down and put a nitroglycerin tablet under your tongue. Let it dissolve completely. Don't stand up right away because you may feel dizzy.

• "Take up to three tablets—one every 4 to 5 minutes—if necessary. Record each dose. If the pain doesn't go away after 15 minutes, call your doctor at once or go to the nearest hospital emergency department.

• "If you feel a headache or your face flushes after taking a tablet, don't be alarmed. These effects are common. However, if they persist call your doctor. He may want to lower your dosage. (See *Nitroglycerin precautions.*)

• "Keep your tablets in their original bottle, but remove the cotton. Store the tightly capped bottle in a cool, dry place away from direct heat and sunlight. Don't store it in the refrigerator or bathroom medicine cabinet because moisture may affect the tablets' potency.

• "When taking a tablet, pour several of them into the bottle cap, select one, and pour the rest back. Don't hold them in the palm of your hand because they'll pick up moisture and crumble.

• "Always have a supply of tablets with you. Nitroglycerin is available in different strengths, so don't lend tablets or borrow them from anyone else."

Nitroglycerin patches

Guidelines to give your patient

The transdermal nitroglycerin patch changed long-term treatment of angina pectoris when it came on the scene a few years ago. Since then, some things about the patch have changed. Here's an update.

Patches now come in three brands—Nitrodisc, Nitro-Dur, and Transderm-Nitro—each releasing a constant stream of nitroglycerin into the bloodstream over a 24-hour period.

Therapy usually begins with a dose of 5 mg/24 hours. The dose increases gradually until the drug controls angina. The ideal dose reduces resting blood pressure as much as possible without producing orthostatic hypotension.

The patient may use one or more patches to deliver his daily dose. He may even mix and match different brands, thanks to recent label standardization. All three brands now tell how much nitroglycerin they release over 24 hours. So if a patient's dose is 7.5 mg/24 hours, he can use a 5 mg/24 hours patch from one company and a 2.5 mg/24 hours patch from another.

N

Tell the patient to apply the patch to his chest, upper leg, back, or upper arm at the same time each day, using a different site each day. Warn him not to apply it to his lower leg or arm because these areas don't permit adequate drug absorption. To make sure the patch adheres properly, tell him to place it on a clean, dry, hairless site, avoiding skin that's scarred, callused, or irritated. Warn him not to cut the patch to reduce the dose. If the patch falls off, he should apply a new one.

Remind your patient that the patches help prevent angina, but won't treat acute attacks. To relieve an attack, he should carry sublingual nitroglycerin with him. (See *Nitroglycerin: tablets*.)

Transdermal nitroglycerin patches cause few adverse effects; the most common is headache.

To prevent complications during cardioversion or defibrillation, remove your patient's transdermal nitroglycerin patch before the procedures. The patch's backing, made from aluminum or an aluminized plastic, can conduct electricity, causing an explosion during defibrillation or cardioversion. More importantly, the patch could prevent successful cardioversion.

Nitroglycerin precautions

Ensuring safe use

The most common adverse reaction to nitrates is a pounding headache. Because sublingual nitroglycerin is short-acting, the headache usually passes quickly. Longer-acting nitrates, especially if they're used in high doses to stabilize the patient, can cause an enduring headache that may require acetaminophen (Tylenol). Other common adverse reactions include light-headedness and dizziness, either of which could be hazardous and might require a decreased dosage or stopping the drug.

Noncompliant patient: care

Getting your patient to comply

Here are a few suggestions to get your patient to comply with treatment.

• First, make sure the patient understands the general outline of his treatment and shares the staff's therapeutic goals.

• Next, talk to him about his noncompliance. Explain why compliance is important, and find out why he won't comply. Maybe he has a problem accepting authority.

• Finally, set explicit rules for achieving treatment goals, enlisting his help as much as possible to accomplish difficult tasks.

If the patient's committed himself to the therapeutic goals and understands the general outline of his treatment, the staff has implicit authority to employ the means to achieve those goals.

If you want to devise games, however, make sure the patient participates. He should help choose the rewards, too, such as extra TV time, or the chance to spend more time with a staff member.

Noncompliant patient: consent

When your patient refuses treatment

Your first step is to stop briefly and think about why a particular patient is refusing treatment. Maybe he doesn't really understand it. Ask yourself: Could he have misunderstood the terms the doctor used in his explanation? Has he made any comments that indicate he doesn't?

Perhaps the patient's physical condition or the medications he's received have made him confused. A depressed patient may believe, rightly or wrongly, that his case is hopeless. His adamant "No more tests" may be another way of saying "What's the use?"

Also, if he's had the procedure before, listen carefully to his comments. A muttered complaint ("I got real sick after that test" or "Nothing's worth that much pain") may partly explain why he's refusing.

Does he have any health problems—for example, allergies—that he fears the treatment may aggravate? If he's ever had a drug dependency, is he afraid the prescribed sedatives may reactivate his addiction?

The patient may be desperately trying to keep some control over his life by refusing treatment. Perhaps he's feeling overwhelmed by his illness and becomes angry when asked to replace his routine with the hospital's. This may lead to stalling, noncompliance, and ultimately, refusal of treatment. Comments such as "I'm tired of being awakened for this or that," "Can't I have a little peace?" or "There's no privacy here" can tip you off to potential problems. (See also *Noncompliant patient: care.*)

Nosebleed: emergency care

Steps to follow

If your patient has a severe nosebleed, quickly take his vital signs. If you detect tachypnea, hypotension, or other signs of hypovolemic shock, have another nurse notify the doctor immediately. Insert a large-gauge I.V. for rapid fluid and blood replacement, and attempt to control bleeding by pinching the nostrils closed. (However, if you suspect a nasal fracture, don't pinch the nostrils. Instead, place gauze under the nose to absorb the blood.) Have the hypovolemic patient lie down and turn his head to the side to prevent blood from draining down the back of his throat, which could cause aspiration or vomiting of swallowed blood. If the patient isn't hypovolemic, have him sit upright and tilt his head forward. Check airway patency and if his condition is unstable, begin cardiac monitoring and attempt to give supplemental oxygen by mask, as ordered.

If your patient isn't in distress, take a history.

Continue the physical examination by inspecting the patient's skin for other signs of bleeding, such as ecchymoses and petechiae, and noting any jaundice, pallor, or other abnormalities. For a trauma patient, assess for associated injuries, such as eye trauma or facial fractures. Be prepared to assist the doctor with a nasal examination to visualize the bleeding site. (See *Nosebleed: packing.*)

Nosebleed: packing

Controlling a nosebleed

When direct pressure and cautery fail to control nosebleed, prepare for *anterior* packing if the patient has severe bleeding in the anterior nose. In this procedure, the doctor will insert horizontal layers of petrolatum gauze strips into the nostrils near the turbinates.

If the patient has severe bleeding in the posterior nose or if anterior bleeding starts flowing backward, prepare for *posterior* packing. This

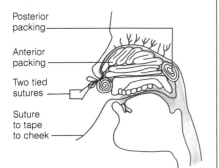

Posterior packing
Anterior packing
Two tied sutures
Suture to tape to cheek

consists of a gauze pack secured by three strong silk sutures. After anesthetizing the nose, the doctor

will pull the sutures through the nostrils with a soft catheter, positioning the pack behind the soft palate. He'll tie two of the sutures to a gauze roll under the patient's nose, which will keep the pack in place, and tape the third suture to the patient's cheek. (Anterior packing may also be inserted for extra traction and to avoid pressure on the nostrils.)

If the patient has nasal packing, remember these important nursing considerations:
• Watch for signs of respiratory distress, such as dyspnea, which may occur if the packing slips and obstructs the airway.
• Keep emergency equipment (flashlights, scissors, and hemostat) at the patient's bedside. Be prepared to cut the cheek suture and remove the pack at the first sign of airway obstruction.
• Avoid tension on the cheek suture, which could cause the posterior pack to slip out of place.
• Keep the call bell within easy reach.
• Monitor the patient's vital signs frequently. Notify the doctor if you detect signs of hypoxia, such as tachycardia and restlessness.
• Elevate the head of the patient's bed, and remind him to breathe through his mouth.
• Administer humidified oxygen, as ordered.
• Instruct him not to blow his nose for 48 hours after the packing's removed. (See *Nosebleed: emergency care.*)

Nurturing

Supporting yourself and others

When you feel stress building, try these techniques:
• List the problems you're having and decide which ones you'd try to solve if someone else mentioned them to you. This will help you see your right to nurturing.

• Give yourself decompression time—15 minutes or more to unwind from your home life and work life—before you dive into your next role.
• Do something fun every day, if only for a few minutes.
• Stay healthy by eating and sleeping wisely and taking care of any health problems you develop.

We've all learned the importance of mutual support and nurturing, but we forget quickly if the lesson isn't reinforced frequently. To help your colleagues remember, try these techniques:
• Get together with your colleagues for coffee once in a while. Find someone you can trust enough to say, "I'm having a rough day, I need someone to hug me." And offer the same kind of support to others. We know how soothing and supportive touch is to our patients—let's offer that same support to our colleagues.
• Use gentle humor to help someone recognize behavior that's irritating to others. (See *Humor.*)
• Offer your ears more than your mouth. Most people can solve many of their own problems if someone will help them express their needs. If a colleague has serious personal problems such as alcoholism or marital problems, encourage her to see a professional counselor.
• Guard each others' confidences. Let others on the staff learn they can depend on you—not only to listen but also to keep what they've said confidential.
• Learn to enjoy your colleagues and develop supportive relationships by joining an exercise class, bowling league, or some other activity that has nothing to do with nursing.
• Celebrate each others' birthdays on the unit. Make a chronological list of the birthdays, and give copies to everyone. Each person on the list could bring in a cake for the next person's birthday.
• Try talking instead of writing. Stay late or come in early occasionally

N

so you can talk to nurses on other shifts instead of writing notes. If note-writing is essential, be sure you write a few thank-you's. One of our most common non-nurturing behaviors is to pick up our pens to write only complaints about the previous shift. If you have a problem with someone on another shift, talk to her in person, so you can communicate your support of her despite your displeasure with her behavior.

• Plan special events for the nursing staff. If your hospital won't pick up the tab, collect enough money from each nurse to pay for the event. (See also *Stress.*)

Nutrition

When your patient won't eat

A common professional frustration is having a patient who desperately needs nutrition persist in refusing food. Three times a day—or more—you face defeat, and the frustration mounts. Is there *anything* you can do? Yes—start by identifying the problem as either *physical* or *emotional*.

If a physical problem makes eating unpleasant or difficult, offer routine, practical support. For example, if the patient has trouble chewing or swallowing, tell him to order food that's easy to chew, to cut his food into bite-size pieces, and to take his time. Perhaps the trouble is mechanical—he has difficulty holding utensils. If so, ask the occupational therapist for special equipment like scooper plates, swivel spoons, or universal cuffs.

But what if you can rule out physical causes and the problem is emotional—then where do you start? Start by exploring the patient's feelings about eating and why he's choosing not to eat. Consider these common reactions:

• *Control.* Hospitalization robs a patient of his independence; your patient may be looking for a way to

control what's happening to him. Claims of nausea or poor appetite give him some sense of making his own decisions.

• *Anger.* He may be displacing his anger on you or his family. Using mealtime as a battle arena, he can easily draw opponents into the ring.

• *Depression and despair.* Your patient, like so many others, may be temporarily depressed and have lost his appetite. Or he may be in deep despair about an overwhelming illness or long-term rehabilitation plans. Refusing food is one way of throwing in the towel.

Once you have your patient talking about these feelings, you can help him understand them. Such a discussion can provide him with insights that lessen his anxiety and increase his confidence, particularly if you acknowledge and accept any fears he expresses. Sometimes, just explaining his treatment will help.

What else can you do? Recognize when you must alert other members of the health care team. When a patient's depressed or in despair, counseling or even drug therapy may be in order; you're the one who must intervene and make the connection.

When you've exhausted conventional means of persuading a patient to eat, total parental nutrition or tube feeding may be necessary. Don't be surprised if your patient resists these alternatives as much as he's resisted eating; again, counseling may be needed.

Remember, however, if the patient is in possession of his faculties, the decision to eat remains his. You may feel frustrated and defeated if he won't eat, and you may question his rejection of your help: "Why didn't he like me well enough to eat for me?" "Why couldn't I make him feel life was worth living?" Recognize that these are very human reactions, that you did all you could, and that you let the patient know

you wanted him to eat and to live. After that, the decision was his. (See also *Nutritional supplement.*)

Nutritional disorder

Teaching someone with a decreased appetite

Advise your patient to make sure his diet includes the four basic food groups.

Meat group
Your patient should have two or more servings of meat per day. For example, 2 or 3 ounces of lean, cooked meat, poultry, or fish would constitute a serving. Or as an alternative, one egg, ½ cup cooked dry beans or peas, or 2 tablespoons of peanut butter in place of half a meat serving.

Milk group
The amount of milk your patient needs per day depends upon his age:
• child (age 8 or under)—two to three servings
• child (age 9 to 12)—three or more servings
• teenager—four or more servings
• adult—two or more servings
• pregnant woman—three or more servings
• nursing woman—four or more servings.

A serving of milk consists of 8 ounces of fluid milk, 1⅓ ounces of cheddar cheese, 1⅓ cups of cottage cheese, 1 cup yogurt, or 1⅔ cups of ice cream.

Fruit and vegetable group
At least four servings are recommended of either ½ cup dark green or deep yellow vegetables or fruit (apple, banana, half a grapefruit, half a cantaloupe).

Bread and cereal group
Your patient should have four or more servings per day. A serving consists of 1 slice of whole grain or enriched bread, 1 ounce of dry cereal, or ½ to ¾ cup of cooked cereal, pasta, or rice. (See also *Nutritional supplement.*)

Nutritional status

Evaluating it

If your patient has an excessive weight loss or gain, you can help assess his nutritional status by measuring his skinfold thickness and midarm circumference and by calculating his midarm muscle circumference. Skinfold measurements reflect adipose tissue mass (subcutaneous fat accounts for about 50% of the body's adipose tissue). Midarm measurements reflect both skeletal muscle and adipose tissue mass.

To measure the triceps skinfold, locate the midpoint of the patient's upper arm, using a nonstretch tape measure. Mark the midpoint with a felt-tipped pen. Then grasp the skin with your thumb and forefinger about 1 cm above the midpoint. Place the calipers at the midpoint and squeeze them for about 3 seconds. Record the measurement registered on the handle gauge to the

Measuring triceps skinfold

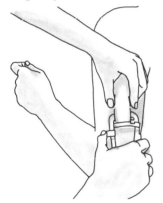

nearest 0.5 mm. Take two more readings and average all three to compensate for any measurement error.

A triceps or subscapular skinfold measurement below 60% of the standard value indicates severe depletion of fat reserves; a measurement between 60% and 90% indicates moderate to mild depletion; and above 90% indicates significant fat reserves. A midarm

circumference of less than 90% of the standard value indicates caloric deprivation; greater than 90% indicates adequate muscle and fat. A midarm muscle circumference of less than 90% indicates protein depletion; over 90% indicates adequate protein reserves.

To measure the subscapular skinfold, use your thumb and forefinger to grasp the skin just below the angle of the scapula, in line with the natural cleavage of the skin. Apply the calipers and proceed as you would when measuring the triceps skinfold. Both subscapular and triceps skinfold measurements are reliable measurements of fat loss or gain during hospitalization.

To measure midarm circumference, return to the midpoint you marked on the patient's upper arm. Then use a tape measure to determine the arm circumference at this point. This measurement reflects

Measuring midarm circumference

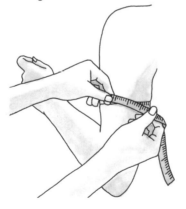

both skeletal muscle and adipose tissue mass and helps evaluate protein and caloric reserves. To calculate midarm muscle circumference, multiply the triceps skinfold thickness (in centimeters) by 3.143, and subtract this figure from the midarm circumference. Midarm muscle circumference reflects muscle mass alone, providing a more sensitive index of protein reserves.

Then express the three measurements as a percentage of standard by using this formula:

$$\frac{\text{actual measurement}}{\text{standard measurement}} \times 100 = \underline{\quad}$$

Standard anthropometric measurements vary according to the patient's age and sex and can be found in a chart of normal anthropometric values.

Nutritional supplement

A good recipe to give your patient

When a patient needs a high-calorie, high-protein nutritional supplement but is tired of the same old thing, teach him this recipe:

"Mix one of the following combinations in equal amounts:
• strawberries, whipped cream, and vanilla Sustacal pudding
• chocolate Sustacal pudding and whipped cream
• vanilla liquid Sustacal, whipped cream, and several drops of peppermint extract.

"Add pieces of banana, apple, or other fruit, according to your preference. Then pour the mixture into 30-ml medicine cups, place a toothpick in the center of each cup, and put them in the freezer. When the mixture is frozen, remove the medicine cup, and you have a frozen nutritional ice pop.

"These supplements keep well in the freezer, so you can enjoy a tasty 'nutripop' whenever you want." (See also *Nutritional disorder.*)

O

Ommaya reservoir

Preparing the patient for insertion

The doctor may implant an Ommaya reservoir beneath your patient's scalp to administer drugs directly into the cerebrospinal fluid, thus avoiding a spinal tap; to measure cerebrospinal pressure; or to obtain cerebrospinal specimens.

Barring complications, the reservoir can remain in place permanently. Follow these guidelines:
• Carefully prepare the insertion site beforehand. Wear a mask and have the patient wear one, too.
• Explain the procedure. Tell him he won't need a local anesthetic because he won't feel pain.
• Help him into the proper position as ordered.

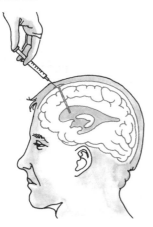

• After insertion, have the patient lie down briefly.
• Monitor him for postinsertion nausea, vomiting, headache, and dizziness. Notify the doctor if these symptoms persist.
• Tell the patient to immediately report these signs and symptoms of possible infection: tenderness, unusual warmth, redness, or drainage at the reservoir site; a fever of 101° F. (38° C.) or more; neck stiffness; and headache with or without vomiting.

Ophthalmoscope

Examining your patient's eyes

First, seat your patient in a room that you can darken partially or completely. As you know, a darkened room will cause your patient's pupils to dilate, exposing more of his peripheral retina. (Place a lamp near his chair, so you'll be able to see after the room's darkened.)

Now, darken the room. Sit or stand facing your patient at his eye level.

To examine your patient's right eye, position yourself on his right side. Hold the ophthalmoscope up to your right eye with your right

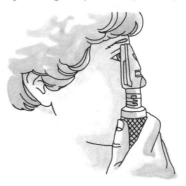

hand, and illuminate it. Set the ophthalmoscope lens at 0 (unless contraindicated).

Next, ask your patient to focus on a stationary object at eye level. Hold the ophthalmoscope about 12" (30 cm) in front of him, and direct the beam of light at your patient's right pupil.

Slowly move the ophthalmoscope closer to your patient until you're about 6" (15.2 cm) from his right eye. (You should be at a 25-degree angle to his right side.)

Looking through the lens aperture, you'll see an orange glow, known as the red reflex, on his pupil. If you don't see the red reflex, your patient may have corneal lesions or a complete retinal detachment. Notify the doctor.

Now, move the ophthalmoscope toward your patient's eye until you visualize the optic disc. If all's well, the optic disc will be yellowish, and round or oval in shape.

Look for the optic disc cup, which is a white, central depression one third the size of the disc. As you probably know, the nasal edge of the cup will be less distinct than the temporal edge. You may also see a white crescent around the tem-

poral edge. Suppose the optic disc appears out of focus. Rotate the lens selection disc (white dial) until you can clearly visualize the disc.

Get ready to examine the fundus. Study a photograph of a normal fundus so you know what to look for. Begin by observing the color, clarity of the optic disc's outline, and the elevation and condition of the blood vessels.

If the optic disc appears enlarged and gray (with white edges), your patient may have glaucoma. Recommend that he see a trained professional to have his intraocular pressure measured.

Suppose the optic disc's obscured and you see flame-shaped hemorrhages (some near disc edges), and tufts of exudate. Your patient may have hypertension. Notify the doctor.

Now, locate the macula, which is about 3 mm from the optic disc's temporal edge. The macula, which normally has no blood vessels, should appear darker than the surrounding areas.

Suppose the macula is spotted with white exudate and the retinal edges have irregular vessels, with small aneurysms, hemorrhages, and patches of white exudate. Your patient may have diabetes. Notify the doctor.

Next, inspect the peripheral areas of the fundus by instructing your patient to look up, then to one side, and then toward his nose. Note any capillary hemorrhages, white patches, opacities, or dilated vessels.

Repeat the entire examination on your patient's left eye.

Orders, sliding scale

Deciding how much analgesic to give

For sliding-scale analgesic orders, you need to use your nursing judgment to decide how much medication the patient should receive. To

avoid harming him—and incurring liability—follow these guidelines:
• Assess the patient carefully. Note the severity of his pain and how he describes it. (See *Pain detection.*)
• If this isn't his first dose, note what helped him most in the past—the higher dose or lower dose? How long was it effective? Then use that information to determine future doses.
• Support your decision in your nurses' notes. (See also *Analgesia administration.*)

Orthopedics: inspection

Knowing what to look for

While inspecting and palpating each area of a patient's body, look for symmetry, swelling, deformity, or increased limb size. Palpate muscles for spasm, masses, and painful areas; joints for swelling, tenderness, stability, crepitus, and warmth; and bones for abnormal shape or junction with other bones.

Don't forget to check extremity pulses and limb temperature—poor circulation, rather than an orthopedic problem, may cause limb pain.

If you think palpation of one area may cause the patient pain, skip that area until the end of the assessment. Approach the painful area cautiously and tell the patient you're about to touch it.

Observe how the patient moves his arms and legs and spine. Of course, you wouldn't assess range of motion if the patient has a possible cervical spine injury, neurologic signs that suggest instability of the cervical spine, or a possible fracture or dislocation.

To test muscle strength, apply maximum force to the extremity while the patient pushes against your fixed resistance. (See *Neurologic exam: muscle strength; Orthopedics: patient history.*)

Orthopedics: legs

Assessment technique

Follow this procedure:
1. Ask the patient to lie down. Measure each leg from the anterior iliac spine to the medial malleolus.
2. To test hamstring tightness, first stabilize his pelvis with your hand. Then raise his leg, keeping his knee straight.
3. Next, test his hips. To test flexion, first bend his knee, then bend his hip as far as possible. Place his leg back on the bed, making sure his hip isn't flexed.
4. To test adduction and abduction, first stabilize his pelvis with your hand. Move his leg across the body's midline, then away from the midline.
5. To test external and internal rotation, ask him to flex his knee and hip. Rotate his hip away from his body's midline, then toward the midline.
6. Now test his knees. To test flexion and extension, ask him to bend his knee as far as possible, then straighten it.
7. To test for a torn meniscus, check for McMurray's sign. (See *McMurray's sign.*)
8. Next, test his feet. To test plantar flexion and dorsiflexion, bend his foot downward as if he were going to stand on his toes. Then bend his foot upward.
9. To test eversion and inversion, hold his ankle steady. Move his foot

Eversion and inversion

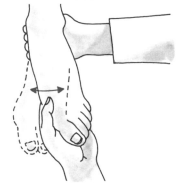

away from the body's midline, then toward the midline.
10. Document your findings. (See also *Orthopedics: patient history.*)

Orthopedics: patient history

Getting all the details

Start your musculoskeletal assessment by taking a history of the patient's problem. Identify his chief complaint, when it started, the pain or disability it causes, and what helps relieve it. Review his past medical history as well as his family and social history.

As you take the patient's history, check his general appearance for clues to his overall condition. For instance, look at how he sits in his chair or lies in bed. Does he sit to one side? Support an affected limb? Shift constantly to get comfortable?

If the patient can stand, ask him to do so. Note whether he has any trouble getting up from the sitting or lying position. For example, does he protect a limb or his back? As he's standing, look for unusual lesions, scars, deformities, or poor posture.

Ask him to walk so you can observe his gait pattern. As he does, look for abnormalities, such as a limp, a wide-based gait, a lateral shift of the torso (a lurch), or a slow and apprehensive step. Most abnormalities occur during the stance phase when the foot is on the floor, because that's when the leg is under the most stress.

An abnormal gait may be caused by a neurologic deficit, muscle weakness, pain, a shortened leg, congenital abnormalities, or ankylosed joints.

Tell the patient to walk on his toes, his heels, then to stoop down like a baseball catcher for a preliminary assessment of his legs. (See *Orthopedics: inspection.*)

O

Orthopedics: spine and arms

Assessing them correctly

Here are 13 steps to follow:

1. After the patient is comfortably seated on the edge of the bed or examining table, ask him to look straight ahead. Tell him you're going to test his neck. To test rotation, ask him to look over each shoulder.

2. To test lateral flexion, ask him to touch his ear to his shoulder.

3. To test flexion and extension, ask him to touch his chin to his chest, then put his head back as far as he can.

Flexion and extension

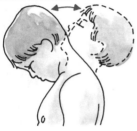

4. Next, test his shoulders. To test abduction and adduction, have him put his arm out to his side and raise it as far as it can go. Then have him put his arm behind his back.

5. To test flexion and extension, ask him to put his arm out in front of him, first next to his body at the side, then next to his body behind him.

6. To test external and internal rotation, have him place his elbow

External and internal rotation

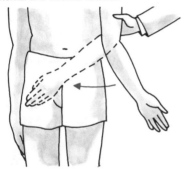

at his side and rotate his arm outward, then place his forearm over his abdomen.

7. Now test his elbows. Test extension and flexion by having him put his arm straight out in front of him, and then bending his elbow as far as possible.

8. To test supination and pronation, have him place his elbow at his side and turn the palm up toward the ceiling, then down toward the floor.

To measure the exact range of motion more precisely, have him hold a pencil while turning his palm. If the pencil is parallel to the floor during supination and pronation, you'll know the patient can complete normal range of motion.

9. Next, test his wrists. To test flexion and extension, ask him to bend his wrist as much possible, then extend it as much as possible.

10. To test ulnar and radial deviation, have him move his wrist away from the body's midline, then toward the midline.

Ulnar and radial deviation

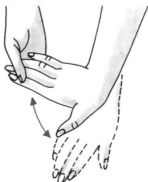

11. Then test his hands. To test flexion of the MP (metacarpophalangeal), PIP (proximal interphalangeal), and DIP (distal interphalangeal) joints, ask the patient to flex his fingers into a fist.

12. To test abduction, ask him to straighten out the fingers, then spread them apart.

13. To test opposition, have him touch his thumb to his little finger.

Orthopedics: torso

Examination guidelines

Follow these steps when examining your patient:

1. Ask the patient to stand. To measure his chest expansion, first ask him to exhale, then place a tape measure around his chest at the nipples. Write down this measurement. Now ask him to inhale, and note this measurement. The difference in the two measurements equals his chest expansion.

When measuring a woman's chest expansion, place the tape measure directly under her breasts.

2. Then test his spine. To test rotation, place your hands on his hips

Spine rotation

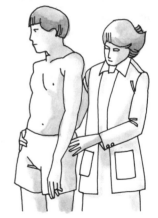

to stabilize his pelvis, then ask him to twist to the right and left.

3. To test lateral flexion, stabilize his pelvis, then ask him to bend to each side.

Lateral flexion

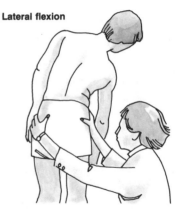

While the patient's standing, check for scoliosis: look for asymmetry in his back, waistline, or shoulders.

4. To test for scoliosis and flexion, have the patient bend forward facing you and touch his toes. Look for asymmetry of the rib cage, especially a rib hump in the lumbar area. Next, look at him from the side for kyphosis (round back). Finally, to test extension, have him stand up and bend backward as far as possible.

Osteoporosis

Preventive measures to give your patients

Osteoporosis affects 15 to 20 million people in the United States. Women—especially postmenopausal women—are at highest risk. Here's what to tell your patients about preventive measures:

• "Make sure you get an adequate supply of calcium—from 1,000 to 1,500 mg daily—during the years before menopause. Foods that are especially high in calcium include milk; plain yogurt; Gruyere, Swiss, and Parmesan cheeses; sardines; and salmon. Although taking calcium supplements is controversial, many doctors recommend them for people who don't get enough calcium in their diet.

• "Maintain an adequate supply of vitamin D (it helps with calcium absorption)—especially if you don't get much sunlight. But, because high doses of vitamin D are toxic, don't consume more than 600 to 800 units daily.

• "Perform weight-bearing exercises, such as walking, jogging, bicycling, or aerobics, to help increase bone density.

• "If you have a high risk of osteoporosis (because of premature menopause, for example), your doctor may recommend estrogen replacement therapy. Estrogen retards postmenopausal bone cell loss, but because it's associated with endometrial cancer, estrogen replacement therapy isn't indicated for all women."

Ostomy: bathing

Patient-teaching strategies

Tell your patient that unless the doctors gives specific instructions about wearing the pouch while bathing, it's a matter of personal preference. Water won't hurt your patient's stoma, as long as the shower stream isn't hitting it full force. Tell him to rinse well, lest soap residue prevent the bag from adhering properly. If he feels uncomfortable about drainage leaking into the bath or shower, he may want to wear his pouch. If he does, tell him to make sure the adhesive seal is watertight. He can ensure this by applying extra tape around the edge of the pouch opening.

Ostomy: clothing

Teaching guidelines to give your patient

Begin by having your patient dress in his street clothes and stand before a full-length mirror. Realizing that he can hardly detect the stoma under his clothes may improve his outlook.

Chances are, he won't need to alter his outer clothing to accommodate an ostomy pouch. Male patients should wear briefs that aren't too tight. And depending on the stoma's placement, suspenders might be more comfortable for him than a belt.

If a female patient asks about wearing a girdle, suggest an Ostobinder; this is a garment made especially for ostomy patients who need more abdominal support. A heavy, tight girdle may injure the stoma or cause drainage to pool around it, loosening the adhesive seal.

Ostomy: diarrhea

Good advice on protecting your patient's skin

When an ostomy patient has continuous diarrhea, how can you keep the skin around his stoma from getting contaminated while you're changing the pouch? Here's one suggestion:

Take the cardboard tube from a roll of toilet paper and stuff it with toilet paper. Place the tube over the patient's stoma, and have him hold it perpendicular to his abdomen. For

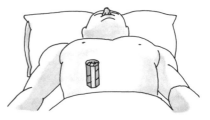

a custom fit, cut and tape the end of the tube so its diameter is the same as the stoma's. The toilet paper will absorb the fecal material, and the tube will keep it away from his skin. (See *Ileal conduit.*)

Ostomy: diet

Advising your patient

Explain to your patient that the doctor may put him on a low-residue diet for the first few weeks after surgery to give his bowel a rest.

If he was on a special diet before surgery (such as one for diabetes), tell him he'll return to it after surgery. Also, tell him foods that caused digestive problems before surgery will probably continue to do so. Stress the importance of chewing his food thoroughly and limiting his intake of hard-to-digest foods, such as whole corn, nuts, and sunflower seeds.

Advise him which foods may cause foul-smelling gas—such as

O

onions, eggs, cabbage, and beans. Tell him to consume smaller portions of these foods or to avoid them entirely.

Advise your patient to avoid foods that cause gas, such as beer, carbonated drinks, cucumbers, radishes, and dairy products. Also, tell him to try using a disposable or reusable pouch without a gas filter. Tell him to open the clip at the bottom of it and drain the contents. This lets gas escape.

Ostomy: odor control

Patient-teaching guidelines

If your patient cleans his reusable pouch or changes his disposable pouch on a regular schedule, he probably won't have odor problems. But for additional security, suggest a pouch deodorant. Be sure to remind him to notify his doctor if he develops an extremely foul stool odor. Although the odor may be diet-related, it could also indicate an infection. Here are some alternative methods for odor control.

Tell your patient to put a few drops of lemon-scented dishwashing liquid in his ostomy bag. The lemon scent masks the odor, and the liquid lubricates the bag so the stool slides to the bottom. Cleaning the bag will be easier, too, since the soap is already in it.

Another method your patient could use is to saturate a small wad of tissue with vanilla extract and then place it in the bottom of his appliance.

Ostomy: physical exertion

Patient-teaching pointers

Your patient can probably return to work as soon as he regains his strength. If his occupation requires heavy physical labor—such as construction work or meat packing—he may have some limitations, so have him check with his doctor.

The doctor may advise avoiding rough contact sports, such as wrestling and football. He may also prohibit certain individual sports, such as weight lifting. These sports strain abdominal wall muscles and may cause a hernia in the stomal area.

If your patient plans to swim, warn him to eat lightly, empty and clean his pouch, and seal it securely before entering the water. Suggest also that he wear an Osto-binder for additional support. (See *Ostomy: bathing.*)

Ostomy: travel

Guidelines to give your patient

With advance preparation, your patient can travel. However, recommend that he always keep his ostomy equipment with him, in case his luggage gets lost. Also advise him to take along enough ostomy supplies for the entire trip, if possible. If he wears a reusable pouch, advise him to pack some disposable pouches as a precaution.

He can find out in advance where to buy supplies elsewhere in the United States by referring to the manufacturer's catalog. It lists pharmacies and medical supply stores carrying their products.

Before any long trip, he should check with his doctor, who may want to prescribe medication for possible diarrhea or constipation.

If he's among the small percentage of patients who irrigate their ostomies, warn him to use only potable water. If that's not available, he should buy bottled water.

Otoscope

Using one correctly

When the patient reports an earache, use an otoscope to inspect ear structures closely. Follow these techniques to obtain the best view and ensure patient safety.

Inspecting young children
To inspect an infant's or young child's ear, grasp the lower part of the auricle and pull it down and back to straighten the upward S-curve of the external canal. Then gently insert the speculum into the canal no more than ½″ (1 cm).

Inspecting adults
To inspect an adult's ear, grasp the upper part of the auricle and pull it up and back to straighten the exter-

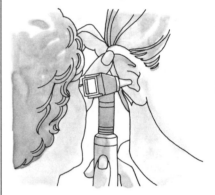

nal canal. Then insert the speculum about 1″ (3 cm). Also use this technique for children over age 3.

Oximetry

How to use it

Until recently, nurses had to rely on arterial blood gas (ABG) measurements to sound the alarm when acute hypoxemia threatens a patient's life. But many hospitals are now using a new, improved version of an old procedure—oximetry—to provide continuous monitoring of arterial oxygen levels in patients with cardiorespiratory disorders.

An oximeter monitors your patient's oxygen saturation continuously, so it rapidly (within 6 seconds) detects any trend in his oxygenation status—unlike ABGs, which you can measure only periodically. And, because oximetry's a simple, noninvasive procedure, you don't need to be specially trained to do it.

An *ear oximeter* measures a patient's arterial oxygen saturation by monitoring the transmission of two light waves through his earlobe's vascular bed. Light emitters and

Ear oximeter

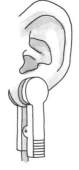

sensors are contained in an ear probe that you clip to your patient's earlobe. A heater in the heat probe's tip maintains the skin's surface temperature at 98.6° F. (37° C.), dilating the arterial vascular bed to enable more accurate readings. A cable conducts the ear probe's electrical signal to the oximeter, which calculates oxygen saturation and displays the values on a digital-readout on the front panel.

If low cardiac output causes insufficient arterial perfusion in your patient's earlobe—preventing an accurate determination of oxygen saturation with an ear oximeter—you can use a *pulse oximeter*. This is a receptacle you slip over your patient's fingertip (no heater is required) that measures the wavelengths of light transmitted through a *pulsating* arterial vascular bed.

Pulse oximeter

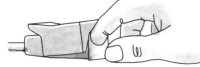

You can't use the fingertip receptacle on a patient who has any condition that significantly reduces peripheral vascular pulsations (such as hypothermia or hypotension) or who's taking vasoactive drugs. Instead, you'll use a nasal probe that fits around your patient's septal an-

terior ethmoid artery, where vascular pulsations are less easily disrupted.

Oxygen-delivery systems

Types and considerations

Five major types of oxygen-delivery systems are available. The first four are low-flow systems; the last, high-flow.

Nasal cannula
• Remove and clean the cannula every 8 hours with a wet cloth. Give good mouth and nose care.
• If the patient is restless, explore other methods of oxygen delivery.

Nasal cannula

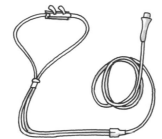

• Check for reddened areas under his nose and over his ears. Apply gauze padding, if necessary.
• Moisten his lips and nose with water-soluble jelly, but avoid occluding the cannula.

Simple face mask
• Place the pads between the mask and your patient's bony facial parts.
• Wash and dry his face every 2 hours.

Simple face mask

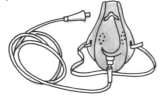

• For adequate airflow, maintain a flow rate of 5 liters/minute.
• Remove and clean the mask every 8 hours with a wet cloth.

Partial rebreather mask
• Never let the bag totally deflate during inhalation. Increase liter flow if necessary.

Partial rebreather mask

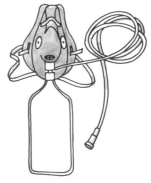

• Avoid twisting the bag.
• Keep the mask snug to prevent inhalation of room air.
• To initially fill the bag, apply the mask during exhalation.

Nonrebreather mask
• Never let the bag totally deflate.
• Avoid twisting the bag.
• Keep the mask snug to prevent inhalation of room air.

Nonrebreather mask

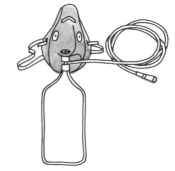

• Make sure that all rubber flaps remain in place.
• Watch the patient closely for signs of oxygen toxicity (see *Oxygen toxicity*).

Venturi mask
• Check arterial blood gas measurements frequently.
• Soften the skin around the patient's mouth with petrolatum to prevent irritation.

O

Venturi mask

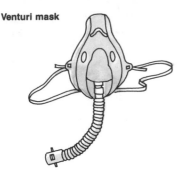

• Remove and clean the mask every 8 hours with a wet cloth. (See *Airway, esophageal gastric tube; Breathing devices.*)

Oxygen toxicity

Early warning signs

Be alert for these early signs of oxygen toxicity: retrosternal distress, dyspnea, paresthesias in the arms and legs, lethargy or restlessness, and anorexia. Intervening promptly when you first detect these signs may save the patient from an extended hospital stay.

Oxygen tubes

Checking patency

If your patient is receiving oxygen, it may be delivered through an MA-I volume-cycled ventilator, from wall units, or from a cylinder. Whatever source is used, the oxygen must flow through a tube.

Is the tube patent? If you're working with humidified oxygen and the tube is working properly, you'd see signs of moisture, either as droplets within the tubing or as mist within the face mask.

You should hear a hiss, usually very quiet (but present nevertheless), somewhere within the system. Also, when oxygen is delivered through a closed system of tubing (for example, through the MA-I), built-in alarm systems tell you if the tube isn't patent and the preset amount of oxygen isn't reaching your patient.

If the patient is assisting the ventilator, when you disconnect the endotracheal tube from the ventilator tubing to suction the patient, you should feel air escape. Place your hand or ear near the endotracheal tube. Do you feel or hear air escape on expiration? Can you see the patient's chest expand and contract? After suctioning, reconnect the tube to the ventilator. Does the air intake and output increase after suctioning? Auscultate the chest and trachea for air movement to further ensure that the tube is patent. (See also *Breath sounds: ventilator patient.*)

Pacemakers: discharge teaching

What to tell your patient

Ideally, discharge teaching of a pacemaker recipient is a team effort, including the doctor, nurse, and staff member from the outpatient pacemaker clinic. In reality, it often falls entirely to the nurse. Regardless of who does the teaching, certain key topics should be covered: immediate and long-term restrictions, plus the many ways the pacemaker is monitored.

Movements are usually restricted only for the first 6 weeks after surgery. During this time, any vigorous activity of the arms and shoulders could dislodge the electrode. After 6 weeks, your patient can be as active as his capabilities allow—including sexual intercourse. Long-term, the patient should avoid activities that could result in chest trauma (for example, contact sports).

Clothing restrictions are minimal: Your patient shouldn't wear anything that puts pressure on the incision or the pulse generator. This means women should avoid tight bra straps or heavy shoulder purses. Warn your patient to notify the doctor if the incision starts oozing or becomes tender, red, or swollen. (See also *Pacemakers: safeguards.*)

Pacemakers: postop care

Monitoring the patient after insertion

Keep a close watch on the patient's heart rate, his waveform pattern, and the position of the pacer spikes. Take his vital signs every 2 hours for the first night and every 4 hours thereafter.

Pay special attention to preventing the electrode in his right ventricle from dislodging. It'll take 48 to 72 hours for enough fibrous tissue to form around the electrode so it's secured to the endocardium. During that time, keep your patient on bed rest. Elevate the head of his bed, but not more than 30 degrees. Because the electrode usually settles near the septum, don't let him lie on his right side.

After 24 hours, the dressing over the incision will probably be removed. Assess the wound every shift. Once your patient can take fluids—usually on the day after surgery—he'll probably be switched to oral antibiotics. Be sure they're administered properly.

When your patient increases his activity, his heart may be monitored by telemetry. He'll also continue having his pacemaker checked regularly.

After 72 hours—assuming no problems have arisen—your patient will be taken off the cardiac monitor and be allowed to walk, with help if needed. (See *Pacemakers: discharge teaching.*)

Pacemakers: preop teaching

What your patient needs to know

Explain that the pacemaker has two components: a pulse generator that houses the battery and the electric circuitry, and a lead with an electrode at its far end. Let the patient handle a demonstration model of the pacemaker. Also, show him an X-ray of a patient with a pacemaker so he'll know how it'll be positioned in the chest.

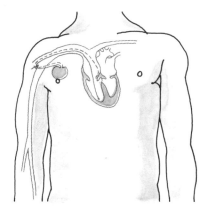

Explain that insertion procedure, emphasizing that it's simple, requires only a local anesthetic, and takes less than an hour. Point out the incision site (usually the right deltopectoral groove) and explain that while it may feel sore initially, it shouldn't be painful. Once the bandage over the incision is removed—usually after 1 day—a bulge may be visible, depending on the size of the pulse generator and the amount of fatty tissue at the insertion site. Later on, the bulge can be easily obscured by wearing loose clothing or a scarf.

Assure him that pacemakers rarely malfunction. Even so, he'll be watched very closely for the first few days after the insertion. Before going home, he'll be thoroughly instructed in how his pacemaker works and what he can do to help keep it working. After he goes home,

he'll have scheduled examinations at his doctor's office or the pacemaker clinic. If necessary, he'll receive a special monitoring device that allows his pacemaker to be checked by telephone at any time.

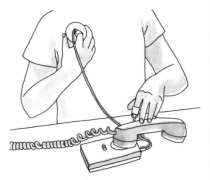

In the unlikely event that his pacemaker does malfunction, he'll experience a return of the symptoms he had before the unit was inserted. Though serious, these symptoms rarely endanger a patient's life.

Explain that the pacemaker battery can last up to 10 years. During that time, the doctor will check the battery periodically and the patient will check it himself by taking his pulse once a day. If the battery's getting weak, he'll notice a slight drop in his pulse rate—nothing dangerous, just an early warning that the time's approaching to replace the pulse generator. The replacement procedure is even simpler than the initial insertion procedure because the lead to the heart is usually left in place.

Finally, since you may not have time to cover everything before the pacemaker's inserted, assure your patient you'll continue your discussions after his pacemaker's in place. (See also *Pacemakers: discharge teaching*; *Pacemakers: safeguards*.)

Pacemakers, rate-responsive

Monitoring their function

First, find out where the rate-responsive pacemaker has been

placed. If in the atrium, the pacing spikes will appear before the P waves. If in the ventricle, the spikes will precede the QRS complex.

You should also know the lower- and upper-rate limits programmed for your patient, so you can compare them with the heart rate calculated from the electrocardiogram. Usually, the lower-rate limit is 60 pulses/minute and the upper-rate limit is 150 pulses/minute for adults. Remember that the pacing rate will vary between these limits. So don't interpret this variation as a malfunction of the pacemaker.

Finally, you'll want to make sure the patient and his family understand how a rate-responsive pacemaker works and how to detect malfunctions. (See *Pacemakers: discharge teaching.*)

Pacemakers: safeguards

Instructions about self-care

Before your patient's discharged, teach him (and a family member or companion) how to take his apical or carotid pulse. Once he's home, he should take his pulse daily. If he notices he's gradually losing beats, his pacemaker battery is probably getting weak. He should tell his doctor, who'll judge how soon the battery needs replacing. If the slowed pulse is accompanied by a sudden return of prepacemaker symptoms, the pulse generator has probably developed a defect in its circuitry. This rarely happens and is almost never fatal, but the doctor should be notified immediately anyway.

Daily pulse taking, while important, may seem scant security to some pacemaker recipients. Reassure him that he'll also be scheduled for regular visits to his doctor or a pacemaker clinic after he's discharged. Stress the importance of these visits—not only for periodic checks on the pacemaker and the patient but also for reprogramming the pacemaker's rate or impulse strength, should it be necessary.

Still another safety net is the telephone monitoring device. This usually consists of bracelet-type wrist leads connected to a telephone transmitter (they look like expansion watchbands) and a transmitter with a receptacle for a telephone receiver. Check whether your patient will receive such a device when he's discharged and, if so, explain how it works.

The patient will call his monitoring station—usually at a hospital—and say he wants to have his pacemaker checked. He'll be told to slip one lead onto each wrist and to place the telephone receiver in the receptacle on the transmitter. The monitoring station's equipment will then read the printout of his ECG, his pulse rate, his R-R interval, and the location of the pacer spikes in the cardiac cycle. These findings will be compared with his previous records to determine if his pacemaker's functioning properly. Telephone monitoring—whether done on a regular schedule or at the patient's request—offers the security of on-the-spot checkups 24 hours a day, without the patient having to leave his home. (See also *Pacemakers: discharge teaching; Pacemakers: preop teaching.*)

Pain, intractable

Being sensitive to your patient's pain

Your anxiety or frustration about relieving your patient's intractable pain may make you tend to avoid him. This will only increase his anxiety—and possibly his pain. Try to reduce his anxiety level by concentrating on his needs. Show him that you're interested in him and care about how he feels. As you listen to his complaints, stand close to him. And look him straight in the eye when you speak.

He's apt to wonder if you believe how much pain he's experiencing. How can you convince him that you believe him? First avoid labeling him as a problem patient. Instead, develop a personal perspective on his complaint of pain by asking questions that focus on his activities, not on his pain. ("Have you been up in the chair today?" or "Were you able to eat some of your lunch?") Focusing on his activities will also help both of you recognize when he's making progress—maybe he couldn't sit up in the chair yesterday, but today he can. Even such small victories can offset a patient's anxiety about his pain.

When a patient's in pain, he needs to know that you'll check on him regularly and give him the help he needs. If he constantly turns on his call light, tell him he won't need to do this anymore because you'll definitely check on him every 10 minutes, half hour, or hour. Then do it.

A patient in pain may strongly resist sitting up in a chair, exercising, or doing other painful procedures that his doctor has ordered. If so, spare both of you the frustration of "I can't!" by breaking up painful tasks into smaller, more manageable ones.

Try a creative approach to pain relief medication by showing the patient how to determine his own medication needs. Help him chart the intensity and duration of his pain and of the relief his medication provides. Together, you'll be able to see when and how often he needs his medication. (The chart will also be available to show the doctor if the medication fails to provide relief despite your interventions. And it will ease any concern you have about overmedicating the patient.) Keep your patient calm and oriented by giving him a list identifying each medication, describing its purpose, and pointing out its place in his medication schedule. He can keep the list at his bedside and cross off his medications as he receives them.

Fear of the unknown can be a big factor in a patient's pain. Do your teaching after the patient's had some relief from his pain. He simply can't concentrate on what you're saying when pain's all he can think about.

A patient may refuse to consider alternative methods for relieving his pain because this gives him a feeling of control. To avoid a power struggle, neutralize his resistance in advance by wording your suggestions so he thinks *he's* made it. Here's an example: "I'm sure you've already thought about other ways to manage your pain, such as relaxation techniques." (See also *Relaxation techniques.*) This will let him show his knowledge—another way he can feel in control—and it opens the way for him to accept other pain management methods. (See also *Orders, sliding scale.*)

Pain, low back

Exercises to relieve it

Tell the patient:

"If you have chronic low back pain, these exercises may help relieve your discomfort and prevent further lumbar deterioration. When you perform these exercises, keep in mind the following points:
• "Breathe slowly, inhaling through your nose and exhaling completely through pursed lips.
• "Begin gradually, performing each exercise only once per day and progressing to 10 repetitions.
• "Exercise moderately; expect mild discomfort, but stop if you experience severe pain."

Back press
"Lie on your back, with your arms on your chest and your knees bent.

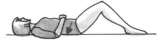

Press the small (lower portion) of your back to the floor while tightening your abdominal muscles and buttocks. Count to 10, then slowly relax."

Knee grasp

"Lie on your back, with your knees bent. Bring one knee to your chest,

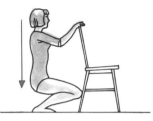

grasping it firmly with both hands; lower your knee. Repeat with the other knee—then with *both* knees."

Knee bend

"Stand with your hands on the back of a chair for support. Keeping your back straight, slowly bend your

knees until you're in a squatting position. Then return to your starting position."

Sit-up

"Lie on your back, with your arms at your sides. Using your abdominal muscles, slowly sit up and reach for your toes, touching them if you can." (See also *Laminectomy, lumbar*.)

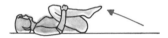

Pain, postop

Steps to take before administering an analgesic

During the first 48 hours after surgery, the patient's pain will range from moderate to severe. He'll need narcotic analgesics, such as morphine and meperidine (pethidine), to relieve it. After that time, his pain will lessen and a nonnarcotic analgesic may suffice.

Before administering a narcotic analgesic postoperatively, determine the cause of the patient's pain. If it's from his incision, give the medication. But if it's remote chest or leg pain, the narcotic analgesic

may mask a complication; if it's gas pain, the narcotic analgesic may aggravate it. If the medication is not effective or makes the patient extremely lethargic or somnolent, notify the doctor. He may want to change the order.

The risk of addiction to pain medication rarely exists postoperatively. During the first 24 to 48 postoperative hours, administer the narcotic analgesic every 3 to 4 hours, if needed. That'll ensure that the patient receives the medication before his pain becomes severe. If he requests pain medication, give it to him promptly. Remember, minutes can seem like hours to someone in pain.

Administer analgesics so that they take effect before the patient must perform any activities that may be painful. For instance, he should be pain-free when you encourage him to deep-breathe, cough, turn, or walk. Of course, as with any medication, watch for adverse reactions, such as bowel spasms, decreased peristalsis, nausea and vomiting, respiratory and cough depression, and hypotension, especially with narcotic analgesics.

Remember that other measures can also prevent or relieve postoperative pain. For instance, to prevent pain when the patient turns or gets out of bed after abdominal surgery, encourage him to use his limbs rather than his abdominal muscles. Controlled breathing and relaxation techniques can also relieve pain by reducing anxiety and distracting attention from his pain. These techniques also help him to relax his muscles and give him some control over his pain. (See also *Orders, sliding scale*.)

Pain and anesthesia

Postop medication

Knowing which drug or combination of drugs the patient received intraoperatively, its effects, and the

administration time will help you decide how much of a postoperative narcotic analgesic to give and when to give it. Some general guidelines to keep in mind:

• If your patient received droperidol, the standard dose of the narcotic analgesic should be reduced by one-half to one-third during the first 8 to 10 hours postoperatively (because of droperidol's potentiating effects on narcotics).

• If he received meperidine or morphine, administer a postoperative narcotic analgesic 1 to 1½ hours after the intraoperative administration time.

• If you're a recovery room nurse and your patient received naloxone (Narcan) to reverse respiratory depression caused by an intraoperative narcotic, you may have to administer a postoperative narcotic analgesic within 15 to 30 minutes of his arrival in the recovery room. This is because naloxone is a pure narcotic antagonist that acts very quickly (within 2 minutes of I.V. administration), and if the patient doesn't receive a narcotic analgesic soon after the naloxone takes effect, he'll be in a great deal of pain. (See also *Orders, sliding scale*.)

Pain detection

Doing it properly

The patient's bodily reactions give clues to the presence, severity, duration, and location of his pain. Watch for these reactions:

• *Restlessness* indicates impending pain or increasing pain.

• *Immobilization* of a certain part of the body or the whole body is one way a patient minimizes pain. For instance, after massive physical trauma, a child may immobilize his entire body. Or if he has a minor injury to a toe, he may hold his entire foot still.

• *Position* also indicates the type of pain the patient feels. For instance, if he has visceral pain, he'll hardly move at all because visceral pain depresses most behavior responses. This immobility is an appropriate reaction to pain from within.

• *Purposeless* or inaccurate body movements is another way to detect pain. The patient may tremble, flail his arms, or flutter his eyelids. He may reach for a glass and inadvertently knock it over.

The patient's first response to pain is usually the "flight or fight" reaction: The patient may try to pull away from a venipuncture or attack the person inflicting the pain. Think of the child who kicks when you try to do a procedure that will hurt him. This reaction is less overt with an adult patient, but even he may try to push your hand away when you're palpating a tender area.

Using a rhythmic or rubbing movement also indicates pain. A baby may rub his ear if he has otitis media. An adult may rub his head if he has a headache. A patient with abdominal pain may draw his feet up to his abdomen and rock.

Pain relief: abdomen

Helping your patient relieve abdominal pain

Abdominal pain and general discomfort will probably make it difficult for the patient to stay in any position for very long. Still, you have to try your best to keep him on some kind of regular turning schedule to promote peristalsis. Be as gentle as possible.

Not surprisingly, the pain will also disrupt the patient's normal sleeping pattern. He will tend to sleep fitfully for short periods, so you need to plan your care accordingly, doing what you can without waking him when he finally does fall asleep.

The patient will usually feel best right after a morning bath with warm water. He'll probably feel most comfortable with the head of his bed raised 45 degrees or more. Or you can place him on his side

with a pillow between his knees, another one behind his back, and another under his abdomen—again, with the head of his bed raised.

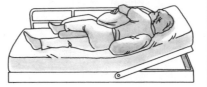

Pain medication is controversial because it may mask other important signs and symptoms. If it is ordered, it will most likely be meperidine (Demerol) or another synthetic analog. Most doctors won't order morphine, which would only further decrease intestinal motility and risk increased nausea and vomiting. As a precaution, you should question any pain medication order, especially if the patient is being seen by more than one doctor.

Pain relief: distraction

Effective techniques

Distraction is a kind of "sensory shielding." By directing the patient's attention to something other than his pain, he's unconsciously shielding himself from full awareness of his pain and increasing his tolerance of it.

Characteristically, relief lasts only as long as the distraction lasts. Then the patient will usually feel tired and suddenly more aware of his pain. Then he may understandably ask for an analgesic or some other pain reliever that will allow him to rest.

Here's how to distract a patient from pain.

1. *Tall tales.* Encourage the patient to give you a detailed account of an exciting ball game or stimulating book. This is the simplest form of distraction and is particularly effective for brief, mild pain.

2. *Active listening.* Ask the patient's family to provide a battery-operated tape recorder, earphones

or headset, and a cassette of fast, loud music the patient likes.

Then tell him to emphasize the rhythm of the music while listening to it: tap his finger or foot, slap his thigh, or nod his head.

Or he can keep his finger on the volume control. As his pain increases, he should increase the volume. As the pain decreases, he can decrease it.

This kind of distraction blocks out all other sounds, providing a demanding auditory stimulus for the patient without disturbing others. It's so easy to learn and do that even a patient who's tired, sedated, or passive can use it successfully. And it allows the patient to respond to varying intensities of pain.

Patients who don't like music can substitute a recording of a comedy routine, an intriguing story, or an exciting ball game.

3. *Sing and tap.* Distract the patient with a rhythmic singing exercise. This can work well with children and adults. Tell the patient to sing and tap his hand or foot faster when the pain intensifies and slower when the pain subsides.

4. *Rhythmic breathing.* If he needs a more structured distraction technique, have the patient try slow, rhythmic breathing. Tell him to concentrate on the "feel" of his breathing as he slowly inhales and exhales. He might want to close his eyes and try to picture the air going in and out of his lungs, or picture a restful scene, such as a meadow or a quiet beach. If he feels breathless, tell him to breathe more slowly or take a deep breath.

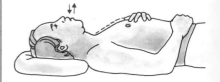

If rhythmic breathing alone isn't sufficient, make the technique more complex. Suggest that he massage part of his body with stroking or circular motions as he breathes. Or that he inhale through his nose and exhale through his mouth. Or raise his head as he inhales and lower it as he exhales.

Pain relief: drug addiction

Dealing with the known addict

Depriving a patient of pain relief is never an option. In fact, most doctors who specialize in pain control and substance abuse would allow a patient to have as much narcotic as he asked for, unless it threatened his physical well-being (say, if he has a drop in respiratory rate from 14 to 8 breaths per minute).

Because of an addicted patient's probable drug tolerance, very large doses may be both safe and necessary to achieve pain relief. But as long as the patient can converse and breathe satisfactorily, the health care team should respect his request for more narcotic.

If the patient hasn't been admitted for substance abuse treatment, setting a goal of rehabilitation is inappropriate and perhaps even dangerous. Although narcotic withdrawal is rarely life-threatening, it may put a very ill patient at greater risk for complications. An addicted patient in pain should get enough narcotic at least to prevent the extreme discomfort of withdrawal.

If the patient is willing, the health care team may try to detoxify him (gradually decrease the narcotic dose) before discharge and arrange for nonnarcotic pain relief after discharge. The patient may also want information about local drug rehabilitation programs.

The decision to take pain medications should always be the patient's, not the health care team's.

If your patient has participated in a substance abuse program in the past, advise him to contact his counselors for advice and support.

True, most substance abuse programs advocate abstinence from all medications that affect consciousness. But their intent isn't to make the recovered addict suffer needless pain. Most programs suggest alternative methods for handling pain relief such as these for postoperative pain:
• infiltration of the surgical site with a long-acting local anesthetic just before wound closure
• transcutaneous electrical nerve stimulation (TENS) (See *TENS.*)
• 100 mg of indomethacin (Indocin) administered rectally q8h for 24 to 72 hours, or another drug such as choline magnesium trisalicylate (Trilisate), 1,500 mg P.O. twice a day.

Whether your patient is a drug abuser or not, you have to respect his report of pain and help manage it effectively. Only then are you truly giving him the care he deserves. (See also *Pain, intractable.*)

Pain relief: massage

Using ice massage

Research has shown that ice massage provides quicker and longer-lasting pain relief than either a cold or hot pack for musculoskeletal pain.

You apply a small block of ice directly to the patient's skin over the painful area—usually until the pain disappears, but for no longer than 10 minutes. During that time, he will experience four stages of sensation: cold, burning, aching, and numbness. Pain relief lasts from 10 minutes to as long as 3 hours.

The only contraindications are previous frostbite in the area being treated or hypersensitivity to cold. Be careful about using the technique for pain that's been traced to vascular problems. If the pain is caused by poor circulation, you don't want to add to the pain by applying something cold. Also, don't use ice massage anywhere around

the throat because of the chilling effect on blood vessels there.

Patients suffering from cervical pain accompanied by muscle spasms can get temporary relief, as can those with rheumatoid arthritis or osteoarthritis. This technique helps relieve muscle cramps, stump pain, certain types of chronic cancer pain, pain from acute trauma, and pain of a bone marrow aspiration. The ice can't be applied directly to the bone marrow aspiration site because it would interfere with the procedure. But knowing that both sides of the body influence pain impulses passing through the spinal cord, apply the ice contralaterally—and it will work. The patient feels nothing during the procedure—only the ice and pressure.

To do an ice massage, you need towels and an ice cake measuring approximately 4″ × 6″ (10 cm × 15 cm). You can use a plastic food storage container, margarine tub, or large paper cup as a mold.

Your patient can be in any position—sitting, standing, or lying down as long as he's comfortable and the painful area is exposed.

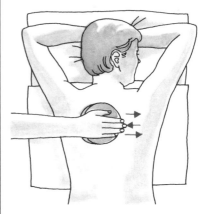

Begin by emphasizing that the procedure is safe and that the skin will not freeze.

Next, place a towel under the area you'll be treating. If you're treating more than one area, drape towels over the patient, exposing only one area at a time. Divide large areas into several 6″ sections, and massage each one separately.

P

Place a cloth or paper towel over the ice to protect your hand and absorb water runoff. Warn the patient just before you apply the ice so he's not surprised. With firm but not heavy pressure, rub the ice directly on the skin, using either a circular or back-and-forth motion. Ask him to tell you which way feels more comfortable. At first, he may experience an aching, throbbing, or burning sensation—that's normal. But stop immediately if the skin turns unusually red or he reports unusual or severe pain. Remember, he'll feel tender over the bones, so be especially gentle there and avoid bony prominences if possible.

After 5 to 10 minutes, the treated area should be numb. Because of the threat of frostbite, however, the ice massage should definitely be stopped after 10 minutes. Afterward, dry the patient's skin with a towel. Ice massage can be used again on the same patient after an hour.

Palpation

How to palpate your patient properly

Remember that touching a patient is apt to elicit fear, embarrassment, and other strong emotions. Be sure to explain what you're doing and why, as well as what he can expect—especially if it's discomfort. Make sure your hands are warm. Try to get your patient to relax because muscular tension or guarding can interfere with the performance and results of palpation. Instruct the patient to breathe deeply through his mouth. If you know he has tender areas, palpate them last.

Part of the skill of palpation is in knowing which areas of your hands and fingers to use. This is because your hands and fingers are not equally sensitive to all sensations—such as temperature. For example, you might suspect that your patient has an elevated surface temperature over a sprained ankle, or

a lowered surface temperature in his hands from poor circulation. To investigate these and similar suspicions, use the backs of your hand or fingers because the skin there is thinner and more sensitive to temperature. You may find it helpful to palpate the suspect area with the back of one hand, while palpating an unaffected area with the back of the other. Then switch hands to confirm the differences you perceive between the two areas. For discriminating skin surface textures, first use your fingertips, to detect general differences, then use the backs of your hands and fingers for finer distinctions. Use the pads of your fingertips to determine the position, form, and consistency of structures—to palpate lymph nodes, for example. For determining muscle and tissue firmness, as well as joint positions, use your thumb and index finger to grasp the body part. To detect vibrations (such as thrills or fremitus), use the palmar surface of the metacarpophalangeal joints—the ball of the hand.

Pancreas transplant

Monitoring your patient after surgery

The first 2 to 4 days after surgery are critical. The patient's vital signs, central venous pressure, urine intake and output, and nasogastric drainage must be monitored closely. He may have a three-lumen catheter for administering total parenteral nutrition (TPN) and drawing blood samples. And he'll receive I.V. fluids as well as immunosuppressive and antirejection drugs. He'll need TPN and insulin if he can't take anything by mouth within 1 week. Usually, though, he should be off insulin and have a normal blood glucose level a few days after the transplant.

Watch for complications: Elevated temperature accompanied by pain or tenderness at the graft site could

indicate an infection or rejection. If he's had the bowel procedure (anastamosis of the pancreas to the bowel), a rise in his glucose level could mean the new organ is being rejected. Or it could mean thrombosis of the graft, preventing blood flow to the transplanted pancreas. Similarly, a decreased urine amylase level signals rejection if he's had the bladder procedure (anastamosis of the pancreas to the bladder).

He'll be discharged in about 2 to 3 weeks. Once he goes home, he'll need laboratory tests twice a week to check the function of the pancreas and the effect of immunosuppressive drugs. Tell him to avoid straining and heavy lifting for 90 days. After that time, he should start an exercise program of walking, biking, or swimming, but he'll always have to avoid contact sports.

Pancreatitis

Summary and priorities for acute cases

Initial assessment of the patient may have revealed these signs and symptoms of acute pancreatitis:
• an acute onset of severe epigastric pain, possibly radiating to his back and occurring within a few hours after a large meal or excessive alcohol intake
• nausea
• restlessness
• vomiting
• abdominal tenderness, rigidity, and distention
• Cullen's or Grey Turner's sign (See Cullen's sign.)
• a history of alcoholism, biliary tract disease, or hyperlipidemia.

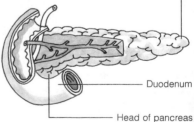

Tail of pancreas

Duodenum

Head of pancreas

An I.V. is established for fluid and medication access, and blood is drawn for complete blood count, electrolytes, alkaline phosphates, blood glucose, bilirubin, and serum amylase studies. Abdominal X-rays, ultrasonography, or a CT scan may be done to show diffuse or local enlargement of the pancreas.

Priorities

Your patient may suffer acute plasma volume depletion from hemorrhage or as a result of fluid sequestered in his abdomen, bowel, and other extracellular spaces. Your first priority, then, is to maintain his hemodynamic status. Infuse colloids and crystalloids I.V., as ordered, to replace lost fluid volume, and insert a Foley catheter, as ordered, to aid in accurate output measurements. Type and crossmatch the patient's blood in case a transfusion is necessary. Give the patient nothing by mouth—not even ice chips. You want to prevent *all* gastric stimulation because gastric activity increases pancreatic secretions and makes pancreatic edema worse. Insert a nasogastric tube, as ordered, and connect it to intermittent suction to remove the patient's stomach contents. Start a detailed intake and output record.

Pancuronium therapy

Caring for the patient

Ventilating a patient with acute respiratory failure can reduce lung compliance. High-peak ventilatory pressure, which increases PaO_2, may limit the patient's ventilation and increase his risk of complications. To prevent such problems, the doctor may order pancuronium (Pavulon), a neuromuscular blocking agent. By inducing complete skeletal muscle relaxation while maintaining a fully alert central nervous system, pancuronium improves the patient's response to mechanical ventilation.

Pancuronium induces paralysis in less than 3 minutes. The doctor will probably order an initial dose of 4 to 8 mg, administered by I.V., then 2 to 8 mg in 30- to 90-minute intervals.

When caring for a patient receiving this potent drug, follow these special guidelines:
• Explain the drug's effects to the patient and his family. Reassure and reorient the patient frequently during therapy. Remember, although he's paralyzed, the patient can hear your conversations.
• Administer a sedative, as ordered, to diminish the patient's perception and recall of paralysis.
• Double-check ventilator connections.
• To prevent corneal abrasions, tape the patient's eyes shut. Remove the tape every 2 to 4 hours and instill artificial tears.
• Monitor his fluid intake and output (renal dysfunction may prolong the drug's duration of action).
• Closely monitor his pulse and respiratory rate.
• Check electrolyte levels regularly and compare them with baseline measurements (an electrolyte imbalance may increase pancuronium's neuromuscular effects).

Panic attacks

Dealing with acute anxiety

Your first step is to make sure the patient's not having a heart attack. Examine him carefully. Listen to his description of the onset and the course of his signs and symptoms. The doctor will examine him to rule out hypoglycemia, pheochromocytoma, hyperthyroidism, caffeinism, drug withdrawal, amphetamine use or abuse, and prepsychotic states.

Try to understand his fear and reassure him, if you can. Stay with him, or have a family member stay with him, to prevent him from feeling alone and helpless.

He may begin to calm down while he's telling you how the panic attack

came about. To help allay his fear, explain that anxiety is an extreme form of nervousness, which can cause the signs and symptoms he's feeling. If a precipitating event brought on the attack, explore its significance. Try to show him how emotions can cause physical problems, and how those problems, in turn, can increase anxiety.

If he's hyperventilating, instruct him to breathe into a paper bag. Suggest that he keep a bag handy in the event of future attacks. Before he leaves, check with a doctor to see if he should be referred for some form of psychiatric treatment, such as supportive therapy, behavior modification, or insight-oriented psychotherapy. (See also *Anxiety: assessment; Anxiety: counseling; Anxiety: detection.*)

Parkinson's disease: care measures

What to do

Your patient should sit in chairs with arms so he'll have support when sitting down and getting up. Also suggest tying a sheet to the foot of his bed so he can help pull himself to a sitting position. If he's experiencing orthostatic hypotension, instruct him to rise slowly from a lying or sitting position.

To help him maintain his balance and a forward momentum, teach him to walk with a wide-based gait and to swing his arms. If appropriate, show him how to use a weighted cane or walker. Teach him how to unlock a position if he becomes fixed in it. Some common unlocking techniques include turning the head, opening the mouth, placing an arm behind the back or across the chest, tapping a leg with the hand, bending the knees slightly, or raising the toes. But he must take care not to lose his balance while using some of these techniques.

To prevent falls, recommend removing throw rugs and unstable furniture and placing furniture against the walls to create wider traffic paths. Also tell him to wear sturdy shoes with good support and traction.

Explain the importance of daily bathing because of increased skin oiliness and perspiration. Advise him to avoid oil-based soaps or lotions, and tell him to use an antiperspirant on his hands if he has sweaty palms.

If he experiences urinary urgency, tell him to remain near a bathroom or to keep a urinal nearby. Suggest having a raised toilet seat and grab bars installed in the bathroom if he has difficulty sitting and standing.

If dressing's a problem, advise him to wear clothing with zippers or Velcro strips rather than buttons. Loafer-style shoes solve the problem of tying and untying shoes. If he has dysarthria, instruct him to take his time pronouncing each word. If his voice is too soft, tell him to breathe deeply before beginning each sentence. Reading aloud and singing can help his articulation and voice projection.

Tell the family to watch for signs of depression in the patient (see *Depressed patients*), such as anorexia, insomnia, and disinterest in his surroundings. Tell them to encourage his participation in family discussions, even though facial rigidity may make him look disinterested. Also urge them to encourage the patient's independence and continued social contacts.

Stress the importance of wearing a medical identification bracelet or necklace at all times. Finally, refer the patient and his family to a support group for more information.

Parkinson's disease: diet

What to tell the patient

Tell your patient to avoid a high-protein diet. Excess protein can af-
fect the action of levodopa, an amino acid used to treat Parkinson's disease. But caution him against following a low-protein diet; this may cause nutritional imbalance. Also, tell him to avoid caffeine, which may worsen his symptoms. And because intestinal motility may decrease in Parkinson's disease, advise him to drink adequate amounts of fluid and to eat more high-fiber foods if he's troubled by constipation.

If the patient has difficulty chewing or swallowing, recommend semisoft foods (such as applesauce, mashed potatoes, or solid foods prepared in a blender) to help ensure adequate nutrition and minimize the risk of aspiration. Suggest freezing liquids to a slush or mixing them with other foods, such as cereals, to prevent choking. For the same reason, instruct him to sit up straight, move food to the back of his mouth, tilt his head slightly forward, and then swallow.

Remind him to keep a supply of napkins on hand to absorb excess saliva. If he has severe tremors, advise using an arm brace for steadiness. He should try using flexible straws or cups with lid spouts (such as travel cups) to help make drinking easier. Also, using utensils with built-in handles will give him a better grip.

If your patient takes a long time to eat, advise eating small, frequent meals and keeping foods on a warming tray. If he's obese, discuss a weight-reduction diet. Explain that his weight affects his mobility, which in turn, affects the absorption of his medications.

Parkinson's disease: exercise

Patient-teaching pointers

Stress the importance of moderate exercise to help improve mobility, decrease the risk of contractures, improve respiration and circula-
tion, promote bowel function, lessen rigidity, and increase strength. Encourage the patient to perform range of motion exercises if possible. (Passive exercises can be done if necessary.) Tell him to exercise daily when movement is easiest—such as in the late morning or early afternoon, and soon after he takes his medication.

Review specific exercises with him, using pictures when helpful and providing a checklist so he can do them in order. Caution him to avoid excessive exercise because fatigue will interfere with his other daily activities. Instruct him to start his program slowly, gradually increasing his level of exercise.

Parkinson's disease: medication

What to tell your patient

Stress to your patient that he should never stop taking his medication abruptly because this may precipitate a parkinsonian crisis, intensifying the signs and symptoms of the disease. Explain that as Parkinson's disease progresses, the doctor may increase the medication dosage. But caution the patient against increasing the dosage on his own, because toxicity could result.

Initially, your patient's medication may cause nausea and vomiting. Reassure him that these adverse reactions will disappear in a few months. Suggest taking medication after meals to decrease nausea.

If he has a cognitive impairment or memory difficulties, instruct him and his family to premeasure his medication doses for the day in separate containers, each marked with the scheduled administration time.

If he has difficulty swallowing, tell him to crush pills and to open and mix the contents of capsules with a food that's easy to swallow, such as applesauce.

Parkinson's disease: surgery

What to expect

If medication fails to control your patient's tremors, stereotaxic thalamotomy may be used to relieve or eliminate them if they're unilateral. To prepare your patient for this type of surgery, tell him that his head will be shaved and cleaned and that a metal frame will be attached to his head to hold it still and to guide the surgeon during the procedure.

Tell your patient that after he's given a local anesthetic, the surgeon will make a burr hole in his skull and create a surgical lesion in the thalamus on the side *opposite* the tremors. (Explain that the right side of the brain controls the left side of the body, and vice versa.) This lesion will block the transmission of nerve impulses that cause the tremors.

During surgery, he'll be asked questions to test his speech and memory, and he'll be asked to follow commands, such as raising his arm. Tell him that he'll experience some discomfort when the doctor applies the head frame and that he may have a headache after surgery.

Patient care: introductions

Introducing yourself to patients

To make sure patients know who you are and when you're available, give them an index card. On it write your name, shift hours, and a brief message encouraging them to call you if they need help or have any questions. This will help you establish a good relationship with all of your patients.

Patient care, nighttime

Checking on patients

Working on the night shift and doing rounds, you can't always tell whether the patient in the dark room is breathing unless you turn on the light or shine a flashlight on his chest—and this almost always wakes him up. Try pointing the flashlight at

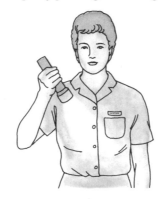

your uniform instead. The reflected light will let you see the patient's chest without waking him.

Patient care conference

Making it work

Anyone taking part in a patient's care or a family member can request a patient care conference. Designate a leader, for example, the primary nurse or any health care worker who's familiar with the patient's and family's needs. Let's say you're the primary nurse chosen to be a conference leader. Overall, you're responsible for planning and conducting the conference and for notifying others about decisions.

Planning the conference
Your first job is to establish the conference objectives. Typically, objectives are centered around meeting the patient's treatment needs and planning his discharge.

After setting objectives, make a list of the participants. An ideal number is 10 or fewer and includes only those people directly involved with meeting the conference objectives. If appropriate, invite the patient and his family.

Next, after checking with everyone, pick a convenient date, time, and place. Finally, choose someone to be the conference recorder.

Conducting the conference
Start the meeting by reviewing the objectives, and briefly go over the patient's history. Next, ask each person to summarize his involvement to date with the patient and his family as well as his treatment and anticipated discharge objectives.

Document decisions and plans
At the end of the patient care conference, review the important points discussed, then schedule another meeting to determine whether the objectives have been met. The decisions and plans should also be incorporated into the nursing care plan.

Your next step is to discuss the outcome of the conference with the patient and his family. Document their responses in the patient's chart. When the conference members meet again for a progress report, they can decide if a follow-up conference is necessary.

A well-planned patient care conference can help you communicate better with your patient and his family. The result? Everyone benefits—the patient, his family, and the health care workers involved in his care.

Patient falls

Determining who's at risk

Once you know which patients are most apt to fall, you can help protect them. To determine who they are, consider *why* they fall. Reasons include:

• the patient's illness and the medication he's receiving may make him less aware of his surroundings.

P

• the complex diagnostic and therapeutic procedures he's undergoing may make him less aware of his surroundings.

• the unfamiliar environment, without the usual protection of family and friends, may also confuse him or put unexpected stumbling blocks in his path.

Add to these problems the crucial factor of the patient's age. In or out of the hospital, elderly patients are most likely to fall, and when they do, they're likely to suffer serious consequences. Most falls occur in patients between ages 60 and 69. Certain changes resulting from the aging process account for this high incidence. For instance, decreased visual acuity and difficulty in distinguishing color can compound the problem of being in an unfamiliar environment. Moreover, even if an elderly patient's proprioception is only slightly affected, a move out of bed may lead to a stumble.

Also, time of day may be significant. Many falls result when the patient gets out of bed to use the bathroom. Sleepiness, darkness, and an unfamiliar environment can lead to poor footing and a fall.

Now, how can you protect these patients? Try this three-part protection plan:

1. *Consciousness raising.* Consider providing a checklist of safety precautions, such as keeping side rails up, beds in low position, wheelchair brakes locked, and night-lights on after dark. Also, display posters reminding your colleagues about these basic safety measures.

2. *Specific nursing practices.* During your admission interview with the patient, pay special attention to questions concerning bowel and bladder habits, mobility, and mental orientation. Information about past hospitalizations is especially important.

At the end of the interview, take time to thoroughly familiarize the patient with his room and immediate environment.

During the hospitalization, assign a nursing assistant to offer the high-risk patient a bedpan or urinal every 2 hours during the night if he's awake. Place a luminous sticker on the foot of his bed as a day-and-night warning for the staff: This patient needs careful watching and extra protection against falls.

3. *Nursing education.* Ask nursing administration to add a review of the physiology of aging to its in-service offerings. This review should include problems in gait, frequency and urgency of urination, postural hypotension, central nervous system changes, hearing, and vision problems.

Of course, you want to do all you can to prevent patient falls. Sometimes, though, the patient's need for individuality and independence will result in a fall despite your best efforts. But a combination of consciousness raising, specific nursing practices, and ongoing education may be the best "no-fall insurance" you can offer your patient. (See *Legal risks: patient falls.*)

Patient satisfaction

How to achieve it

Knowing what patients value in personal care makes it easier to ensure their satisfaction. But what can busy nurses do? Here are 10 ideas:

1. As much as possible, organize your work load around your patients' requests and preferences rather than around your duties, policies, and protocols.

2. Develop relationships with your patients.

3. Let your patients know you think of them as individuals rather than as diseases or conditions. And be sure others treat them that way, too.

4. Take at least 5 minutes a day to sit with each patient to determine his needs, wants, and priorities. By sitting in a nearby chair or on his bed, you'll communicate that you care. And he'll feel that he's getting more

time and attention from you than if you just talk to him on the run or while you're doing other tasks. (See *Listening to patients.*)

5. Listen to your patients' comments and suggestions about their comfort, convenience, and nonmedical preferences. When their basic needs for caring, safety, hunger, and thirst are met, they'll respond to your nursing interventions.

6. Don't get defensive about your patients' suggestions for improving their care. They know what they want and need more than you do, and they'll let you know if you're willing to listen.

7. Make your patients' priorities for food and drink your priorities. Just asking if someone would like a cup of coffee between meals and then getting it may help more than any pain medication.

8. Provide the service your patients want quickly and courteously. Don't be afraid to challenge old ways of doing things.

9. Keep your patients informed about what's happening with them—and with you. Tell them if you'll be busy somewhere for a while, and ask if you can get anything for them before you leave. Some patients push their call light just to find out where you are and to remind you not to forget them. But by keeping in touch with them, you can increase their sense of security, decreasing the number of unnecessary flashing call lights.

10. Review comments from patient satisfaction surveys regularly. Don't be afraid to change protocol based on these comments. (See also *Patients' trust.*)

Patients' possessions

Legal precautions

When a patient refuses and the doctor insists on a search of a patient's possessions, do the following:

• Get the doctor's written order to search.

- Notify the nursing supervisor, hospital administration, and possibly the hospital attorney of the search.
- Fully document your explanation to the patient, his reactions, and the fact that you notified the proper authorities.
- Take along another nurse to serve as a witness.

Patients' trust

Earning it

Here's how to gain your patient's trust:

1. *Call the patient by name.* Put yourself in his position. He's just been admitted to a hospital, a scary and unfamiliar place. He's not sure if anyone even knows who he is. If you call him by name, you'll put him more at ease.

Use his name as much as possible throughout his hospital stay. This will assure him that you recognize him as an individual, not just as "the patient in 409."

2. *Tell him your name.* This can go a long way toward developing a trusting relationship. Routinely introduce yourself to patients during rounds or between shifts. Once a patient knows who you are, he'll feel more comfortable with you the next time you go into his room. (See *Patient care: introductions.*)

3. *Consider your attitude.* Your attitude will contribute toward his ability to trust you.

For example, do you consider certain patients to be chronic complainers or overly demanding? If so, that attitude will reveal itself, however subtly, when you're with them. Through something you do or say, they'll sense that you have reservations about them, and that perhaps you'd rather be assigned to an "easier" patient.

4. *Explain why you're there.* Let your patient know that you're there to help. Explain that you'll be the nurse caring for him for the next 8 hours, and that you'll bring him

medications and perform certain procedures. But don't promise him something you can't deliver. You'll lose his trust this way.

If you have a demanding patient, he may behave that way because he's afraid you won't respond to his needs. On the other hand, if he knows what he can expect from you and sees that you're prepared to make him as comfortable as possible, he'll start trusting you. He'll also stop being so demanding.

5. *Talk about procedures first.* If you walk into a patient's room carrying equipment for a procedure and he has no idea what's up, he'll be understandably anxious. And he's not going to trust you to have his best interests at heart.

Leave the equipment you'll need outside the patient's room. Then go in a talk to him for a few minutes. (Remember to call him by name.) Carefully explain what you intend to do and why. Tell him you'll be as gentle as possible; this will help things go more smoothly. Answer any questions he might have. Then get the equipment and carry out the procedure. Be sure to keep talking to him during the procedure, explaining every step and letting him know when you're almost done.

6. *Keep your appointments.* If you've arranged to do something with a patient at a certain time, don't break the appointment unless something really urgent comes up. If you must do so, let him know you can't do it at the scheduled time. Then be sure to set up another time.

If the patient asks to change an appointment, try to be as accommodating as possible—but let him know if you won't be able to change it. Then set up another time.

7. *Be honest.* Honesty is the most important element in any trusting relationship. Don't tell a patient you'll return if there's a chance you won't. If you don't know the answer to a question, don't try to bluff him with clinical double-talk. If you tell him you'll find out the answer and get back to him, make sure you do. (See also *Patient satisfaction.*)

Patient-teaching checklists

Using them to motivate your patient

Using a checklist will give you and the patient clear evidence of what learning goals he's achieved and what ones need more work. Follow these tips:

- Make the list concise but wide-ranging enough to cover all aspects of the activity being evaluated.
- Limit the items on the checklist to a group of related activities, such as the steps in tracheostomy care or the facets of a cardiac rehabilitation plan. Arrange the items in a logical order—sequentially, chronologically, or in order of importance.

Drawing up insulin

Yes	No	
☑	☐	Disinfected top of vial thoroughly.
☑	☐	Inserted needle into vial without contamination.
☑	☐	Injected air into vial.
☑	☐	Withdrew proper amount of insulin.
☑	☐	Expelled air from syringe.
☑	☐	Retained exact dose of insulin in syringe.
☑	☐	Replaced cap on needle without contamination.

- Identify the *essential* steps of the activities you're evaluating.
- Make the checklist items relate to the patient's learning goals and to your teaching methods.
- Use only one idea or concept in each item.
- Phrase each item concisely and accurately.
- Test your checklist on at least two patients before adopting it.
- Use the checklist along with other evaluation tools to avoid giving it undue importance.

Patient-teaching errors

Avoiding common ones

Here are several mistakes to avoid when teaching patients:

• *Not confirming information with the patient.* One such example is giving printed material to a patient who's illiterate.

• *Failing to reassess the patient throughout his hospitalization.*

• *Refusing to work within the restrictions of the patient's situation.* Consider possible lack of family support, the patient's educational level, his financial situation, or his cultural or ethnic background.

• *Territoriality or "owning" the patient.* You can fall into this trap when you invest a lot of time and effort in teaching patients. No one owns the patient. He's personally responsible for his own behavior.

• *Denying or overlooking the patient's right to change his mind.* This mistake occurs when you've over-invested yourself in the patient and his progress.

• *Inability to learn from your mistakes.* Nurses can be task-oriented and believe there's only one way to do things.

• *Using medical jargon* with patients who are clearly unable to understand it.

• *Failure to negotiate goals.* Acknowledge any discrepancy in goals, and recognize that the patient's goals supersede yours.

• *Duplication of teaching effort.* Although repetition *can* be a useful teaching device, it should be planned, not haphazard.

• *Overloading the patient with information.* Keep teaching sessions short. Shorter sessions will let the patient integrate new information and formulate questions for the next teaching session—something he couldn't do if you taught everything in one long session.

Watch for signs that a patient is saturated: inability to answer questions regarding the material, fidgeting, yawning, and glazed, staring eyes. When you see these signs, tell the patient to prepare questions for the next session and, if appropriate, leave printed information with him.

• *Poor timing and inattention to the patient's stress level.* This problem is usually caused by focusing on *your* needs, not the patient's.

Just as patients under stress aren't good candidates for teaching, neither are patients in denial.

Sometimes the length of the patient's stay is too short for adequate teaching.

• *Failure to arrange for feedback and evaluation.* Ask for a return demonstration or verbal feedback, and frequently you'll be surprised by how little the patient has actually absorbed. (See *Patient-teaching feedback.*)

Another part of this problem is providing inadequate time for patients to ask questions.

Skill building is an important aspect of the teaching/learning process to consider when planning time requirements. The patient must practice skills requiring physical manipulation alone and in your presence to master them.

• *Using materials that you haven't reviewed or using media exclusively.* Relying totally on media is an inadequate approach to patient education. This makes it impossible to individualize patient teaching, allow the patient to ask questions, or gather feedback from him. (See also *Elderly patients: discharge planning; Legal risks: patient teaching.*)

Patient-teaching feedback

Giving it effectively

Make your comments helpful, not hurtful. Share information and present alternatives, rather than dictate rules. And avoid using absolute words, such as "always" and "never."

Be sure to focus on the patient's behavior, not on his progress or personality. And discuss his *current* behavior, not his past.

First give the patient positive feedback to reinforce desired behavior. Then discuss the points that he still needs to master. Otherwise, the negative comments are probably all he'll hear and remember.

Give feedback as soon as possible after you observe behavior. The longer the patient continues with an undesirable behavior, thought, or attitude, the more comfortable he'll become with it and the greater difficulty he'll have changing it.

Offer specific suggestions for improvement along with the rationale. If the patient understands why something needs to be done, he'll more easily remember to do it—and do it correctly.

And make sure he understands the feedback you've given him. If he's perfecting a technique, have him repeat it at once, so you can check his efforts. If he's attempting something less tangible, such as changing an attitude, you might ask him to rephrase your feedback, to see if he's really listening. Also, look for other clues in his facial expressions and his offhand remarks.

Comment on situations that the patient can change, not ones beyond his control. For instance, if your colostomy patient has limited financial resources, don't emphasize the advantages of using more expensive disposable equipment.

Move at the patient's pace, not yours. Keep in mind his needs and abilities and the amount of information he can handle.

Patient-teaching techniques

Teaching children and adolescents

Teaching children demands ingenuity and an approach very different from that of teaching adults.

Always consider their physical, emotional, and intellectual levels. They have a short attention span and a great need for support and nurturing. Keep teaching sessions short, and consistently offer praise and show affection.

Children learn more easily through active participation than adults. This means you'll undoubtedly use play to teach them about their illness or disease. That'll help them assimilate what you teach. But don't just use it before a procedure or when explaining a disease. Use it also *after* a procedure to help children understand what happened. This follow-up will let them work through unresolved feelings and questions they need to ask.

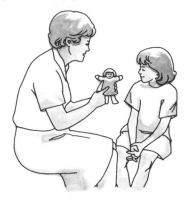

Have parents present when you teach children, so they can provide emotional support during the session and can later reinforce what you taught.

Allow adequate time for children to assimilate information and ask questions. Meet with parents alone to give them more detailed information and answer their questions.

When teaching adolescents, remember that they're different from children. The ability to think abstractly and to reason deductively starts to develop around age 12. Their thought processes are similar to adults', so you'll teach them much the same as adults.

However, two main aspects of their development are different from adults': their social development and the importance of their peers. They develop their identity in re-

lation to their peers and in opposition to their parents. So don't teach them with their parents present. And don't assume that they have more knowledge about their anatomy and physiology than they actually do. Use illustrations as much as possible to enhance what you teach.

Finally, be honest with adolescents. Adequately prepare them if their body image will change because of surgery or disease. Because they want to be "one of the gang" and look like everyone else, adolescents who face a change in appearance feel especially threatened. They'll need your help to hide or camouflage the change whenever possible. (See also *Patient-teaching errors.*)

Patient-teaching timesavers

Helpful shortcuts

Here are some guidelines to save time when teaching patients:
• Before you begin, have the patient review any available written materials, audiocassettes, or videotapes to gain a basic understanding of his disorder.
• Use diagrams, charts, and other visual aids during your teaching sessions to speed comprehension.

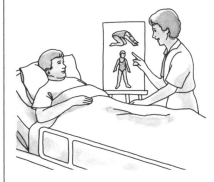

• Rely on support staff to augment your teaching. For example, have the dietician discuss meal plans or ask the respiratory technician to explain spirometry.

• If the patient's family will participate in his home care, schedule his teaching sessions during their visits.
• Teach the patient while you give routine nursing care. Let his questions guide your teaching.
• If you're teaching a short-stay patient who'll be visited by a home health nurse, stress only major points in your teaching and leave the rest for the home health nurse.
• Document your teaching to avoid duplication of instruction.
• Document a patient's repeated resistance to teaching and move on to another patient.
• Give the patient preprinted information and instructions to take home, rather than write new ones yourself.
• Once you've developed a teaching plan for a specific disorder, file it for reuse or adaptation.
• Constantly evaluate your teaching to find the methods that work best for you. Then use them.

You can save staff time by doing the following:
• For same-day surgery patients, assign a nurse to the preadmission testing staff to handle preoperative and postoperative teaching.
• Use group-teaching sessions for patients with similar teaching needs, such as instruction on diabetes, hypertension, cardiac rehabilitation, and postnatal care. (See *Communication: group; Patient-teaching checklists.*)

PEG tube

Assisting the doctor

If your patient needs long-term nutritional support—because he's lost his ability to swallow, for example—he may be a good candidate for percutaneous endoscopic gastrostomy (PEG). In this procedure, a feeding gastrostomy tube is placed endoscopically, so the patient must have an intact, unobstructed gut.

The patient's stomach must be empty, so discontinue all oral, duodenal, or gastric tube feedings for at least 8 hours before the procedure. Place him in the supine position. To lower his risk of aspirating oral secretions, elevate his head 20 to 45 degrees and have suction equipment ready.

Monitor vital signs closely during the procedure.

After the procedure, apply a topical antibiotic ointment at the tube's insertion site. Check the site daily for signs of infection. Mark the tube with indelible ink at the point where it exits the abdomen so you'll know if the tube has moved. If it does, withhold the tube feeding until the doctor checks the tube's position. Administer tube feedings as ordered.

Pericardiocentesis

Monitoring your patient during an emergency

If the doctor suspects your patient has cardiac tamponade, he may perform emergency pericardiocentesis. (This procedure is also used to diagnose pericardial effusion.) Pericardiocentesis involves inserting a 16- or 18-gauge intracardiac needle into the pericardial sac to aspirate fluid and to relieve intrapericardial pressure.

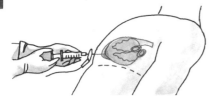

Pericardiocentesis may cause life-threatening complications, such as ventricular dysrhythmias, bleeding from the myocardium, and coronary artery laceration. A precordial lead, attached to the needle's hub, lets the ECG monitor reflect needle position. If the needle contacts the patient's myocardium inadvertently, causing bleeding and ventricular irritability, you'll see abnormal waveforms—large and erratic QRS complexes. Elevated ST segments indicate that the needle's contacted the ventricle; prolonged PR intervals indicate that it's touched the atrium.

Monitor your patient's ECG, blood pressure, and central venous pressure constantly. Make sure, too, that emergency resuscitation equipment's on hand.

After the procedure, monitor his vital signs every 5 to 10 minutes. His blood pressure should rise as the tamponade is relieved.

Be alert for signs and symptoms of recurring tamponade because pericardiocentesis will need to be repeated. (See *Cardiac tamponade.*)

Peripheral disorders: patient teaching

Useful pointers

If your patient has chronic peripheral arterial occlusion, suggest these guidelines to relieve symptoms and prevent further complications:
• Avoid all tobacco products.
• Avoid extreme heat or cold. If you must go outside in cold weather, dress warmly (taking special care to protect your feet). If your feet become cold, don't apply heat to warm them. Instead, use lukewarm water or another warming agent that's below body temperature.
• Follow this daily foot-care regimen: Wash your feet with mild soap and water. Examine them carefully for cuts, blisters, ulcers, or infections. Lightly powder them with talc if they're sweaty; apply hydrous lanolin ointment if they're dry or scaly. Wear only clean cotton socks.
• Protect your feet from injury by never walking barefooted and by having a doctor trim your toenails and shave any corns or calluses. Always wear shoes that fit properly and that have soft tops and thick soles.
• If you have foot or toe pain at night, sleep with your head elevated and your feet below heart level (for example, by placing 6″ to 12″ [15 to 30 cm] wooden blocks under the head of your bed).
• Try to walk a total of 1 to 2 miles each day in 6 to 10 sessions. Stop if leg pain develops.

Peritoneal dialysis: doctors' orders

Proper interpretation

Suppose you've been assigned an acute renal patient who'll be undergoing peritoneal dialysis (PD) for the first time. Unlike the chronic renal patient, this patient's dialysis may end with one or two treatments. He probably won't receive an indwelling (Foley) catheter, which is typically inserted in an operating room setting. Instead, a PD trocath setup will be used.

Before you do anything else, review your hospital's procedure manual for specific instructions.

Then, assess the patient's and family's response and understanding of the procedure. If you can't answer their questions, refer them to a co-worker or the doctor.

Next carefully read the doctor's orders. Typical ones might include:
• Peritoneal dialysis—24 exchanges
• Each exchange—2,000 ml
• 18 exchanges—1.5% dialysate
• 6 exchanges—4.25% dialysate
• Add KCl, 6 mEq, and heparin, 500 units, to each exchange
• Dwell time—20 minutes
• Culture PD drainage after first and last exchange.

Considering the procedure's length, these orders aren't very complicated. But they do need some explanation.

A closer look
The most commonly used volumes for an adult patient are 1,500 ml or 2,000 ml. Certain volumes, however, are better for certain patients.

Specified percents for the dialysate refer to the amount of dextrose it contains—1.5%, 2.5%, or 4.25%

dialysate is more concentrated and thus removes more water.

The orders don't include length of "fill time"—you simply fill the abdomen as fast as the dialysate goes in. Most patients can tolerate a wide-open rate, but someone who has a new incision may be more comfortable with a slower fill rate.

The "dwell time" is specified—20 minutes usually—because it's the actual treatment time. "Drain time" is as long as it takes for the fluid to run out in a steady stream after you open the clamp to the drainage bag. When the drainage slows to a drip rate, start the next exchange. (See *Peritoneal dialysis: preparation.*)

Peritoneal dialysis: exchange

Carrying it out

To begin peritoneal dialysis, let an exchange bag empty into the abdomen; clamp the tubing off when the bag completely empties. Check your watch, then wait about 20 minutes before opening the drainage clamp to let the fluid drain out. When the drainage slows to a drip rate, clamp off the drainage tubing, and begin the next exchange by opening the drainage clamp on the second dialysate bag.

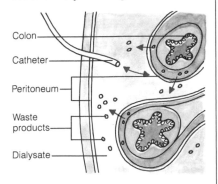

Colon
Catheter
Peritoneum
Waste products
Dialysate

Measure and empty the drainage bag, just as you would a Foley bag. Repeat this fill-dwell-drain sequence until you're finished. (See *Peritoneal dialysis: record keeping; Peritoneal dialysis: termination.*)

Peritoneal dialysis: patient preparation

Step-by-step procedure

First, weigh the patient. You'll compare that baseline weight with his weight after the last exchange. Expect to see a loss; a patient receiving a higher concentration of dialysate will have a greater weight loss.

Usually a patient in renal failure won't have urine in his bladder, but insert a Foley catheter just in case. Making sure the bladder is empty (not pushing up high in the abdomen) will reduce the risk of damage to it and adjacent organs from the stylet used to insert the peritoneal catheter.

Explain what you're doing. After providing for privacy, lower the head of the patient's bed and have him lie flat on his back. Drape the area and set up a sterile field.

Each nephrologist or surgeon has his own insertion technique, but he might do the following: Select the proper site, avoiding areas of previous surgery or scars. Prep the abdomen with povidone iodine (Betadine) and inject Xylocaine to numb the insertion site. Insert the stylet and peritoneal catheter.

Once the catheter is in place, the doctor will ask you to attach it to the tubing. As you do, check that the catheter is well secured. It's taped in place, rather than sutured, because it'll be removed at the end of the treatment. Apply Betadine ointment to the insertion site, cover it with a sterile occlusive dressing, and tape the dressing. (See *Peritoneal dialysis: exchange.*)

Peritoneal dialysis: preparation

Setting up

Once you've read the orders, collect the necessary equipment. A dis-

posable peritoneal dialysis (PD) trocath set normally comes from central supply with nearly everything you'll need: tubing, insertion equipment, $4'' \times 4''$ gauze pads, and lidocaine (lignocaine, Xylocaine).

You'll have to order the dialysate bags. You might specify 2,000-ml bags—18 of the 1.5% concentration and 6 of the 4.25%. Have both the heparin and the I.V. solution of KCl ready.

You'll want to instill the dialysate at body temperature (or as close to that as possible). Otherwise, it could cause intolerance, cramps, or even hypothermia. If the dialysate comes in glass bottles, you can simply place them in a warm water bath. However, most hospitals now use bags for the dialysate. These, like I.V. bags, are permeable, so

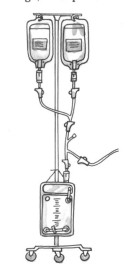

never immerse them without their protective outer wrappers—or you'll risk introducing bacteria from the nonsterile water.

Another piece of equipment you'll need, for the very end of treatment, is a Deane prosthesis (sometimes called a PD button).

The procedure will establish a direct route from the outside into the peritoneal cavity. That makes infection, particularly peritonitis, a constant threat—and perfect sterile technique an absolute necessity.

When opening the PD kit, you'll note that the tubing has a Y connec-

P

tor setup. Connect two bags, which you should have already warmed, to the tubing for your first two exchanges. Add the medications to the bags, if needed, and number each bag. (The doctor may ask you to administer the bags in a certain order; for example, three bags of 1.5% dialysate, followed by one bag of 4.25% dialysate, and so on.)

Hook the drainage bag to the bed. Then, open the clamps to prime the tubing and expel the air, just as you would with any I.V. line.

Clamp off everything. The PD equipment is now set up. Prepare the patient. (See *Peritoneal dialysis: patient preparation.*)

Peritoneal dialysis: record keeping

Paperwork and calculations

Here's a word about the record keeping you should do during peritoneal dialysis (PD). Some hospitals use special PD flow sheets to help you monitor how the treatment is going. Any type of sheet can work, as long as it lets you keep track of the inflow and outflow at a given time. For instance, if you instill 2,000 ml, but only 1,800 ml drains out, you're behind 200 ml. But, if on the next exchange, you instill 2,000 ml and get back 2,400 ml, you're now ahead 200 ml—and the total is cumulative.

At the start of dialysis, fluid tends to pool in the abdomen, so you're likely to be behind at first. But drainage improves as the treatment progresses. (See *Peritoneal dialysis: termination.*)

Peritoneal dialysis: termination

Ending the treatment

To determine when the peritoneal dialysis (PD) treatment should be

over, add the times for each fill-dwell-drain step. For instance, an order of 2,000 ml of dialysate usually needs a fill time of 10 to 15 minutes; dwell time is 20 minutes; and drain time is about 15 to 20 minutes. (Typically, more fluid comes out than goes in.)

However, to simplify things here, figure that each exchange takes about 1 hour. So the 24 exchanges should take about 24 hours. When you do this yourself, you'd calculate the time more exactly to determine which nursing shift and probable time the dialysis would end.

After putting on gloves (some hospitals may require you to wear a mask), remove the dressing. Clean the area with povidone-iodine solution and slowly withdraw the catheter from the abdomen.

Your last step is to insert the Deane prosthesis, or PD button. (Some hospitals, however, consider this a medical procedure.) Lubricate the button with sterile normal saline solution. Again with absolutely sterile technique, insert the lubricated button, pushing it downward until its round top is lying flat against the skin. (If you feel any resistance, stop and call the doctor.) Then, cover the button with an occlusive dressing. The button will keep the insertion site open if another treatment is needed; it will also prevent any fluid remaining in the abdomen from leaking out.

Peritoneal tap and lavage

Nursing responsibilities

Keep these points in mind if the doctor's ordered peritoneal tap or lavage for your patient:
• If ordered, assist with nasogastric tube insertion before the procedure, to decompress the stomach.
• Have the patient void before the procedure, or insert an indwelling (Foley) catheter as ordered.

• Maintain a sterile field and strict sterile technique during the procedure.
• To allow fluid to flow back into the container, make sure the I.V. tubing doesn't have a nonbackflow filter. If you're using an I.V. bottle setup, break off the air vent's plastic tubing so a water seal doesn't form.
• Apply an antibiotic ointment and sterile dressing after trocath removal.
• After the procedure, observe for complications, such as bowel or bladder perforation and free air in the peritoneal cavity.

Peritonitis

Intervention

Be alert for the following signs and symptoms of peritonitis:
• sudden abdominal pain, which may be localized or diffuse but is most intense in the area of the patient's primary GI disorder
• abdominal distention and rebound tenderness
• increased temperature (103° F. [39.4° C.] or higher), with chills
• signs of shock (weakness, pallor, diaphoresis, tachycardia, and decreased blood pressure)
• shallow, rapid respirations (due to diaphragmatic irritation).

If you note any of these signs and symptoms, notify the doctor immediately. Remember, peritonitis can develop very rapidly.

Diagnosis

The doctor will order a complete blood count to determine if the white blood cell count is elevated ($20,000/mm^3$ or more). He'll also order abdominal X-rays, which may show a paralytic ileus, edema, distention of the small and large bowel, and upward displacement of the diaphragm. He may also perform paracentesis to check for bacteria, exudate, pus, blood, or urine in the patient's abdominal cavity.

Treatment involves three steps:
• Identifying the underlying cause and treating it.

• Treating the infection.
• Correcting dehydration and paralytic ileus.

Your patient may need surgery to remove or seal off the source of peritoneal contamination, or he may have an incision to drain the area if the infection is localized.

Nursing interventions

Expect to start antibiotics promptly. Start an I.V. for fluid and electrolyte replacement, and insert a nasogastric tube, as ordered, to aspirate the patient's stomach contents (see *Nasogastric tube: patient care*). Give the patient nothing by mouth until his bowel sounds return and his gastric aspirate becomes scanty. Administer analgesics, as ordered.

Phototherapy: diapers

Making a bikini diaper

For an infant who needs phototherapy, try making a bikini diaper

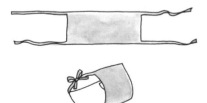

using a four-string, disposable face mask with the metal nosepiece removed. This allows maximum skin

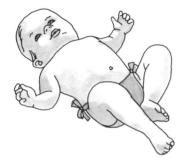

exposure to the lights, while protecting the infant's genitals. (See *Phototherapy: eyepads.*)

Phototherapy: eyepads

Making them for newborns

When jaundiced newborns need phototherapy, you can make pads to protect their eyes. First, put a piece of polyurethane dressing (for example, Op-Site, Bioclusive, Tegaderm), about 1½″ (4 cm) long, on each of the infant's temples. These pieces of dressing will remain in place throughout phototherapy. Next, cut an adult-sized eye pad in half to fit over the infant's eyes, and tape these halves together. Attach another piece of tape to the outer edge of each pad and attach the pads to the dressings on the infant's temples. (The tape only touches the dressing—not the skin.) Turn the ends of the tape under for easy grasping and removing. Now, you can remove the pads easily to change them, give eye care, and provide visual stimulation without applying and reapplying tape to the infant's delicate skin.

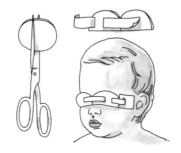

Here's another way to make comfortable, *tapeless* eye pads for newborns. Cut a disposable face mask across the width—½″ (1 cm) above and below the elastic band—and cover the edges with paper tape to prevent fraying. Then cut an adult-sized eye pad in half, lay the halves on the inside of the mask, and secure them to the mask with doubled paper tape. Adjust the elastic band to fit the infant's head by tying a knot in the band. (See also *Phototherapy: diapers.*)

Pin care

Performing it

Once your patient has a pin in place—for skeletal traction or an external fixation device—the doctor will order pin care. (See *Fixation devices, external; Traction patients.*) Specific procedures vary according to hospital protocols. Here are some general guidelines to follow when giving it:
• Examine the patient's skin around the pin for tautness, pain, tenderness, and redness from inflammation and infection.
• Note any crusted serous drainage around the pin site. *Gently* remove the crust to prevent it from obstructing wound drainage.
• Give skin care every 4 hours.
• Note any signs and symptoms of pin looseness—such as increased or purulent drainage or free turning of the pin in the patient's skin.
• Don't prod the patient's skin around the pin—you may cause additional pain or skin abrasions that can lead to infection.
• Clean the pins once or twice a day, using povidone-iodine solution or hydrogen peroxide, as ordered. For an external fixation device, work proximally to distally on one side, then on the other. Afterward, wipe the device's frame with a sterile cloth moistened with sterile water. Cover the pins' ends with pin caps, corks, or rubber plugs from blood sample vials.

Placenta previa

Nursing priorities

If your patient's hemorrhage is severe and fetal age is more than 37 weeks, your patient will be transferred to surgery, where the doctor will perform a vaginal examination using a "double setup": The operating room will be prepared so that either a vaginal delivery *or* a cesarean section can be performed. The doctor will examine the position of the placenta and, if it doesn't cover the cervical os, he may rupture the patient's membranes and induce labor. If the placenta *does* cover the os, the doctor will perform a cesarean section to deliver the fetus. Before surgery, insert an I.V. line and an indwelling (Foley) catheter, and prepare the patient as ordered.

Complete placenta previa

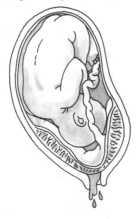

If your patient's bleeding isn't severe and fetal age is less than 37 weeks, the doctor may ask you to give the patient supplemental oxygen and I.V. fluids and to place her on bed rest so the fetus has more time to mature. (If the bleeding becomes severe and can't be stopped, the doctor will perform a cesarean section, and the baby will be maintained in the intensive care nursery.) Monitor fetal heart tones. If the fetus isn't in distress, the doctor may ask you to administer betamethasone, which may improve the fetus' chances of survival. After you give betamethasone, monitor fetal heart tones every 5 minutes. (See *Fetal monitoring, external electronic.*) At the first sign of fetal distress, notify the doctor immediately.

Record the number of perineal pads the patient uses and the time required to saturate them, and roll your patient over occasionally to check whether blood has pooled under her. (If it has, try to estimate its contribution to her blood loss.)

Monitor your patient's vital signs closely, watching for any indication of internal hemorrhage or impending shock.

If she develops any of the signs or symptoms of shock, call the doctor immediately. At the first signs of fetal or maternal distress, the doctor will transfer the patient for an emergency cesarean section. (See *Shock: intervention; Shock: recognition.*)

Planning, personal

Focusing on actions to achieve personal goals

Follow these steps to develop more effective goals:
• Set up goal categories, such as career, financial, personal, and so on. (See *Career strategies; Job change: planning.*) Achieving one goal may meet your needs in two categories. For example, getting your MSN might meet a personal and a career goal.
• Write the specific goals you want to attain in each category. Next to each goal, write a target date for accomplishing it. For example, "Finish MSN by the end of next year."
• Write the actions you plan to take to meet each goal and any interim steps necessary to reach your goal, with target completion dates. For example, if your goal is to finish your MSN, you might write, "Take two courses over summer; complete by August 20th" as your interim steps.
• Keep a calendar listing your target completion dates. Reward yourself whenever you meet one of these goals.

Planning: priorities

Becoming more efficient

As you plan activities, write down one or two nursing priorities for each patient. Then promise yourself to satisfy those priorities.

You can't always begin the shift with a full assessment of each patient, so learn to make spot assessments and observations: Focus on the body part or body system most closely associated with the patient's illness or injury.

Also think of tasks that you want to do for your patients—for their safety and comfort and for your own peace of mind. A back rub, a shampoo, extra teaching, or a quiet, reassuring talk should go on your list of important priorities, too.

Each time you accomplish a prioritized task, cross it off your list. You'll be more satisfied when you review all that you've accomplished by the end of your shift. If you didn't complete your list, determine why. Did you underestimate the time a procedure would take? Were you called to another unit for an hour? Was the task something that could have been postponed?

How could you have completed prioritized tasks that didn't get done? Better planning? More help? Knowing more about the task or procedure? Setting more realistic priorities? Even on the best of days, infiltrated I.V.s and malfunctioning nasogastric tubes interrupt you. Don't expect to accomplish everything, just the most important things.

Pneumothorax

Managing the different types

Recognizing and managing thoracic injuries takes some fine-tuned assessment skills. Here's what to look for and do.
Closed (simple) pneumothorax
1. Assess the patient's airway, breathing, and circulation, and intervene as necessary.
2. Place him on a cardiac monitoring device.
3. Start I.V. fluids, and administer oxygen at a high flow rate.

P

4. Place him in the semi-Fowler's position, if possible.

Closed pneumothorax

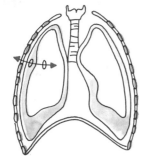

5. Prepare him for chest tube insertion.

6. Obtain a blood sample for arterial blood gas (ABG) studies.

Open pneumothorax

1. Assess the patient's airway, breathing, and circulation (ABC), and intervene as necessary.

2. Cover the sucking wound with sterile occlusive dressing.

3. Place him on a cardiac monitoring device.

4. Start I.V. fluids, and administer oxygen at a high flow rate.

5. Observe for signs of tension pneumothorax. If signs are present, relieve pressure of occlusive dressing.

6. Prepare him for chest tube insertion. (See *Chest tube insertion.*)

7. Obtain a blood sample for ABG studies.

Hemothorax

1. Assess the patient's ABC, and intervene as necessary.

Hemothorax

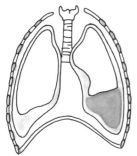

2. Place him on a cardiac monitoring device.

3. Start I.V. fluids, and administer oxygen at a high flow rate.

4. Apply medical antishock trousers (unless contraindicated by hospital policy). (See *MAST suit.*)

5. Prepare him for chest tube insertion.

6. Obtain a blood sample for ABG studies.

7. Prepare him for surgery, if indicated. (See also *Chest wound, sucking; Pneumothorax, spontaneous; Pneumothorax, tension.*)

Pneumothorax, spontaneous

Detecting a recurrence

Your patient with a spontaneous pneumothorax has a 60% chance of experiencing a recurrence on the same or opposite side. Pneumothorax may recur a few days after the initial pneumothorax—or up to 20 years later. However, it usually recurs within 2 to 3 years.

To prepare your patient for a recurrence, explain the risk and answer any questions he and his family may have. Emphasize the importance of detecting telltale signs and symptoms early and of seeking medical attention immediately. Instruct him to watch for:
• sharp, stabbing chest pain
• shortness of breath
• anxiety or restlessness
• increased pulse and respiratory rates.

Pneumothorax, tension

What to do immediately

One of your patients just had a CVP (central venous pressure) catheter inserted and suddenly develops respiratory distress and pain. Breath sounds are absent on the left side of the chest. You suspect tension pneumothorax.

Page the patient's doctor to return to your patient's room; she needs to have a chest tube inserted at once. (See *Chest tube insertion.*) Reassure the patient that she's going to get immediate help, and put her into the Fowler's position. Check her vital signs continuously, especially her pulse. Be prepared to call a code.

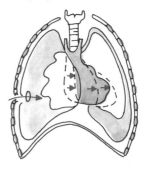

Begin giving 100% oxygen through a nonrebreather mask. If she doesn't already have a peripheral I.V. line in place, insert one so emergency drugs can be administered if necessary.

Have someone get a thoracotomy tray, chest tube, and chest drainage system while you stay with the patient. Open the tray so it'll be ready when the doctor arrives. If you have time, swab povidone-iodine on the patient's anterior chest along the mid-clavicular line. The doctor will insert the chest tube in the second intercostal space.

When the doctor arrives, brief him on the patient's status while he inserts the chest tube. (He may first choose to do a needle thoracotomy—as a temporary measure only—by inserting a 12- to 16-gauge needle into the chest.)

While the doctor inserts the chest tube, set up the chest drainage system as you continue to monitor the patient's condition. (See *Chest drainage system: preparation.*) After he connects the chest tube to the drainage system, he'll probably suture it to the patient's chest to secure it. Then you'll apply a dressing.

Tape the dressing to the patient's chest, then tape all junctions of the drainage tubing. Coil the tubing and pin it to the patient's bedclothes, allowing slack for her to move.

P

The patient needs a chest X-ray now—to check placement of the CVP catheter and chest tube and to confirm that the pneumothorax has been resolved. Maintain the infusion through the CVP line at a keep-vein-open rate until placement is confirmed, then adjust the rate, as ordered.

What to do later

Auscultate the patient's lungs and assess her vital signs, then record your findings. Since she didn't suffer an arrest, her condition should improve as quickly as it deteriorated. Assess her need for oxygen, and draw a blood sample for arterial blood gas analysis if her condition warrants it. Be sure the chest drainage system is operating properly. Then record what happened on the patient's chart.

Poisoning, carbon monoxide

Emergency care

In home health care, you might someday encounter a case of carbon monoxide poisoning, as from a kerosene heater. You'll find a patient confused and apt to have a headache, with a slightly elevated pulse and respiratory rate.

If possible, stop the source of carbon monoxide, and help the patient into another room, next to a window. Open this and all windows wide, and open the outside doors as well to get in as much fresh air as possible. Cover the patient with coats and blankets and explain why the windows must be kept open.

Call the fire department, if appropriate, and give the address and a brief description of the problem. Fire department personnel will want to examine a kerosene heater, for example, and check for any other sources of carbon monoxide leakage.

When the rescue squad arrives, give a full report of your findings, including when you discovered the

patient and what his most recent vital signs were. Fill them in on his medical history, current medications, and his doctor's name.

Rescue personnel will begin administering 100% oxygen through a tight-fitting face mask. They'll also hook up the patient to a cardiac monitor, and they may start an infusion of D_5W. Once in the emergency department, samples will be drawn for analysis of arterial blood gases, electrolytes, blood urea nitrogen, and creatinine as well as a complete blood count.

Document everything, including the time you called the fire department. Check on the patient's condition. Then take a minute to review the facts about carbon monoxide.

When inhaled, carbon monoxide combines with hemoglobin, the oxygen-carrying pigment in red blood cells, to produce carboxyhemoglobin. Thus, hemoglobin can no longer carry oxygen to the cells. Organs needing the most oxygen (the heart and the brain) are the most severely affected. Any increase on the body's demands for oxygen (fever, physical exertion) will speed up the poisoning process.

The signs and symptoms you'll see depend on the percentage of carboxyhemoglobin in the victim's blood:

• 10%—dyspnea on mild exertion, headache
• 20%—dyspnea on mild exertion, throbbing headache, nausea, vomiting
• 30%—headache, irritability, impaired thought processes, severe nausea and vomiting
• 40% to 50%—severe headache, confusion, syncope, sinus tachycardia with ectopic beats
• 60% to 70%—loss of consciousness, seizures, respiratory failure
• greater than 70%—rapid death.

Also, a cherry red coloration of mucous membranes and blood is a traditional indicator of carbon monoxide poisoning. It's usually a poor prognostic sign. (See *Poisoning: inhalation.*)

Poisoning: ingestion

Detection and emergency intervention

Signs and symptoms of poisoning include constricted or dilated pupils; altered state of awareness, including unconsciousness; foaming at the mouth; abnormal pulse; nausea or vomiting; diarrhea; stomach or abdominal pain; abnormal respirations; convulsions; coughing; burns in and around mouth (if a corrosive substance was ingested); and distinctive breath odors (for example, the odor of bitter almonds indicates cyanide poisoning; odor of coal gas, carbon monoxide poisoning; odor of pears, chloral hydrate poisoning; odor of violets, turpentine poisoning).

First seek medical advice from a doctor, a poison control center, or an emergency department.

If the victim is conscious, dilute the poison by giving him a glass of water or milk if he's not having convulsions. When the victim is transported send the poisonous substance and its container and any vomitus with him. If a caustic substance is on his skin, flush with water.

If the victim is or becomes unconscious, maintain his airway, call for the emergency medical squad, and administer CPR if necessary. (See *CPR: technique.*) Don't try to give fluids or induce vomiting. If vomiting occurs, position him by turning his head to the side or rolling him to his side so that vomitus drains from his mouth. (See *Poisoning: medication.*)

Poisoning: inhalation

Taking swift action

The signs and symptoms may vary depending on the source of poisoning. Usually they include dyspnea, coughing, abnormal pulse, and eye irritation. The lips and skin may appear cherry red in carbon monoxide poisoning.

First, remove the victim from the dangerous environment. If he's in a closed room or space, take a deep breath and hold it before entering. Cover your mouth and nose with a wet towel. Try to move the victim into fresh air or allow fresh air into the area.

Call an emergency squad immediately; tell them oxygen will be needed. Loosen the victim's clothing. Maintain airway and initiate CPR if necessary. (See *CPR: technique.*) Induce vomiting when he is conscious and has not swallowed strong acids, alkalies, strychnine, or camphor. The product container may not have correct instructions regarding vomiting. To be safe, call an emergency department for instructions.

Never induce vomiting when a victim is stuporous or comatose, has seizures, has no gag reflex, has a possible myocardial infarction, has ingested corrosives, or has ingested silver nitrate, strychnine, or camphor.

Beware of these oxygen-occlusive gases:
- carbon monoxide
- ammonium gas
- chlorine gas
- smoke (mixture of toxic and air-occlusive gases)
- propane.

Carbon monoxide causes more poisoning deaths than any other inhaled substance. Also beware cases of cyanide gas poisoning. Oxygen will help the victim, but he'll also need an antidote. (See also *Poisoning, carbon monoxide; Poisoning: ingestion.*)

Poisoning: medication

Pediatric emergency measures

Ever get a phone call from a mother saying her child has accidentally taken medication? It could happen, and you'll need to know exactly what to do.

Find out how much time has passed since the child took the medication, how much he weighs, whether he's showing any signs and symptoms, the name and strength of the drug he took, the maximum dose that could have been taken, the child's name, and the home telephone number. Take care to warn his mother not to induce vomiting but to wait until you call her back.

Then, call the poison control center in your area; the number should be listed on the first page of your telephone directory. Give the poison information specialist all of the information you got from the mother. Also, tell him if the mother has tried to induce vomiting.

If the specialist tells you that the overdose could be fatal, the mother should not waste time trying to induce vomiting. Instead, she should take the child to an emergency department (ED), where he can be given gastric lavage under medical supervision. Also, the child can be monitored in the ED for at least 6 hours after he's treated, during which time his vital signs and cardiac rhythm should be assessed continually. They'll admit him if he develops dysrhythmias or any other adverse reactions, and he'll have to stay in the hospital at least 24 hours after these adverse reactions subside.

Call the mother back and urge her to take the child to a hospital's ED immediately. Again, tell her not to induce vomiting, briefly explaining why. Ask if she knows where the nearest hospital is. If she doesn't, tell her which one is closest, and give her directions if necessary.

Call back the poison control center and tell the specialist which hospital the child is going to. He'll call the ED to alert the staff there and to give treatment information. (See *Poisoning: ingestion; Poisoning: inhalation.*)

Positioning, patient

Using pillows to position a patient on his side

When you're positioning a patient on his side in bed and you prop a pillow behind his back, does the pillow slip away? If so, untuck the drawsheet and place the pillow un-

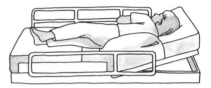

der the drawsheet. Then tuck the sheet back under the mattress. The pillow won't slip, and the patient will stay on his side. (See *Bed positioning; Bedridden patients.*)

Postanesthesia recovery

Essentials of care

When your patient arrives, and at intervals throughout his stay in the recovery room, assess his physiologic status. Write down his arrival time, your observations, and any actions you take. Enter them on the recovery room record, the flow sheet, or in your nurses' notes.

1. First, check his airway, making sure it's patent. If oxygen is to be administered, start it at the flow rate ordered. Note the rate, depth, and quality of his respirations.

2. Note the presence or absence of protective throat reflexes.

3. Take his pulse and blood pressure every 15 minutes until they're stable, then every half hour. Note both the rate and quality of your patient's pulse. The vital sign readings you record must be compared with the preoperative and intraoperative readings. Also monitor ECG, arterial line, or Swan-Ganz catheter readings, if present.

P

4. Ascertain your patient's level of consciousness by testing his responses to various stimuli.

5. Note the condition of his skin and the color of his nail beds and lips. Report cold, clammy, or hot, dry skin.

6. Observe I.V. infusions. Note the position of needle, condition of site, type and amount of fluid being infused, and rate of infusion. If blood is being transfused, watch for signs of an adverse reaction. (See *Blood transfusion reaction.*)

7. Note the presence and condition of any drains and tubes, including a urinary catheter. Be sure they aren't kinked or clamped and are properly connected to suction or a drainage bag. Observe the color, odor, amount, and consistency of drainage. Label the tubes to properly identify drainage. (See *Drains: guidelines.*)

8. Assess any dressings and, if they're soiled, note the color, type, odor, and amount of drainage. Describe the amount in a measurable term—for example, "dime-sized."

9. Note the presence and type of any irrigant. Record not only the amount infused and returned, but also the color and type of the return.

10. Observe anything relevant to the patient's specific surgical procedure.

11. Take his temperature.

Perform suctioning as needed. An intramuscular antiemetic and an I.V. narcotic for pain may be ordered once vital signs have stabilized. Have the patient deep-breathe three to four times each time you check his vital signs; turn and move his legs every hour; and cough, if appropriate, every 30 minutes. (See also *Anesthesia, general; Postop hazards.*)

Postop exercises

Teaching them

Before a patient has surgery, you should teach, demonstrate, and supervise the exercise program he'll follow postoperatively. First, teach him deep breathing and coughing. Tell him he'll do these exercises at least five times an hour after surgery to get air into his lungs and to improve venous return to his heart. Patients at risk for developing atelectasis and pneumonia after surgery will do these exercises even more often. Such patients include the elderly and smokers as well as those with respiratory conditions, chest or abdominal incisions, and those who will be immobilized postoperatively.

To teach your patient deep-breathing exercises, have him sit down or lie on his back with his knees slightly flexed. Tell him to inhale slowly through his nose, hold his breath for 3 seconds, then exhale slowly through his mouth. His abdomen should rise when he inhales and fall when he exhales. To make sure he's doing the exercise correctly, suggest he place his hands on his abdomen and watch them rise and fall.

Next, teach him how to cough to clear secretions that collected in his tracheobronchial tree during anesthesia. Teach him *cascade coughing*, *huff coughing*, or *augmented coughing*. To teach *cascade coughing*, tell him to take a deep breath and hold it for a moment, then to cough repeatedly while exhaling until he has no more air left. To teach *huff* coughing, tell him to take a deep breath with his mouth open and to huff repeatedly as he exhales until he has no more air left. (See *Cough technique.*) To teach *augmented* coughing, tell him to exhale completely, then inhale completely and hold his breath for a moment before coughing forcefully.

Splinting the incision

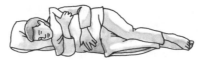

If he's scheduled for chest or abdominal surgery, teach him how to splint his incision. Suggest he place his hands, a small pillow, or towel over his incision to minimize movement during deep breathing, coughing, or turning.

Then tell him he'll need to turn hourly to improve his circulation and loosen respiratory secretions. Splinting his incision and placing a pillow between his legs will help reduce pain when he turns from side to side. Have him practice turning before surgery.

Teach him leg exercises to improve his circulation. Alternately extend and flex his hip, knee, and ankle joints. Rotate his ankle as though tracing a circle with his toes.

Leg exercises

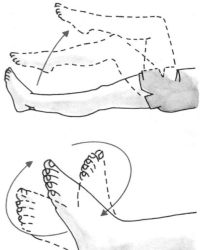

Then ask him to move his legs as if he were riding a bicycle. He may do similar exercises with his shoulders, elbows, and wrists. Immediately after surgery, help him with these exercises. Within a day or so, he should be able to do them while you observe and document his progress.

Postop hazards

Guarding against them

You can prevent postop complications by watching for the following:
• *Obstruction* can occur anywhere along the respiratory tract, though

it's most common in the pharynx or larynx. Your patient's tongue is his worst enemy, since it can easily slide back and obstruct his airway. But obstructions can also come from secretions, edema, blood, mucus plugs, and, particularly, vomitus.

• *Active vomiting* is hazardous, but not as dangerous as *passive regurgitation*, which happens with little noticeable gagging movement. If vomitus is aspirated into the trachea and bronchi, it may cause severe pulmonary complications and even death. So be alert for any signs of gagging, and if you notice your patient is starting to regurgitate, turn his head to the side. Medications that control postoperative nausea and vomiting include benzquinamide, droperidol, prochlorperazine, promethazine, and trimethobenzamide.

• To manage *respiratory distress*, first identify what type it is. Is the problem an obstruction, or is it laryngospasm, bronchospasm, or laryngeal or subglottic edema? Is it an anesthetic or narcotic overdose, a reaction to the anesthetic agent, incomplete reversal of the muscle relaxant, or splinting?

Laryngospasm, which you'll recognize by audible "crowing," occurs in both children and adults. (See *Laryngospasm.*) It results from intubation irritation or the presence of other foreign bodies, such as blood, mucus, or the tube itself. Bronchospasm is characterized by wheezing. Preexisting respiratory disease, such as asthma or emphysema, can set these spasms off. To counteract drug-induced hypoventilation, find out what medications and anesthetics were given and their effects.

• Watch for any *abnormal respiratory patterns*: noisy respirations, aberrant movements, and altered behavior. In the patient who's had upper abdominal or thoracic surgery, be alert for splinting. The closer to the thorax the incision is, the shallower his breathing will be as he tries to protect himself against pain from chest movements. (A dressing that's too tight may also have the same effect.)

Postop hypertension: fluids

Keeping alert for postop fluid overload

In the postanesthesia recovery room, you must carefully monitor a hypertensive patient's fluid balance. To treat intraoperative hypotension, the anesthesiologist will frequently give significant volumes of fluids. Stay alert for fluid overload.

A patient with a diseased heart may not be able to handle this overload. So if your patient has known or suspected compromise of left ventricular function, carefully monitor him for fluid overload by central venous pressure (CVP) or pulmonary artery catheter.

Signs and symptoms of fluid overload will vary with the degree of imbalance. Early signs might be rapid pulse and dyspnea; periorbital edema; and normal to high blood pressure. Later signs might be excessive oral secretions and moist crackles. A chest X-ray might show pleural effusion, infiltrates, or frank pulmonary congestion. The patient's hematocrit value may be lowered.

If you suspect fluid overload, decrease I.V. fluids and keep precise intake and output records. Add intra-arterial and CVP monitoring flush-fluids to these records. Chart urine output hourly as well as the CVP readings or the pulmonary capillary wedge pressure.

Postop hypertension: oxygen

Postop recognition and correction

In the postanesthesia recovery room, you may see two respiratory problems that cause hypertension: hypoxemia or hypercapnia. Some patients develop both.

Hypoxemia probably occurs more frequently in postanesthesia recovery than anyone imagines. The most common cause is chronic obstructive pulmonary disease.

Hypoxemia may result indirectly from splinting the chest wall, fluid excess, or the type of dressing applied. It may also result directly from surgery on the thorax, head, or neck, or simply from the drugs used before and during surgery.

Recognizing hypoxemia in the sedated patient is difficult because the signs are subtle. First, there are those of sympathetic stimulation, such as hypertension and tachycardia—probably already present from pain. Then you might also observe that the patient is restless, confused, irritable, somnolent, lethargic, vague, or facetious.

If you note these signs, obtain an order for an arterial blood gas (ABG) study. Confirmation of hypoxemia comes from a low PO_2 with a normal or reduced PCO_2.

Treatment consists of giving the patient oxygen or, if he's already receiving it, giving higher inspired levels by mask or intubation and mechanical ventilation. Correct the cause of hypoxemia as well.

Hypercapnia, an elevation of PCO_2, results from hypoventilation. The clinical diagnosis of hypercapnia, like hypoxemia, is difficult and based largely on suspicion. Hypercapnia does cause sympathetic stimulation, so the patient is usually diaphoretic and hypertensive. He may also be restless, confused, irritable, or particularly somnolent.

You can roughly evaluate expiratory flow at the nose and mouth to see if the patient is hypoventilating, or you can attach a spirometer (see *Lung volumes*) to a well-fitted oxygen mask for an accurate measure of tidal and minute volume. Or you can get an ABG sample (see *Arterial puncture*).

Treatment of hypercapnia is based on its cause and the level of

P

CO_2 retention. With an immediately reversible cause, such as narcotic ventilatory depression or residual neuromuscular weakness, restoration should be fairly quick. With a long-term cause, you'll have to begin adequate ventilation by mechanical means and continue to check the PCO_2 level until the underlying problem is improved or corrected.

Postop hypertension: pain

Recognition and management

A patient's need for postoperative analgesia can be greatly reduced by preparing him psychologically, reassuring him that he won't suffer needlessly.

Not only his mental state but also the operative site determine the amount of analgesic he'll need. Pain usually originates from the incision itself, but don't overlook other causes, such as a distended bladder.

To check for pain, look for increased heart and respiratory rate; pallor; dilated pupils; clenched jaws or hands; grimacing; a cold sweat; and increased blood pressure. Nausea can also be a symptom. Restlessness and anxiety may indicate pain, *or* they may signify cerebral oxygen deficiency, so monitor your patient closely.

Before giving analgesics, you can try other pain relief measures, such as positioning him to avoid stress on his incision, applying an ice bag, and giving reassurance.

Before giving analgesics or narcotics, take the patient's vital signs, check him for allergies, and evaluate the patient's need. It's always safer to give a second small dose of narcotic than a large initial one, which may reanesthetize him. (See *Orders, sliding scale.*)

When giving narcotics to block pain, remember that I.V. titration has proven superior to intramuscular injection. Opiate receptors in the central nervous system are more susceptible to I.V. doses.

Perhaps the most effective current method of providing analgesia is epidural spinal nerve block. This is because in most cases the relief is total. (See *Pain and anesthesia; Postanesthesia recovery.*)

Postop hypertension: temperature

Methods for maintaining postop normothermia

Because of many contributing factors in the operating room, you'll find a hypothermic patient intensely vasoconstricted in the postanesthesia recovery room. This results in poor peripheral perfusion and metabolic acidosis and may contribute to dysrhythmias and hypertension as well.

Shivering, which increases muscle metabolism, commonly occurs when a patient emerges from general or regional anesthesia.

You'll recognize hypothermia because the patient will be vasoconstricted and shivering, feel cool to the touch, and have goose bumps. His respiratory rate and tidal volume will be lowered; his temperature will be below normal. Plus, his urine output will have dropped because of reduced renal blood flow.

To care for him, do the following:
• Provide oxygen until his temperature returns to normal.
• Monitor his heart rate and rhythm.
• Record his urine output hourly.
• Measure his vital signs at least once an hour. Take rectal, not oral, temperatures.
• Provide an electrically controlled hypothermia blanket.
• Warm any blood transfusions that may be required. (See *Blood transfusion preparation.*)

Postop infections

Prevention techniques

Hand washing is the single most effective way to prevent spread of infection. If your staff members aren't washing their hands as often as they should, suggest a meeting to find out why. The reason may be as simple as a stopped-up soap dispenser or an irritating or unpleasant-smelling soap. Also list specific times for hand washing (for example, before changing a patient's dressing or before suctioning him). Post eye-catching reminders in appropriate places.

Using incentive spirometry protects your patient from the number one postoperative pulmonary complication—atelectasis—and helps reverse abnormalities that atelectasis produces. (See *Incentive spirometry: adults; Incentive spirometry: children.*) By encouraging sustained maximal inspiration, incentive spirometry reinflates collapsed alveoli, improves oxygen transport, and prevents mucus accumulation. Together, these results reduce the possibility of pulmonary complications.

If possible, teach your patient how to use incentive spirometry *before* his surgery. Chances are, that's when he'll be free of pain, unencumbered by tubes and dressings, and he'll able to concentrate on your directions and practice the exercise. Depending on his postop condition, encourage him to start using incentive spirometry shortly after he returns to his room. Monitor him for the first few times, then he should be able to do the exercise on his own.

Also give plenty of fluids. Keeping his kidneys thoroughly flushed will greatly limit, and may even prevent, bacterial growth in the urinary tract—the most common site of nosocomial infection. Fluids also promote tissue healing, speed up recovery time, and help eliminate the dehydration caused by preoperative preparations.

Devise a specific fluid plan for your patient. For example: 7 a.m. to 3 p.m., 1,500 ml; 3 p.m. to 11 p.m., 1,000 ml; and 11 p.m. to 7 a.m., 500 ml. If a round-the-clock plan disturbs your patient's sleep, build one around his waking hours.

Use aseptic wound care. Preventive measures include using sterile instruments and dressings, aseptic technique, and effective and frequent hand washing. Also, never allow the dressing to become moist; this provides an excellent medium for bacterial growth and breaks the protection barrier that the dressing is meant to provide. Have the proper equipment on hand for each dressing change. If someone else changes the dressing and you know this person doesn't always use proper technique, have another staff member offer to assist. (See also *Wound care dressings: changes.*)

Assess your patient and his wound frequently. Note the color, odor, and amount of drainage, as well as the progress of tissue granulation. As always, document your findings and report any significant changes to the doctor.

Posturing

Applying a painful stimulus to an unconscious patient

When you apply a painful stimulus to your unconscious patient's supraorbital notch, his motor response indicates his neurologic status. Normally, he will reach above his shoulder level toward the pain stimulus. Remember, a focal motor deficit, such as hemiplegia, may prevent a bilateral response.

As the patient's brain stem function deteriorates, he may respond by assuming one of the following postures. Each posture suggests advanced deterioration:

• *Flexor (decorticate) posturing.* The patient flexes one or both arms on his chest and may stiffly extend his legs.

Flexor (decorticate) posturing

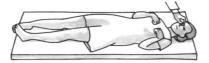

• *Extensor (decerebrate) posturing.* The patient stiffly extends one or both arms and, possibly, his legs.

Extensor (decerebrate) posturing

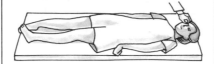

• *Flaccid.* The patient displays no motor response in any extremity.

Prednisone

Preventing bruises

Some patients who take prednisone develop bruises on their arms when they do housework or yard work. So, suggest they wear white sport socks (with the feet cut off) on their arms. The socks will cushion any impact and are easily hidden under long-sleeved shirts and blouses. (See also *Steroids.*)

Pregnancy

When your patient suffers abdominal trauma

When caring for a pregnant patient with abdominal trauma, intervene as ordered, following the same priorities as for a nonpregnant patient. However, keep these special nursing considerations in mind:

• Initiate continuous fetal monitoring. (See *Fetal monitoring, external electronic.*) Abdominal trauma complications include fetal distress, fetal skull and long-bone fractures, and fetal death. Decreased fetal heart rate may also appear as the first sign of maternal internal injury and shock because the patient compensates for hypovolemia by reducing uterine perfusion. Fetal heart rate below 120 beats/minute warrants immediate action; below 100 beats/minute indicates significant hypoxia.

• Administer drugs cautiously, and avoid vasopressors, which constrict uterine blood flow.

• Replace fluids rapidly and generously.

• Apply medical anti-shock trousers if the patient has hypotension or is in shock, using care when inflating the abdominal section. (See *MAST suit.*)

• Give high-flow oxygen (maternal hypoxia compromises utero-placental blood flow).

• Place the patient in the left lateral position to avoid supine hypotension syndrome. If injuries rule out this position, place pillows beneath her right hip or manually displace her uterus to the left. Avoid Trendelenburg's position, which may compromise cardiac and respiratory function.

• Assess the patient frequently for signs and symptoms of disseminated intravascular coagulation.

• Administer tetanus prophylaxis, as ordered, if the patient has a vaginal or uterine injury.

• Administer preoperative antibiotics, as ordered, early in your care.

• Take steps to reduce the patient's anxiety (anxiety increases catecholamine release, which in turn decreases uterine blood flow).

• Whenever possible, shield the fetus before diagnostic X-rays.

Pregnancy, ectopic

Nursing considerations

The patient with an ectopic pregnancy probably has a history of one

P

or two missed menstrual periods. She may not have known she was pregnant. If she was initially examined by the doctor before the ectopic pregnancy ruptured, she probably had some of these signs and symptoms:

• scant, dark red vaginal bleeding
• lower abdominal pain, which might be sharp or dull, constant or intermittent, or referred to the right shoulder
• the usual signs of early pregnancy (amenorrhea; soft, blue cervix; swollen, tender breasts; and enlarged uterus)
• a palpable crepitant mass in one of the lower quadrants on pelvic examination
• severe abdominal pain in response to any movement of the cervix during a pelvic examination.

Common sites

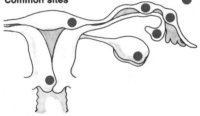

Surgery is the only treatment for an ectopic pregnancy, so your initial priority is to stabilize your patient until the operating room is ready. Replace lost blood volume with I.V. fluids or blood, as ordered, and titrate the I.V. infusion to match her urine output. Monitor her pulse and blood pressure carefully, particularly if her vaginal bleeding is profuse. If her pulse rate increases and her blood pressure decreases, be sure to notify the doctor immediately. He may ask you to increase the I.V. infusion rate or to begin transfusing blood if you haven't done so already.

Prepare your patient for surgery as ordered. Expect to give preoperative pain medications and to insert a nasogastric tube (and—if you haven't yet inserted one—a Foley catheter, as ordered).

Pregnant nurse: infection risks

Protecting yourself from infection

As a nurse, you risk everyday health hazards on the job—infectious diseases, exposure to radiation, antineoplastics, and other drugs and chemicals. And there's always the risk of injuring yourself while turning a patient or pushing a bed.

Any of these things could harm your health or, more likely, your fetus'. But there are precautions you can take to protect yourself and your fetus while you're working.

When you first learn you're pregnant, discuss your job in detail with your obstetrician. This will alert him to any potential risks you might encounter. Then meet with your employee health nurse and perhaps the nurse manager on your unit to decide whether to make any changes in your day-to-day responsibilities.

Don't try to keep your pregnancy a secret. Tell your co-workers as soon as it's confirmed. Remember that the fetus is most vulnerable during the first 3 months—before you start showing. If your co-workers know you're pregnant, they can keep an eye out for you and make sure you're not taking any unhealthy and unwise chances.

Patients with infectious diseases pose a significant threat to your fetus. Yet, how many times have you learned a patient had a communicable disease *after* you'd already been in contact with him? Don't wait; be prepared.

If you're planning a pregnancy, get a rubella titer and take the rubella vaccine if the titer is low. Remember, though, that after you're vaccinated you must wait at least 3 months before trying to conceive—the vaccine itself can harm the fetus.

As an added precaution before becoming pregnant, get vaccinated for hepatitis B. This disease is associated with an increased incidence of spontaneous abortion, premature labor, and stillbirth. The hepatitis B virus can be transmitted in utero or during delivery, and the infant may be born with active hepatitis.

No matter how busy you are, take the time to study your patients' charts before assuming their care. Read the orders, history, physical exam results, progress notes, lab values, and X-ray results. Otherwise, you could be in for an unpleasant surprise.

Exposure not only to hepatitis B and rubella but also to herpes simplex virus, herpes zoster, and cytomegalovirus can be ominous for the fetus, too. Hospital policies vary as to whether pregnant workers should care for patients with these diseases. (See *Infection control; Pregnant nurse: medication hazards.*)

Pregnant nurse: medication hazards

Precautions to take

Many medications are known or suspected teratogens. Antineoplastic agents, for example, are an obvious hazard. Hospital policies vary as to what role a pregnant nurse should play in caring for patients receiving these drugs.

Regardless of the policy at the hospital where you work, assume that you can't be too careful about exposure to antineoplastics, and ask that you not be assigned to patients receiving them. If necessary, ask your co-workers to be careful when they prepare antineoplastics. (See *Antineoplastic drugs: handling.*)

Many other medications can also harm your fetus. Repeated, prolonged, or concentrated contact can lead to systemic absorption, so wear gloves when you're preparing or giving medications.

Also stay away from chemicals, such as hexachlorophene, the sterilizing agent ethylene oxide, and anesthetic gases. These can all cause congenital abnormalities of the fetus, as can other substances you may not be aware of—paint, insecticides, and industrial cleaning agents, for example.

Pregnant nurse: physical demands

Limiting physical exertion

Nursing is physically demanding work. If you're pregnant, be especially careful not to strain yourself.

Because adequate rest is so important during pregnancy, always take your allotted breaks and lunch periods. And avoid working overtime. You need to sit from time to time during your shift so you can elevate your legs. (Remember to wear support hose.)

If you find you can't take breaks or lunch when needed, you may need to change jobs or consider taking leave.

By following these precautions, you should (if you choose) be able to continue working full-time on your unit up until your due date. (See also *Pregnant nurse: infection risks.*)

Pregnant nurse: radiation hazards

Safeguards to follow

Exposure to radiation can cause miscarriages and congenital deformities. So never assist with any radiologic procedures while you're pregnant. In fact, leave the area when they're being done—and don't let anyone talk you into staying.

Besides staying out of areas where you might be exposed to radiation, never enter the room of any patient who has a radioactive im-

plant or is taking radioactive iodine. And be cautious about caring for patients who've recently undergone nuclear medicine procedures, such as brain, bone, or liver scans. Avoid contact with their excreta for the specified length of time after the injection (for example, avoid contact with a patient's stool for 96 hours after he's had a gallium scan and with his urine for 24 hours after he's had a bone scan). (See *Radiation precautions: implants; Radiation precautions: nuclear; X-rays.*)

Prenatal testing

When reality shatters parents' dreams

Prenatal tests can reveal a problem with the fetus—such as polyhydramnios, chromosomal abnormalities, or open neural tube defects. How can you help parents when tests reveal an abnormality? You must give them all the facts they need to make their decision whether to have an abortion. Yet, you must not be afraid to show your feelings.

Amniocentesis

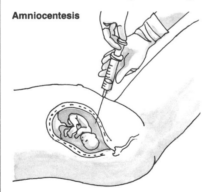

Because perinatology is an imprecise science, you may not know all the facts yourself. If a couple decides to take a chance and have their infant despite abnormal prenatal test results, emotional support may be the only thing you can offer.

Each couple must sort through their shattered dreams. Expect different expressions of grief—tears, anger, or silence. Some couples will

prefer to be left alone, and you must respect that choice.

Many people, however, want to talk about their experience. Explore what the family's growth means to the couple. Was this a planned pregnancy? How long did it take to conceive? What were their expectations for this pregnancy, for this child?

Be alert for guilt feelings. Most couples will wonder what they did to cause the defect. Explore myths and correct misinformation.

If the defect was preventable (for example, related to drug use during pregnancy), empathize with the tremendous psychological burden the couple must be carrying. You can explore prevention strategies with them later.

Help the couple identify family members and friends who can support them during their crisis. Offer strategies for explaining their situation to others, but assure them that they needn't discuss it with everyone who asks.

Also, keep in mind that the couple is made up of *two* people, whose reactions may be very different. Discuss the marital tensions that may follow pregnancy loss—such as sexual disinterest or dysfunction, communication problems, financial concerns, and physical symptoms. You might also encourage the couple to join a parent support group.

Years ago, couples who lost an infant during pregnancy were told to go home and try to forget the experience. Today, the emphasis is on validating the event. To help the couple, you must first recognize that the event *is* meaningful.

Whenever possible, offer the couple tangible reminders of the pregnancy (such as fetal monitor strips, footprints, or sonograms). Some couples will refuse such reminders when you first offer them, only to ask for them later. Create a storage file for mementos. If the couple lost their infant late in the pregnancy, always ask them if they'd like to see or hold the infant.

Parents who undergo prenatal testing in which an anomaly is dis-

P

covered need to integrate what's happened into a story that has a beginning, middle, and end. Couples start developing the story at different stages of their experience. Some start when they learn the diagnosis. Others start several months postpartum. You might have to review clinical events to help them understand how it all began. Go over the procedures, test results, and delivery data. This would also be the time to bring up any prevention strategies that must be discussed (for example, avoiding drug use during pregnancy).

When reviewing the sequence of events with them, you can help the couple put things in order from the beginning of the story, with its fears and unknowns, to its end, where there is acceptance of the loss. (See also *Grief.*)

Pressure cuff

Operating a Thrombo-Gard cuff

The Thrombo-Gard pressure cuff system is designed to reduce the incidence of deep vein thrombosis (DVT) in immobilized patients during surgery and throughout the postoperative period in patients with chronic venous disease and other patients at risk for DVT (see *Thrombosis: prevention*). Wrapped from ankle to knee on each leg, the cuffs imitate normal leg pumping action by sequentially inflating and deflating a series of air cells from the ankle proximally.

To operate the pressure cuffs:

1. Connect the tubing to the first cuff; attach the ankle connector to the two tubes on the cuff marked *ankle*, and attach the knee connector to the two tubes on the cuff marked *knee*. Now, connect the tubing to the second cuff the same way. Both cuffs must be connected before use. If you're applying one cuff to an amputee, place vinyl caps

over the unused connectors to prevent a hissing noise.

2. Place the first cuff on the patient's leg so its shortest cell is at his ankle, its padding is against his leg, and its connector is on the side of the leg. To avoid securing the cuff too tightly, place two fingers between the patient's leg and the cuff before fastening it. Then, put on and fasten the second cuff. Repeat the procedure for the other leg.

3. Put the Thrombo-Gard into a grounded outlet and turn it on.

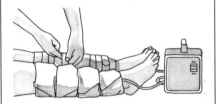

4. Observe cuff filling for at least the first two cycles (approximately 3 or 4 minutes), to ensure correct operation. Only one cuff should fill at a time, in this order: first cell (closest to ankle), second cell, third cell, fourth cell (closest to knee). Then, all cells should deflate simultaneously. The second cuff then follows the same sequence. If the sequence isn't correct and you're sure the cuffs have been properly applied, remove the cuffs and have the system checked for malfunction. Also, remove the cuffs and check for malfunction if the pump indicator light goes on at any time.

5. At least once every 8 hours, check the patient's skin color, temperature, sensation, and ability to move. If you notice any significant changes, remove the cuffs and notify the doctor immediately.

Professionalism

Improving nursing's image

Part of your problem in conveying a true picture of nursing is to undo the damage television has done. The best way to handle this is to ask

people about the impression they have of nurses based on what they've seen on TV. Ask them to think about the situations portrayed. How realistic do they seem? How realistic do the nurses seem? Why has TV chosen to show nurses as sex objects and fools? Your questions may encourage people to be more critical of such portrayals in the future. Educate them on what nursing can do for them, since they're probably not interested in nursing as a career.

Your own professional image starts in the mirror. Good grooming and a well-fitting, dignified uniform or suit will increase your own self-confidence as it builds the image of all nurses. More tips:

• *Watch your behavior at work.* You're never really off duty when you're in uniform or at the hospital. Are you careful to avoid loud laughter, inappropriate remarks, sloppy posture, and gum chewing—even when you're talking informally with other nurses? These behaviors all say "unprofessional" to bystanders.

• *Welcome people to your unit.* Show them you're in charge and ready to help them. Introduce yourself to strangers who come on the unit, look them in the eye, and give them a firm handshake. Greet people you know with a smile and a handshake.

This tactic has a remarkable effect on angry or rude people. When a doctor comes on the unit barking orders, say good morning and offer your hand. He may stop in his tracks, wish you good morning, and continue in a more respectful tone.

Prostactectomy: complications

Detecting problems after transurethral resection

To detect hemorrhage after transurethral resection, check the return flow from the patient's irrigation infusion. Irrigation may be performed through suprapubic and Foley catheters or a three-way Foley catheter alone. If the infusion is continuous, with the clamp wide open, and the return flow remains red, the patient is hemorrhaging from an artery or vein. (Moderate bleeding, causing pinkish returns, is normal during the first few hours after surgery.) Arterial bleeding will cause tachycardia and hypotension; the return flow will be bright red and viscous, with many clots. Report such returns immediately because the patient will need emergency surgery to control arterial bleeding and to clear the bladder of clots.

If the irrigation returns are dark red and not so viscous, the patient is bleeding from a vein. The doctor may try to control the bleeding by applying gentle traction on the Foley catheter for 2 or more hours. (He'll apply traction immediately after surgery if he suspects that venous bleeding may develop.)

Urinary obstruction will result if blood clots, mucus plugs, or clumps of tissue block the catheter or if the catheter kinks or becomes displaced. To prevent this complication, make sure the catheter (or catheters, if the patient has a suprapubic catheter, too) is patent. Check it every 15 minutes for the first 2 hours after surgery, every half hour for the next 2 hours, and then every hour for the next 20 hours.

Remember that urinary obstruction may cause the patient's bladder to become distended. This, in turn, can cause a hemorrhage by straining freshly coagulated blood vessels; it can also lead to a urinary tract infection. To detect bladder distention, stop the infusion of the irrigating solution and palpate the lower abdomen for abnormal swelling (see *Bladder distention*).

If the bladder is distended, the doctor may tell you to irrigate the catheter. Use a syringe filled with 30 to 50 ml of normal saline solution to try to clear the obstruction. If this doesn't relieve the distention, notify the doctor. He may have to insert a new catheter.

Septicemia can occur if bacteria in the urine enters the vascular system during the resection. Watch for signs and symptoms of this complication, such as a fever of 101° F. (38.3° C.) or higher and shaking chills. Report them immediately because septicemia can develop into life-threatening septic shock.

Prostatectomy: patient teaching

Giving your patient instructions after surgery

Tell the patient that the night before surgery, his doctor may order an enema or suppository to clear his bowel. This way, after surgery he won't have to strain to pass a stool, which could cause bleeding.

If he's scheduled for open surgery (any type of prostatectomy except a transurethral resection), a nurse will wash and shave the incision site the morning of surgery. He may have a urinary catheter inserted into his penis before he goes to the operating room.

After surgery, the urinary catheter will still be in place and his bladder may be flushed constantly to reduce the chance of blood clots forming. The fluid draining out of his bladder may be bright red after surgery. This is normal. It will gradually become lighter until it's pink. He'll have an I.V. infusion running in his arm.

After the urinary catheter is removed, he may experience some difficulty passing urine. This is normal. He may again experience feelings of urgency and possibly some dribbling of urine. These will gradually diminish. If necessary, the doctor may suggest exercises to help him regain full control of his bladder.

Prostatectomy: postop care

Important guidelines to follow

When caring for a patient who's had a prostatectomy, follow these important guidelines:
• If the patient has a continuous bladder irrigation system in place (to maintain catheter patency), make sure the sterile solution flows at a rate that keeps urine pink. Carefully monitor fluid intake and output to ensure adequate urine output. Assess urine color and immediately report any bright red bleeding to the doctor. (See *Prostatectomy: complications.*)

When the catheter's removed (usually 2 to 4 days postoperatively), warn the patient to expect urinary frequency and burning on urination. Encourage him to drink at least 2 quarts (1,900 ml) of fluid daily to dilute the urine and reduce the burning sensation. Closely monitor his urinary pattern for the first 24 hours; notify the doctor if the patient can't urinate or has other urinary problems.
• If the patient lacks urinary control, recommend exercises that contract the abdominal, gluteal, and perineal muscles. Reassure him he'll probably regain control eventually and provide positive reinforcement as his control improves.
• To relieve constipation and straining at stool—which may cause bleeding from the operative area—give stool softeners and laxatives, as ordered.
• To help prevent postoperative hemorrhage, avoid giving enemas, inserting suppositories, or using a rectal thermometer.
• To relieve postoperative pain—usually associated with bladder spasms—administer an antispasmodic drug, as ordered. For a patient with back discomfort from the dorsal lithotomy position required

P

for transurethral prostate resection, administer an analgesic, as ordered.

Transurethral resection

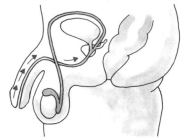

• Perform meticulous skin care if your patient's had a perineal prostatectomy. Clean the incision site several times a day and immediately after any bowel movement. To help relieve pain and promote healing, have the patient take sitz baths after the removal of any incisional drains.

• Be aware that lower pelvic surgery and the exaggerated lithotomy position required for perineal prostatectomy increase the risk for thrombophlebitis. To reduce this risk, encourage the patient to walk, as ordered, and to use support stockings. Assess leg circulation frequently.

• Remember that genitourinary surgery may make the patient anxious about his sexual performance. If he's had transurethral prostatic resection, for example, he'll have "dry orgasm" caused by retrograde ejaculation (backward semen flow into the bladder) from incomplete bladder neck closure during ejaculation. Show sensitivity to his concerns by reassuring him that this probably won't impair his ability to have an erection, intercourse, or orgasm. Also warn him that he may have cloudy urine in the first voiding after sexual activity.

• Before discharge, make sure the patient understands his medication regimen as well as measures to prevent hematuria. Instruct him to avoid lifting objects weighing more than 20 lb (9 kg) for 6 weeks and

to avoid driving for 2 weeks. Warn him that he may experience slight bleeding for 10 days after surgery. Instruct him to get plenty of bed rest and to drink adequate fluids.

Prosthesis, eye

Patient teaching for removal and insertion

Tell your patient:
"Your prosthesis has been custom-designed just for you. Learning how to properly remove and insert it will ensure a comfortable, pleasing appearance."

Removing the prosthesis
"Always wash your hands first and place a towel on the hard surface you will be working over to protect the polished surface of the prosthesis.

1. "To begin, lift your head slightly downward. Using your fingertip, gently depress the lower lid backward and downward toward your cheekbone. This will break the suction that holds the prosthesis in place.

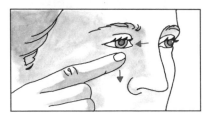

2. "Now cup your other hand under the prosthesis to catch it when it slips out. Don't let the prosthesis fall on a hard surface.

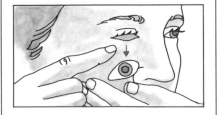

"If you can't remove the prosthesis, contact the doctor or an ocularist to obtain a specially designed suction cup to help you."

Inserting the prosthesis
"Stand in front of a mirror and place a towel on any hard surface you're working over. Moisten the prosthesis with lukewarm water. (Don't insert a dry prosthesis since friction makes insertion difficult.)

1. "Hold the prosthesis with the painted side facing out and the narrow end toward your nose.

2. "Use the index finger on your opposite hand to secure the upper lid against the bony surface above

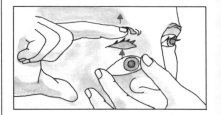

the socket. At the same time, slide the prosthesis upward into the socket under the upper lid until it's seated at the top of the socket.

3. "Now pull the lower lid downward and then push slightly upward

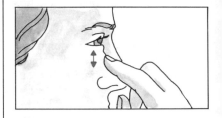

to enclose the lower edge of the prosthesis."

Prosthesis, leg

Making undressing easier

A patient who has a leg prosthesis usually has to remove his pants to get his prosthesis on or off. To eliminate this bother, suggest that he put a zipper on the inside seam of his pant leg (so the zipper opens at the *bottom* of the pant leg). Likewise, a patient who has an arm prosthesis can put a zipper in the

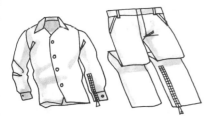

sleeve of his shirt. This will make putting on and taking off the prosthesis a lot easier—a real zip.

Psoas sign

Eliciting it in an adult who has abdominal pain

You can use two techniques to elicit a psoas sign in an adult with abdominal pain. With either technique, increased abdominal pain is a positive result, indicating psoas muscle irritation from an inflamed appendix or a localized abscess.

The first technique. With the patient supine, instruct him to move his flexed left leg against your hand

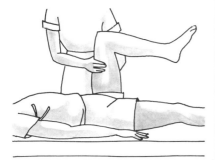

to test for a left psoas sign. Then perform this maneuver on his right leg to test for a right psoas sign.

The second technique. To test for a left psoas sign, turn him on his

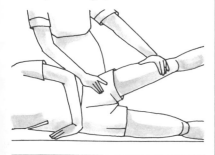

right side. Then instruct him to push his left leg upward from his hip against your hand. Next, turn him onto his left side and repeat this maneuver to test for a right psoas sign.

Psychotic patients

Managing them and preventing injury

A patient who displays psychotic behavior may be terrified and unable to differentiate between himself and his environment. To manage him and prevent injury to the patient, staff, and others, you'll need to act calmly and quickly. Follow these guidelines:
• Remove potentially dangerous objects, such as belts or metal utensils, from the patient's environment.
• Help him discern what is real and unreal in an honest and genuine way.
• Be straightforward, concise, and nonthreatening when speaking to him. Discuss simple, concrete subjects and avoid theories or philosophical issues.
• Positively reinforce his perceptions of reality, and correct his misperceptions in a matter-of-fact way.
• Never argue with him. However, don't support his misperceptions.
• If he's frightened, stay with him.
• Touch him to provide reassurance only if you've tested this before and know that it's safe.
• Move him to a safer, less stimulating environment.
• Provide one-on-one nursing care if his behavior is extremely bizarre, disturbing to other patients, or dangerous to himself. (See also *Violent patients.*)

PTCA

Preparation, monitoring, and aftercare

Prepare the patient for percutaneous transluminal coronary an-

gioplasty (PTCA) by reinforcing the doctor's explanation of the procedure, including its risks and alternatives. Tell him that a catheter will be inserted into an artery or vein in the groin area and that he may feel pressure as the catheter moves along the vessel. Also explain he'll be awake during the procedure and may be asked to take deep breaths to allow visualization of the radiopaque balloon catheter. He may also have to answer questions about how he's feeling during the procedure and will have to notify the cardiologist if he experiences any angina. Advise him that the entire procedure lasts from 1 to 4 hours and that he'll have to lie flat on a hard table during that time.

Explain to the patient that a contrast medium will be injected to outline the lesion's location. Warn him that during the injection he may feel a hot, flushing sensation or transient nausea. Check his history for allergies; if he's had allergic reactions to shellfish, iodine, or contrast medium, notify the doctor.

Tell the patient that an I.V. line will be inserted. Explain that the groin area of both legs will be shaved and cleansed with an antiseptic and that he'll experience a brief stinging sensation when a local anesthetic is injected.

Restrict the patient's food and fluid intake for at least 6 hours before the procedure or as ordered. Ensure that coagulation studies, complete blood count, serum electrolyte studies, and blood typing and crossmatching have been performed. Also palpate the bilateral distal pulses (usually the dorsalis pedis or posterior tibial pulses) and mark them with an indelible marker to help you locate them later. Take vital signs and assess the color, temperature, and sensation in the patient's extremities to serve as a baseline for posttreatment assessment. Before the patient goes to the catheterization laboratory, sedate him as ordered and put a 5-lb sandbag on the bed, to be used later for the application of direct pressure on the arterial puncture site.

Catheter insertion

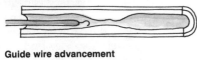

Guide wire advancement

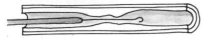

Balloon inflation

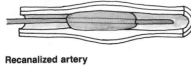

Recanalized artery

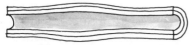

Monitoring and aftercare

When the patient returns from the cardiac catheterization laboratory, he may be receiving I.V. heparin or nitroglycerin. In addition, he'll have the sandbag over the cannulation site to minimize bleeding and hemorrhaging until the arterial catheter is removed. He'll require continuous arterial and ECG monitoring.

To prevent excessive hip flexion and migration of the catheter, keep his leg straight and elevate the head of his bed no more than 15 degrees; at mealtimes, elevate the head of his bed 15 to 30 degrees. For the first hour, monitor vital signs every 15 minutes, then every 30 minutes for 2 hours, and then hourly for the next 5 hours. If vital signs are unstable, notify the doctor and continue to check them every 5 minutes.

When you take vital signs, assess the peripheral pulses distal to the catheter insertion site and the color, temperature, and capillary refill time of the extremity. If pulses are difficult to palpate because of the size of the arterial catheter, use a Doppler stethoscope to hear them. (See *Stethoscope, Doppler ultrasound.*) Notify the doctor if pulses are absent.

Assess the catheter insertion site for hematoma formation, ecchymosis, or hemorrhage. If an ex-

panding ecchymotic area appears, mark the area to determine the rapidity of expansion. If bleeding occurs, apply direct pressure and notify the doctor.

Monitor cardiac rate and rhythm continuously and notify the doctor of any changes or if the patient reports chest pain; it may signal vasospasm or coronary occlusion.

Give I.V. fluids at a rate of at least 100 ml/hour to promote excretion of the contrast medium, but be sure to assess the patient for signs of fluid overload (distended neck veins, atrial and ventricular gallops, dyspnea, pulmonary congestion, tachycardia, hypertension, and hypoxemia).

The doctor will remove the arterial catheter 6 to 12 hours after the procedure. Afterward, apply direct pressure over the insertion site for at least 30 minutes. Then apply a pressure dressing and assess the patient's vital signs according to the same schedule you used when he first returned to the unit.

Home care instructions

• Instruct the patient to call his doctor if he experiences any bleeding or bruising at the arterial puncture site.

• Explain the necessity of taking all prescribed medications and ensure that he understands their intended effects.

• Tell him he can resume normal activity. Most patients experience an increased exercise tolerance.

• Instruct him to return for a stress thallium imaging test and follow-up angiography, as recommended by his doctor.

Public speaking: gaming

Making your presentations more interesting

When giving a presentation to a group of patients, try to make it more interesting by playing a game.

Divide the group into two teams. Each team member takes a turn picking an index card from a pile of cards with typed questions on them. The team member tries to answer the question on the card. If he can't answer it, his team pitches in and tries. If they can't answer it, the other team gives it a try.

The team that answers the question correctly scores a point. When all the cards have been picked and all questions answered, the team with the most points wins the game.

Besides adding an element of fun to the presentation, the game will prompt a lot of interesting, informative discussions.

Public speaking: visual aids

Tips on using a flip chart

Let's say you want to tell your staff about a new, innovative staffing schedule. You realize an oral explanation alone might make it sound too complicated, so you decide to use a flip chart to clarify your idea. To make the chart more helpful (and more visually appealing), try these techniques:

• *Make sure your chart is readable.* Letters should be at least 1½" (4 cm) high, and you should leave 2" (5 cm) between lines. Use as few words as possible, and center your message, leaving the bottom one third of the chart page blank so people sitting in the back can read it.

• *Brighten the chart's visual appeal.* Underline and box key words. Use color, graphic designs, and geometric shapes. If you can't draw, cut out descriptive pictures from magazines.

• *Use flip chart pages to record information.* For example, during a brainstorming session, quickly write key words that reflect contributors' ideas. Use different colored marker pens and two different charts—one for the pen-written agenda and one for contributors' comments, questions, and ideas.

• *Try these self-help tips.* So that pages tear off easily, score them before the meeting. Pencil in notes to yourself that the audience can't see. And flag specific chart pages for easier access during the presentation. (See also *Visual aids: patient teaching.*)

Pulmonary artery catheter, dislodged

Guarding against a possible crisis

When a pulmonary artery (PA) catheter becomes dislodged, act quickly so the patient doesn't go into cardiac arrest or hypovolemic shock, or develop an air embolus or catheter embolus.

Apply pressure at the insertion site and call for help. Watch the monitor for ventricular tachycardia or fibrillation, and observe the patient for signs of angina. Ask whoever responds to page the patient's doctor and check that the defibrillator and emergency drugs are ready.

Make sure the patient has a patent peripheral intravenous line for emergency drugs if needed. If he doesn't, ask someone to insert one while you maintain pressure on the insertion site for 5 to 10 minutes. Once the bleeding is controlled, cover the site with sterile dressing.

While doing all this, keep your eye on the monitor. Reassure the patient that the situation is under control; calming him will reduce the sympathetic stress response and decrease the likelihood of dysrhythmias. Continue to monitor his vital signs, heart rhythm, level of consciousness, and degree of pain. Check the insertion site dressing.

When the doctor arrives, brief him on the patient's condition and tell him what drugs, if any, were being given through the catheter. Report the last pulmonary artery pressure reading. Depending on the patient's condition and medication needs, the doctor will decide whether to insert a new catheter immediately or leave the catheter out. He may order a chest X-ray and arterial blood gas studies.

If the doctor decides to insert a new PA catheter, prepare the patient for the procedure and assist as needed. (See *Pulmonary artery catheter: insertion.*) Observe the patient's vital signs and heart rhythm closely: Inserting the catheter will irritate an already irritated endocardium, increasing the risk of dysrhythmias. Continue to inspect the old insertion site for bleeding, and check for hematoma formation. Assess the patient for cardiovascular, respiratory, and neurologic changes.

Finally, because this is an uncommon event, determine how the patient pulled out the catheter. Was the tubing properly sutured and taped in place? Should the patient have been sedated? Then document the incident.

Pulmonary artery catheter: insertion

Assisting the doctor

You'll need a standard pulmonary artery (PA) catheterization tray, plus the following items: a local anesthetic, heparinized solution, antibacterial solution, syringes, needles, and the PA catheter. (See *Pulmonary artery catheter: preparation.*)

1. The doctor will moisten the outside of the catheter with heparinized solution and flush all the lumens. He will also test the catheter balloon by inflating it with 0.7 to 1.5 cc of air, according to the manufacturer's recommendations.

2. The doctor will then prepare the insertion site. The veins most commonly used are the brachial, femoral, jugular, and subclavian.

3. After the doctor's performed either a percutaneous puncture or a venous cutdown and introduces the catheter into the vein, attach the high-pressure I.V. tubing to the catheter's distal port using aseptic technique. This end of the catheter is now considered unsterile, so keep it out of the sterile field during the rest of the procedure.

4. Watch the monitor as the catheter is advanced. You should see the right atrial pressure reading appear on the monitor about when the catheter reaches the 40 cm mark, depending on where it was inserted.

When the monitor shows the catheter has entered the right atrium, the doctor will gently inflate the balloon by injecting air into the balloon port. Blood flow can then help the catheter advance through the right atrium, right ventricle, pulmonary artery, and into the pulmonary artery branch.

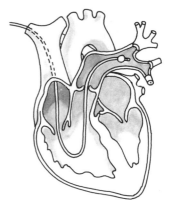

5. Record all pressure readings and waveforms. After you record the final reading, slowly deflate the balloon by removing the syringe from the balloon port. Don't draw back on the syringe, lest you break the balloon. The pulmonary artery pressure reading should appear on the monitor as the balloon floats back in the pulmonary artery.

6. The doctor will then suture the catheter in place and order a chest X-ray to confirm that it's positioned correctly. Apply an antibiotic ointment and sterile dressing to the site.

P

The dressing, tubing, and solution should be changed every 24 hours, and the site inspected for swelling, soreness, inflammation, and discharge every shift. (See *Central line: dressings.*) The patient's vital signs should be monitored, and he should be observed for developing complications, including dysrhythmias, pulmonary infarction, thromboembolus, infection, endocarditis, and pneumothorax. Observe also for signs of balloon rupture and knotting of the catheter.

Pulmonary artery catheter: preparation

Equipment and supplies

After the doctor has explained the procedure, review it with the patient to be sure he understands it before he signs the consent form. Measure and record his vital signs, and check placement of the ECG electrodes.

See that the following equipment and supplies are assembled: the pulmonary artery catheter monitor, I.V. pole, high-pressure tubing, stopcocks, a pressure infuser, a transducer, dead-end unvented caps, a collapsible plastic I.V. bag containing 500 ml of normal saline solution, heparin sodium solution, a sterile needle and syringe, and a syringe containing sterile water. Also, be sure a defibrillator and emergency drugs are close at hand.

Insert the bag of saline solution into the pressure infuser and hang it on the I.V. pole. Be careful not to apply pressure to the bag. Add 500 to 5,000 units of heparin to the solution, following hospital procedure, then label the bag accordingly.

Next, use a sterile needle and syringe to remove air from the bag through the medication port. With the roller clamp closed, insert the high-pressure tubing into the bag. Open the clamp and gently com-press the drip chamber until it's about one-third full. (The amount of solution will increase after the system is pressurized.)

Place the transducer into the fitted bracket on the I.V. pole. Using a sterile syringe, place a few drops of sterile water on the transducer head to ensure a proper seal. (Use sterile water instead of normal saline solution, which forms a crust when it dries.) Tighten the transducer dome firmly onto the head, being careful to maintain sterility.

Open the roller clamp to slowly fill the tubing with the heparinized solution. Then slowly flush the system by gently pulling the gross flush mechanism on the pressure infuser. Gently tap or flush the dome or tubing to dissolve any bubbles. You may need to turn the dome or tubing to get air to rise from a particular spot.

Flush each port as follows: Remove the stopcock port cover, turn the stopcock off, hold the stopcock port upright, pull the gross flush mechanism, and run the solution through to clear out the air. Then cover the port with a sterile dead-end unvented cap and turn the stopcock off to the port. Each stopcock port should remain capped and turned off to the port when it's not in use to ensure a closed, sterile system.

Apply 300 mm Hg of pressure to the I.V. solution by turning the pressure infuser handle; pull the gross flush mechanism at the same time to avoid putting excess pressure on the transducer head, which could become damaged.

Attach the transducer cable to the monitor's receptacle. Turn on the monitor and allow it to warm up for at least 15 minutes. Then level the transducer to the patient's mid-axillary line at the fourth intercostal space (the level of the right atrium).

Calibrate the monitor according to the manufacturer's instructions. (See *Pulmonary artery catheter: insertion.*)

Pulses, peripheral

Evaluating them

The rate, amplitude, and symmetry of peripheral pulses provide important clues to cardiac function and the quality of peripheral perfusion. To elicit these clues, palpate peripheral pulses lightly with the pads of your index, middle, and ring fingers—as space permits.

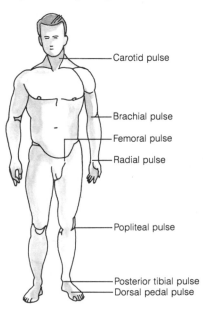

- *Rate.* Count all pulses for at least 30 seconds (60 seconds when recording vital signs). The normal rate is between 60 and 100 beats/minute.
- *Amplitude.* Palpate the pulses during ventricular systole. Describe pulse amplitude as follows:

    4+ bounding
    3+ normal
    2+ difficult to palpate
    1+ weak, thready
    0   absent

Use a stick figure to easily document the location and amplitude of all pulses.
- *Symmetry.* Simultaneously palpate pulses (except carotid) on both sides of the patient's body, and note any inequality. Assess peripheral pulses methodically, moving from the arms to the legs.

Pulsus paradoxus

Checking for cardiac tamponade

Always check a patient with a cardiac injury for pulsus paradoxus— a sign of cardiac tamponade. Pulsus paradoxus refers to a marked decrease in systolic blood pressure on inspiration. To assess for it, inflate and then slowly deflate the blood pressure cuff until you hear the first systolic sound at expiration. Slowly continue to deflate the cuff until you hear sounds both on inspiration and expiration. The difference between the two readings is called the paradox. A difference greater than 10 mm Hg indicates pulsus paradoxus. (See *Cardiac tamponade.*)

Pupillary reaction

Using a penlight

To check for pupillary reaction to light, use a penlight. Bring the penlight in from the side of one eye and watch the pupil on that side to see if it constricts under the light—a direct response. At the same time check the other pupil to see if it also constricts. This is called a consensual response. The other pupil constricts even though the light's not shining directly on it. Both eyes must be assessed for direct and consensual responses.

Normally, you'll see both responses, although the speed with which the pupils respond can vary. If the room is very bright, you might

Reaction to light

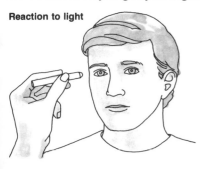

want to turn the lights off; you can assess constriction easier in a darkened room than in a well-lit one.

If your patient is alert enough to follow a verbal command, you can also check for pupillary accommodation. To do this, ask him to look at an object across the room. Looking at a distant object will usually cause the pupils to dilate. Ask your patient to look at your index

Accommodation

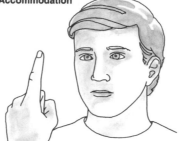

finger, which you hold about 6″ (15 cm) from his nose. Look for the normal responses—pupillary constriction and convergence of the eyes.

If all pupillary responses are normal, document your findings in the nurses' notes or on a neuro flow sheet as "PERRLA." If there's an abnormality, describe it clearly. (See *Pupil size.*)

Pupil size

Grading it

To ensure an accurate evaluation of pupillary size, compare your pa-

Pupil size scale

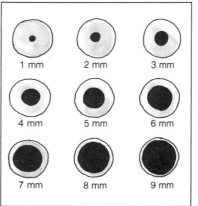

1 mm 2 mm 3 mm
4 mm 5 mm 6 mm
7 mm 8 mm 9 mm

tient's pupils to the scale shown here. Keep in mind that maximum constriction of the patient's pupils may be less than 1 mm and maximum dilation greater than 9 mm. (See *Pupillary reaction.*)

Queckenstedt's sign

Checking for it

If an obstruction in the spinal subarachnoid space is suspected, you may be asked to help the doctor as he tests for Queckenstedt's sign. After inserting the spinal needle, the doctor will take an initial cerebrospinal fluid (CSF) pressure reading and then ask you to compress one or both of the patient's jugular veins with your fingers for 10 seconds. Doing so will obstruct blood flow from the patient's cranium, increasing his intracranial pressure and, in the absence of a subarachnoid block, cause his CSF pressure to rise also. A partial subarachnoid block may cause the patient's CSF pressure to rise sluggishly; a complete block will prevent it from rising at all.

Normally, the fluid column in the manometer should rise after 10 seconds of compression, then fall to the patient's initial pressure within 30 seconds. CSF pressure is recorded every 5 seconds from the time you begin compression until the pressure returns to baseline.

Because the patient runs the risk of developing cerebellar tonsillar herniation or medullary compression, he should not be tested for Queckenstedt's sign if he shows signs of increased intracranial pressure.

Q
R

Quinsy

Special considerations

Key symptoms of quinsy (peritonsillar abscess) include severe throat pain, occasional ear pain on the same side as the abscess, and tenderness of the submandibular gland. Dysphagia causes drooling. Trismus may occur as a result of edema and infection spreading from the peritonsillar space to the pterygoid muscles. Other signs and symptoms include fever, chills, malaise, rancid breath, nausea, muffled speech, dehydration, cervical adenopathy, and localized or systemic sepsis. Follow these guidelines:

• Be alert for signs of respiratory obstruction (inspiratory stridor, dyspnea, increasing restlessness, or cyanosis). Keep emergency airway equipment nearby.

• Explain the drainage procedure to the patient and his family. Since the procedure is usually done under a local anesthetic, the patient may be apprehensive.

• Assist with incision and drainage. To allow easy expectoration and suction of pus and blood, place the patient in a semirecumbent or sitting position.

After incision and drainage:

• Give antibiotics, analgesics, and antipyretics, as ordered. Stress the importance of completing the full course of prescribed antibiotic therapy.

• Monitor the patient's vital signs, and report any significant changes or bleeding. Assess pain and manage accordingly.

• If the patient can't swallow, ensure adequate hydration with I.V. therapy. Monitor fluid intake and output, and watch for dehydration.

• Provide meticulous mouth care. Apply petrolatum to his lips. Promote healing with warm saline solution gargles or throat irrigations for 24 to 36 hours after incision and drainage. Encourage adequate rest.

Rabies

Guidelines for prophylaxis

When caring for a victim of an animal bite, don't forget to assess his need for rabies prophylaxis. As you know, untreated rabies is invariably fatal—so take every precaution to protect your patient.

If your patient was bitten by a dog or cat, and the animal is healthy during 10 days of observation, rabies prophylaxis is not needed. If the animal is rabid, or suspected to be rabid, administer both rabies immune globulin (RIG) and human diploid cell (HDC) vaccine. If RIG isn't available, expect to administer antirabies serum.

If your patient was bitten by a stray dog or cat and you're uncertain if the animal is rabid, consult public health officials; if treatment's indicated, give RIG and HDC vaccine.

If your patient was bitten by a wild animal (for example, a raccoon, skunk, bat, or fox), consider the animal rabid unless proven negative by laboratory tests on the captured animal. Administer RIG and HDC vaccine.

If the animal bite was from livestock, rodents, or rabbits, consider the animal individually and consult public health officials. Rodent and rabbit bites rarely cause rabies in humans. (See *Bite, dog; Bite, human.*)

Radiation monitoring

Using detection devices

You can be sure you don't exceed a safe exposure level to radiation by wearing a radiation monitor that tracks the amount of radiation you've been exposed to.

One of the most popular monitoring devices is the film badge, which resembles a credit card and is clipped to your uniform. The badge contains a film that is developed and read for the amount of exposure. If you routinely work with radiation or if you care for patients who are undergoing therapeutic nuclear radiation, you should wear a badge. Usually, your hospital radiation department supplies these badges and monitors employees' exposure to radiation.

Film badge

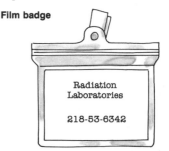

Radiation
Laboratories

218-53-6342

Besides film badges, ring badges and dosimeters monitor radiation exposure. Worn on the finger, the ring badge works on the same principle as the film badge. It's used primarily by hospital employees who handle radioactive isotopes that may expose their hands to higher levels of radiation than the rest of the body.

The dosimeter, a 6"- (15-cm) tube that clips onto a pocket, has an ionization chamber inside. To read it, look inside and see a needle that measures the amount of ionizing radiation you've been exposed to. It's used mainly by employees exposed to high levels of radiation for short periods.

To ensure accurate monitoring with a radiation badge, follow these guidelines:

1. Wear the badge at all times inside the hospital. Don't wear it outside or take it home.

2. Don't expose the badge to intense light, heat, or moisture because this can make the monitoring tape inactive and cause inaccurate readings.

Q
R

3. If you lose or damage your radiation badge, request a replacement badge from your radiation protection supervisor immediately.

4. Replace your badge every month.

Radiation precautions: implants

Useful guidelines

Radioactive implants emit higher levels of radiation than many other procedures. Your exposure can occur while the radioactive material is in the patient or while it's being inserted or removed. With radioactive implants, only the source, not the patient, is radioactive. Once the source is removed, you're no longer at risk.

The amount of radiation emitted and your exposure level depend on the radioactive substance used, the amount used, and its half-life (the time required for half the atoms of a radioactive substance to disintegrate).

Radiation safety

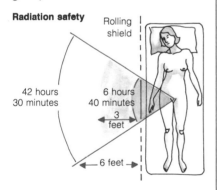

Rolling shield

42 hours 30 minutes

6 hours 40 minutes

3 feet

6 feet

For example, suppose you're taking care of a patient with an intrauterine implant of 100 mg of radium. If, during the entire course of her treatment, you stay at her bedside for a half hour and within 3′ of her bed for 1 hour, you'll be exposed to a cumulative dose of 150 millirems. As a nonradiation nurse, you shouldn't exceed a radiation dose of 500 millirems per year. So, following the recommended limitation, you can spend the same amount of time with no

more than three radioactive-implant patients a year.

Here are additional guidelines for caring for patients who've received radiation implants:

• Provide a private room.

• When giving nursing care, wear a film badge. Use portable bedside lead shielding, when available. (Lead aprons are ineffective protection against radiation from implants and other high-energy emitters.)

• Limit the amount of time you spend with these patients while the radioactive material is in place. Omit bed baths and avoid giving perineal care during the treatment period, but change the patient's perineal pads frequently, as ordered by the doctor. (Of course, you should tell patients beforehand that you'll be spending less time with them after they receive the implant—to minimize your exposure. But assure them you'll still be providing necessary nursing care.) If possible, rotate nursing assignments with co-workers to minimize everyone's exposure.

• Carefully check linens, clothing, and bedpans to make sure radioactive tubes or needles haven't been dislodged. If you find an implant tube or needle, don't touch it. Place a moist towel over it. Or pick it up with long-handled forceps and put it in a special lead-lined container provided by the radiation therapy department. Then notify the doctor and the radiation protection supervisor. Soiled linens that may be contaminated should be scanned with a radiation detector before being sent to the laundry.

Radium tube

Radium needle

• Only the doctor should change patients' dressings.

• Place a visible tag marked "Radiation precautions" on each pa-

tient, his bed, his chart, and the nursing Kardex.

• Don't worry about taking special precautions with vomitus, sputum, urine, feces, or eating utensils from these patients—this is unnecessary.

• If you frequently assist in the operating room during implant surgery, wear a film badge. And limit the amount of time you spend with these patients in the recovery room.

• If you're pregnant or think you might be, avoid taking care of these patients. (See *Pregnant nurse: radiation hazards.*)

Radiation precautions: nuclear

Proper procedure

In metabolized therapeutic treatments (such as radioactive iodine treatments for thyroid cancer), the doses of clear radiation are higher—and more hazardous—than those used in diagnostic testing.

In this type of nuclear therapy, radioactive isotopes are given either orally or intravenously in the form of tumor-seeking drugs. Because these isotopes circulate freely in the blood and are metabolized by the body, all body fluids can become radioactive. So, by handling patient secretions and excretions, you could be exposed to radiation.

Follow these precautions:

• Provide a private room.

• When giving nursing care, wear a film badge and use portable bedside lead shielding. (Lead aprons are minimally effective against radioactive iodine.)

• Limit the amount of time you spend with these patients by avoiding informal visits and curtailing nonvital procedures, such as bathing, shaving, or hairdressing. (Of course, you should tell patients beforehand that you'll be spending less time with them after they receive nuclear radia-

Q R

tion—to minimize your exposure. But assure them you'll still be providing necessary nursing care.) If possible, rotate nursing assignments with co-workers to minimize everyone's exposure.

• Wear waterproof gloves when handling urine, feces, blood, vomitus, or any other secretions from patients who've had radioactive isotopes. Discard gloves and wash hands thoroughly afterward. If you must collect specimens, use a special container provided by the laboratory.

• Wear waterproof gloves when cleaning bedpans, urinals, or any other items that might come in contact with radiation-contaminated secretions or excretions.

• Provide these patients with disposable eating utensils. Place all disposable items that may be contaminated in a container supplied by the radiation protection supervisor.

• Soiled linens that may be contaminated should be scanned with a radiation detector before being sent to the laundry.

• Place a visible tag marked "Radiation precautions" on each patient, his bed, his chart, his Foley catheter collection bag, his I.V. line (if used), and the nursing Kardex.

• If you're pregnant or think you might be, avoid taking care of these patients. (See *Pregnant nurse: radiation hazards*.)

Radiation reactions

Relieving indigestion and nausea

Indigestion or nausea usually begins 1 to 6 hours after a radiation treatment and peaks within 12 hours. Daily treatments may cause continuous indigestion or nausea.

When you talk to the patient before a radiation treatment, don't deny or overemphasize that indigestion or nausea may occur. The power of suggestion alone may precipitate or intensify these symptoms. A simple factual statement should suffice: "Some people experience indigestion or nausea from radiation treatments, but others don't."

If indigestion or nausea does occur, tell the patient to take an antiemetic 1 to 2 hours before a treatment, then every 4 to 6 hours for at least 12 hours. Use a positive approach when you offer the antiemetic: "This will help your indigestion or nausea."

Since the patient may not want to eat, offer these dietary tips to minimize indigestion or nausea:

• A high-protein, high-calorie liquid supplement will help provide the protein and calories he needs. Serve the supplement cold, and suggest sipping it slowly.

• Cold foods or foods at room temperature, such as sandwiches and salads, may be better tolerated than warm or hot foods, which tend to aggravate indigestion and nausea. Bland foods, such as applesauce and crackers, may also be well tolerated. The same holds true for sour foods, such as lemons or sour hard candies.

• Clear liquids, such as apple juice or ginger ale, may help relieve indigestion or nausea. These liquids should be cold, and the patient should sip them slowly.

• Foods that are sweet, fatty, salty, or spicy should be avoided. So should foods with strong odors.

• The patient shouldn't eat or drink for 1 to 2 hours before and after a radiation treatment. Instead, he should eat a large meal 3 or 4 hours before one, then eat very light meals for the rest of the day. Or he can eat five or six light meals throughout the day.

To specifically prevent or reduce nausea:

• Advise always eating and drinking slowly.

• Move all objects that might make him nauseated, such as emesis basins, from the patient's view. Make sure his room is free of unpleasant odors.

• Encourage him to listen to music, watch a favorite television program, or read a book for distraction during periods of nausea.

• Suggest that he rest when nausea's most likely to develop. For instance, if the patient's usually nauseated when he wakes up, he could take an antiemetic and rest in bed for a half hour before rising. (See also *Nutritional disorder*.)

Radiation safety

Protecting yourself

To limit your exposure to radiation, remember the key principles of time, distance, and shielding. When you work near a radioactive source:

• Spend as little time as possible near the source.

• Put as much distance as possible between you and the source.

• Place adequate protective shielding (a lead barrier, for example) between you and the source. (See *Radiation precautions: implants*.)

Radiation wounds

Irrigating them

Cancer patients can get shallow excoriated lesions from radiation therapy. Daily irrigation with equal parts of hydrogen peroxide and

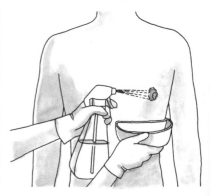

sterile water can be cold and messy for the patient—when you use traditional irrigating equipment. So try using a sterilized spray bottle instead—the kind used for spray-on glass cleaner. You can deliver an adequate amount of solution with a minimum of dripping and a maximum of comfort for your patient.

Radioactive iodine

Teaching patients about therapy

Radioactive iodine therapy is an alternative treatment for Graves' disease if thyroid hormone antagonists are ineffective. (See *Graves' disease.*) If your patient is scheduled for this treatment, explain that it decreases production of thyroid hormone by destroying thyroid tissue. Reassure him that the procedure is painless and won't harm other body tissue. But be sure he understands the risk of hypothyroidism, which can result from excessive destruction of thyroid tissue.

Tell him that the procedure for radioactive iodine therapy involves drinking a tasteless, colorless, radioactive solution or swallowing a radioactive capsule. Review the precautions he'll need to take after the procedure. For example, tell him to avoid close contact with pregnant women, infants, and children for 1 week. During the first 48 hours after the procedure, he should flush the toilet immediately after urinating and use disposable plates and silverware because his urine and saliva will be temporarily radioactive. Be sure to warn family members to avoid contact with the patient's body fluids, such as saliva, during this time. Reassure the patient and his family that the radioactive iodine poses no hazard after 48 hours.

Inform your patient that symptoms of Graves' disease should subside 3 to 4 weeks after therapy begins. If they don't, he may need a second round of therapy after several months.

Rape: assessment

Examining the victim

Your first priority is to give your patient a private room and continuous emotional support during your assessment and emergency interventions. If you can't stay with her, find someone who can. If she's physically unstable from trauma associated with the rape, start an I.V. line and provide oxygen, as ordered. Cover any severely bleeding wounds with pressure dressings, immobilize any fractures, and get X-rays. Then, with your patient's physical stability ensured, begin a thorough assessment and examination, following your state's laws for collecting evidence and your hospital's protocols for caring for a rape victim. Remember, although your patient may not want to prosecute her attacker initially, she may change her mind. Unless you've collected objective evidence of sexual intercourse and a history of force, prosecution will be impossible.

Before you begin your assessment, ask someone to bring you a sterile speculum and a rape collection kit containing such items as capped and labeled laboratory tubes, glass slides, a clean comb, a nail scraper, and paper bags for clothing.

Make your patient feel as safe and comfortable as possible by explaining the examination that you and the doctor will conduct and by assuring her that you'll stay with her. Encourage her to ask questions about anything she doesn't understand. Start by taking a history of the incident, recording the patient's own words whenever possible. She's likely to be ashamed to tell you what happened and even more ashamed to have you write it down. To ease her embarrassment, ensure complete privacy during this time, and explain that you need the information to plan her care. Offer nonjudgmental emotional support during the history, and let her vent her feelings as she tries to relate the incident.

After you've recorded a history of the incident, collect a sexual history, including what birth control measures, if any, she uses (if she's sexually active) and the date of her last menstrual period. Take a medical history, including any medications she's taking and any allergies or chronic diseases she has. Before the physical examination begins, help the doctor obtain necessary consent, and witness the patient's signature.

Help your patient remove her clothing, and save it to be analyzed for semen and bloodstains. (See *Rape: specimen collection.*) Circle any suspected blood or semen stains on the clothing with a laundry marker, and place each piece of clothing in a paper bag. (Don't use plastic bags: An airtight bag will stimulate bacterial action that may alter the evidence.) Record any bruises, scratches, and other injuries on your patient's body.

Rape: specimen collection

Ensuring accuracy

Collect scrapings from underneath your patient's fingernails because these may contain skin or blood specimens that will help identify the attacker. Put specimens in capped laboratory tubes, and label each tube with your initials, the date, and the patient's name and hospital number.

During the doctor's examination, hold your patient's hand, talk to her, and comfort her. Assist the doctor in the following procedures:
• Collect an aspirated or scraped specimen from any of the patient's orifices that may contain sperm or seminal fluid (pharynx, vagina, rectum, or urethra). These specimens will also be cultured for gonorrhea. (Remember that use of a lubricant

Q
R

may make analysis of specimens impossible; so use only water or saline solution on the speculum.) Semen specimens will dry out quickly, so have someone take the properly labeled specimens to the laboratory immediately and wait for them while the lab technician records the number of sperm per high-power field. (For permanent smears, the doctor will order a Pap smear, a methylene blue test, or a Gram stain.)

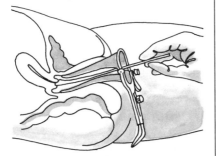

• Comb your patient's pubic hair to collect foreign hairs—or let her do this herself. Place all the hairs collected in a labeled container. Then ask your patient's permission to clip a few of her pubic hairs for comparison. Put these in a labeled container as well.
• Draw blood for syphilis testing.
• Send blood and urine samples for pregnancy testing, a toxicology screen, and a blood alcohol level. Remember that failure to label and seal specimens will break the chain of evidence necessary to use the specimens in a trial. *Don't* let any specimen leave the examination room without a label, the initials of someone present during the examination, and a sealed lid. *Don't* leave the room until the next person in the chain collects the evidence and until you've both signed for each item.

Reagent strips

Cutting costs

Tell patients they can save money by cutting reagent strips in half

when they test their blood or urine at home. Even cut in half, each strip

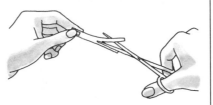

has enough reagent to give an accurate reading. (See *Glucose monitoring*.)

Rectal exam

Inspection and palpation

You'll use both inspection and palpation when performing a rectal exam. First, position the patient on his left side, with his knees up and his buttocks close to the edge of the examining table. (If he's ambulatory, ask him to stand and bend over the examining table.)

To inspect, spread his buttocks to expose the anus. Expect rectal skin to be darker than the surrounding area. Check for inflammation, lesions, scars, rectal prolapse, tumors, fissures, and external hemorrhoids. Ask him to strain as though to defecate while you check for internal hemorrhoids, polyps, rectal prolapse, and fissures.

To palpate, ask the patient to strain again. Using a disposable glove and lubricant, palpate with

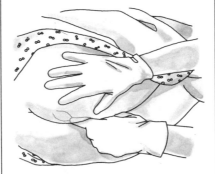

your index finger for weak anal outpouchings, nodules, or tenderness on movement.

Explain that you'll insert your gloved finger a short distance (usually 2¼″ to 4″ [6 to 10 cm]) into his rectum and that this pressure may make him feel as though he needs to move his bowels. When the anal sphincter relaxes, insert your finger gently and rotate it to palpate the rectal wall. Palpate for nodules, irregularities, tenderness, and fecal impaction. In men, assess the prostate's lateral lobes and median sulcus as you palpate the anterior rectal wall—it should feel firm and smooth. Test any fecal matter adhering to the glove for occult blood.

Reflex, corneal

A simple way to check it

To elicit the corneal reflex, have the patient turn his eyes away from you to avoid involuntary blinking during the procedure. Then approach him from the opposite side, out of his line of vision, and brush his cor-

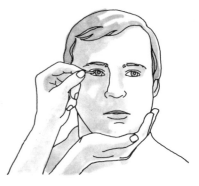

nea lightly with a fine wisp of sterile cotton. Repeat this procedure on his other eye.

Reflexes: documentation

Documenting deep tendon reflexes

Record the patient's deep tendon reflex scores by drawing a stick figure

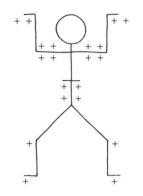

and entering the grades on this scale at the proper location:
• 0 for absent
• + for hypoactive (diminished)
• + + for normal
• + + + for brisk (increased)
• + + + + for hyperactive (clonus may be present).

Reflexes: testing

A method for deep tendon reflexes

Use a percussion hammer to test each reflex bilaterally as follows:
• *Biceps reflex.* Rest the patient's elbow in your hand. Position your thumb over his biceps tendon. Then

Biceps reflex

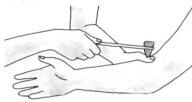

percuss your thumbnail and watch for forearm flexion.
• *Triceps reflex.* Flex the patient's arm slightly, using your hand to steady his arm. Percuss the tendon

Triceps reflex

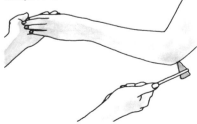

right above the back of his elbow. Watch for elbow extension.
• *Brachioradialis reflex.* Ask the patient to rest his hand on his thigh with the palm down. Percuss the radius about 1″ to 2″ (3 to 5 cm) above the wrist, and watch for forearm flexion and supination.

Brachioradialis reflex

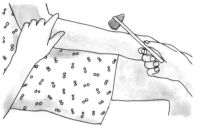

• *Patellar reflex.* Have the patient sit on a table with his legs dangling freely (or have him cross his legs). Percuss the tendon right below his patella. Watch for leg extension at the knee.

Patellar reflex

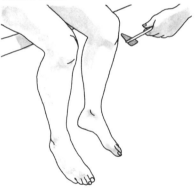

• *Achilles reflex.* Support the patient's foot in your hand. Rotate his

Achilles reflex

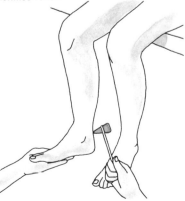

foot and leg outward and percuss the Achilles tendon. Watch his ankle for plantar flexion.
• *Plantar reflex.* With a sharp object, such as a pen or the blunt end of bandage scissors, stroke the lat-

Plantar reflex

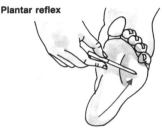

eral aspect of the sole of his foot from heel to ball. Watch for flexion of his toes.

Relaxation: breathing exercises

Helpful techniques

Proper breathing is the key to relaxation. You may laugh at the notion of "learning to breathe," but chances are, if you're tense, you breathe incorrectly. Proper breathing uses the muscles of the abdomen, not the chest, and gives slower, deeper responses, with an increased tidal volume. To learn deep breathing required for relaxation:

1. Sit or stand in a comfortable position with your eyes closed. "Comfortable" means maintaining good posture without rigidity.

2. Breathe in through your nostrils to the count of 4, keeping your mouth closed. Let your stomach expand like a balloon.

3. Exhale through your mouth to an unrushed count of 8. (If you find counting to 8 distracting when you're just learning to use your abdominal muscles, one possible alternative is to breathe out slowly and completely to the count of 4.)

4. Place the palms of your hands on your abdomen to sense the regular, rhythmic breathing. Once you've felt the "in" and "out" breaths grow longer and deeper, try

Q R

placing your hands around your rib cage. This will give you a tactile sense of how the rib cage expands and contracts as you breathe in and out. The lungs operate much like a bellows; but this rib cage action is a by-product of deep abdominal breathing, not an isolated action. (See also *Relaxation techniques at work.*)

Relaxation: concentration

Eliminating distractions

Concentration will contribute to your sense of being centered, poised, and in better control of your own thoughts and actions. To promote concentration:

1. Look fixedly at a small object, such as a safety pin, a pencil, or a paper clip. Keep your eyes open, and think only of that object: its size, shape, color, texture. Think about the whole object. Distracting thoughts will probably intrude during the exercise. Set such thoughts aside, and refocus on the object.

2. Count breaths—which is another means of concentrating. As a variation, count to 4 on the inhalation and on the exhalation say the word "relax" as slowly as you can.

3. Try to develop a detached attitude toward the random thoughts that come to mind. Do not use any force either to hold or to reject them. Picture the thoughts as birds flying in the sky of your mind: now coming into view, now disappearing.Thoughts that disappeared seem to return after the relaxation session, but in a clearer form.

Relaxation, progressive

Learning

You can control your response to stress by using progressive relaxation, self-coaching, and guided imagery. And you can teach your patient how to use them.

Progressive relaxation involves tightening and relaxing muscle groups systematically, beginning with your face and finishing with your feet. This usually takes 15 to 30 minutes.

When you do progressive-relaxation exercises, wear loose clothing and remove your shoes and glasses (if you wear them). Sit or recline comfortably with your neck and knees supported. Don't lie completely flat. Close your eyes or stare at a distant spot and take in a slow, deep breath. Then exhale slowly. Continue breathing slowly and rhythmically. Feel the tension leave your body with each breath.

Next, relax each of your muscle groups. To do this, breathe in and tense your muscles, then relax them as you breathe out. Use the following tension-relaxation combinations (tension techniques are in parentheses):
• face, jaw, mouth (squint eyes, wrinkle brow)
• neck (pull chin to neck)
• right hand (make a fist)
• right arm (bend elbow in tightly)
• left hand (make a fist)
• left arm (bend elbow in tightly)
• back, shoulders, chest (shrug shoulders up tightly)
• abdomen (pull stomach in and bear down on chair)
• right upper leg (push leg down)
• right lower leg and foot (point toes toward body)
• left upper leg (push leg down)
• left lower leg and foot (point toes toward body).

Practice progressive relaxation slowly. End the session by counting to 3, inhaling deeply, and saying, "I'm relaxed."

Self-coaching is a stress management technique that can help you understand and respond to signs of anxiety, such as increased heart rate or sweaty palms. When these signs occur, coach yourself to relax.

For example, when you get anxious, think: "I'm upset about this situation, but I can control my anxiety. I'll take this one step at a time, and I won't focus on my fear. Instead, I'll focus on taking slow, deep breaths. I'll think about what I must do to finish the task. This situation won't last forever. I can manage until it's over."

Guided imagery, another stress management technique, lets you use your imagination to achieve relaxation and control. Concentrate on an image and picture yourself involved in the scene. Think about something pleasurable and relaxing, such as lying on a warm beach.

Choose a scene that will involve at least two of your senses. Then begin rhythmic breathing and progressive relaxation. Mentally travel to the scene. How does it look? Sound? Smell? Feel? Practice using the scene to relax. End the session by counting to 3 and saying, "I'm relaxed." A specific ending is important. If you don't use one, you may become drowsy and fall asleep.

Relaxation guidelines

Effective lessons

Start checking the tension in your shoulders, neck, and jaw. Here are some ways to release that tension:

1. Part your lips slightly and rest your tongue on the floor of your mouth. Then let your mind tell the tension to drain from these areas while you breathe deeply.

2. Release tightness in your throat by swallowing and deliberately letting the muscles in that area become soft and relaxed.

3. Holding your upper body straight, yet comfortably, drop your chin onto your chest. Return your head to its normal upright position. Let your head fall back; then return to an upright position. Repeat these movements, synchronizing them with the "in" and "out" of your rhythmic breathing.

Q
R

4. Keeping the same upright body position, let your head drop toward your right shoulder, as though trying to touch your ear to your shoulder. Return your head to its upright position. Then let your head move toward your left shoulder and return to its upright position.

5. Drop your head to your chest and gently move it clockwise making as full a circle as possible. Then gently move it counter-clockwise. Coordinate these motions with regular, rhythmic breathing.

6. Check for any remaining tension in your head and neck. Picture the tension as knots in a rope. Imagine untying the knots one by one and releasing the tension.

Because the head and neck area serves as the switching station for so many nerves and muscles, the relaxation achieved here permits other areas of the body to become more relaxed.

Relaxation techniques

Teaching your patient

If your tense patient's a willing pupil, plan a graduated schedule of relaxation exercises and set specific times for him to practice. In this planning, be sure to collaborate with other members of the health care team to keep the patient's program consistent and regular, whether you're available or not.

Once you've tailored a set of exercises to your patient's needs, give him a 10- to 15-minute teaching session so he'll have a true understanding of what he's supposed to do. Ask him to verbalize his reactions: Does he feel the abdominal breathing, the tension draining from his neck and shoulders, his hands growing warmer? Direct him to practice his prescribed exercises one to four times a day on his own. Ask him to summarize for you what

he's going to do in his own practice sessions. Also suggest that the patient use his deep breathing to overcome anxiety during treatments or special procedures. He can decrease his anxiety on the way to such procedures by breathing deeply and regularly rather than tightening his jaw and breathing slowly. He can help himself further by saying silently, "I am relaxed. I am relaxed." Before discharge, tell the patient he can use these same exercises at home and make them an integral part of his everyday life.

Relaxation techniques at work

Learning how to relax before patient care

You can share the benefits of relaxation with your patient in two ways: one, by giving better bedside care; two, by teaching him the skills you've learned yourself.

To help relax, try this simple centering exercise for 5 to 10 seconds before entering a patient's room:
• Close your eyes; let the tension leave your forehead, your eyes, and your jaws. Take a few slow abdominal breaths, counting "in 2, 3, 4; out 2, 3, 4."
• Scan your body for tension, starting at your scalp and traveling down to your toes. Sense how the tension's draining away.
• Empty your mind of all thoughts; close your eyes and think of the darkness as a great, free space. Turn thoughts away gently as they enter your mind.
• Lower your shoulders, which often hunch up with tension.
• Take one last deep breath, in and out; you should now feel a sense of relaxation and be ready to care for your patient.
• The short time this exercise takes can enhance the quality of your time with your patient.

Renal calculi assessment

Recognition and intervention

Initially, the patient has some or all of these signs and symptoms:
• excruciating pain in his flank, abdomen, or groin

Pain with left-sided calculus

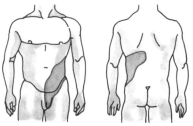

• abdominal distention
• nausea and vomiting
• fever and chills
• hematuria
• sudden interruption of his urine stream
• urinary frequency and urgency.

Get a urine sample for urinalysis to test the patient's urine pH and to detect hematuria, pyuria, crystalluria, and casts. A kidney, ureter, and bladder X-ray and an I.V. pyelogram will be ordered to determine the size and location of the patient's renal calculi. Blood will be drawn for a complete blood count and for calcium, phosphorus, blood urea nitrogen, creatinine, glucose, uric acid, and electrolyte levels.

Your most urgent priority is to assist with efforts to eradicate the calculi. Expect to insert a large-bore I.V. catheter immediately and to begin infusing large amounts of fluids (2,000 to 3,000 ml). This will increase the patient's urine output, dilute his urine, and possibly flush out the calculi so they can pass through his genitourinary tract. Expect to give a narcotic analgesic, such as meperidine (Demerol) or morphine, to relieve your patient's

Q
R

pain. If urinalysis reveals an accompanying urinary tract infection, expect to give broad-spectrum antibiotics, too. You may also need to prepare your patient for emergency surgery to drain accumulated urine to prevent hydronephrosis.

Renal calculi prevention

Guarding against recurrence

Advise your patient to follow these steps for preventing calculus recurrence and future hospitalization:
• "Drink plenty of liquids—enough for your body to produce 1½ to 2 liters of urine each day.
• "Exercise regularly to keep your urine moving. Exercise may also prevent calcium (which can cause stones) from accumulating in your urine.
• "Stick to the diet your doctor has recommended. Some foods contain chemicals that promote stone formation. (You'll need to find out the kind of calculi your patient had to know which foods he should avoid.)
• "Take your medication according to the doctor's orders. The medication keeps your urine at a pH level that discourages stone formation. (If necessary, explain that urine pH refers to the urine's acidity or alkalinity. Also, teach him to monitor urine pH with reagent strips.)
• "Watch for signs of urinary tract infection—for example, cloudy, foul-smelling urine. If you think you might have an infection, call your doctor right away."

Renal failure

Helping your patient recover

To support the recovery of a patient with acute tubular necrosis (ATN), follow these guidelines:
• *Monitor his fluid balance.* Maintain a scrupulous fluid intake and output record, and weigh him daily. Watch for 24- to 48-hour patterns of loss or retention. Because fluid retention raises blood pressure and causes edema, check blood pressure every 4 hours and watch for generalized edema in dependent body parts (for example, the presacral area). Check his respirations and breath sounds every 4 hours, too, for crackles and other signs of pulmonary edema. Because he's susceptible to fluid retention and overload, give all I.V. fluids with an infusion pump.
• *Monitor his electrolyte levels.* Watch particularly for signs and symptoms of hyperkalemia, such as bradycardia; also monitor his laboratory values for hypocalcemia and hyperphosphatemia. If any of these imbalances develop, notify the doctor immediately.
• *Correct acidosis.* Regularly check the patient's serum pH levels, watching for signs and symptoms of acidosis, including fatigue, headache, central nervous system changes (such as confusion, seizures, or coma), hyperventilation (Kussmaul's respirations), and signs of myocardial depression. Be alert, too, for hyperkalemia—which may accompany acidosis.

As ordered, correct symptomatic acidosis with sodium bicarbonate via I.V. bolus. Then maintain a safe serum pH with oral sodium bicarbonate and dialysis, as needed. Although all ATN patients become acidotic, not all experience the symptoms of acidosis. The doctor may not treat asymptomatic acidosis.
• *Monitor the patient's blood urea nitrogen (BUN) levels and correct uremia.* Uremic symptoms appear when the patient's BUN level rises above 100 mg/dl. Early signs and symptoms include lethargy, confusion, nausea, vomiting, weight loss, muscle wasting, skin changes (pruritus, yellowish color, dryness, and ecchymoses), uremic fetor (azotemic breath odor), edema, and stomatitis.
• *Provide adequate nutrition.* Because appetite loss and vomiting accompany uremia, this is more easily said than done. Fluid and dietary restrictions (including limited protein intake) also work against adequate nutrition—all at a time when your patient's nutritional needs are higher than normal because of his hypercatabolic state.

Your goal is to supply essential amino acids (to minimize muscle tissue breakdown from hypercatabolism) and plenty of calories. Provide small meals at frequent intervals; if the patient can't eat enough to supply his nutritional needs, administer total parenteral nutrition, as ordered. Make sure that dietary levels of sodium, potassium, and protein are adjusted for his condition to avoid exacerbating his uremia and electrolyte imbalances. Also give multivitamins and folic acid, as ordered. Explain his dietary restrictions to the patient's family, so they don't give him inappropriate snacks.
• *Prevent infection.* Perhaps the most dangerous ATN complication your patient faces, infection may develop because uremic toxins reduce phagocytosis and inhibit the immune response. Minimize infection risks by maintaining adequate nutrition and keeping BUN levels under 100 mg/dl. Obtain urine specimens for culture on admission and throughout treatment, as ordered. Avoid unnecessary invasive procedures, too. If the patient must have a Foley catheter or an I.V. line, observe strict aseptic technique. Be sure to maintain his skin integrity. (As you know, the skin is the first line of defense against infection.) If possible, keep him away from visitors and patients who may have infections.
• *Check his hematocrit values for signs of anemia.* ATN inhibits the kidneys' production of erythropoietin, a hormone that stimulates production of red blood cells (RBCs) and helps prolong their life. The resulting anemia will worsen if the patient's underlying condition causes blood loss or if he develops bleeding during recovery (for ex-

ample, from a stress ulcer). If ordered, administer packed RBCs, folic acid, and iron supplements.

• *Provide emotional support.* Your patient has undergone a frightening change from health to an acute illness from which he may never fully recover. To help him cope, keep in mind that the stages of his emotional adaptation are similar to those of the classic grieving process: denial, anger, bargaining, depression, and acceptance. And encourage him to share his feelings with you and his family. Explain all procedures fully, and answer his questions frankly. Provide special support for his family, especially if he's critically ill or unlikely to recover fully. Regularly assess how well he's coping with his condition; if necessary, refer him to the psychiatric nurse liaison for additional help.

Reports, shift

The best way to give a good report

A thorough shift report includes the following information:

• *Identification of patient.* Give each patient's name, room number, and bed designation—for example, "Mr. Winthrop, Room 304, Bed A." This will help ensure that one patient isn't confused with another. And the information will be especially helpful for nurses who have been on vacation or have floated from other units.

• *Reason for admission.* Always include this information so staff members don't lose site of the patient's original complaint and medical diagnosis. Amid a flurry of tests, consultations, complications, and even transfers, this information can get lost unless it's repeated at report.

• *Nursing diagnoses.* Read the nursing diagnoses and all protocols for each patient. Reviewing the nursing diagnoses emphasizes the main nursing concerns; reading the protocols reminds the staff of the nursing care required for each patient during the upcoming shift.

• *Changes in patient's condition or protocols.* Note any significant changes in the patient's condition. Obviously, nurses on the next shift must know about any change for the worse so they can monitor the patient appropriately. But they should also be told about any improvement in the patient's condition, so they know their hard work has paid off.

• *Patient's emotional status.* Knowing the patient's reaction to his condition will help determine nursing care strategies. Report the family's reactions, too, since they greatly influence a patient's emotional status.

• *Additional information.* Depending on your unit, you may want to include additional information in your shift reports. Psychiatric nurses, for instance, may discuss reports from group therapy sessions; critical care nurses may note blood gas levels or electrocardiogram patterns.

You should also decide what not to include. For instance, you and the other nurses on the unit may feel that giving such information as normal temperatures, pulses, and blood pressures just takes too much time.

To determine what to leave in and what to leave out, analyze the needs of the typical patients on your unit. What are the most important nursing problems resulting from their illnesses, diagnostic procedures, and treatments? These are the problems you want to address in your shift report.

Respiratory exam: anterior chest

Auscultation landmarks

The first important landmark here is the sternal notch, located at the top of the sternum. The clavicles extend from the sternal notch. Two or three fingerwidths below the sternal notch, you'll feel the elevated ridge known as the sternal angle. This is where the second rib joins the sternum.

Locate the second rib, then slide your finger down to the second intercostal space. From here you can count up or down to find the other ribs and intercostal spaces. Don't try to count the ribs and intercostal spaces by sliding your fingers down along the sternum: The ribs are too close together at the lower sternum. Instead, move your fingers diagonally away from the sternal angle.

The anterior chest has two other important landmarks—the midclavicular lines. These imaginary lines begin at the midpoint of the clavicles and run straight down the thorax.

Once you're familiar with the anterior chest landmarks, you can readily locate the lung lobes. The apexes of the upper right and left lobes extend just above the clavicles. Keep this in mind during your assessment, and be sure to auscultate above the clavicles. Near the sternal angle, the trachea bifurcates into the two mainstem bronchi. Note that the horizontal fissure between the upper right and middle lobes is located at the fourth rib, on the midclavicular line. The lower right and left lobes begin at the sixth rib, also on the midclavicular line. (See *Breath sounds, normal.*)

Respiratory exam: auscultation

Methods to follow

Before you begin auscultating your patient's lungs, have him sit on the side of the bed with his chest exposed. If he can't sit in this position, help him into high-Fowler's position. Then ask him to lean forward to expand his chest. When he's comfortable, tell him to breathe slowly and deeply through his mouth. This will accentuate breath sounds. Explain to him that breathing slowly will prevent hyperventilation and dizziness.

Use the same approach every time during auscultation you would during inspection. Start with the

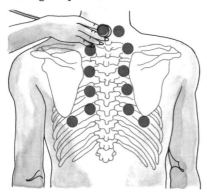

posterior chest, going from one side to the matching area on the other side, checking for symmetrical breath sounds. Then move to the anterior chest, again checking for symmetrical breath sounds.

Here's an auscultation tip: Place the diaphragm of your stethoscope firmly against the thorax. This will create a seal that will eliminate most extraneous noise. If a male patient's chest hair causes too much noise, mat it to the chest with water, then apply your stethoscope. (See *Breath sounds, normal; Stethoscope, acoustic.*)

Respiratory exam: inspection

Proper technique

Begin your assessment of the patient's respiratory status with a systematic inspection. To save time, start it while you're obtaining a brief history and continue it as you auscultate breath sounds.

First, observe the patient's respiratory rate and rhythm and the quality of his breathing. Also, note the patient's posture. If he's having trouble breathing, he'll most likely lean forward when he sits.

His respiratory rhythm should be regular, with expirations taking

about twice as long as inspirations. A prolonged expiratory phase may indicate an obstructive pulmonary disease, such as asthma or emphysema. When a patient's expirations are prolonged, you may also note labored, pursed-lip breathing. Irregular rhythms, such as ataxic breathing or Cheyne-Stokes respirations, are usually associated with central nervous system or metabolic disorders. They require immediate intervention.

Next, observe his anteroposterior (AP) and transverse diameters. Normally, the transverse diameter is about twice the AP diameter. If the AP diameter is as large as (or almost as large as) the transverse diameter, the patient could have emphysema which would cause barrel chest. In an elderly patient, however, such a large AP diameter could be a normal finding.

Barrel chest

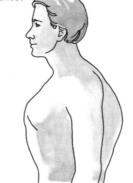

As the patient breathes, watch how his chest moves. On inspiration, his chest should move up and out symmetrically. If one side of his chest doesn't expand as much as the other, he may have atelectasis or an underlying pulmonary disease. Certain thoracic and spinal deformities—kyphosis, scoliosis, and pectus excavatum, for example—may also restrict chest expansion.

Now listen to him breathe without using your stethoscope. Normal respirations are quiet and unlabored. Labored breathing may be accompanied by audible wheezes, gurgling, or stridor (an inspiratory

high-pitched crowing). Any of these sounds requires immediate intervention.

Respiratory exam: palpation

Palpating the posterior and anterior chest

Palpate the patient's posterior chest to assess his thorax, identify thoracic structures, and check chest expansion and vocal or tactile fremitus. Begin by feeling for muscle mass with your fingers and palms (use a grasping action to assess position and consistency). Normally, it feels firm, smooth, and symmetrical. As you palpate muscle mass, check skin temperature and turgor. Note the presence of crepitus (especially around a wound site). Then palpate the thoracic spine, noting tenderness, swelling, or such deformities as lordosis, kyphosis, and scoliosis.

Next, using your metacarpophalangeal joints and fingerpads, gently palpate the patient's intercostal spaces and ribs for abnormal retractions, bulging, and tenderness. Normally, the intercostal spaces delineate a downward sloping of the ribs. In a patient with an increased anteroposterior diameter caused by obstructive lung disease, you'll feel ribs that are abnormally horizontal.

Now palpate the thoracic landmarks to identify underlying lobe structures. To help you identify the division between the patient's upper and lower lobes, instruct him to raise his arms above his head; then palpate the borders of his scapulae. The inner edges of the scapulae should line up with the divisions between the upper and lower lobes.

The inferior border of the lower lobes is usually located at the 10th thoracic spinous process and may descend, on full inspiration, to the 12th thoracic spinous process.

To locate the lower lung borders in a patient lying laterally, palpate the visible free-floating ribs or costal margins; then count four intercostal spaces upward for the general location of the lower lung fields.

Palpate for symmetrical expansion of the patient's thorax (respiratory excursion) by placing your palms—toward the spine—flat on the bilateral sections of his lower posterior chest wall. Position your thumbs at the 10th-rib level, and grasp the lateral rib cage with your hands. When he inhales, his posterior chest should move upward and outward, and your thumbs should move apart; when he exhales, your thumbs should return to midline and touch each other again. Repeat this technique on his upper posterior chest.

Palpating for respiratory excursion

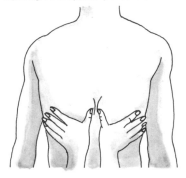

Palpate for vocal or tactile fremitus by using the top portion of each palm. To check for vocal fremitus, ask your patient to repeat "99" as you proceed. Palpable vibrations will be transmitted from his bronchopulmonary system, along the solid surfaces of his chest wall, to your palms and fingers.

Note the symmetry of the vibrations and the areas of enhanced, diminished, or absent fremitus. (Remember, fremitus should be most pronounced in the patient's upper chest, where the trachea branches into the right and left mainstem bronchi, and less noticeable in the lower regions of the thorax.)

You can estimate the level of his diaphragm on both sides of his pos-

terior chest by placing the ulnar side of your extended hand parallel to the anticipated diaphragm level. Instruct him to repeat "99" as you move your hand downward. The level where you no longer feel fremitus corresponds approximately to the diaphragm level. To palpate his anterior chest, begin by using your palms. Feel for areas of tenderness, muscle mass, and skin turgor and elasticity. Note any crepitus during your palpation, especially around wound sites, subclavian catheters, and chest tubes.

Palpate his sternum and costal cartilages for tenderness and deformities and then, using your metacarpophalangeal joints and fingerpads, palpate his intercostal spaces and ribs for abnormal retractions, bulging, and tenderness. Remember to proceed to the lateral aspects of the thorax.

Next, palpate the thoracic landmarks used to identify underlying structures.

To assess for symmetrical respiratory expansion, place your thumbs along each costal margin, pointing toward the xiphoid process, with your hands along the lateral rib cage. Ask the patient to inhale deeply, and observe for symmetrical thoracic expansion. Now palpate for vocal or tactile fremitus, remembering to examine the lateral surfaces and to compare symmetrical areas of the patient's lungs. (If your patient is a woman, you may have to displace her breasts to examine her anterior chest.) Remember that fremitus will usually be decreased or absent over the patient's precordium.

Respiratory exam: percussion

Performing it properly

To learn the density and location of such anatomic structures as the patient's lungs and diaphragm, you

must identify five percussion sounds: flat, dull, resonant, hyperresonant, and tympanic. Start by percussing across the top of each shoulder. The area overlying the lung apexes—approximately 2″ (5 cm)—should be resonant. Then percuss downward toward the patient's diaphragm, at 2″ intervals, comparing right and left sides as you proceed. Remember to avoid his scapulae and other bony areas. The thoracic area (except over the scapulae) should produce resonance when you percuss. At the level of his diaphragm, resonance should change to dullness. A dull sound over the lungs indicates fluid or solid tissue. Hyperresonance or tympany over a patient's lung suggests pneumothorax, massive atelectasis, or large, emphysematous blebs. A marked difference in diaphragm level from one side to the other is an abnormal finding.

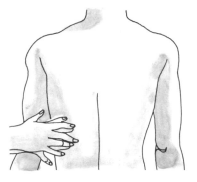

Next, measure diaphragmatic excursion. Instruct the patient to take a deep breath and hold it while you percuss downward until dullness identifies the lower border of the lung field. Mark this point. Now ask him to exhale and again hold his breath as you percuss upward to the area of dullness. Mark this point, too. Repeat this entire procedure on the opposite side of his chest. Now measure the distances between the two marks on each side. Normal diaphragmatic excursion measures about 1¼″ to 2¼″ (3 to 6 cm). (A person's diaphragm is usually slightly higher on his right side.)

Percussing the patient's anterior chest allows you to determine the location and density of his heart, lungs, liver, and diaphragm. Begin by percussing the lung apexes (the supraclavicular area), comparing right and left sides. Then percuss downward in 1¼″ to 2″ (3- to 5-cm) intervals. You should hear resonant tones until you reach the third or fourth intercostal space (ICS), to the left of the sternum, where you'll hear a dull sound produced by the heart. This sound should continue as you percuss down toward the fifth ICS and laterally toward the midclavicular line. At the sixth ICS, at the left midclavicular line, you'll heart tympany over the stomach. On the right side, you should hear resonance, indicating normal lung tissue. Near the fifth to seventh ICS you'll hear dullness, marking the superior border of the liver.

To percuss his lateral chest, instruct the patient to raise his arms over his head. Percuss laterally, comparing right and left sides as you proceed. These areas should also be resonant.

Respiratory exam: posterior chest

Auscultating landmarks

Starting with the posterior chest, the first landmark vertebra you'll need to locate is C7. This is the most prominent spinous process. You'll find it at the base of the neck when the patient lowers his head. From C7, you can slide your fingers down the spinal column, moving from T1 to T12. Each of these spinous processes articulates with a rib. Below each rib is the corresponding intercostal space.

While palpating the posterior chest, be sure you locate the spinous processes T3 and T10. You'll need these key landmarks when auscultating your patient's posterior lung fields. T3 marks the point

where the major fissures dividing the upper and lower lung lobes begin. From this point, the fissures arc down laterally, behind the scapulae. Note that on the posterior chest the trachea branches into the left and right mainstem bronchi at T4. T10 usually marks the lower border of the lungs. On inspiration, though, the lower border descends to T12. (See *Breath sounds, normal.*)

Restless patients

Keeping them covered

When a patient is restless or confused and kicks off his covers, protecting his modesty becomes a problem. How can you keep him covered?

Just put another hospital gown on him—but put his legs through the armholes of this one. (The bottom edge of the second gown extends to the patient's chest.) Tuck the gown's sides under the patient, and you'll spare him, his visitors, and staff members the embarrassment of an unintended view.

Restraints: padding

Proper procedure

When a patient needs limb restraints, use a piece of eggcrate-like foam rubber to pad the restraints. Cut each piece about 3″ (7.5 cm) wide and long enough to fit around the patient's arm or leg. Place the smooth

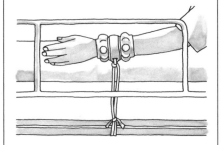

side of the foam against the patient's skin, with the egg-shaped side facing outward. Apply the restraint over the

foam in the channels between the egg-shaped protrusions. The eggs keep the restraint secure, while the foam cushions the skin and keeps the restraint from becoming too tight when it's pulled. (See *Legal risks: restraints; Restraints: precautions.*)

Restraints: precautions

Avoiding pitfalls

When a patient must be kept in a vest or limb restraint, use these guidelines:
• Cross the vest flaps so that the V is in the front. (Some vests have "front" marked on the piece of fabric that should cross over the chest.) Don't cross the vest flaps so that the V-shaped opening is in the back. If the patient tries to squirm out of a vest that's on backward, he could choke.
• Make sure you can fit your fist between the vest and the patient, so you know that the vest isn't too tight.

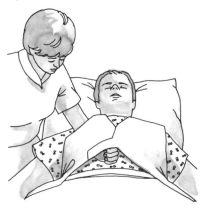

• Flex the patient's arm or leg slightly before securing a limb restraint. Leave as much slack as possible—at least 1″ (3 cm) to provide room for movement and to prevent locked or dislocated joints. Palpate the pulses below the restraint to make sure it isn't too tight. Don't tie the restraint so tightly that it restricts the patient's breathing or blood flow. A tight restraint can cause skin trauma.

• Tie the restraint to the bed frame or wheelchair frame, safely out of the patient's reach. Don't tie the restraint to the side rails of the bed; the patient could be injured if the rail were pulled down.

• Use a knot that can quickly be released when securing the restraint to the bed frame—a magnus hitch, clove hitch, or loop. Use a reverse clove hitch to tie the limb restraint to the patient. Don't use a regular knot to tie the restraint; you wouldn't be able to release it quickly in an emergency.

• Release the restraint at least every 2 hours so you can change the patient's position and inspect his skin. (See *Legal risks: restraints; Restraints: padding*.)

Resumés

Self-advertising

A good resumé advertises your experience, education, and career path. If you want the customer to buy, your ad has to be good.

In a resumé, employers want to see clarity, conciseness, career-directedness, knowledge, and skills.

To give prospective employers what they're looking for, follow these guidelines:

• Start with the basics—name, address, and telephone number.

• State your career objective: either a specific job or the skills you'd like to use.

• List previous employment, starting with the most recent position. After each position, list the skills you used and the responsibilities you had, in order of their importance in the position you're now seeking. Use active verbs, such as plan, coordinate, and manage.

• Then give other important information you haven't covered: your RN license number and certificates you've earned, for example. You

might also list any published articles, teaching activities, and special appointments.

• When you're done, double-check your grammar, spelling, and punctuation. Remember, careless mistakes undermine your credibility. And reinforce your professional image by having your resumé printed on high-quality paper, not duplicated on a copying machine. (See *Career strategies; Job change: planning*.)

Resuscitation manikin

Replacing the body

When a resuscitation manikin wears out, here's how to replace the body. Remove its head and shoulders and disengage its chest mechanism. Then make a small slit inside the shoulder insert. Through this slit, tightly stuff polyester batting (purchased at a local upholstery store) into the manikin's arms, legs, and abdominal area. After replacing the chest mechanism, continue stuffing the manikin until it's filled. Put a vinyl patch over the slit in the shoulder to seal it securely.

Finally, reattach the manikin's head and neck band, and it's as good as new—but at a fraction of the cost of a new body.

Retarded patients

Reducing their fears

Like most of us, a mentally retarded patient fears what he doesn't understand. And he probably doesn't understand his strange new environment—the hospital. That means you'll spend part of your care time allaying his fears.

Begin by orienting him to his surroundings. Make sure he understands where he is and why he's

there. He may think a hospital is a place where people go to die.

Take time to explain procedures. Be sure your explanation is geared to his level of understanding. He may be unfamiliar or uncomfortable even with such simple procedures as taking blood pressure. If he isn't prepared for a procedure, it may frighten him. And because he may not deal with fear effectively, he may disrupt the procedure.

Perhaps the most important thing you can do is give him plenty of understanding and loving care. Chances are, he has a poor self-image. But by showing him you care, you'll be helping him to improve it.

When you provide hands-on care, move slowly to avoid frightening him. Explain what you're doing and be gentle. He may be uncomfortable with touching or being touched. But usually, if you speak calmly and don't pose a threat, he'll let you touch him.

Some mentally retarded patients seem to want to touch others constantly. Such behavior usually indicates a need to feel accepted and loved. If your patient exhibits this type of behavior, you can help fulfill these needs. But limit the type of touching he does. For instance, encourage him to greet you and other staff members with a handshake, not a bear hug.

You're likely to find that caring for a mentally retarded patient requires a lot of your time. But try to be understanding. If you can't spend time with him when he wants, tell him when you *can* come back. Usually, you should relate this to an event—for example, say you'll return after he's eaten dinner.

Caring for a mentally retarded patient isn't routine. It takes extra time, patience, and concern. But, of course, the rewards aren't routine, either. When you help a mentally retarded patient get through a difficult time, you know you've met a special challenge.

Q R

Retinal reattachment

Keeping the patient comfortable after surgery

After retinal reattachment surgery, a patient may have to lie prone for 24 to 48 hours. To help her maintain this position without developing neck stiffness, facial irritation from the sheets, or boredom, try this:

Remove the headboard from her bed and put an overbed table between the wall and the bed (leave some space between the table and bed). Pad the table with a towel and position her with her forehead resting on the table so she'll be facing the floor.

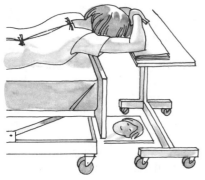

Place a mirror on the floor beneath her face; this way, the mirror will reflect the wall-mounted television screen or other room activity. Visitors can make eye contact with the patient by looking into the mirror. When her eye needs to be examined, just raise the bed a bit, so the nurse or doctor can squat down—and look up.

Reye's syndrome

Nursing intervention

Reye's syndrome is an acute illness that occurs in children, usually after a viral infection. Rapid liver decompensation and encephalopathy occur. Here are the stages of treatment.

Stage I
Vomiting, lethargy, hepatic dysfunction
• Monitor vital signs and check level of consciousness for increasing lethargy. Take vital signs more often as the patient's condition deteriorates.
• Monitor fluid intake and output to prevent fluid overload. Maintain urine output at 1 ml/kg/hour, plasma osmolality at 290 mOsm, and blood glucose levels at 150 mg/dl. (The goal is to keep glucose levels high, osmolality normal, and ammonia levels low.) Also, restrict protein intake.

Stage II
Hyperventilation, delirium, hepatic dysfunction, hyperactive reflexes
• Watch for seizures and maintain seizure precautions.
• Immediately report any signs of coma that require invasive, supportive therapy, such as intubation.
• Keep the head of the patient's bed at a 30-degree angle.

Stage III
Coma, hyperventilation, flexor posturing, hepatic dysfunction
• Monitor intracranial pressure (should be <20 mm Hg before suctioning) or give thiopental I.V., as ordered; hyperventilate the patient as necessary.
• If the patient lapses into a coma, immediately give dextrose 50% in water I.V., as ordered.
• When ventilating the patient, maintain PCO_2 levels between 23 and 30 mm Hg and PO_2 levels between 80 and 100 mm Hg.
• Closely monitor cardiovascular status with a pulmonary artery catheter or a central venous pressure line.
• Give good skin and mouth care, and help the patient perform range-of-motion exercises.

Stage IV
Deepening coma; extensor posturing; rigidity; large, fixed pupils; minimal hepatic dysfunction
• Check the patient for loss of reflexes and signs of flaccidity.
• Provide extra support for the family.

Stage V
Seizures, loss of deep tendon reflexes, flaccidity, respiratory arrest, serum ammonia levels above 300 mg/dl
• Help the family prepare for the patient's death.

Ring removal

How to do it safely

A few feet of string is all you need to remove a tight ring from a swollen finger. Slip a few inches of string under and through the ring toward the patient's wrist. Then wind the

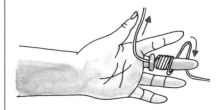

long end tightly down the finger until you reach the top. Finally, take the short end of the string and pull

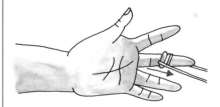

it toward the patient's fingertip. As the coiled string unwinds, the ring will come with it.

Safety

How to maintain it in the hospital

• Stop any suspicious-looking person on your unit, and ask to see his identification. If he won't comply, call your security department—don't take any further action yourself.

• Call hospital security if you see someone destroying hospital property, having a serious argument, or carrying a suspicious package anywhere in the hospital. Again, don't take any further action yourself.

• Check the identity of any private duty nurse you don't know; call the agency to verify employment.

• Report all thefts and losses to hospital security.

• Lock desks, cabinets, and offices at the end of the day or anytime you'll be leaving them unattended. Assign one person in your area to be in charge of this.

• Lock away purses, wallets, and other personal property.

• Ask patients to leave valuables at home or to deposit them in the hospital safe.

• Lock away all supplies not currently being used, and have the charge nurse keep the key.

• Introduce yourself to your patients, show them your identification (ID) badge or name tag, and tell them to call the nurses' station if anyone without proper identification tries to care for them.

• Be especially alert when caring for infants or children involved in custody battles. Know which family members have visiting privileges, and call security if someone not on the visitor list arrives on your unit.

• Alert hospital security if a staff member on your unit is threatened by a patient, a visitor, or even a spouse. Ask for a description of the threatening person, and watch out for him.

• Alert hospital security if one of your patients was a victim of a violent crime. Screen all visitors, and isolate the patient as soon as possible. Some hospitals write fictitious names and room numbers on the front of such patients' charts. Use these same precautions with patients who are well known to the public.

• Don't broadcast patients' vulnerabilities by posting signs on their doors such as "Blind." This only invites theft.

• Dispense all drugs in unit doses, so you won't have to store excess drugs on your unit.

• Be alert for dramatic changes in a co-worker's behavior that might indicate drug use or drug stealing—for example, depression, inability to concentrate, or an erratic work schedule with high absenteeism. (See *Alcoholic nurse.*)

• Go on walking rounds every shift instead of taking reports in a conference room. You can do a security check at the same time.

• Ask a security officer to escort you to and from your car after dark or if your hospital's in a high-crime area.

• Ask to have a security alarm installed at the nurses' station, especially if you work alone on the night shift.

• Wear your photo ID badge at all times, and remind other staff members to wear theirs. If your hospital doesn't have photo IDs, suggest that they get them.

• Enlighten your whole staff, not just the other nurses. Encourage nursing assistants and clerical staff to report any security risks.

• Ask hospital security to hold a seminar for your unit if you have a special concern.

• Notify your union if your hospital ignores requests for increased security. Unions can pressure administrators.

• Trust your sixth sense: If you feel uneasy about someone or something, ask security to check it out. (See also *Kidnapping.*)

Salem sump tubes

Irrigation technique

To irrigate through the main lumen, simply disconnect the tube from

suction, remove the connector, and instill 30 ml of normal saline solution into the tube. Then reattach the main lumen to suction, and instill 10 to 20 cc of air into the vent lumen.

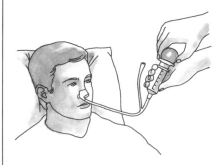

To irrigate through the vent lumen, and so irrigate the sump lumen, leave the Salem sump attached to suction and simply inject the irrigant into the vent lumen. Then instill 10 to 20 cc of air.

Gastric contents sometimes leak out through the vent lumen. This is called reflux, which occurs when the vent lumen or collection strap is improperly placed or when the suction-drainage lumen is clogged. To prevent reflux, place the vent lumen above the level of the patient's midline and the collection bottle below it. To prevent clogging of the suction-drainage lumen, irrigate it as described earlier.

When using a Salem sump tube with continuous suction, use the lowest level of suction that pulls drainage through the tubing into the collection bottle. If using intermittent suction from a thermotic pump, such as Gomco, set the suction on a high setting. But if you're using intermittent suction from a central suction source, set the suction at a low level, as with continuous suction. Remember to keep the vent lumen open when applying suction regardless of the source and the suction setting used. Closing the vent lumen halts the sump action, causing mucosal damage. (See also *Drains: guidelines.*)

S

Seizures: classification

Recognizing the different types

If your patient has a seizure, it's important to be able to characterize what type he's having.

Generalized seizures

• *Generalized tonic-clonic seizure* (formerly called a grand mal seizure). The tonic phase involves generalized stiffening of the muscles (especially muscles in the arms, legs, and jaw, and the intercostal muscles). It usually lasts less than a minute. Then the clonic phase, characterized by rapid jerking, begins. The patient is unconscious during both phases of the

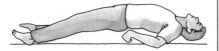

seizure. Because this type of seizure affects the entire brain, he doesn't feel or see anything during the seizure and won't remember anything about it afterward. (See *Seizures, generalized motor.*)

• *Absence seizure* (formerly called a petit mal seizure). Characterized by loss of consciousness, this type of seizure usually lasts less than 15 seconds, usually with no other visible changes. However, the patient may blink his eyes or smack his lips.

• *Myoclonic seizure*. This type of seizure involves generalized jerking of the extremities and lasts less than 5 seconds, usually with a brief period of unconsciousness that can easily be missed by others. Myoclonic seizures may occur in clusters—that is, several in a row or several in one day. (Each patient tends to develop his own characteristic pattern.)

• *Atonic seizure* (formerly called "drop attacks"). This type of seizure involves a paroxysmal loss of muscle tone, usually resulting in a fall. In most cases, the patient will also lose consciousness.

Partial seizures

• *Complex partial seizure* (formerly called a psychomotor seizure or temporal lobe epilepsy). It's characterized by unusual stereotypical behaviors, such as staring, fumbling with clothes, lip smacking, and automatic hand movements (patting a leg, for example), and accompanied by a change in or loss of consciousness.

When the patient regains consciousness, he'll be tired and confused, so tell him briefly what happened. Clean his mouth, checking his tongue to see if he bit it. Give him a bed bath if he's uncomfortably sweaty. Then raise the head of his bed slightly and let him rest. Make sure the side rails are up and padded, and have oxygen and suction equipment set up at his bedside. Assess him as needed.

Now, record what happened, including your interventions. (See also *Seizures: precautions.*)

• *Simple partial seizure* (formerly called a focal motor or focal sensory seizure). This kind of seizure is characterized by a stereotypical, paroxysmal sensation or movement, which occurs during every seizure. An example of a paroxysmal sensation would be a sudden feeling of pain, a sudden perception of a foul odor, or a sudden feeling of nausea. Simple partial seizures don't affect consciousness.

Seizures, generalized motor

Managing them effectively

What do you do if your patient exhibits signs of a generalized tonic-clonic seizure? First, call for help, but do it discreetly. One assistant is all you need, not a crowd of health care professionals. Then, have the unit secretary call the patient's doctor.

Next, protect the patient from injury by putting up the side rails and lowering the head of his bed. Remove any pillows from under his head; use them and blankets to pad the side rails. Turn him on his side to help keep his airway patent, and loosen tight clothing. Remember to protect yourself also; he may flail his arms during the seizure.

Then, observe him and note the pattern of the seizure so you can document it later. Assess his airway and breathing. Because a generalized motor seizure usually lasts only from 3 to 5 minutes, the patient won't be apneic the entire time. But if the seizure is prolonged or repeated, he may need oxygen to breathe and suctioning to remove secretions or vomitus. See that oxygen and suction equipment is ready to use.

If the patient develops repeated or prolonged seizures, you'll have to keep his airway open until anticonvulsant drugs can be given. Place your thumbs at the angles of his jaw, and gently but firmly push upward. This will raise his tongue off the back of his oropharynx, ensuring a patent airway. Administer oxygen by nasal cannula (an oxygen mask could frighten the patient and precipitate vomiting). Be sure the oxygen tubing doesn't wrap around his neck as he's moving about.

Don't try to insert a bite-block, a padded tongue depressor, or an oral airway. If his teeth are clenched, prying them open could injure them or your fingers. Also, the tongue depressor or airway could stimulate his pharynx, causing vomiting and subsequent aspiration.

After the seizure, the patient may be unconscious for 15 to 30 minutes. Keep him on his side to prevent aspiration of secretions. If he was incontinent, clean him up quickly but quietly, so as not to stimulate him. (See also *Seizures: precautions.*)

S

Seizures: home care

Emergency technique

The signs and symptoms of a seizure include muscular rigidity, usually lasting from a few seconds to half a minute, followed by jerking movements. While rigid, the victim may stop breathing, bite his tongue, and lose bladder and bowel control. He may have cyanosis of the face and lips and may be drooling and foaming at the mouth.

Your top priority should be to protect him from bodily injury and to maintain his airway. First, lower him to the floor at the first sign of a seizure, supporting his head and neck. Move away objects that may endanger him. Don't force a blunt object between his teeth. (It could break and obstruct the airway.) Observe the pattern of the seizure—when it started, how it progressed, and the signs accompanying it. The doctor will want this information to help with diagnosis.

Loosen clothing around the victim's neck. If possible, keep him lying down, but turn his head to the side or roll him onto his side to allow vomitus and saliva to drain from his mouth. Maintain his airway and monitor his pulse.

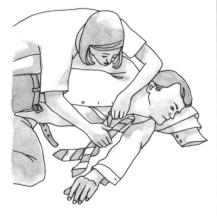

After the seizure, cover him and allow him to rest or sleep. Don't question him immediately. He may be disoriented and confused for about 2 to 4 hours. Check for incontinence and clean him as needed. Reassure him that you're doing all you can to help him. Try to find out the cause of the seizure. Counsel and make referrals, as needed. If repeated seizures occur, call for medical help or take him to a hospital.

Seizures: patient history

Asking the right questions

Make sure you ask the following questions when taking a history from a patient at risk for seizures:
• "What type of seizure do you normally have? Have you had more than one type? (If the patient has had more than one type of seizure, ask about each type.) (See *Seizures: classification.*)
• "Are you aware of anything that can cause you to have a seizure (for example, such external causes as loud noises or bright lights and such internal causes as a cold, the flu, constipation, or emotional stress)?
• "Are there any warning signs (such as an aura) before the seizure starts?
• "What's the first thing you notice when a seizure starts? What happens next?
• "What's the first thing I would notice about you during a seizure?
• "How often do you have them?
• "When was your last one?
• "After a seizure, do you know that you've had one?
• "What happens afterward? Are you confused, sleepy, or frightened?
• "How long does it take before you feel like yourself again?
• "What helps you during or after a seizure? What doesn't help?
• "What was your longest seizure-free period?
• "What medication do you take to control your seizures?
• "When do you take it?
• "Are you having any adverse reaction to this medication?

• "Are you allergic to any seizure medications?
• "What other medications are you taking?"

Ask these questions of the patient's family and friends. They may have witnessed one of his seizures and should be able to give you more information.

Also check the patient's chart to see his seizure history. You'll want to know if he's ever had status epilepticus.

Seizures: patient teaching

Practical pointers

Teaching should cover the factors that trigger seizures and the importance of strict compliance with drug therapy. Remember to include the patient's family members in your teaching, too, so they'll know how to help him during a seizure.

Tell the patient that he may experience more than one type of seizure and that during the initial phase of a seizure he may notice an aura—a sensory phenomenon, such as seeing stars or smelling roses.

Tell him to eat regular meals and to check with his doctor before dieting. Maintaining adequate blood glucose levels provides the necessary energy for neurons to work normally. Skipping meals or dieting may lead to decreased glucose levels (hypoglycemia), triggering a seizure. Teach the symptoms of hypoglycemia, so he'll know to eat a snack when needed.

Make sure the patient understands that anticonvulsant drugs can't cure his seizures but will control them. Advise him to take his medication exactly as ordered. Explain that his doctor will regulate drug dosage according to his blood levels, so the dosage may change periodically. And the drug regimen may change. If illness prevents him

S

from taking his medication, he should have a caregiver contact his doctor immediately. The doctor may decide to administer medication by another route.

Emphasize that he'll need to strictly adhere to his drug regimen. Overmedication may cause increased adverse reactions, and undermedication can increase the duration, frequency, and number of seizures.

Tell your patient what to do if he misses a dose, but caution him not to apply these same instructions to any other drug he's taking; instructions vary according to each drug's mechanism of action.

Stress that withdrawal seizures are possible if he abruptly stops taking his anticonvulsant drug. Even if he doesn't have a seizure for years, he shouldn't stop taking his medication unless ordered by his doctor. The length of time he'll require an anticonvulsant drug (a few years or for life) depends on many factors, such as the cause of his seizures and his age.

Help your patient identify factors that can trigger a seizure; they may include stressful situations and, in some people, flashing lights on video games, computer screens, and sights and sounds associated with highway construction.

Encourage your patient to pursue his normal activities if possible, but remind him that fatigue can trigger seizures. For his own safety, warn him to avoid activities that require complete alertness until his seizures are under control. The same rule applies to operating any equipment that could cause an injury. If he has a driver's license, tell him to notify the Department of Motor Vehicles of his condition.

Make sure his family knows what to do if a seizure occurs. If your patient's a child, instruct his parents to notify day-care or school authorities of his condition.

Stress the importance of wearing a medical identification bracelet or necklace at all times. Also encourage the patient to contact the Epi-

lepsy Foundation of America for additional information, and refer him to a local support group.

Seizures: precautions

When you know your patient's at risk

To prepare for a seizure, you need to ask yourself certain questions about your patient and his situation. For example, how will you know if your patient is having a seizure? Does he usually experience an aura beforehand? If so, instruct him to call you as soon as he begins to experience an aura so that you can take appropriate action.

The patient's roommate (if he has one) may be the first person to notice something unusual. You don't want to make the roommate responsible for the patient's safety. But if he's alert and receptive to the idea, it wouldn't hurt to have someone else keep an eye on the patient.

If it's likely that the patient will have a seizure during his hospital stay, his room should be near the nurses' station, and he should be checked frequently—at least every 15 minutes. Simply looking in on the patient isn't enough. You have to speak to him to check his responsiveness.

You'll also need to have certain equipment on hand. A padded tongue depressor should never be used on an epileptic patient. It's not effective in managing a generalized seizure because if you try to force a tongue depressor into his mouth, you might break his teeth. Aspirated teeth are far more dangerous to the patient than a chewed tongue.

Using a tongue depressor is equally pointless with partial seizures because teeth clenching doesn't even occur.

Now here's what you *will* need:
• *suctioning equipment*. You may need to suction a patient who has had a generalized tonic-clonic seizure. This type of seizure may cause the patient to salivate and vomit.

• *oxygen*. You may need to administer oxygen if your patient has had a generalized tonic-clonic seizure. Some doctors order 6 liters of oxygen given by nasal cannula or face mask in compromised patients (such as the elderly or those with decreased lung capacity). Clarify this beforehand with the doctor.
• *heparin lock*. If it's likely that a patient will have a seizure, you may want to keep a heparin lock in place. This will ensure prompt administration of an I.V. antiepileptic drug.
• *seizure medication tray*. Again, depending on the likelihood of a seizure, you may want to set up a tray with a few syringes, I.V. medications (such as phenytoin [Dilantin], diazepam [Valium]), and heparinized solution (for a heparin lock).

Finally, check with the doctor to make sure you understand how he wants to respond to a seizure. Some doctors may want to be called immediately. Others may not want to be called right away; instead, they'll leave orders for another dose of medication to be given after a first seizure. (See *Seizures, generalized motor.*)

Self-esteem

Improving it

How you feel about yourself is usually how others will feel about you. Improve your self-image by taking the following measures:

1. *Give yourself pep talks.* Have you ever stopped to think about your successes and the helpful influence you've had on many peoples' lives? Do you give yourself credit for those things? If you don't do this very often, start now.

Consider the tasks you do well—for example, inserting I.V. lines or patient teaching. Then, write them on index cards for ready reference when your self-esteem wilts. Every day, review them to reinforce their positive "charge."

Soon you'll be adding other accomplishments.

2. *Envision future successes.* Regularly relax and concentrate totally on a vision of yourself achieving an important goal (for example, getting your BSN or a promotion). This will program you to actually achieve it. Freely enjoy the pleasurable feelings of this vision of achievement—but don't accept them as a substitute for the real thing. They're just the appetizer, not the whole meal.

3. *Change false-negative ideas about yourself.* With the help of trusted family members or friends, examine the negative ideas you have about yourself. Chances are, you'll discover that some of them are simply false. For example, maybe you've always thought of yourself as selfish, but your family members or friends may recall many instances when your kindness or thoughtfulness has helped them. Once you've identified false-negative ideas, mentally throw them away—and watch your self-esteem blossom.

4. *Appreciate the humor in everyday events.* A good laugh can lighten almost any burden. Next time a situation turns tense—for example, when a doctor gives you an order with a condescending flourish and you'd like to let him know he's offended you—don't react in knee-jerk fashion by verbally attacking him. Instead, mentally see yourself viewing the situation from a distance. From that vantage point, chances are you'll be able to see something funny in it—and comment accordingly.

5. *Give compliments generously—and receive them graciously.* Try to notice the good things your co-workers are doing and to compliment them accordingly. And prepare yourself to receive compliments from others with a pleased smile and a gracious "Thank you." When you're trying to raise your self-esteem, what could be more appropriate than accepting the compliments you've earned?

Self-extubation

Emergency intervention

Here's what to do when a patient has forcibly removed his endotracheal tube.

Call another nurse and ask her to contact the doctor and a respiratory therapist. Place the patient in high Fowler's position to improve oxygenation. Draw blood for a stat arterial blood gas (ABG) analysis. Ask the other nurse to administer 40% humidified oxygen through a mask until you get the ABG results and the doctor arrives.

While you're waiting for the results, assess the patient's respiratory status. Note the rate, depth, and pattern of his respirations. Check for signs of respiratory distress, such as increased respirations, stridulous breathing, flaring nostrils, and blood in his sputum. Observe his chest movement; he may begin using accessory muscles to help him breathe. Also note his skin color.

When you get the ABG results, continue the 40% humidified oxygen through a mask, as needed. To clear secretions, carefully suction the patient's oropharynx. You don't want to induce gagging, coughing, or vomiting, all of which could increase his intracranial pressure. Explain your interventions to calm him.

The doctor may order two medications: a beta-adrenergic agent, such as isoetharine hydrochloride (Bronkosol), as a bronchodilator and hydrocortisone sodium phosphate (or a similar steroid) to decrease tracheal inflammation.

Over the next 4 hours, you'll monitor the patient every 15 minutes for signs of respiratory distress. You may have to suction him nasotracheally to ensure a patent airway. Again, be careful. Make sure his oxygen mask fits correctly, and provide skin care to prevent excoriation. Oral care is important, too. Evaluate his level of consciousness to see if he should be placed in restraints. Before his family visits, let them know what has happened.

Tell the patient to expect a hoarse voice and sore throat for several days. Make sure he has adequate gagging and swallowing reflexes, then give him a throat lozenge.

Self-improvement

Tapping into your strengths

First, determine what your goals are and how you can reach them. Do you want to become a manager? A clinical specialist? Figure out which positions will bring you closer to the one you ultimately want and what other education you may need. By doing that, you'll gain insight into yourself, and that knowledge will give you power.

Next, package yourself as a person with power. One part of your package is attire. You probably know that the way you look can affect how others feel about you. But as a nurse, you face a tricky problem. Many people don't view a person in a white uniform as powerful. To overcome this misconception, wear a clinical lab coat over your street clothes. Or, if you must wear traditional nursing attire, dress meticulously. Buy a tailored uniform and blazer, and wear only simple jewelry.

Another part of your package is body language. (See *Communication, nonverbal.*) For example, when you keep your back straight and plant your feet firmly on the ground (whether you're standing or sitting), you communicate strength.

Finally, learn to adapt your behavior. Depending on whom you're dealing with, you may have to be assertive, aggressive, submissive, or whatever. To effectively use your power at work, you'll need to develop different ways of interacting with your supervisor and your subordinates.

S

Self-inflicted injury: prevention

Breaking the cycle

You can offer your patient these patient-tested guidelines for breaking the cycle of deliberate self-harm:
• "Avoid alcohol and drugs." These substances contribute to conflict with others, worsen feelings of distress, and can cause mood shifts so that a patient who feels tired may turn angry—as always, at himself.
• "Avoid isolation." As tension mounts during this cycle, the impulse to go off alone may become irresistible. Suggest that your patient seek out the company of others, even if he doesn't feel like interacting with them. Find out about his interests, then try to get him involved in a scheduled weekly activity—an adult education class or exercise class, for example. Just going shopping or taking a long bus ride may help.
• "Avoid locations where self-injury has previously occurred." Many of these patients keep instruments for self-harm—razor blades or matches, for example—stored at such locations. Advise him to have someone throw these out.
• "Keep in mind that these feelings will pass." Although his distress may seem unendurable, it will dissipate if he lets time pass while shopping or otherwise keeping busy.
• "Learn a relaxation technique (such as yoga, deep muscle relaxation, or visualizing a relaxing scene), and practice it regularly." Reducing tension will reduce your patient's need to hurt himself.

Self-inflicted injury: treatment

Giving emotional first aid

Patients with self-inflicted injuries are usually young women and are frequently categorized as manipulators and attention-seekers. But, in most cases, self-harm is a means of escape from unbearable distress. These tormented patients need your sympathy and supportive care. Follow these guidelines:

1. *Assess and treat her injuries.* This is your first priority, but not your most important one—because her injuries probably aren't serious. Remember, the patient's trauma is more emotional than physical. You can probably take care of her injuries quickly, then attend to her complex emotional needs.

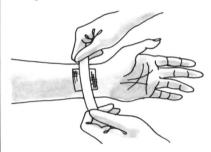

2. *Assess her motivation.* Although these patients typically don't intend to kill themselves, be aware of the possibility of suicide. Be particularly alert to a possible suicide attempt if this is the patient's first self-inflicted injury, if she has injured a different part of her body than in the past, or if this injury is more severe than previous ones.

Ask the patient if she was *trying* to commit suicide, but don't necessarily trust her answer. So no matter what she tells you, obtain a thorough assessment by requesting a psychiatric consultation.

3. *Offer support.* Some doctors and nurses withhold emotional support from these patients, concerned that such attention will reward the self-harming behavior and provoke further episodes. But let's consider why the patient probably harmed herself:
• She feels rejected or abandoned, typically by an important person in her life.
• She hopes someone in the hospital will meet her physical and emotional needs.
• She hopes that coming to the hospital will cause the important person to come back to her.

If you can express your care and concern for the patient, you may be able to start her on the road to a healthier outlook about herself and her reactions to stress. Don't say anything judgmental, such as "Can't you control this?" or "This must really upset your parents."

If your patient appears angry, withdrawn, or sad, tell her she looks that way to you, and ask if she views herself the same way. From this small start, she may go on to accept the therapy she so desperately needs.

4. *Try to prevent future episodes.* If your patient's able to go home, ask her how she thinks she'll feel when she gets there. If she has injured herself before, ask her to think about the aftermath of that experience: What happened when she went home? Was anyone supportive? Did she do added harm to her original injury, such as ripping out sutures? When did stress begin to build up again? What were the circumstances? Try to help her think of healthier ways to respond to stress, of how she might have used them then, and of how she can use them to prevent future self-mutilation.

Before your patient leaves, be sure a family member or friend has arrived to go home with her—and that she won't be left alone at home. Or find a halfway house that will take her; again, make sure someone comes to take her from the hospital. Then, before she leaves, make sure she has the name of a therapist, and set up a definite appointment. Give her the telephone number of a 24-hour crisis intervention line, too, if your community has one.

If you can't find anyone to go home with the patient, keep her in the hospital—a psychiatric consultation is one plausible reason. Don't send her home alone.

Septic shock

What to do

Let's say a paraplegic man is brought to your emergency department (ED) with complaints of lethargy, no appetite, and fever. He also has a 1″ (3 cm) sacral decubitus ulcer that looks infected. He tells you he's been running a fever of 100° to 101° F. (37.8° to 38.3° C.). His skin is warm, slightly flushed, and dry. Within 30 minutes, you note that his level of consciousness has decreased. His condition *has* worsened: Rectal temperature is up to 104° F. (40° C.); heart rate has jumped to 106; respiratory rate remains at 24; and blood pressure has dropped to 86/48. His skin is now clammy. What you're seeing are signs of septic shock.

Alert the ED doctor. Begin giving the patient oxygen by nasal cannula at 2 liters/minute. Then, using a large-bore catheter, start an infusion of dextrose 5% in 0.45 sodium chloride solution at 100 ml/hour. Take a 12-lead ECG, and set up the cardiac monitor to observe for dysrhythmias. As ordered, obtain an arterial blood sample for analysis of arterial blood gases, being careful to maintain sterile technique.

Obtain venous blood samples as well for culture and sensitivity testing. The doctor will order a broad-spectrum antibiotic, such as cefazolin, cephalothin, or cefoxitin. Start the antibiotic at once (after checking for drug allergies) because the laboratory will need at least 24 hours to identify the pathogens.

Decreasing the patient's fever is also a high priority. Administer acetaminophen, either orally or rectally, and place the patient on a hypothermia blanket. Be sure to use a rectal probe to assess the blanket's effect. Insert an indwelling (Foley) catheter to monitor urine output, taking a urine sample for culture and sensitivity testing as you do so.

The doctor may request other tests to confirm septicemia and detect complications. Be prepared to carry out orders for a portable chest X-ray, wound and sputum cultures, coagulation studies (to help diagnose disseminated intravascular coagulation), and cardiac and liver enzyme studies. As you perform the necessary procedures, explain to the patient what you're doing. Try to group similar procedures together to ease his anxiety and minimize their effects on him.

What to do later

After the patient is stabilized, he'll be transferred to the ICU. There he may have an intra-arterial line inserted for monitoring blood pressure and obtaining specimens. A pulmonary artery line may also be placed to monitor left- and right-sided heart function.

The ICU doctor will probably order steroids (to restore and maintain hemodynamic status and metabolism) and vasopressors (to improve blood pressure and tissue perfusion). Antibiotics will be administered around the clock.

Sex after childbirth

Vaginal exercises to teach your patient

After childbirth, women—especially primiparas—commonly experience reduced vaginal sensation during sexual intercourse. During delivery the vaginal muscles were stretched, decreasing both muscle tone and sensation. To help a woman improve this condition after childbirth, teach her the following exercise:

1. "Get in a comfortable position, close your eyes, and imagine there's a tampon in your vagina.

2. "Breathe normally and try to squeeze it as tightly as possible for a count of five.

3. "Release for a count of five, while breathing normally."

Tell your patient to do at least 20 repetitions several times a day. (See also *Incontinence, urinary.*)

Sex after mastectomy

Helping your patient adjust

Here's how to help your patient cope with a mastectomy:
• Observe her reactions before surgery. Appropriate behavior includes crying, feelings of anxiety or panic, and an inability to concentrate. But if she seems overly concerned about her appearance, she may have difficulty adjusting later.
• Help her express her fears and her feelings of grief, loss, or anger. She may think she'll be less attractive to her husband.
• Explain to her husband that she'll need support and reassurance. Suggest that he touch her, hold her hand, and tell her that he loves her as often as possible.
• After the surgery, encourage her to look at her incision and to assist with dressing changes. This will help her accept her altered body image.

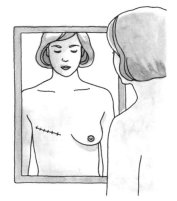

• Ask her husband to help too. Show him how to massage her arm gently, to restore lymphatic circulation and to provide reassurance.
• Encourage the couple to discuss their sexual desires with each other. Assure them that sexual intercourse probably can be resumed when the patient goes home. Suggest sexual positions that will leave the affected area untouched until it heals.
• Encourage the patient to join a support group, too. *Reach to Recovery* sends women who've had

S

mastectomies to counsel new patients and their families. Check with your local chapter of the American Cancer Society, or write to the American Cancer Society, 777 Third Avenue, New York, N.Y. 10017.

• If she's a likely candidate, suggest that the patient explore with her surgeon the possibility of breast reconstruction. It could promote more positive attitudes about herself and her sexuality and reduce feelings of loss and anxiety about sexual functioning. (See *Mastectomy, bilateral; Mastectomy: flap necrosis; Mastectomy: incisions; Mastectomy: phantom sensations; Mastectomy, radical.*)

Sex after pelvic radiation

Ways patient can avoid painful intercourse

If a woman who's having pelvic radiation therapy complains about painful intercourse, give her these suggestions:

• "Resume sexual intercourse as soon as possible after the full effects of radiation subside. Early resumption of intercourse will help keep your vagina flexible and can also benefit you emotionally.

• "Once you resume sexual intercourse, try to engage in it at least once a week. Regular intercourse will make you feel better about your own sexuality and will ensure vaginal flexibility, minimizing discomfort. (A patient without a regular partner can keep her vagina flexible by using mechanical or manual dilation.)

• "Explain to your partner that foreplay and arousal will help reduce your discomfort. The pleasant sensations will provide a distraction and help relax the perineal muscles.

• "Use a water-soluble lubricant. Try applying it with your partner as a part of foreplay. Artificial lubrication is necessary because radiation impairs the vagina's ability to produce natural lubrication.

• "Find the most comfortable position for sexual intercourse. Typically, the male superior position is most comfortable—if the man is gentle. The female superior, although it may cause more discomfort, gives more control."

Sex and cardiac disease

Advice to give your patient

Most people's heart rate and blood pressure don't change significantly during sexual activity when they're in a position that involves isometric exercise. So you needn't tell cardiac patients to avoid positions involving isometric exercise. Instead, advise them to assume positions that were familiar and comfortable before the onset of their heart problems. These positions will help them avoid undue stress. Here are some other tips to pass along:

• "After eating a large meal or drinking alcohol, wait at least 3 hours before engaging in sexual activity.

• "Make your environment as pleasant as possible. Don't engage in sexual activity in an environment that is very hot or very cold.

• "Avoid sexual activity if you feel rushed, fatigued, or angry."

Sex and COPD

Advising your patient

Explain how sexual activity makes demands on the heart and lungs: Heart rate, respiratory rate, and blood pressure all rise for a short time, but they quickly return to baseline levels. And the energy expended during orgasm is about the same as the energy required to climb stairs or take a brisk walk.

So, your chronic obstructive pulmonary disease (COPD) patient can engage in sex safely if you give him the following precautions.

• "Engage in sexual activity when you feel rested. The best time may be the early afternoon after a nap or in the morning, unless your respiratory tract is usually congested at these times. A word of caution, though: Don't change your habits if doing so will cause stress.

• "Engage in sexual activity in pleasant surroundings. Be comfortable—if you're too hot or too cold, you won't be relaxed.

• "Don't try new positions if they make you or your partner nervous. But use positions that require less energy: side-lying, either facing each other or with the man behind the woman.

• "If you become extremely short of breath during sexual activity, pause to take slow, deep, diaphragmatic breaths.

• "If sexual activity routinely causes shortness of breath or wheezing, take one or two puffs of your prescribed bronchodilator inhaler before sexual activity. (See *Inhalers.*)

• "If you use oxygen at home, use it during sexual activity.

• "Avoid sexual activity after a heavy meal.

• "Avoid sexual activity after drinking alcohol, lest it decrease your sexual function.

• "Don't engage in sexual activity during times of stress (if you're angry, for example). Stress would make breathing even more difficult.

• "If you're taking medications that decrease your sex drive or sexual function, consult your doctor about these adverse reactions."

Sex and dialysis

Advising the kidney dialysis patient

If the patient is a man, you can help him by explaining that timing is critical in planning sexual activity. A man who's impotent most of the time because of his renal problems is less likely to achieve and maintain an erection before a dialysis treatment than after it. That's be-

S

cause the level of uremic toxins in the body is highest just before dialysis, causing sexual feelings to diminish. And for about 4 to 6 hours after the dialysis treatment, a patient is usually lethargic. So he'll probably find sexual activity most satisfying after a rest period following dialysis.

Tell both male and female patients that continuous ambulatory peritoneal dialysis (CAPD) may improve their sex lives. Men undergoing CAPD claim they're more capable of maintaining an erection than they were before starting CAPD; women report the return of menstruation. These changes may result from elevated hematocrit levels or from stabilization of the body's chemical processes produced by CAPD.

Encourage dialysis patients and their partners to use other means of sexual expression besides intercourse. Touching, stroking, and caressing can not only be mutually satisfying in themselves, but they may also lead to spontaneous sexual intercourse. Patients may also want to explore new patterns of sexual activity, since old patterns can contribute to anxiety about performance failure.

And of course, as in any relationship, the partners should talk openly so that they understand each other's expectations. Unresolved feelings of resentment, anger, or guilt will interfere with a healthy sexual relationship.

Sex and Foley catheter

Patient-teaching pointers

Intermittent catheterization is ideal for patients who have indwelling catheters from urine retention or spinal cord damage or whatever reason. But if your patient has an indwelling (Foley) catheter, here's how to instruct her or him to have intercourse.

A *woman* should first drain the bag and tubing, then anchor the catheter away from the vagina. If she chooses to keep the drainage system intact, it should have an antireflux valve. If she chooses to disconnect the system, she should clamp the catheter and cover the ends of the catheter and the drainage system. After sexual intercourse, she must cleanse both ends, reconnect them as soon as possible, and unclamp the catheter.

A *man* also begins by draining the bag and tubing. Then, after an erection occurs, he doubles the catheter back over his penis. Next,

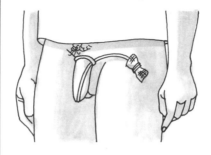

he anchors the catheter on his abdomen and slips a condom over his penis and part of the catheter. The condom will provide security and comfort during sexual activity. A man can also choose whether he wants to disconnect the drainage system.

After having sexual intercourse, a woman or a man who has a Foley catheter must check that the system is draining properly. Because of the high risk of urinary tract infection, the patient should also carefully cleanse the genitals after intercourse and drink extra fluids. (See *Foley catheter problems; Foley catheter techniques.*)

Sex and multiple sclerosis

Helping with possible problems

A patient with multiple sclerosis (MS) faces many sexual problems.

Here are some examples:
• A male patient may become impotent, especially in the later stages of the disease. He also may have premature or delayed ejaculation and impaired fertility.
• A female patient may lose her orgasmic ability because of impaired genital sensation. She may be able to conceive children, but pregnancy may exacerbate her disease.
• Both male and female patients may have less interest in sex because of decreased energy levels and poor body image. Finally, they may have problems related to muscle contractures or spasms, bowel and bladder incontinence, and poor lubrication.

Here's how to help:
• Get a sexual history from your patient and his partner to find out what problems they're having, then make appropriate referrals. (See *Sexual history.*)
• You might mention alternative methods of sexual arousal. A male patient may need a vibrator or oral or manual stimulation to achieve a reflex erection. He may also need an external sheath for penile stiffness—or a penile implant in some cases. Encourage both male and female patients to explore their bodies for erotic areas other than the genital areas. Suggest visual aids for stimulation. Above all, encourage them to freely discuss their sexual wishes and concerns with their partners.
• Advise your patient and his partner that certain positions will be difficult or painful because of muscle weakness or spasms. The side-lying or prone position may be most comfortable. Pillows can be used to support weak limbs. Couples should try different positions to find what's comfortable for them.
• If your patient's incontinent, tell him to empty his bowel and bladder before having intercourse.
• Give contraceptive counseling to patients of childbearing age.

S

Sex and ostomy

Practical advice

If your patient's sex life was satisfying before surgery, it can be satisfying afterward. Emphasize that the stoma can't be injured by the close physical contact. And the ostomy pouch, if applied correctly, won't interfere with intercourse. You may want to recommend emptying the pouch first and using a pouch cover, or wearing an opaque or decorative pouch.

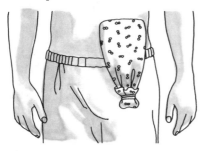

Rarely will female ostomy patients develop a sexual dysfunction. But some men will experience temporary impotence, and others (who had an ostomy because of rectal cancer) may have permanent nerve damage. A woman with an ostomy can become pregnant and have a normal pregnancy. However, she should discuss the prospect with her doctor before becoming pregnant. The doctor may recommend waiting a year or so after an ostomy. (See *Ostomy: physical exertion.*)

Sex and spinal cord injury

Counseling technique

If a patient asks about his sexual capabilities soon after his injury, explain that they may improve once spinal shock subsides but that only time, patience, and experimentation will tell fully.

Tell him and his partner that spinal cord injury precludes some spontaneous sexual activity. If he needs intermittent catheterization, for example, he'll need to empty his bladder before engaging in sexual intercourse. (See *Sex and Foley catheter.*)

Explain that he may have to change his sexual priorities. Because sexual intercourse may be difficult for a man with a spinal cord injury, satisfying his partner may be a more realistic goal than experiencing an orgasm himself.

You should encourage the patient to experiment with his partner to find ways that will satisfy his sexual needs. Perhaps if his partner assumes a more active role, he will be able to take pleasure in sex. Finally, if appropriate, give the male

Semirigid penile prosthesis

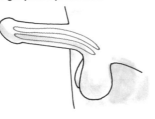

patient information on penile prosthesis implantation.

Sex and stroke

Encouraging your patient

After suffering a stroke, a patient may think his sex life has ended forever. But most patients can return to their previous level of sexual activity if they want to. And many of them do want to.

Encourage your stroke patient to discuss his sexual concerns. Here are some suggestions:
• First, get a sexual history. To start the discussion, you may ask, "How important was sexual activity to you and your partner before your stroke?" This will acknowledge his concerns and let him know you're open to discussing them. If he indicates that sexual activity isn't important to him, don't pursue the discussion. (See *Sexual history.*)

• Find out the frequency and type of sexual activity he engaged in before the stroke, especially during the previous year.
• If sexual function has recently become a problem for the couple, find out if something besides the stroke is involved, such as aging, antihypertensive medication, or diabetes. If medication or a medical condition was contributing to the problem, refer the patient to his doctor.
• Finally, help the patient and his partner recall the intimacy of touching, holding, and sharing feelings during sexual intercourse.

If the couple still has sexual problems despite your efforts to help, suggest professional counseling.

Sexual attraction

When you're attracted to a patient

Acknowledge that you're only human and that such feelings are normal. You'll occasionally feel sexually attracted to someone—even when you don't want to.

Remember, your first responsibility is to the patient. If the attraction you feel makes it difficult to give quality care, have another nurse care for him.

But as a professional, you'll probably feel obligated to at least try to cope with the problem. If so, don't keep it to yourself. Discuss your feelings with a friend or a colleague you can trust. Consider various options—for instance, avoiding intimate contact with the patient, removing all sexual overtones from what you say and do, and being careful about where and how you stand or sit.

If, after taking these steps, you can't cope with your feelings, talk to your supervisor about having another nurse care for the patient. Explain that you're having a personality conflict with this patient, making it clear that the problem is a result of *your* personality. Such an admission shouldn't reflect

S

negatively on you. Nurses are not machines.

Sexual history

Taking one effectively

Your patient may feel reluctant to discuss his sexual activity. Try to put him at ease by establishing a forthright, matter-of-fact tone. Explain that direct, complete answers will help you evaluate his health problems. Ask the following:
• "Are you currently having sexual relations with anyone? (If not, ask about his past sexual relationships and how he's meeting his current sexual needs.)
• "Is your partner a man or woman? (If the patient expresses a same-sex preference, ask about bisexual activities, too.)
• "Are you having sex with more than one partner?
• "How many sexual partners have you had during the past year?
• "Do you find sexual activities satisfying?
• "Do you have difficulty becoming sexually aroused? (Ask a male patient about his ability to achieve and maintain an erection.)
• "Do you experience pain or discomfort during or after sexual activities? (If so, describe it.)
• "Have you ever contracted a sexually transmitted disease? If so, what was it and how was it treated?
• "How do you protect yourself (and your partners) from sexually transmitted diseases?
• "Do you use birth control? If so, what type?" (See *STD: history taking.*)

Shampooing: arthritic patient

Avoiding unnecessary discomfort

Washing an arthritic patient's hair can be difficult because she can't tilt her head back to keep the water and shampoo from getting into her eyes and ears. To help her, cut a big circle out of the top of a plastic shower cap. Put the cap on her head, pulling her hair through the cut-out circle. The elastic rim is now above her eyes and ears. Simply flip down the remaining plastic to protect her face. Now she won't have to

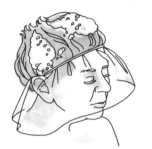

move her head at all, and she won't get any water or shampoo in her eyes and ears. (See *Arthritis aids.*)

Shampooing: bedridden patient

Doing it more easily

Here's a neat and easy way to wash a bedridden patient's hair:
Position her near the head of her bed and put incontinence pads under her shoulders and upper back. Then drape a large plastic bag over the head of the bed. Open the bag,

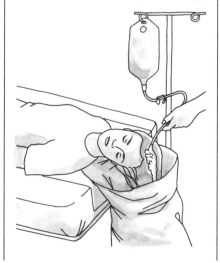

fold the lower open edge onto itself to make a lip, and place the patient's head on the lip.

Next, fill an enema bag with water and hang it on an I.V. pole. Use the bag's tubing as a hose to direct the flow of water onto the patient's head. (Adjust the clamp to control the flow.) One bag of water is usually enough for a shampoo and rinse.

This no-mess method of hair washing leaves the bed and patient dry—most of the excess water drains into the open bag. The remainder is caught in the lip of the bag and you can brush it into the bag with your hands. (See *Shampooing: preparation.*)

Shampooing: patient on Clinitron unit

Practical pointers

Ask another nurse to help you with this procedure. Position the patient on his back, with the bed in the fluid position. (Only a little padding is needed because the bed dries itself when turned on.)

With your assistant helping, place a basin or clean bedpan under the patient's head. To do this, each person should support the patient's head and neck with one hand and plunge the basin into the bed with the other. Then, turn the bed to the freeze position or have the patient do it if he can.

Place a small, rolled towel over the basin's edge to relieve pressure

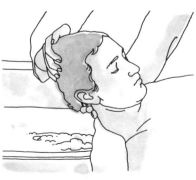

S

on the patient's neck. Support his neck with one hand while shampooing. If he seems uncomfortable, you may need to place the basin deeper into the bed.

You'll need to empty the basin several times during the shampoo. To do so, keep the bed in the freeze position, remove the basin, and empty it. Replace the basin in the indented space. (See *Shampooing: preparation.*)

Shampooing: patient on Stryker frame

Using the proper method

Be sure to cover the mattress with underpads, and place the patient in the prone position. Spread a bath blanket or underpads on the floor. Place a small trash can or basin beneath the patient's head to collect the rinse water.

Then, cover the headrest with underpads, and start the shampoo and rinse. If the patient is in cervical traction, follow the shampoo with pin care. (See also *Pin care.*)

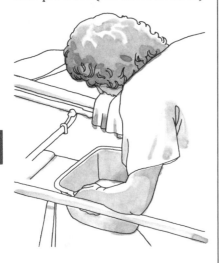

If the patient is able, he can hold the basin himself to catch the rinse water. (Push the headrest up to the end of the frame.)

Shampooing: patient with cervical collar

Helpful tips

First, you'll need to remove the bed's headboard and pad the bed well with underpads. Then, slide a large, open plastic bag under the patient's head to the middle of his collar or

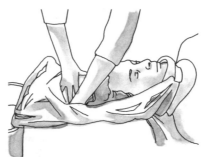

brace. If the patient can help you, let him.

Next, secure the edges of the bag to the front of the collar or brace. You can tape it or ask the patient to hold it.

Place a trash can under the sealed end of the bag. Cut a hole in this end so that water can drain through to the trash can. Now shampoo and rinse. Water tends to collect in depressions, especially between the mattress and bed frame. To speed rinsing and the emptying of runoff water, depress the bag into the mattress. Placing a hard, flat surface (such as a clipboard with the clip turned down) under the bag will help. (See *Collars, cervical.*)

Shampooing: patient with halo vest

The best procedure

Place a clean bedpan between the posts of the halo vest. (You'll find it fits perfectly.) Place a rolled towel behind the patient's neck to keep the sheepskin liner dry.

As an alternative, set up a shampoo basin to empty into a trash can. This eliminates the need to constantly remove the bedpan to empty it. When you use a shampoo basin,

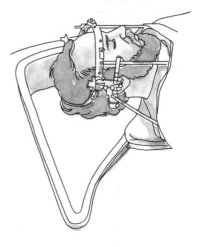

though, be sure to place the bed in a deep Trendelenburg position. (Because the halo vest elevates the patient's upper torso, water is more likely to run down his neck.)

Place a rolled towel behind the patient's neck, shampoo, and rinse. Then perform pin care. (See *Halo vests; Pin care.*)

Shampooing: preparation

Setting things up properly

Washing a patient's hair, especially if he's immobilized, can be an exhausting and time-consuming experience for everyone. But it doesn't have to be if you think creatively and improvise.

You'll need two towels (or more), bath blankets, shampoo, conditioner (if necessary), underpads (to protect the bedclothes), a shampoo basin (or a clean bedpan or large, heavyweight plastic garbage bag), a container for pouring water (for example, a clean urinal), and a container for collecting water (for example, a trash can or basin that can be easily emptied during the procedure). A blow-dryer is optional;

you may find it easier to use than towels for some patients.

While you must adapt your shampooing techniques to each patient, the general procedure remains the same. Explain to the patient what you're going to do, then cover his bed and bedclothes with underpads. Next, position him. The Trendelenburg position is best because it promotes water drainage. But if this position is contraindicated, keep the bed flat and use extra padding to keep it dry.

When positioning the patient, take into account the nature of his illness or injury, the type of bed or immobilization device he has, and his ability to participate in the procedure. Some patients may want to lather their hair themselves, whereas others may be able to help by holding a basin or towel.

Place the trash can or basin where it can catch the rinse water. Then fill the water container, making sure the water temperature feels comfortable. Protect the patient's face and clothing with towels. Now you're ready to wet his hair, shampoo, rinse thoroughly, and dry.

If the patient's hair is matted with blood, use hydrogen peroxide to dissolve clots, then rinse with saline solution. Be sure to tell him that the peroxide won't bleach his hair, but it will feel warm and bubbly.

Shaving

Doing it smoothly and quickly

Before shaving a patient who has a coarse beard or sensitive skin, try coating his face and neck with lubricating gel. Let the gel stand a minute or so, apply shaving soap or cream, then shave and rinse as usual. This will soften the patient's skin and hair and let the razor blade glide more smoothly over his face. However, don't use the gel with electric razors.

Shock: complications

Recognizing the patient at risk

You'll need to watch for hypovolemic shock if your patient:
• has lost a lot of blood in surgery or a lot of fluid through vomiting or diarrhea.
• has lost circulating blood volume because of pooling in the extravascular space—the trauma patient with long-bone or pelvic fractures, for example.
• has impaired venous return—the aneurysm patient with vena cava obstruction, for example.

You'll need to watch for septic shock if your patient:
• is very old or very young (because of immune system deficiencies).
• is immunosuppressed.
• is chronically ill.
• is undergoing an invasive gastrointestinal or genitourinary procedure.

You'll need to watch for cardiogenic shock in any patient with impaired cardiac function (such as myocardial infarction or contusion). (See *Cardiogenic shock detection.*)

Be safe, not sorry: Assume your patient's in shock if you're getting a mixed picture early on. If you see all the classic signs and symptoms of shock, your patient's already in trouble.

Make the most out of your time because you don't have much of it. You have more time with hypovolemic shock, less time with septic shock, and almost no time at all with cardiogenic shock. (See also *Hypovolemic shock intervention; Septic shock.*)

Shock: emotional support

Helping the patient cope

A patient who's in shock will be frightened by the flurry of activity around him. And his anxiety will put even more stress on his body systems. Support him emotionally.

If he asks you if he's going to die, you could say "We're working so that doesn't happen." But some nurses would answer more aggressively than that. Some might say "no," believing that the patient needs that extra confidence at that moment.

His family needs reassurance as well. They see people and equipment flying into the room. They don't need to hear that he's in critical condition. They need to know that he's receiving the best care possible, that they'll be getting information at certain intervals, and that staff members are constantly with him. Families are terrified that their loved one may die alone.

So get the family into the room as soon as possible, especially if your patient is critical. They need to say "We're here" and touch the patient. Too many families say, "He never knew we were here. We didn't get to see him before he went to the operating room...before he died." You don't want to leave them with unnecessary guilt feelings or with a sense of "incompleteness" about the death. These feelings would interfere with the grieving process.

Even if you just get the family in for seconds, that time is important. Don't worry about the equipment or the clinical atmosphere. These will be like a blur around what's most important to them—the patient himself. (See *Communication: family.*)

Shock: intervention

What to do for the patient

Follow these steps:
1. Stay with the patient. Call for help.
2. Tell the unit secretary to send the patient's chart to you.
3. Unless the patient is in cardiogenic shock, lower the head of his bed and, depending on his blood pressure, raise his legs. Don't put

his head below body level. Tell him, "I'm removing the pillow so you'll be able to breathe more easily."

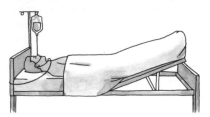

4. Administer oxygen.

5. Open a vein.

6. Place him on a cardiac monitor.

7. Cover him with a blanket to prevent heat and fluid loss.

8. Work calmly and efficiently. The patient needs to have confidence in you.

9. Don't alarm him. Say, "Your pulse is up for some reason, so just to play it safe, I want you to stay still and not talk now. Let me do all the work. I'm having your doctor and other staff people called, but I'll be staying with you." Just seeing you in action should tell him you know what you're doing.

10. Continue assessing him, and give him updates, such as "Your pulse has slowed," "It's still up there," and so on. Ask only questions that require minimum talking by the patient.

Remember, anxiety and pain will increase the sympathetic nervous response. This can put a patient further into shock. So assess the need for pain medication against changes in vital signs. A vasodilator can change vital signs—for example, decrease blood pressure.

Shock: recognition

Knowing what to look for

To recognize subtle changes in your patient, you'll need an accurate baseline assessment. Review the chart to see what's been happening with him. And if he's new to you, ask another staff member to look at him too. Here's what to note:

• *level of consciousness.* A change in level of consciousness is, in many cases, the first clue to impending shock. Restlessness may hint that cerebral perfusion is decreasing, and it changes to confusion as the brain becomes more hypoxic. In the final stages of shock, the patient may be totally unresponsive or comatose.

• *pulse.* You'll see pulse changes before blood pressure ones. So tachycardia is one of the first clues to impending shock; increasing tachycardia means shock is progressing.

• *blood pressure.* In the early stages of shock, both systolic and diastolic pressure may rise as a result of compensatory mechanisms. As shock progresses and cardiac output decreases, the systolic pressure also begins to fall. Diastolic pressure remains elevated because of continued vasoconstriction. So with progressive shock, pulse pressure narrows.

• *skin.* Initially, the skin may be warm, dry, and pink, but as compensatory mechanisms start working, signs of vasoconstriction and decreased cardiac output appear. The skin becomes cool, pale, and clammy. One exception to this is septic shock, in which initial changes of vasodilation will cause hot, flushed skin ("pink shock"). Only in the later stages of septic shock will the skin become cold, mottled, and ashen.

• *respiratory status.* The patient will hyperventilate. Progressive lung congestion produces crackles, wheezes, and dyspnea, as well as hypoxia, hypercapnia, and uncompensated metabolic acidosis. As respirations gradually become shallow and ineffective, the patient will be cyanotic and dyspneic.

• *urine output.* Initially, urine output may remain within normal limits. As shock progresses, urine output decreases and may be negligible with hypoperfusion of the kidneys. And in spite of decreased urine output, the patient will complain of thirst because fluid has moved from the extravascular to the vascular space.

As you use these assessment guidelines, keep looking for trends: Don't rely on one reading. And keep comparing these trends with baseline values. (See *Shock: complications.*)

Shoes

Keeping them clean

To keep your new shoes white, apply a coat of clear floor wax before wearing them. The wax will help prevent scuff marks, so you won't have to polish them as often.

To keep your old shoes looking like new, use baby powder. First apply white shoe polish as usual and wait until it's just about dry. Then liberally sprinkle the powder on the shoes. When the polish is dry, gently buff the shoes until they look as white and clean as new.

Put laces in a bowl or jar of warm water and add some dishwasher detergent. Agitate them in the solution, let them soak for 1 or 2 hours, then rinse and air-dry. Your laces will look as white and clean as your shoes.

Here's another suggestion for spotless shoes: Try wiping them with an alcohol prep pad. This removes surface dirt and smudges instantly.

Shunt, arteriovenous

What to do when it ruptures

What do you do when a patient has developed a sudden, rapidly spreading subcutaneous hemorrhage, presumably from a ruptured aneurysm on his internal arteriovenous (AV) shunt? You must act quickly because the hemorrhage could cause hypovolemia, which quickly progresses to shock and could lead to cardiopulmonary arrest. Rapid intervention will control the bleeding, and blood transfusions will replace the lost blood, averting hypovolemia.

Internal arteriovenous shunt

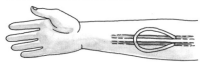

First, call for assistance. Then tie a tourniquet above the AV shunt site. If a tourniquet isn't readily available, an inflated blood pressure cuff will work just as well. Next, apply a pressure dressing to the site and elevate the patient's arm. (If the patient had an external AV shunt, you would see two bulldog clamps attached to the Ace bandage. You'd attach these clamps to the shunt to stop the bleeding.)

Ask someone to bring you a large-bore intravenous catheter and an infusion bag of normal saline solution. As you're inserting the catheter and starting the infusion, have someone call the doctor, who will insert a central line. (See *Central line: insertion.*) Elevate the patient's legs and begin administering oxygen at 2 liters/minute through a nasal cannula.

The doctor will instruct the unit secretary to call the operating room staff, who will remain on stand-by. Obtain a blood sample for a stat hemoglobin and hematocrit study so that you'll have a baseline measurement. Obtain samples also for blood typing and crossmatching and for routine preoperative studies. Be sure to alert the blood bank that you may need O-negative blood sent up stat before type and crossmatch results are available. Continually monitor the patient for signs of shock. As ordered, administer blood transfusions according to hospital protocol.

A ruptured AV shunt can produce a massive hemorrhage in an exceptionally short time. So don't release the tourniquet, even if it's been in place for more than 15 minutes. It

will be released in the operating room under controlled conditions.

Don't let the patient have anything to eat or drink, and prepare him for surgery. Continually reassure him; don't leave him alone. Remember that because he's already in renal failure, he has fluid and electrolyte problems. Watch closely for signs of pulmonary edema (dyspnea, increased respiratory rate, moist-sounding respirations), and monitor his central venous pressure.

Once the blood transfusions and fluid infusions have reversed hypovolemia, the patient's doctor may order a dopamine drip to maintain blood pressure and prevent possible pulmonary edema secondary to fluid overload. Maintain a strict record of the patient's intake and output.

What to do later

After the patient returns from surgery, draw blood samples every 4 to 6 hours for hemoglobin and hematocrit testing. Keep his doctor informed of the results. Remember that the patient's potassium level will rise as the blood cells that leaked into the subcutaneous tissue break up and are reabsorbed. So observe him closely for related complications, and obtain blood chemistry tests, as ordered.

Some of the subcutaneous hemorrhage may have been drained when the shunt was repaired, but the patient will still have a hematoma. To reduce the swelling and ease the pain, elevate his arm, apply cold compresses, and administer pain medication as ordered. Monitor circulatory, motor, and neurologic functions below the level of the hematoma.

Shunt insertion

Postop positioning

To drain excess cerebrospinal fluid (CSF) from the ventricles of the brain, a neurosurgeon may insert a shunt. This is a flexible tube that transfers CSF from the ventricles to

another part of the body—usually the peritoneal cavity—where it will be reabsorbed.

After this procedure is performed, place the patient on his nonoperative side to avoid putting pressure on the shunt valve. Also, make sure the head of his bed is flat. This helps ensure that CSF doesn't drain too rapidly, which could cause a sudden, dangerous reduction in intracranial pressure and a shifting of intracranial contents. If the size of the ventricles decreases too fast, the cerebral cortex could pull away from the dura and tear the small interlacing veins, producing a subdural hematoma.

Sickle cell crisis

Nursing considerations

First, begin hydrating your patient to minimize the risk of vaso-occlusive complications.

Expect to insert a large-gauge I.V. catheter and to begin infusing normal saline solution at twice the normal rate. This will increase his hydration, decrease his blood viscosity, and prevent additional cell sickling.

Quickly assess your patient for signs and symptoms of dehydration, such as poor skin turgor (see *Skin turgor*) and dry mucous membranes, and ask whether he's had any illness recently that caused fluid loss through diarrhea or vomiting. If dehydration triggered your patient's sickle cell crisis, he'll need even more aggressive fluid replacement.

After you've intervened to increase your patient's hydration, give a narcotic analgesic (such as morphine or meperidine [Demerol] intramuscularly), as ordered, to relieve his severe pain. Insert an indwelling (Foley) catheter to monitor his urine output accurately. Perform a complete physical assessment, and take his history. Your goals are to discover the extent of his disease and to iden-

S

tify what precipitated his sickle cell crisis so that you and the doctor can intervene appropriately to correct it.

SIDS

Helping families survive

All parents whose infants die of sudden infant death syndrome (SIDS) will have two problems: First, they'll be confused about their infant's death and its cause; and second, they'll need to cope with a wide range of emotions—anger, hurt, and guilt. If you see them in the emergency department, try to take them to a quiet room, where they'll avoid the staring eyes of people in the waiting room and start to sort out what happened.

Don't assume that the parents know their child is dead. If resuscitation began at home and continued on the way to the hospital, they may expect to hear that their infant survived. In fact, one of a nurse's most difficult tasks is accompanying the doctor when he tells the parents their infant is dead. But your presence is essential.

While the parents may not be able to fully understand the doctor's explanation, they need this information to begin mourning their dead infant and to help them deal with their emotions. Be prepared for their reactions. Let them express their feelings. Because the death was sudden and unexplained, they may be stunned and react with disbelief and denial. Reinforce the fact that SIDS is unpreventable. That'll help alleviate their feelings of self-blame and distrust of themselves and others.

Above all, listen to them. They may feel overwhelming guilt and ask themselves, "What could we have done to prevent the death?" Reassure them that they weren't to blame.

If they wish, let the parents see and hold the dead infant so they'll know that he's whole and peaceful.

Let them say goodbye in their own way. This will help them grieve.

An autopsy may be required to rule out other causes of the infant's death. Laws governing the need for one after a sudden infant death vary from state to state. If an autopsy is mandatory, the coroner or medical examiner will conduct one. But if your state doesn't require one, encourage the parents to allow one. It will substantiate the cause of death and help them know they didn't cause it and couldn't have prevented it.

Remember, these parents were completely unprepared for their infant's death. Their grief may be almost unbearable. Don't let them leave the hospital until you arrange for professional counseling. Refer them to the social services department or to a visiting nurse who will visit them within a week or two after the infant's death. You can also arrange to have other parents who've lost infants to SIDS contact the couple. (See *Death; Death, child; Grief.*)

Sinuses: palpation

Assessing for sinusitis

When your patient reports postnasal drip, assess his sinuses for swelling and tenderness—telltale signs of sinusitis. Carefully press up

Palpating frontal sinuses

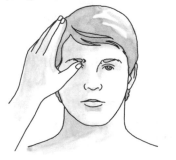

with your thumb on his eyebrow and on his cheekbone directly below his eye. Avoid placing pressure on his eyes.

Tenderness and swelling beneath the middle of his eyebrows may in-

Palpating maxillary sinuses

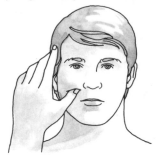

dicate frontal sinusitis; over his cheeks, maxillary sinusitis.

Sinuses: transillumination

Proper technique

Transillumination of frontal and maxillary sinuses can determine the source of a nasal discharge. First, darken the room. Then, gently press a penlight under the patient's right or left brow, close to his nose, and shield the light with your hand.

Transilluminating frontal sinuses

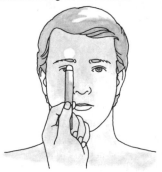

You'll normally see a dim red glow through the air-filled frontal sinus; if you don't, suspect secretions or thickened mucosa. Repeat this procedure for the other brow.

If the patient wears an upper denture, have him remove it. Then ask him to open his mouth wide. Tilt his head back slightly as you shine a penlight downward, on his right or left cheek, just below the inner aspect of the eye. Look through his open mouth at the hard palate. A red glow indicates his sinus is clear;

Transilluminating maxillary sinuses

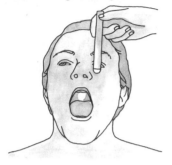

its absence suggests secretions or thickened mucosa in the maxillary sinus. Repeat this procedure on the other cheek.

Skin lesions

Measuring them accurately

When you need to measure a skin lesion, and your measuring tape isn't handy, here's a good substitute.

At your leisure, measure some of your own accessible body parts —such as the nail bed of your little finger—with a ruler and memorize these measurements.

This measuring equipment is easy to remember, water-resistant, and portable. It never gets lost—and is always *right at hand.*

Skin mottling

Observation techniques

If your patient's skin is mottled over his elbows and knees, or all over, and is pale, cool, and clammy, suspect hypovolemic shock. (See *Hypovolemic shock intervention.*) Quickly take his vital signs, noting tachycardia or a weak, thready pulse. Observe for flat neck veins. Does he appear anxious? If you find these signs and symptoms, place him supine in bed with his legs elevated 20 to 30 degrees. Then notify

the doctor immediately. (See *Shock: intervention.*) What about localized mottling in a pale, cool extremity that the patient says feels painful, numb, and tingling? This may signal acute arterial occlusion. Immediately check his distal pulses: If they're absent or diminished, notify the doctor at once. Insert an I.V. line in an unaffected extremity, and prepare the patient for arteriography or immediate surgery, as ordered.

Skin protection

When dressings need to be changed frequently

Stomahesive can be used to protect the skin of a patient who has a central venous or Hickman catheter line and a dressing that needs to be changed every 48 hours. Cut out the middle of a 4″ × 4″ piece of Stomahesive, leaving just a thin, square frame. Apply the frame to the patient's skin around the insertion site.

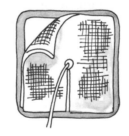

Then apply the dressing as usual, and tape the dressing right to the frame. When you change the dressing, just pull the tape from the frame—not from the patient's tender skin.

Skin test results

Interpreting them

About 48 hours after an intradermal injection, evaluate the erythema and induration produced by each skin test reaction and record the results. In most cases, where there's erythema, there's induration; the two signs nearly always occur to-

gether. Induration is more significant clinically, but to keep the information in the patient's chart complete, always note the degree of erythema.

To evaluate induration, use the three-finger method. This allows you to measure the size of the induration and to grade it according to palpability and visibility. Here's how to do it:
• Locate the injection site.
• Holding your index, middle, and ring finger together, stroke the patient's skin firmly in a downward motion. If induration is present, you'll feel the difference in the skin thickness after a few strokes. (You may even be able to see the induration.)
• Measure the diameter of the induration horizontally, then vertically, in millimeters. To make this step easier, gently mark the skin with your fingernail where the induration begins and ends. (You can use a pen or marker, if you wish, but make sure you wipe the skin with an alcohol sponge afterward.)
• Record both diameters in millimeters, always noting the horizontal diameter first.
• Grade the degree of erythema and induration. Use this scheme: Erythema is graded tr (trace discoloration) to + + + + (vesiculation/necrosis). Red is + +. Induration is graded as tr (barely palpable) to + + + + (vesiculation/necrosis). Easily palpable and visible is + +.

Mastering the three-finger method takes practice. When you're not sure where the induration begins and ends, try the ballpoint pen method:
• Clean the injection site with alcohol or soap and water. Let the skin dry.
• Hold the ballpoint pen at a 90-degree angle to the skin, about 1″ (3 cm) away from the margin of the test reaction.
• Using only moderate pressure, slowly draw a straight line on the skin toward the center of the reaction.

S

• Stop when you feel resistance. This is caused by the pen encountering the edge of the induration.
• Repeat the procedure on the opposite side of the induration, then on all the lines. The distance between opposing lines, horizontally and vertically, is the size of the induration.
• Record the size of the induration.

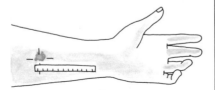

Then grade the degree of erythema and induration as you would with the three-finger method.
• Remove the pen markings with an alcohol sponge.

The following notation is an example of a properly recorded skin test reaction:

$$14 \times 16 \; \frac{++}{+}$$

It indicates an induration measurement of 14 × 16 mm in diameter (horizontally and vertically), with a "++" degree of erythema (red) and a "+" degree of induration (palpable but not visible to the naked eye). Note that the degree of erythema always appears above the degree of induration.

In the tuberculin skin test, an induration of less than 5 mm in average diameter indicates a negative result; 10 mm or more in average diameter indicates a positive result. If the average diameter of the induration falls between 5 and 9 mm, the result is too ambiguous to be meaningful. (See *Skin test site; Skin test technique.*)

Skin test site

Choosing one

For patients over age 60, don't use the traditional injection site (the volar surface of the forearm). In such patients, loss of skin turgor could contribute to bruising or to extravasation of the testing solution. Instead, inject the antigen into the area over the trapezius muscle, just

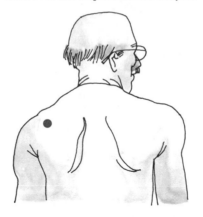

below the acromial process. Using this site will give you more accurate results. (See *Skin test results; Skin test technique.*)

Skin test technique

Using proper methods

Before performing an intradermal skin test, check the patient's chart for a history of hypersensitivity to any of the antigens. If no such hypersensitivity is noted, ask him whether he's had a skin test before and if so, what his reaction was. If this question also fails to uncover a history of hypersensitivity, you can go ahead and perform the test with medium-strength antigens. Report any previous reaction to the doctor. He may want to cancel the test or order weaker antigens. (If you perform the test with weaker antigens, note it in the patient's chart.)

Sometimes a patient assumes that an intradermal skin test is a form of treatment. To avoid any such misunderstanding, always explain the purpose of the test. Tell him that administering a panel of antigens takes about 10 minutes and that reactions should appear in 24 to 72 hours. Also, tell him that if the test results are negative, stronger antigens may have to be given.

If you're performing the test on an outpatient, tell him to return at the appointed time so the test results can be interpreted. With the tuberculin skin test—the test most often performed on outpatients—inform him that a positive reaction appears as a hard, red, raised area at the injection site and that, though it may itch, he shouldn't scratch it. Emphasize that a positive reaction doesn't always indicate active tuberculosis.

If you're drawing up more than one antigen, put strips of adhesive tape on the syringes and label them immediately. That way you won't have to guess what antigen it is when you're ready to perform the injections. Don't draw up antigens until 10 minutes before you're ready to inject.

The ideal site for an intradermal skin test is the upper third of the volar aspect of the forearm. If both forearms are diseased (from atopic dermatitis, for example), you can use the medial aspect of the thigh or the upper back. (See *Skin test site.*) Always clean the injection site with povidone-iodine and, to prevent stinging, let it dry before you administer the antigen.

Just before performing the injection, flush the needle to ensure that you'll be delivering a full 0.1 ml (the standard dose) of the antigen. Then, holding the syringe nearly parallel to the skin, insert the tip of the needle—bevel up—just under the surface. Stop when the bevel is embedded *but still visible*. Now, inject the antigen, using firm, steady pressure.

A pale wheal (6 to 10 mm in diameter) should form over the needle tip as soon as you start the injection. If not, you gave the injection subcutaneously and you'll have to repeat it at another location.

Don't inject the antigen into the belly of a muscle, which would make it difficult to measure the induration afterward, or into a vein, which would cause bleeding and a possible generalized response to the antigen. If you're giving more than one injection, space them at least 2″ (5 cm) apart to prevent reactions from overlapping.

Instead of labeling injection sites with a pen or marker, note the locations of the injection sites and the antigens administered on the patient's chart. Include a drawing of the arm, showing all the injection sites. Drawing circles on the patient's arm will not only make him look like he just came out of a tattoo parlor, but the ink could interfere with an accurate reading of the test results. (See *Skin test results*.)

Skin turgor

Assessing it quickly

To assess skin turgor in an adult, pick up a fold of skin over the sternum or the arm. (In an infant, roll

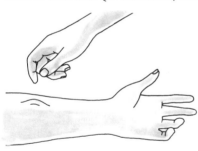

a fold of loosely adherent skin on the abdomen between your thumb and forefinger.) Then release it. Normal skin will return immediately to its previous contour. With decreased skin turgor, the fold of skin will hold for up to 30 seconds.

Skull tongs

Nursing considerations

Skull tongs are a type of skeletal traction device used to immobilize

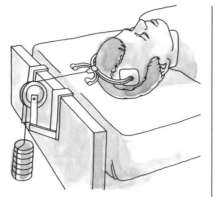

the patient's cervical spine after fracture or dislocation, invasion by tumor or infection, or surgery. Follow these guidelines:
• Reassure the patient and explain the procedure to him.
• Assess his neurologic status, as ordered, with particular emphasis on motor function. (See *Neurologic exam: muscle strength*.) Notify the doctor immediately if the patient experiences decreased sensation or increased loss of motor function: This may indicate spinal cord trauma.
• Be alert for signs and symptoms of loosening pins: redness, swelling, and complaints of persistent pain and tenderness. (Causes include infection, excessive traction force, and osteoporosis.)
• If the pins come out, immobilize the patient's head and neck and call the doctor.
• Take action to prevent pressure sores. Remember, inadequate peripheral circulation can cause sores within 6 hours.
• Make sure the traction weights are hanging freely to maintain proper traction force. Never add or subtract weights unless the doctor orders it. (inappropriate weight adjustment may cause neurologic impairment). (See *Traction patients*.)

SLE: patient teaching

Helping your patient cope

You'll find that teaching a patient who has systemic lupus erythe-matosus (SLE) will probably be an ongoing process. In the early stages, she'll need preparation for the sometimes lengthy diagnostic workup. (See *Diagnostic studies*.) Once the diagnosis is made, you'll focus on the disorder's long-term management, especially the importance of adhering to the prescribed drug regimen, monitoring and reporting warning symptoms, and practicing self-care measures. If your patient is especially prone to flare-ups, you'll have to address any factors that can aggravate her condition, such as excessive activity or stress, and help correct them.

Compliance with the treatment regimen can reduce the risk of complications and improve the quality of life for the patient with SLE. Despite these possible benefits, teaching her may not always be easy: The disorder's chronicity and unpredictability can act as a barrier to learning. Typically, you'll have to help your patient adjust to the prospect of life lifelong treatment and periodic flare-ups before she'll be receptive to your teaching.

Describe the disorder
Begin your teaching by telling your patient that SLE is a chronic disorder that causes structural changes in the connective tissue, the fibers that support many other body tissues. Its unpredictable course includes exacerbations interspersed with long periods of complete or near-complete remission. The disorder may produce only mild effects. However, it may also be life-threatening because of its effects on the heart, blood vessels, kidneys, lungs, and central nervous system.

Explain that the cause of SLE isn't known but that researchers believe antibodies develop against the body's own tissues—mostly deoxyribonucleic acid (DNA), but sometimes ribonucleic acid (RNA), clotting factors, and blood cells. This autoimmune response generates immune complexes, which damage connective tissue and cause inflammation. Tell her that

S

because these immune complexes may be present in any part of the body, she may have different symptoms at different times and with varying severity.

Point out possible complications
Your patient should know that failure to follow the prescribed treatment plan can cause a flare-up, but that even total compliance doesn't rule one out.

Explain that emotional stress and inadequate rest may make her more prone to a flare-up. Exposure to sunlight—including reflected sunlight—may lead to a flare-up, severe urticaria, and bullous lesions. Even brief exposure (20 minutes or less) can produce a rash. Stress the importance of minimizing exposure to infection because the patient has increased susceptibility.

Teach her about tests
Inform her that a definitive diagnosis of SLE may take months of observation, many laboratory tests, and sometimes a trial of drugs. That's why she must provide a precise history of her symptoms to aid diagnosis.

Tell her that blood tests will be performed to evaluate her immune system and to detect certain antibodies. One such test, the antinuclear antibody test, yields positive results in about 95% of SLE patients. Also, a positive lupus erythematosus factor test strongly suggests SLE, especially if clinical symptoms are present. However, the anti-DNA antibody test remains the most specific test for SLE because it rarely gives positive results in other disorders. These blood tests may be repeated periodically to monitor the effectiveness of therapy.

Explain that a complete blood count, an erythrocyte sedimentation rate, a urinalysis, a chest X-ray, an ECG, and renal function tests may be performed to evaluate the effects of SLE. If a renal biopsy is scheduled to determine the extent of renal involvement, tell your patient to fast for 6 hours before the test.

SLE: treatments

Patient teaching

Here's what to teach your patient with systemic lupus erythematosus (SLE):
• *Procedures.* If your patient has life-threatening complications or an acute flare-up that's unresponsive to corticosteroids, a procedure called therapeutic apheresis may be performed. To prepare her, explain that a needle will be inserted in each arm and that her blood will be pumped through a machine to remove the circulating immune complexes that are exacerbating her disorder. Tell her that her pulse rate and blood pressure will be monitored and that she should report any tingling sensations around her mouth or in her hands or feet.
• *Medication.* Drug therapy controls symptoms of SLE. Corticosteroids, for example, form the backbone of treatment to slow SLE's progressive symptoms. Salicylates or nonsteroidal anti-inflammatory drugs may be used to treat fever and arthritic symptoms. Antimalarial drugs may be used to combat skin manifestations and joint involvement. And immunosuppressants may be prescribed when other drugs fail to control the disorder.

Tell your patient that as her condition improves, drug dosages will be lowered gradually. Remind her that any deviations from her prescribed regimen can exacerbate her disorder. (See *Steroids.*)
• *Diet.* Explain that no specific diet will improve or cure SLE but that foods high in protein, vitamins, and iron help maintain optimum nutrition and prevent anemia. If your patient has lost weight, advise her to increase her caloric intake with between-meal snacks or commercially available high-protein, high-calorie supplements.
• *Activity.* Tell your patient that joint stiffness may be relieved with a program of moderate exercise and specific range-of-motion exercises.

Recommend the use of moist or dry heat before exercising to decrease discomfort. Warn her to avoid exercising to the point of fatigue so that she doesn't trigger flare-ups. Advise her to restrict her activity if she's experiencing a flare-up and to resume activity slowly afterward.

Because fatigue commonly occurs in SLE, recommend that your patient sleep 10 to 12 hours each night and rest periodically during the day. Make sure she understands that she should curtail any activities before she tires.

Other care measures
Caution your patient to avoid exposure to sunlight—even sunlight that's reflected from sand or snow. Advise her to use a sunblock or to wear protective clothing. Also recommend wide-brimmed hats, sunglasses, and hypoallergenic cosmetics.

Make sure she understands the need to prevent infection. Advise her to avoid crowds and people with known infections and to consult her doctor about influenza and pneumococcal vaccines. Caution against excessive bathing because it can dry or break down the skin, leaving it vulnerable to infection. However, each day she should clean and pat dry areas where two skin surfaces touch, such as the underarm or genital areas. Tell her to regularly inspect these areas for signs of infection or skin breakdown.

Stress the importance of meticulous mouth care to prevent or treat oral lesions. She should use a soft toothbrush and avoid commercial mouthwashes because of their high sugar content and the irritating and drying effect of the alcohol base. Tell her to call her doctor if she notices white plaques in her mouth; they could indicate a fungal infection. Suggest soft, bland foods if she has open sores. Emphasize the importance of regular dental care to prevent infection.

Be sure she knows that emotional upset and stress can worsen symptoms. Advise her to maintain a calm, stable environment if possi-

S

ble. Also teach her relaxation exercises and other stress-reduction techniques.

If your patient has Raynaud's phenomenon (a common occurrence in SLE), tell her to protect her hands and feet against cold weather to prevent vasospasm. She should avoid cold water and wear gloves when handling cold items, such as frozen foods.

Explain that she may experience menstrual irregularities during flare-ups but will resume her normal cycle during remissions. Advise her to discuss contraceptive methods or pregnancy plans with her doctor. Patients often feel better during pregnancy, but flare-ups can occur postpartum.

Finally, tell your patient to call the doctor if fever, cough, or skin rash occurs, or if chest, abdominal, muscle, or joint pain worsens.

Sleep apnea

Detecting it

How can you recognize that a patient has sleep apnea? Pick up clues while taking his history. Does he complain of excessive daytime sleepiness and fatigue? Is he a restless sleeper, or does his sleeping partner complain of loud snoring alternating with periods of silence? Does he sleepwalk or experience nocturia? Or fall out of bed or wake up to find himself sitting on the side of his bed? Does he sleep upright in his bed or in a chair?

Such activities are his ways of coping with the constant threat to his airway. Sitting or standing clears obstructing tissue.

To support your patient's defenses against sleep apnea, encourage him to continue his usual behavior—such as sleeping upright. Also, be careful if you give him narcotics, sedatives, or soporifics; they can dangerously depress his arousal response.

A patient who has obstructive sleep apnea may undergo a tracheotomy to improve airway patency or surgery to remove obstructions. A patient who has central apnea may use a mechanical ventilator at night.

Sleep deprivation

Recognizing it in the ICU

When a patient doesn't get adequate sleep for 2 to 5 days, you'll start to see signs and symptoms of sleep deprivation: slurred speech, irritability, disorientation, and mood changes—listlessness one minute and combativeness the next. If sleep deprivation continues, he may have delusions and hallucinations and act psychotically. (See *Delusions; Hallucinations.*) Usually, the more sleep he loses, the more severe the signs and symptoms.

Each patient's signs and symptoms depend on the type of sleep he's missing. If he's deprived of the rapid eye movement phase of sleep, you'll probably note hyperactivity, agitation, and a decreased ability to control certain impulses. He may, for instance, lose his temper more quickly and express his anger more forcefully—perhaps by yelling, pounding his fist, or throwing something. Or he may cry more easily than usual.

If, on the other hand, a patient is deprived of the nonrapid eye movement phase of sleep, he'll probably be unresponsive, apathetic, and excessively sleepy. His face might be expressionless, and his eyelids will tend to droop.

Fortunately, the signs and symptoms of sleep deprivation usually disappear after a good night's sleep or a transfer out of the ICU. But remember that not all patients who suffer from sleep deprivation show signs and symptoms. Factors that increase the chances of a patient showing such signs and symptoms include:

• *age.* An elderly person normally takes longer to fall asleep and wakes up more often during the night, so he starts out at a disadvantage. In the ICU, he's likely to show signs and symptoms of sleep deprivation more quickly than a younger adult would.

• *psychiatric history.* Patients with a psychiatric history (such as depression, paranoid schizophrenia, or delusions) tend to show increased signs and symptoms of their illnesses. A depressed patient may cry more easily, and a paranoid patient may have increased feelings of persecution.

• *equipment.* Too many pieces of equipment in a patient's room can produce sensory overload, thus increasing confusion and disorientation.

• *severity of the illness.* The more severe a patient's condition, the more likely he'll be kept awake by pain, fear, and anxiety, as well as by continuous care (such as dressing checks). (See also *ICU noise.*)

Snakebite

When it's poisonous

If you are not close to medical care when you encounter someone bitten on the hand by a poisonous snake, this is what you should do:

• Remain calm. Move the victim and everyone else away from the area; the snake is probably still close by and may strike again.

• Tell the victim to lie down and remain as still as possible. This will help reduce lymphatic flow, which can carry the venom to the systemic circulation. Have someone call for help and tell the dispatcher the victim's age, sex, and weight; when the attack occurred; and the location and number of bites. If possible, also report the species and size of the snake.

• While waiting for help, remove rings, watch, and bracelets; they could occlude circulation if the arm swells. Tie a belt or strip of cloth 5″ to 8″ (12 to 20 cm) above the bite

S

but not around the elbow joint. This band must be tight enough to occlude superficial venous and lymphatic return but loose enough to preserve a distal pulse. You should be able to fit your finger underneath it. Once you've applied the band, don't untie it suddenly, lest the venom enter rapidly into the circulation.

If you have a snakebite kit with you, use it to incise and suction the wound, but only if less than 30 minutes have elapsed since the bite and if you know the hospital is more than 30 minutes away. Make two small, parallel cuts ¼" long and ⅛" deep, starting at the fang marks and extending downward. Pinch a small amount of skin when making each cut to prevent incising a major vessel, tendon, or muscle. Then suction with the device provided in the kit. (Suction by mouth isn't recommended because it would contaminate the wound with oral microflora.) Immobilization will help retard the spread of venom, so immobilize the arm with a splint, keeping it below the level of the heart but not in a completely dependent position. Remember to allow for swelling when applying the splint.

Don't apply ice or a cold pack. Cold could increase ischemia, making amputation necessary. And if someone suggests giving an alcoholic drink to calm the victim, don't—alcohol would enhance absorption of the venom.

If possible, measure the victim's arm circumference 4" (10 cm) and 8" (20 cm) above the bite. Recheck the measurements every 15 minutes. If they increase, you'll know the venom is spreading.

Monitor the victim's pulse and respirations, and observe for signs and symptoms of a reaction: pain, edema, bleeding, erythema, or ecchymosis. Systemic signs and symptoms, which can occur rapidly, may include nausea and vomiting, paresthesia of the mouth and scalp, twitching of the tongue and eyelids, and hypotension.

If you must move the victim again, carry him. Walking would increase absorption of the venom.

Soaks: arms and legs

Methods to use with children

When a child needs to hold a warm soak against his arm or leg, here's a quick and easy way to make one: Put the wet dressing in place and wrap a disposable diaper (absorbent side against the dressing) snugly around it. Then secure the diaper and dressing with the diaper's adhesive tabs.

The diaper will conform to any shape, shield against wetness, retain the warmth, and allow the child to move freely. You can even draw funny faces on the outside of the diaper with a felt-tip marker. (See *Soaks: hands.*)

Soaks: hands

Improvised method

In the busy emergency department, many children need to have their finger or hand wound soaked. But you may run out of basins for the soaking solution.

Use a clean plastic urine container instead. The container is transparent, so you can play finger games with the child to encourage him to move his fingers or hand for a more thorough cleaning. (See *Soaks: arms and legs.*)

Soaks: home care

Saving money

When your home care patient has to soak his hand or foot in a pre- scribed (but nonsterile) soaking solution, suggest this:

"Pour the solution into a clean plastic bag and put your hand or foot into the bag. Loosely fasten the bag with a wide strip of cloth. Place your bagged hand or foot in a bucket of warm water."

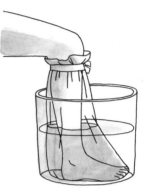

The water will not only warm the solution but also cause it to rise in the bag to the level of the water in the bucket. This way, the patient will use less solution to cover his hand or foot for each soak and will save money.

Spinal cord injury: hypotension

Minimizing risks

Complete cervical injury impairs the sympathetic nervous system, which normally compensates for position changes by regulating heart rate and blood vessel diameter. Thus, the patient loses his ability to accommodate sudden position changes, making him prone to orthostatic hypotension. When the doctor orders a sitting program, take these precautions:
• Wrap the patient's legs with Ace bandages to improve venous return. (See *Bandage, roller.*)
• Apply abdominal binding to facilitate abdominal muscle contraction and venous return.

Explain the procedure to the patient, and ask him to tell you if he starts to feel dizzy. Then, slowly raise the head of the bed—remember, he can't tolerate a rapid position change. If he reports feeling dizzy, stop the procedure until his dizziness clears up. Check his blood pressure with each elevation change. (See also *Blood pressure, orthostatic.*)

Spinal cord injury: motorcycle accident

Managing a suspected injury

Here's how to give first aid to a trauma victim you suspect has a spinal cord injury (SCI).

Suppose you're driving down the street when you see another car suddenly cut in front of a young man on a motorcycle. The cyclist brakes hard to avoid a collision, but his bike rams the car's rear bumper. He's hurled through the air and lands on his back in the middle of the street. A person who suffers a SCI has about one chance in two of walking again *if* he gets proper care in the first hour, so you need to act quickly.

1. Before approaching the victim, inspect the scene for hazards, such as traffic, downed electrical wires, fire, or gasoline leaks. Keep in mind that your safety comes first. You can't help a victim if you're injured. If you can approach the scene, turn off the motor of his vehicle.

Sometimes, it may be safe for you to approach the victim, but he may be in danger—for instance, if he's lying in the middle of the street. In such cases, you must weigh the risks of treating the victim where he is against the risks of moving him. Remember, in a rescue situation, there are no hard-and-fast rules, just many judgment calls.

2. If possible, approach the victim from behind his head. Approaching him from the side may cause him to turn his head to look at you. If you can't approach him from behind, say, "Keep your head still as I speak to you." If possible, lift his helmet face plate so you can observe his face.

Note whether he's conscious and breathing. If he is, immobilize the cervical spine by placing your hands on the sides of his head and spreading your fingers as wide as possible. Usually, you should try to align the neck in the neutral position. But in some cases, you may have to immobilize it in the position in which you find it.

Immobilizing the cervical spine

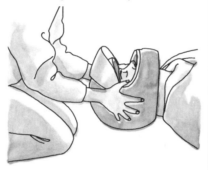

If the victim appears unconscious, quickly check his airway by looking and listening for respirations. Then assess his breathing by observing his chest to see if it's rising and falling. Note the depth, pattern, and rate of respirations. If you see abdominal respirations and diminished chest movement, suspect a cervical spine injury. If the victim isn't breathing, perform rescue breathing. (See *CPR: technique.*) Even if he appears unconscious, introduce yourself and tell him what you're doing.

If you're the only trained person at the scene, maintain cervical spine immobilization and airway patency. As other people arrive, direct someone to contact the emergency medical service (EMS) and have the others assist as needed.

If you suspect a cervical spine injury, don't remove the helmet because of the risk of further cervical damage. Only remove it when the victim's airway is obstructed, when you suspect respiratory difficulty may develop, or when you see evidence of severe bleeding under the helmet.

3. If another rescuer is immobilizing the cervical spine, check the victim's airway and breathing again. Then palpate his carotid pulse. Assess his level of consciousness. Ask him his name, where he is, and what happened. Also ask him what time, day, and year it is. If he answers appropriately, you know his cerebral function is intact.

4. Inspect his head and neck for signs of trauma, such as contusions, bulging neck veins, or brachial deviation. Look for dents in the helmet. Also, observe for blood-tinged cerebrospinal fluid coming from the nose (and the ears, if the helmet is off). Reassure the victim and explain what you're doing as you assess him.

5. Check for impaired motor function by telling him to squeeze and release your hand. Then ask him to move his toes and fingers.

6. Apply enough pressure at various points on his body to stimulate sensory function. Ask if he feels anything. He may feel pain to the touch or complain of warmth, burning, or tingling. Whether you detect any of these symptoms or not, continue treating the trauma victim as though he had a spinal cord injury. Also, check his skin temperature. If his skin is cold and clammy, he may be in shock from bleeding. Cover him immediately. (See *Shock: intervention.*)

With a trauma victim, there's always a risk of vomiting and aspiration. If you see that he's going to vomit, logroll him to one side and immobilize him in that position if possible. If he can't be turned, use your finger to clear his mouth of vomitus and keep his airway patent.

7. Palpate the victim from head to toe, checking for other injuries.

S

If you don't detect a fracture or if the victim is moving his legs, straighten them. If you suspect a fracture or dislocation, report it to the emergency medical technicians (EMTs) when they arrive. Don't try to splint the fracture yourself unless you have the proper equipment and the EMTs won't be arriving right away. What you want to do is keep the victim as still as possible. And the fracture itself will help you. Because of the pain, the victim will be reluctant to move.

If he needs help and you're the only one on the scene, you may have to leave him to call the EMS. However, never leave a victim who's in acute distress. If you think it's safe to leave him for a short time, explain that you must go for help. Then tell him to stay still, pace his breathing with slow, deep breaths, and wiggle his toes or fingers for circulation. Assure him that you'll return as soon as possible.

8. As you wait for the EMTs to arrive, cover the victim with a blanket. Also, place rolled-up towels, scarves, or other suitable material at the sides of his helmet to help immobilize his head and neck.

9. When the ambulance arrives, give the EMTs a brief report on the victim's status; be sure to note his level of consciousness. They may call for a helicopter to speed the transfer. A helicopter also provides a smooth ride—a key consideration for a victim who may have a spinal cord injury.

10. The EMTs will usually apply a rigid cervical collar. Depending on the type of helmet the motorcyclist is wearing, the EMTs may have to remove it before they can apply a collar. If so, one EMT will kneel behind the victim's head with his hands on the sides of the helmet.

11. The second EMT should kneel beside the victim, remove the towels from the sides of the helmet, and unfasten the helmet strap. Next, he should place one hand on the victim's mandible, with his thumb on one side and fingers on the other. Then he should place his other hand at the level of the occiput and hold the victim's head with his fingers.

12. The second EMT should maintain in-line immobilization as the first EMT slowly removes the helmet. He'll raise it, expand it laterally to clear the ears, then slide it out from under the victim's head.

Removing the helmet

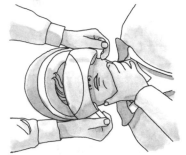

Removing the helmet may not be easy—especially if it's a full-coverage type. A helmet fits snugly even under normal conditions; with blood and sweat underneath it, the fit will be even tighter.

13. Once the first EMT has removed the helmet, he should relieve the second EMT by placing his hands on the sides of the victim's head and spreading his fingers. He shouldn't let the victim's head rest on the ground. From this position, the first EMT should be able to assess for bilateral chest movement, spontaneous limb movement, and any unusual posturing.

14. While the first EMT maintains in-line immobilization, the second EMT should apply an appropriate cervical immobilization device.

15. Now, you and the other rescuers should logroll the victim onto a spine board and secure him to it. One rescuer should place the spine board next to the victim, while two rescuers kneel on the other side of him.

16. When the EMT who's maintaining in-line immobilization counts to three, the rescuers should slowly logroll the victim to minimize any movement of the spine.

17. The rescuer with the spine board should slide it under the victim.

18. On the count of three, the rescuers should logroll him onto the spine board, secure the straps, then

Victim on spine board

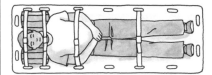

place a folded towel under his head to fill the space between the occiput and the board. Blanket rolls or cervical immobilization devices should be applied to prevent lateral movement. When this is done, the rescuer who's maintaining cervical immobilization can remove his hands from the victim's head.

19. When the helicopter arrives, the EMTs should give a member of the flight crew a brief report on the victim's status. The EMTs and flight crew may also apply an oxygen mask and administer I.V. fluids.

20. The rescuers should then transport the victim to the helicopter.

21. A member of the flight crew should radio the base to give an estimated time of arrival. The trauma team at the hospital will be alerted that the victim is coming. On arrival, he'll undergo X-rays and computed tomography scans. If necessary, he'll have surgery or his cervical spine will be stabilized with a device such as a halo vest. (See *Halo vests.*)

Spinal cord injury: pool victim

Emergency technique

Today, there are more health spas, indoor swimming pools, and backyard pools than ever before. And that means you're more likely to see a water-related injury—no matter what time of year it is.

How should you respond to a water-related injury, such as a diving accident? As a nurse, your first instinct would be to help. But as with any emergency, you should assess the scene before you try to rescue the victim. The first question in *any* water rescue is: Do you have to go in the water to help the victim? Can you throw him something he can float on—an inner tube, a life jacket, or a beach ball? Or maybe he's close enough that you can hold out a pole for him to grab.

Next, you want to determine whether the water is safe for you. If you're at a pool and the victim is facedown in shallow water (that is, water you can wade in), you can go in without endangering yourself. But even if you're a good swimmer, other situations can pose great dangers. If you're at a seashore or lake, for instance, you may have to contend with a strong undertow, rough waves, cold water, unknown water depth, or submerged objects. And, of course, the victim himself can pose a hazard if he's thrashing about.

If you cannot attempt a rescue, carefully note the victim's location before going to contact the emergency medical service (EMS). You might estimate distance and direction from a landmark on shore. Or perhaps you can mark his position with a flotation device. If he sinks, a landmark or marker will help the rescuers to concentrate on a small search area.

Cervical spine injuries

Among the most common injuries resulting from water-related accidents are spinal cord injuries (SCIs). They typically occur when someone dives into shallow water and hits his head on the bottom. The impact causes extreme hyperextension or flexion of the cervical

spine. Almost 97% of all diving-related SCIs involve the cervical spine.

Anytime you find an unresponsive victim in the water, assume he has an SCI. Also, consider that he may have been in the water for a long time, may have suffered a head injury or another traumatic injury besides an SCI, and may be hypothermic or in shock. Head or facial bruises or a loss of motor or sensory function should also make you suspect an SCI.

Any conscious victim who doesn't try to swim, tread water, or even thrash about is probably paralyzed. But movement doesn't rule out an SCI. Remember that someone with an incomplete SCI may be able to move for a short time after the accident.

Taking charge

During a rescue, carefully plan your moves and those of the other rescuers. Tell them and the victim exactly what you want them to do.

If the victim is facedown in the shallow end of a pool, the first thing you want to do is to turn him over, using the proper technique. Next, support his head and neck as another rescuer checks his ABCs—airway, breathing, and circulation. Then you and the other rescuers will place a spine board under him and pull him to the side of the pool.

You'll find that even the heaviest victims are easy to move in the water because they'll float. In fact, obese victims tend to float more easily because adipose tissue is buoyant. Muscular or thin victims don't float as well.

The following instructions will tell you how to rescue an SCI victim who's facedown in the shallow end of a pool. To learn deep-water rescue techniques, we recommend that you take an American Red Cross lifesaving course.

1. If the victim is within range of your voice, tell her that you're a nurse and you can help. Try to calm her by giving simple instructions

such as, "Relax and let your body float." Reassure her that you'll get her out of the water as soon as possible. Send a bystander to contact the EMS.

2. Because the victim may not be able to grab a flotation device or reach for a pole, you'll have to go into the water to help her. Quickly check for hazards, then enter the water feet first—even when you're familiar with a pool, lake, or other swimming area.

3. Approach the victim from the top of her head. Push one of her arms down along her side so it won't hit you or the bottom of the pool when you turn her over. Now place the hand you just used on her spine. Make sure your chest or arm doesn't touch her head.

4. With your other hand, grasp her other arm just below the armpit.

5. Turn the victim faceup by lifting her arm up over her back. To minimize stress on the spine, avoid lifting her arm too high. As you turn her, use your other arm to keep her head and neck in line. You may have to move slowly backward during this maneuver to avoid touching her head with your chest.

6. With the victim faceup, put her arm in the water. Again, be careful not to touch her head.

7. Release her upper arm and place your hand on the base of her skull with your fingers spread. Support her head, being careful not to

Supporting the head

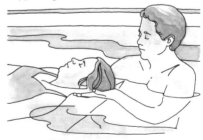

lift it. Keep your other hand in position on her back with your fingers spread.

When you find a suspected SCI victim faceup, support her using the hand positions just described.

8. If another rescuer is present and he's qualified to perform cardiopulmonary resuscitation, he should assess the victim's ABCs—airway, breathing, and circulation. If debris is in her mouth, the rescuer should use a finger sweep to remove it. If the victim isn't breathing, the rescuer should lift her chin without tilting her head, then give rescue ventilations. When the carotid pulse is absent, you and the other rescuers will have to get the victim out of the water as quickly as possible so that you can begin chest compressions on a firm surface.

9. Now, tell two rescuers to bring a spine board toward the victim, approaching her from the side. At least three rescuers (including you) are needed to float the board under the victim and position her on it. This board will support her and keep her head above water.

10. The two rescuers should tilt the board and push the foot of it underwater first. Then they should slide the board under the victim without letting it touch her.

11. The rescuers should position the midline of the board under the victim's spine. Have one rescuer stand on one side of the board and the other rescuer on the opposite side. Now, they should allow the board to rise under the victim. Tell them to center the victim on the board by guiding the board as it rises, *not* by moving the victim.

Victim on spine board with neck immobilized

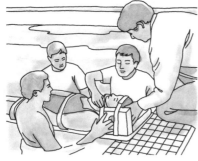

12. As the head of the board reaches the victim's head, slide your hands out from under her. Then stabilize her cervical spine by placing your hands on the sides of her head.

13. The other rescuers should strap her to the spine board. Then the three of you can float her to the side of the pool.

14. When the emergency medical technicians (EMTs) arrive, give them a brief report on the victim's condition. Then the EMTs and initial rescuers should apply a cervical collar and a cervical immobilization device.

15. At least four rescuers should carefully remove the victim from the water. Vomiting is common among near-drowning and head-injury victims, so the rescuers must be prepared to turn the spine board if she vomits.

16. Once the victim is out of the water, the EMTs will assess her condition. Then they may give her oxygen and warm her with a rescue blanket, such as a Mylar wrap.

17. The rescuers should then place the victim on a litter and take her to the ambulance so that she can be transported to the nearest emergency department.

When you're the only rescuer

What if you're alone and the victim isn't breathing? How do you support her and give rescue breaths by yourself? Here's what we recommend:

1. After you turn the victim over, quickly check whether she's breathing. If she isn't, float her to the side of the pool, keeping one hand under her back and the other hand under

One-rescuer breathing and back support

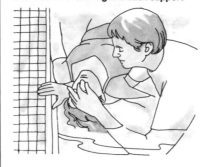

the base of her skull (as described in Step 7).

2. Position her between you and the side of the pool. Then support her by sliding one arm under her neck and shoulders and grasping the side of the pool.

3. Use your other hand to pinch her nostrils shut so that you can give rescue breaths. Periodically, yell for help.

Spiritual comfort

How to help the patient attain it

The patient or his family might ask for your help in arranging certain religious rituals. This may entail some bending of hospital rules.

Don't hesitate to pray with the patient and his family if you feel it's appropriate, even if they're of another faith. Remember, despite different rituals, languages, and customs, our basic spiritual questions and needs are the same. But be careful not to impose your own prayers or rituals. People in spiritual pain need understanding, not preaching.

What if the patient and his family have no faith? Then try to reinforce the things that have sustained them during difficult times—for example, a love of reading or music—and try to let them know you're standing by to help.

Perhaps a disease can't be cured or an accident reversed. But helping the patient (or his family) accept what seems unacceptable or meaningless can give you a sense of accomplishment.

Spirituality

Assessing your patient's needs

When a person needs spiritual comfort, you might try a "spiritual assessment" first. These questions can help you probe three basic aspects of a person's spirituality: religion, meaning, and hope.

Religion

"Do you belong to any specific religion or faith community?

"Is God or religion significant to you? If so, how?

"Is prayer, scripture, music, or reading helpful?

"Are any particular religious practices helpful to you?

Meaning

"How has your illness affected your feelings about God, faith, and yourself?

"What has bothered or upset you the most about being sick?

Hope

"Who (or what) is most helpful to you when you need hope?

"What helps you the most when you feel afraid?

"Do you have any particular hopes or fears?

"Do you have any unfinished business?"

A thorough assessment may take more time than your work load permits. But you can at least find out if spirituality is important to the patient and if he wants to talk to someone—a counselor or another nurse who is comfortable with the subject. (See also *Spiritual comfort.*)

Splenectomy

Preventing postop complications

If your patient has had a splenectomy, your primary responsibility is to watch for signs and symptoms of infection. His temperature may run as high as 100.9° F. (38.3° C.) for 10 days after the surgery. If it goes any higher, that may indicate infection. Watch for chills and a pulse rate over 100 beats/minute.

Also check for adventitious breath sounds and cloudy or foul-smelling urine. Note any complaints of frequency, urgency, or burning on urination. If the patient's skin has a break, inspect it closely for redness, swelling, or unusual drainage. And look for irritation or ulceration inside his mouth.

Closely monitor all laboratory test results. Watch for an elevated white blood cell count and any white blood cells and bacteria in the urine. Report these findings immediately. If ordered, obtain culture specimens of wounds, urine, vaginal and oral secretions, sputum, or blood.

To reduce the risk of infection, make sure the patient maintains a fluid intake of at least 2,500 ml daily, unless contraindicated. Use good hand-washing technique and encourage the patient to do the same. Meticulous aseptic technique during invasive procedures, such as catheterizations, venous and arterial punctures, and injections, will also help minimize infection. Make sure the patient doesn't come into contact with other patients who have infections.

To prevent respiratory tract infection, help the patient turn, cough, and deep-breathe at least every 2 hours if his mobility is limited. And he should use an incentive spirometer just as frequently. (See *Incentive spirometry: adults.*)

Watch for signs of pancreatitis in case the patient's pancreas was injured during the splenectomy—abdominal pain extending to his midepigastric area or back, for example, and possibly increased upper left quadrant pain, fever, or hypotension. (See *Pancreatitis.*)

The patient who has persistent abdominal pain, fever, and an increased pulse rate may have a subphrenic abscess. If so, the doctor will incise the abscess and drain it. Peritonitis is another possible complication. Watch for its usual signs and symptoms: fever, rigid abdomen, severe abdominal pain, rebound tenderness, failure of bowel sounds to return to normal, tachycardia, tachypnea, and decreased blood pressure. (See *Peritonitis.*)

Monitor the patient's platelet count. If it rises above 500,000 mm³,

report the finding. Also report an elevated red blood cell count. Both these findings indicate that the patient is at risk for thromboembolism. Note increasing abdominal distention and pain that may indicate portal system thrombus or mesenteric embolism.

Splenomegaly

How to palpate for it

Detecting splenomegaly requires skillful and gentle palpation to avoid rupturing the enlarged organ. Follow these steps carefully:

• Position the patient supine and stand at his right side. Place your left hand under the left costovertebral angle and push lightly to move the spleen forward. Then press your right hand gently under the left front costal margin.

• Have him take a deep breath and then exhale. As he exhales, move your right hand along the tissue contours under the ribs' border, feeling for the spleen's edge. The enlarged spleen should feel like a firm mass that bumps against your fingers. Remember to begin palpation low enough in the abdomen to catch the edge of a massive spleen.

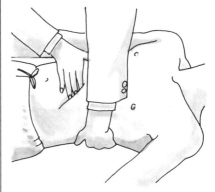

• Grade the splenomegaly as slight (1 to 4 cm below the costal margin), or great (8 cm or more below the costal margin).

• Reposition the patient on his right side with his hips and knees flexed slightly to move the spleen forward. Then repeat the palpation procedure. (See also *Abdominal exam: palpation; Palpation.*)

Splints

Preventing skin irritation

A patient with arthritis or carpal tunnel syndrome who must wear a wrist splint may suffer skin irritation or breakdown under the splint. You can prevent this with a pair of cotton knee socks.

Cut off the toe and make a hole in the heel of each sock. Slip the sock over the patient's hand; put his

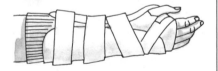

thumb through the hole in the heel and his fingers through the hole in the toe. Then apply the splint.

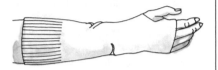

The cotton will absorb perspiration better than knit material or a stockinette. And if you make two protectors from one pair of socks, the patient will always have one to wear while the other's being washed.

Sprains: ligaments

Patient-teaching strategies

Athletic patients don't always heed warnings about resting their sprained ligaments to give them time to heal. So use a teaching aid to help them understand why proper healing needs to takes place.

Use a ½"-wide rubber band with a small cut in the edge to represent a sprained ligament in the ankle. Show your patient that when you

stretch the rubber band, it tears even more—just as a ligament will if overstretched by moving the foot.

This demonstration will show your patient how his ligament will have trouble healing unless he stops exercising for a few days.

Sputum collection: suctioning

Getting enough specimen into the container

When you can't get enough sputum by normal suctioning, try using nonbacteriostatic normal saline solution. You can either instill it into the patient's trachea or rinse the catheter with it. Most microbiology laboratories will allow these techniques so that an adequate specimen can be obtained.

If the laboratory you use doesn't allow these techniques (or your patient's a child), try this: Cut off the top of the suction catheter, using a sterile pair of scissors. Then drop the tip into the specimen cup and

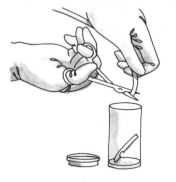

send it to the laboratory. The laboratory technicians can use the tip to inoculate the culture.

Staff management: communication

Helpful techniques

Most supervisors prepare and practice for formal communications. But

when it comes to informal communications—talking to a staff member about her behavior, for example—most supervisors jump right in, unprepared.

If you fit this pattern, try these three steps for better informal communications.

1. Describe the situation that's upsetting you in specific, nonjudgmental terms. Say, "You were late three times last week," not "You're always coming in whenever you please."

2. Describe your reaction to the behavior instead of your interpretation of it. Tell her, "I'm upset by your lateness," not "You're rude, and you obviously don't care about the rest of the staff."

3. Explain exactly what you want. Say, "I'd like you to be here promptly at 6:45 every day next week," not "If you ever come to work late again, you've had it."

Staff management: group dynamics

Getting support from your staff

To rebuild self-confidence, here's a simple and effective technique.

Start an appreciation circle by asking staff to stay an extra 5 minutes after report. Tell them you've noticed that everyone always seems too busy to support each other. Ask

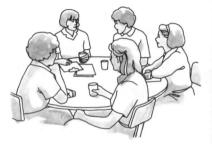

them to try an experiment for the next 2 weeks: Every day after report, go around the group quickly, each person saying something positive about the person to her right.

No one should lie or criticize. At the end of the 2 weeks, you'll all decide whether the appreciation circle has increased your self-confidence and improved unit morale.

Some people will find an excuse not to stay the first day. The second day, some of those people will decide to stay after all—out of curiosity. They'll want to know what good thing someone might say about them. As the days go by, more and more people will stay. And as each person learns what others like about her, she'll feel better about herself, her job, her co-workers, and her profession.

By looking for and finding the good qualities in each other, you'll find yourselves more willing to support each other. As you all feel more valued, you'll begin to trust your own judgment more. (See *Communication: group.*)

Staff management: hiring

Choosing the right people

You can never be absolutely sure that you're choosing the best person for the job. But by following these guidelines you'll have a better chance of doing so:

1. Identify the successful nurses in your hospital. Describe why they're successful, and list the job criteria that led to their success.
2. Screen resumés against those criteria.
3. Interview each candidate for a first impression. (See *Interviewing technique.*)
4. Test each candidate to measure her skills, if necessary.
5. Check references.
6. Hold another interview to check your original impression. Then, make your decision.
7. If the person you hire doesn't meet your expectations, review your decision. The next time, you'll have a better idea of what to look for in a candidate.

Staff management: leadership

Using your influence wisely

Whether you're a new staff nurse or a seasoned manager, your position in the hospital hierarchy gives you authority over some other people. But don't be tempted to use that power to dominate or control. Instead, focus on positive ways to influence your subordinates.
• Promote others' growth. Guide your subordinates' development by clearly indicating your expectations so they don't waste time guessing what you want. Praise them often, and offer constructive criticism when appropriate. Encourage their creativity and commitment to their work by letting them have some say about their job goals. As they grow, so does your power.
• Delegate your authority. Because you have a limited amount of time and energy to do your job, assign tasks to subordinates. When you learn to delegate effectively, your power increases because you're better able to use the available resources to meet your goals.
• Set personal restrictions. To maintain a power position with your subordinates, keep relationships on a professional level. Watch the amount of personal information you share with subordinates, and avoid social relationships, which can weaken your authority. Don't eliminate friendly interactions, just limit them to the workplace. (See *Leadership skills; Leadership strategies.*)

Staff management: morale

Improving attitudes

If you're a savvy nurse-manager, you know that quality patient care can be directly related to high morale and motivation among your nursing staff. Here's what's important for you to do:
• Give your staff a chance to use a wide range of nursing skills.
• Assign your nurses to meaningful roles in projects.
• Whenever possible, allow them to choose how to do their assigned tasks.
• Most important, work with your staff to create an atmosphere of open communication and innovative nursing practice. (See *Staff management: motivation.*)

Staff management: motivation

Getting your staff to do their best

Communication provides the groundwork for successful motivation. For example, *listening* shows people that you care about them—that you want to find out what will increase their satisfaction and comfort. (See *Listening to co-workers.*) Also, pay special attention to *talking*, making sure that everything you say (to individuals, to the staff as a group, even for grapevine consumption) is informative and clear.

Staff members who have a voice in decision making on the unit will usually be motivated to support the final outcome. So, include all appropriate staff members in decisions that would affect them and their patients.

Positive reinforcement strengthens behavior, including motivation. And this is the heart of a positive motivational style: meeting staff members' personal needs for recognition of their achievements and increased self-worth. The rewards needn't always be monetary; recognition and praise can be equally effective. (See *Staff management: morale.*)

S

Staff management: negative behavior

Making it positive

Every leader knows how devastating one nurse's negative behavior can be. But you can counter this behavior.

1. *Be positive and enthusiastic yourself.* Don't let people resign themselves to having a busy, frustrating day. Tell your staff, "Yes, we'll have a busy day, but we'll manage."

Get others involved and committed to the group's goals by asking for their suggestions. When people are actively involved in a project, they're much more committed to it. So encourage your staff to contribute ideas at meetings, and ask for ideas on a one-on-one basis.

2. *Be daring.* If you're in a new supervisory position, use your "newness" to ask questions. Many times, you'll find staff members gasping, "I can't believe she asked that." But when you're learning, you can risk asking questions no one else dares to ask. You'll be "forgiven" more easily than experienced managers, and you'll find out a lot about your staff's needs.

3. *Delegate.* Ask, "Are you interested in this? Would you be willing to try this?" This will give you more free time. And it'll give your staff decision-making power and confidence that they can handle what needs to be done.

4. *Build on others' strengths.* Nothing destroys individual morale quicker than ignoring a staff member's strengths. If patients rave about a nurse's bed baths, don't assign her to retrieve lab reports during morning care. If a staff nurse learns new skills quickly, ask her to teach other staff nurses.

5. *Give positive feedback immediately.* If a staff nurse leads a productive meeting, compliment her on the spot. If a team member comforts a distraught patient, thank her and tell others about her accom-

plishment. Let your staff know you appreciate their accomplishments now.

6. *Finally, put your energy where it will get the most results.* Don't waste 90% of your time and effort trying to change a long-standing problem. Put 10% of your energy there, then concentrate the other 90% on things you can change in a shorter period.

Staff management: orientation

A scavenger hunt to familiarize new staff

Here's a tip to help orient new staff members to the hospital: Stage a scavenger hunt. Make a list of important places and items in the hospital, such as the emergency and pharmacy departments, fire exits, crash carts, I.V. poles, suction equipment, and flashlights. Ask new employees to take a few minutes each day to search for the places and items on the list. As they find each item, they should note its location or some identifying information and check it off the list.

Orientation to unit

1. Crash cart *Nurse's station* ☑
2. Fire exits *Hallway* ☑
3. Suction equipment *Utility room* ☑
4. I.V. poles *Utility room* ☑
5. Flashlights *Medication room* ☑

Also tell them to keep the lists as a reference to use later so that they'll feel sure they know their way around the hospital.

Staff management: problem employee

Helpful techniques

What do you do when you have a subordinate who doesn't listen, un-

dermines authority, or creates problems? Check your hospital's policy on disciplinary steps to follow. Then consider this plan for *progressive* discipline.

1. *Give an oral warning.* Set a time and place to meet privately with the nurse to discuss the problem. Cite specific examples of her problematic behavior, and explain the impact it has on the unit. Tell her that you've counseled her about the problem before and that you're now giving her an oral warning: If her behavior doesn't change, you'll give her a written warning that will also be placed in her personnel file. Encourage her to change her behavior before the situation reaches that point. Make a note of the discussion and keep it with her records.

2. *Give a written warning.* If she doesn't heed oral warnings, document her behavior in a written warning. Meet with her to give her the written warning and to discuss the situation again. Have specific documentation of any incidents. Send a copy of the warning to your immediate supervisor, place a copy in the employee's personnel file, and keep a copy for your records.

3. *Remember the appeal process.* She can take advantage of the appeal process if she thinks you've treated her unfairly. At any point in the disciplinary process, she has a right to take the issue to the hospital grievance board. If the hospital doesn't have such a board and you're blocked in the negotiations, suggest bringing in an impartial third party to evaluate the situation.

4. *Set a penalty.* If her behavior doesn't change, meet with the director of nursing to check the hospital's policy for this stage of the disciplinary process. Let's say the policy recommends suspension without pay for a period of time that you recommend. You and the director might decide that 2 weeks' suspension without pay is a fair penalty.

If the hospital doesn't have a policy, assess the severity of the unacceptable behavior, then apply an appropriate penalty.

But don't be surprised if the nurse hands in her resignation before you have the follow-up meeting. Many problem employees know when you mean business and give up the fight once there's a showdown.

5. *Terminate the employee.* Termination is always an option, and it's obviously the most drastic step. It's usually the last in a series of attempts to make the employee conform to standards. Sometimes, however, behavior is so blatantly unacceptable that it warrants immediate termination. Stealing and patient abuse are examples.

Don't be surprised if the problem employee expresses relief after being fired. Many such employees say, "I'm glad it's over."

When using progressive discipline, you may skip some steps, combine some, or go directly to termination.

Whatever disciplinary action you take, it won't be easy for you. But to be fair to everyone involved, if you follow an employee in a progressive way, you strengthen your chances of remedying problematic behavior. And whether or not your efforts are successful, at least you'll have the satisfaction of knowing that you really tried. (See *Legal risks: wrongful discharge.*)

Staff management: problem solving

A systematic approach

First, be sure at the outset that you *have* a problem, that you have the *right* problem, and that it's *your* problem.

To identify the problem accurately, ask the following questions:
• Does a problem exist?
• Why is the problem a problem? Is it interfering with patient care? Causing staff conflict? Causing new problems?

• Can change make the situation better? If so, who would benefit: the patient, the family, the hospital, or you?
• Is change possible?
• Do you have the people and the resources to help you?
• Does the problem rate a high priority? (To answer this one, you should ask: What will happen if there's no effort to change?)

Assessing the problem in depth
You may find it hard to determine the cause of the problem. Therefore, identify as many conditions relating to the problem as you can. At the same time, probe for what you think could be a starting point for its resolution.

Try to restate the problem in simple, objective terms. If it seems too big to handle as one problem, break it down into smaller problems. Then think of resolving each problem one at a time.

Establishing goals
Try to establish two goals: one, an ideal goal—which might never be reached—and two, a more realistic goal you'd be willing to settle for.

A problem rarely has only one solution. So list all the solutions you can think of—even a few that seem absurd. Now analyze the pros and cons of each until you decide which is most likely to work. Here are some tips to consider:
• Involve a group. The staff members are far more likely to support an idea or plan they've helped to create. In working cooperatively with the group, focus on everybody's participation and contribution.
• Sell your ideas. Support at the administrative level is necessary for the problem-solving process to work. So before you get too far into the project, solicit the endorsement of key management people. Once you have that, the group can proceed more securely and can benefit from the administration's ability to clear away bureaucratic underbrush.
• Determine whether the timing's right for what you're trying to do.

New regulations and restrictions, current hospital politics, or the economic climate can make the finest plans and ideas unworkable for that moment.

Put your plan on paper; that will clarify your own thinking, give you direction, and serve as your documentation—if it's ever called for. It'll also serve as a touchstone to show your progress when you get discouraged.

When you reach the deadline agreed upon at the outset, acknowledge that you're finished. Assess whether you've succeeded partially, totally—or not at all. Whatever the outcome, write down and file recommendations for future action so that groups coming after you can benefit from your groundwork.

Staff management: professionalism

Strategies to increase it in your staff

If you're a manager, try these methods to encourage your staff to be more professional and increase their knowledge:

1. *Set formal learning goals and plans for each nurse.* Write a learning contract that reinforces both the nurse's goals and yours.

2. *Hold weekly case management sessions.* Call a meeting with your staff and ask one nurse to explain a problem she's having with a patient, much as she would in a patient care conference. But don't focus on the patient's illness—focus on the nurse's response and her ability to deal with him. Then help her identify the principal cause behind the problem and possible solutions.

3. *Build learning sequences.* You probably already use basic learning sequences like orientation programs and preceptorships. But you can improve these methods and develop some of your own programs if you know what skills you want to reinforce.

S

4. *Conduct forums.* Programs for all nurses—regardless of levels or units—reduce our tendency to become too specialized and to forget about other nurses and units in the hospital. Forums also help spread news, foster participative problem solving, and develop pride among all nurses in the hospital. Typical formats include lectures, panels, and case studies. Topics can include primary nursing, accountability, peer support, or research. (See also *Professionalism.*)

Staff management: staffing

Guidelines for managers

If you're a manager, understaffing means double trouble: First, you have to deal effectively with today's understaffing problems; second, you have to minimize future problems with careful planning. Take these steps:
• Try to get help immediately. Your options include employing temporary agency nurses, floating nurses from other units, or asking nurses to work overtime.
• Note all your requests for additional staffing in a log or diary. Then, if a patient's injured and a question about staffing arises in court, your lawyer can use the log to show that you tried to staff the unit properly.
• Visit the understaffed unit and assess the situation. Work with the charge nurse, and set priorities for the staff.
• Pitch in as needed. Even if you don't stay on the unit for the entire shift, return periodically to make sure that the staff is concentrating on high-priority tasks.

Advance planning

To avoid having to deal with understaffing daily, plan ahead with these strategies:
• When interviewing a prospective employee, tell her frankly how staffing problems could affect her. For example, explain that you may expect her to work longer shifts occasionally. Then assess her response. If she seems inflexible or resents being asked, you probably won't be able to count on her in a staffing crunch.
• Orient each new employee to at least two units—the one she was hired for and another unit (preferably one she chooses). You can then avoid floating a nurse to an unfamiliar unit. Remember, if you float a nurse to a unit where she has no experience, you could share liability with her if she inadvertently harms a patient. (See *Job assignments.*)
• To reduce the risk for errors, assign less crucial tasks to floating nurses; let the unit's regular staff handle specialized work.
• For efficiency, assign an agency nurse to a fully staffed unit, then float a staff RN from that unit to an understaffed unit. The staff RN will probably be more helpful in the understaffed unit—especially if she's been oriented in advance.
• Prepare a small group of nurses to act as troubleshooters. Orient them to different types of units throughout the hospital so that they can float at a moment's notice.
• Assess all nursing responsibilities, and assign those that don't require special training to LPNs, nursing assistants, or volunteers. Encourage nursing administrators to hire more unlicensed professionals and to delegate responsibilities to them as well. (See *Legal risks: understaffed unit; Staff management: understaffed unit.*)

Staff management: supervision

Ensuring equality among employees

If you're supervising a member of a minority group, these guidelines will help you be fair.

1. Don't let minority stereotypes affect your expectations. Be sensitive to your own prejudices so as to not let them affect your ensuring equality. Give your staff member the benefit of the doubt, and expect the best.

2. Don't treat minority staff members differently. Even if your intentions are good, special treatment can backfire: The rest of your staff nurses may resent your behavior and question your motives. And they may exclude the minority nurse from unit activities.

3. Don't play the "some of my best friends are..." game. Such disclosures are unnecessary, and they'd probably be met with skepticism.

4. Don't overreact if you're charged with mistreatment or discrimination. That would make matters worse. Instead, review the situation carefully. Make sure you know what the staff member's alleging. Then report the situation to your director of nursing for her advice and direction. In many cases, problems result from simple misunderstandings that can be corrected easily.

5. Monitor the minority staff member's progress as you would any other employee. All employees need feedback on whether their performance is acceptable; the minority employee is no exception.

If a minority staff member's performance is below par, focus on what she's not doing as you would for any employee. Outline your unit goals and develop methods to help her meet them.

Staff management: understaffed unit

What to do when you're taking the brunt

If your manager gives you too heavy a caseload or asks you to float to an unfamiliar unit, first tell her why you're uncomfortable and ask her for more staff or a reassignment.

If she denies your request, accept the assignment but document your objection in a brief memo. Mention that when you informed your manager about the problem, she told you that she couldn't do anything about it. Then send copies of the memo to your manager's supervisor and hospital administrators, and keep a copy for your files at home.

Why go to the trouble? Imagine that one of your patients is injured because of a staffing problem. If he sues the hospital and you, your memo shows that you reported the problem to administrators, who were responsible for resolving it.

Don't misunderstand: The memo doesn't necessarily absolve you of liability—that depends on the facts. But it proves that you took steps to protect your patients from a potentially dangerous situation. That's sure to impress any jury. (See *Legal risks: understaffed unit; Staff management: staffing.*)

Staff management: unit relocation

Making the transition easier

Merging your unit with another one can be almost as unsettling as changing jobs. To make the transition easier, open the lines of communication before moving day.

• Start by calling a special meeting for staff members on both units. Ask for their ideas on how to smooth the transition, then give everyone a chance to get acquainted. Combine regular staff meetings, too, until the actual move occurs.

• Hold a separate meeting for each staff to air questions or fears. Let everyone know you'll always be available for advice or support.

• Circulate announcements, memos, and other information between the two units.

• Orient both staffs by rotating them between units, a few at a time. This will help your old staff get oriented to the new physical setup and help both staffs get used to new policies, procedures, and patients.

• Organize some informal activities—breakfast in the hospital cafeteria or a pizza party after work—so that staff members can get to know one another.

After the move, call a meeting to review what you've discussed so far and to determine how everyone's adjusting. Then hold frequent, regular meetings to discuss problems. (See also *Change.*)

Stain prevention

Using pocket savers

To protect your uniform pockets from stains and tears, make a "pocket saver" from a used I.V. bag. Cut away the bottom half of a 1,000-ml bag, then fold the cut edge inside ½″ and staple it securely. The sta-

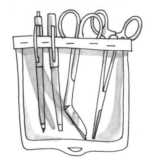

pled edge will be the top of your "pocket saver"; slip it into your pocket and use it to hold your pens, pencils, scissors, keys, money, and so on.

Stains, ink and iodine

Removing them

To remove ink stains on your uniform, spray the stained area with hair spray, then wipe it with a clean cloth. (This will also work for some felt-tip pen stains.)

For iodine stains, try dipping the affected area in milk, and rub gently. Then, machine wash. The stain will disappear after washing.

Status asthmaticus

Prediagnosis and priorities

The patient typically may have most of the signs and symptoms of an acute asthma attack:
• shortness of breath
• wheezing
• use of accessory chest muscles to breathe
• tachycardia
• tachypnea
• restlessness.

He will be treated with drugs, such as epinephrine or terbutaline, and with supplemental oxygen. (See *Asthma.*) Blood will be drawn for arterial blood gas analysis, and an I.V. line will be established. If the patient doesn't respond to the drug, this signals status asthmaticus—a severe asthma attack that's unresponsive to therapy.

If your patient's hypoxemia is severe or he has a history of cardiac disease, connect him to a cardiac monitor. Continue to administer oxygen. Expect to give aminophylline I.V., first a loading dose and then a continuous drip, to "break" his attack. Aminophylline's mechanism of action differs from epinephrine's or terbutaline's, so it may work where initial drug therapy has failed. Also expect to give corticosteroids to decrease inflammation.

Encourage your patient to drink fluids, which will help to thin mucus. However, if his breathing is so labored that he cannot drink, increase the I.V. fluid rate, as ordered. Your patient may also be started on respiratory therapy, such as mininebulizer treatments. Encourage him to breathe deeply during this therapy. He'll receive additional bronchodilators during this therapy. Expect these breathing treatments to be repeated every 4 to 6 hours.

S

STD: counseling

Helping your patient cope

If a sexually transmitted disease (STD) is diagnosed, treatment should consist of more than just a prescription for medication. You'll also need to counsel the patient about his diagnosis and treatment, teach preventive measures to reduce the chance of repeat infections, and provide follow-up care.

If you inform the patient of the diagnosis, be supportive and nonjudgmental. In many cases, he'll react with feelings of guilt, fear, or anger when he hears the diagnosis. He may even deny that he has an STD because of the effect it'll have on his relationships.

Tell him he must inform his sexual partners that they need to be examined and treated. If he asks you to help him make up an explanation about how he became infected, refuse to do so. You can't take part in deceiving his sexual partners. Instead, you should assist the patient in presenting a clear, truthful explanation and suggest family counseling, if necessary.

Give him appropriate information about the prescribed medication, including possible adverse reactions. Also, warn him not to share or save his medication.

Tell him not to engage in sexual activity until a follow-up evaluation shows that he's not contagious. If you think he won't abstain from sexual activity, explain that a condom may prevent the spread of disease. Tell him not to drink alcohol during the treatment period because it can cause genitourinary irritation. It can also interact with certain medications used to treat STDs.

Discuss preventive measures. Explain that the more sexual partners he has, the greater the chance of contracting an STD. Recommend that he avoid having intercourse with people who have many other partners. Teach him to minimize the risk of infection by washing his genitalia and voiding after sexual activity. Explain, too, that good nutrition, rest, and exercise can make him less susceptible to infection.

You may also have to report the patient's name and disease to local public health officials. (Laws concerning which diseases must be reported vary from state to state.) Of course, you'll also have the patient return for laboratory tests to ensure that he's no longer contagious.

STD: history taking

Asking the right questions

Before interviewing a patient with a suspected sexually transmitted disease (STD), find a quiet place to ensure privacy and avoid interruptions. Assure him that the interview is confidential. And remind yourself that no matter what sexual practices he discusses, you need to maintain a nonjudgmental attitude.

As you begin talking, assess his level of understanding—be sure to use terms he understands. Ask open-ended questions about the onset and course of his signs and symptoms. Sometimes neither you nor the patient will know that he has an STD when the interview begins, so be alert for clues that his signs and symptoms are sex-related. Other times the patient will withhold details because of fear, guilt, or anger. You may be able to obtain these details by repeating unanswered questions later in the interview, once you've established a rapport.

After he has described his signs and symptoms, ask if he has experienced anything like them before. Also ask if he has ever been diagnosed as having an STD. If he has, find out when. What treatment did he receive and when did he receive it?

These questions can help you identify a patient who contracts infections frequently and needs intensive preventive counseling. They'll also help you identify a patient who has had ineffective treatment. Some patients who have an STD stop taking their prescribed medication before they're cured. Others treat themselves with leftover antibiotics or home remedies before they seek medical advice.

To determine the kinds of sexual activities the patient engages in, ask direct, nonjudgmental questions. For example, you might say, "Knowing how you got this disease would be helpful. Do you ever have oral or anal sex?" Remember many types of sexual activity—including intercourse, mutual masturbation, oral sex, and anal sex—may transmit sexual disease.

When asking about the patient's sex partners, avoid questions that presume a certain answer. For instance, don't ask a man, "Who was the last woman you had sex with?" You're assuming the relationship was heterosexual and that the patient had only one partner. Instead, ask, "Who were your most recent sexual partners?" Start with these contacts and work backward in time for at least 3 months before the onset of symptoms. Remember, besides treating your patient's STD, you want to contain its spread as much as possible.

STD: physical exam

Searching for signs

When examining a patient for a sexually transmitted disease (STD), put on gloves to protect yourself and the patient. Inspect his mouth and throat for signs of infection. Then have him undress so that you can inspect the area from his abdomen to his thighs. Examine his skin for rashes, lesions, warts, drainage, or signs of trauma. Note any complaints of pain, discomfort, or itching, and look for scratches or burrows from scabies. Observe his body hair and pubic hair for lice or egg deposits, then palpate his lymph nodes for enlargement or tenderness. (See *Lymphadenopathy.*)

If the patient is a man, ask him to stand or lie supine, depending on your preference. Inspect his penis and scrotum for redness, swelling, rashes, lesions, warts, drainage, or

Genital warts

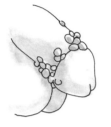

signs of trauma. To examine a woman, place her in the lithotomy position and inspect the perineal area (including the labia, clitoris, and urethra) for the same signs. Then perform a bimanual examination to check for abdominal tenderness. With all patients, obtain the appropriate diagnostic specimens.

Next, examine the patient's anus for signs of sexually transmitted diseases. A rectal culture should be done on a woman because cross-infection can result from vaginal drainage.

Steroids

Instructions for home use

If your patient will continue oral steroid therapy at home, review these important points with him before discharge:
• "Take the drug only as prescribed. Don't alter the dosage or stop taking the drug without consulting your doctor.
• "Take the drug at mealtimes or with snacks to reduce gastric irritation.
• "For alternate-day therapy (common with long-term administration), take twice the usual daily glucocorticoid dosage every other morning—preferably before 9 a.m.
• "For daily therapy, take a higher dose around 8 a.m. and a lower dose in the afternoon or evening to

mimic the body's normal cortisol secretion pattern.
• "Establish baseline blood pressure, weight, and sleep patterns, and continually assess them throughout the steroid administration period.
• "If ordered, eat a high-potassium, low-sodium diet.
• "Notify the doctor if your disease worsens or you undergo severe stress, such as from infection or injury. He may need to adjust your drug dosage.
• "If you have diabetes mellitus, expect the doctor to closely monitor your blood and urine glucose levels.
• "Report any adverse drug reactions, such as excessive weight gain, edema, marked muscle weakness, bone pain, hypertension, depression, headache, polyuria, or infection.
• "Avoid persons with infectious diseases, and notify the doctor if you suspect you have an infection. Also, report any delayed wound healing and any vague feelings of sickness (by suppressing the immune system, corticosteroids may mask infections).
• "Obtain a medical identification bracelet (such as a Medic Alert bracelet) describing your condition, drug, and dosage.
• "Visit your doctor regularly for checkups."

Stethoscope, acoustic

What you need to do

You need a good stethoscope. Its earpieces should fit snugly but comfortably; the binaurals should be angled forward, toward your temples, so that you get the best pos-

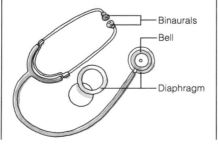

Binaurals
Bell
Diaphragm

sible sound transmission. Make sure the stethoscope has a sturdy 1″ bell and a 1½″ diaphragm. For respiratory assessment, you'll use the diaphragm, which works well for high-pitched sounds, such as breath sounds. You'll use the bell when listening for low-pitched sounds, such as the S₃ heart sound. (See *Heart exam: auscultation; Respiratory exam: auscultation.*)

Stethoscope, Doppler ultrasound

Correct technique

How many times have you been unable to detect a weak pulse you just *knew* was there or been unable to take a systolic blood pressure because the patient was obese or in shock? What you needed was a Doppler ultrasound stethoscope (DUS)—a sensitive, yet easy-to-use, noninvasive instrument that expands your powers of vascular assessment.

The DUS resembles a small transistor radio with a stethoscope headset. It's small enough to be carried in a coat pocket and weighs about 6 oz (170 g). A push button is used to turn the unit on and off, and a knob to adjust the volume.

Check the probe before using the unit to make sure it's wiped clean of old gel and dust. If you hear crackling sounds when you move the unit, it has probably been damaged and should be returned to the manufacturer for repair.

Before using it, plug the headset into one of the two output jacks located next to the volume control. Apply transmission gel either to the patient's skin or to the probe at the tapered end of the plastic case. (The ultrasound beam doesn't travel well through air, and the gel makes an airtight seal between the probe and the patient's skin.) If gel isn't available, soap and water will suffice, but the soap bubbles may create some difficulty in hearing the signals.

S

Don't use K-Y jelly, which contains salts that may damage the probe.

Hold the probe against the skin at a 45-degree angle to the blood vessel being examined. Press the *on* button. You may need to move the probe over the site and to adjust the volume to locate the vessel. Keep the probe in contact with the patient's skin, but don't apply too much pressure or you'll stop the blood flow and obliterate the signal. If this happens, apply more gel and try again with a lighter touch. When you're finished using the DUS, remove all gel from the probe so that the gel doesn't damage the surface. And, of course, remove the gel from the patient.

If the signal still isn't clear, check the unit by trying it on your own arteries. A weak sound can be due to a weak battery. Replace the battery every 6 months or sooner if the unit is used frequently. Use a standard 9-volt alkaline battery, which will last longer than an equivalent carbon-zinc battery. Write the date you replaced the battery on a small adhesive label, and stick it to the case as a reminder.

The typical signal produced by an artery is pulsatile and multiphasic. The typical signal produced by a vein is intermittent, resembles a windstorm, and varies with respirations. The venous signal may be interrupted when the patient's venous return is slowed by a deep breath or Valsalva's maneuver. Because the major arteries and veins lie close together throughout the body, you'll hear the arterial and venous signals simultaneously. You can distinguish the two because of the distinctive pulsatile or pumping quality of the arterial signal.

When arterial flow is weak, as it is distally to a partial obstruction, one or more of the signal components may be absent. Just proximal to an obstruction, the pumping arterial signal usually becomes harsh and pounding. When venous flow is

obstructed, the signal becomes loud and continuous. It does not then vary with respirations.

With a little practice, perhaps with an experienced person listening with you, you can soon learn to distinguish the various signals, just as you did in learning to use a conventional stethoscope.

If you're just learning to use the DUS, remember that the *presence* of

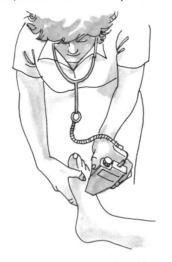

a signal doesn't necessarily mean that circulation and perfusion are adequate to maintain viable tissue. The *absence* of a signal doesn't necessarily mean that blood is not flowing through the vessel. The blood flow may not be detected because it is slower than 6 cm/second. Usually, though, the absence of a signal means that the DUS probe hasn't been positioned properly over the vessel.

Stillbirth

Helping the parents cope

Parents are apt to be unable to think clearly about what steps to take after their infant's death. Planning his funeral or putting away his clothes, for example, will be painful experiences for them; however, such experiences will allow the parents to begin the important process of grieving.

To begin with, tell the mother that if she'd like, you can have her moved from the maternity unit to a medical unit. This will relieve her of the agony of watching other couples cuddling their healthy infants. Ask the parents to think about naming the baby. This would make him real and special.

Next, suggest that they contact their spiritual advisor (or you can do it) to inquire about religious rites. (See *Spiritual comfort.*) They may not know that baptisms are now common for stillborn infants. In fact, besides the clergy, nurses can perform this ceremony, too.

Then, give them the option of planning and attending the funeral. Parents are sometimes under the impression that a stillborn infant isn't given a funeral. If they ask you about prices or funeral homes, make sure your facts are correct. If you don't know, someone from the hospital's social services department can find out.

Another important option is to dispose of the infant's things at home. A well-meaning relative may offer to do it. But the parents may regret not doing it themselves; it can help them realize their infant is dead and is a way of saying a last good-bye.

The most painful option of all is to see and touch their infant, but it may help them face the reality of his death. Even so, many parents of stillborn infants don't want to see their child. To preserve his memory, pictures should be taken of him and kept on file. Initially, the parents may not want to see them, but they may change their minds.

If the parents *do* want to see and hold their infant, you'll need to prepare them for how he may look. For example, if the infant has been dead in the womb for a week or more, the skin will be peeling around his eyes, hands, and feet. Also, the skin will be bluish instead of pink. And he may have an odor and be smaller than expected. If you wrap the infant in a blanket, with just his head showing, the parents can explore him as they wish.

Tell the parents that everything possible was done for their infant and that they're not responsible for his death. Sit when you talk to them. Encourage them to cry, express their loss, and talk. Although these emotions may make you feel uncomfortable, discouraging them will make the parents feel as if their infant never existed (so would being overcheerful or avoiding the subject in conversation). To show respect, refer to the infant by name.

Another source of comfort—maybe not now but later—is self-help support groups.

Knowing what *not* to say is as important as knowing what to say. For example, don't tell the parents, "You can have other children" or "The infant would have been abnormal anyway." The best approach is to simply express your feelings ("I'm sorry" or "I know this is a bad time for you") and offer your help ("Is there anyone I can call?" or "What can I do for you?"). (See *Death: child; Grief; SIDS.*)

Stool specimens

Making collection at home easier

When a patient complains about the difficulty and unpleasantness of collecting stool specimens at home, suggest that he drape a piece of plastic wrap over the toilet bowl (with the lid up), keeping the plastic above the water. Then suggest he tape the sides of the plastic to the outside of the bowl. The stool would then fall onto the plastic wrap, which he could easily lift off the toilet to get the specimen. The remainder of the stool could be flushed away and the wrap placed in a bag for disposal.

Strangulation

Emergency assessment and intervention

Say you're working on the acute care psychiatric unit. During rounds, you enter a patient's room and he's nowhere in sight. Then you turn toward the bathroom door and, through the open door, you see him hanging limply from the shower stall, a bed sheet tied around his neck. He's unconscious from a strangulation injury.

Until you can release the patient, you won't know the extent of his injuries. Their severity will depend on the degree of pressure on his neck and the length of time he was hanging.

A strangulation victim loses consciousness when even minimal pressure on the neck obstructs all four arteries leading to the brain. Compression will also displace the tongue and epiglottis, partially or totally obstructing his airway.

Usually, a strangulation victim's fall won't generate enough momentum to cause a cervical fracture. Still, you should suspect a fracture until you can rule it out by X-ray.

If you don't act quickly, though, your patient could suffer cardiac arrest and die from asphyxiation.

Call for help and turn on the bathroom's emergency light. You'll need at least two other people to get the patient down. In the interim, wrap your arms around his lower trunk and push up to decrease the pressure on his neck.

If you're small and can't support his weight, put a chair under his feet. Wrap one arm around his knees and lock them close to your body. With your other hand, grab the back of his gown to steady him as you push up.

When help arrives, ask one person to climb up on a chair and support the patient's cervical spine. Make sure that person keeps his head and neck in a neutral position, exerting only enough pull to take the weight of his head off the cervical spine. The third person can cut the ligature.

Support the patient's head, neck, and shoulders as you lower him to the floor. Try to position him so that his head is toward the doorway. Assess his airway and breathing. You note that his airway is clear and that he has spontaneous respirations at a rate of 16 breaths/minute. But his breathing is stridulous secondary to edema of the larynx and trachea.

Check his circulatory status. You may not be able to palpate his carotid pulse because the ligature has caused soft tissue damage to his neck. Instead, check femoral pulses and auscultate heart sounds. His pulse rate is 64.

As soon as you can safely move the patient, get him out of the bathroom so that you'll have the room—and equipment—you need to work on him. Administer 100% oxygen through a mask. (See *Airway, oropharyngeal; Breathing devices.*) Insert a cannula, and start an I.V. line at a keep-vein-open rate. Draw blood for arterial blood gas analysis. (See *Allen's test.*) Quickly assess his level of consciousness, then check for soft tissue and skeletal injuries. Report and document any other physical findings. Then transfer him to the intensive care unit.

Stress

When you feel overwhelmed

Follow these eight steps:

1. *Stop and take a few deep breaths and admit that you're feeling overwhelmed.* Acknowledging your feelings is an important step in dealing with them.

2. *Keep your sense of perspective.* You've felt overwhelmed before and survived. You'll survive this time, too.

S

3. *Make a list of your tasks and prioritize them.* Make a mental list, at least, and prioritize the urgent tasks—the ones that can't wait.

4. *Complete one task at a time.* Get moving and prepare those patients for surgery; pass medications; finish your charting. But try to think only about the task at hand. Worrying about everything else you have to do only takes up valuable time and energy you need for what you're doing now.

If a new task arises and you have to do it, add it to your list, prioritize it, and continue on. One sign of professionalism is flexibility.

5. *Ask for help.* Let's face it, you can't do everything alone. But you can't duck out during a crisis, either. So learn to ask for help. Did you ever notice the camaraderie among nurses who've learned to work together and support each other? They know how to ask each other for help.

6. *Take regular breaks from work.* Don't let yourself be bombarded all day by patients, staff, friends, family, telephones, call bells, and deadlines. A few minutes to relax over a cup of coffee or soup can make you feel better—and better able to cope.

7. *Plan ahead to save time.* Don't underestimate the time-saving value of routinely taking certain precautions, such as always checking the crash cart for supplies at the beginning of your shift. Monitor your resources so that you use them efficiently. For example, if you expect several patients back from surgery at the same time, arrange for your staff members to take their breaks before then or afterward.

8. *Learn to say no.* One of the most difficult things about being a nurse is that everyone expects a lot from you—and you expect a lot from yourself. Neighbors may insist that you comment on their medical problems; your supervisor may want you to work overtime; your spouse may ask you to entertain dinner guests; patients want you to meet their every need—and you

want to do it all. But you may become overwhelmed trying to meet everyone's expectations.

How do you say no to people you have to work with every day without offending them? Although you usually help each other, expect that once in a while you'll say no to each other—with good reason, of course. When your colleagues know they can depend on your mature judgment, saying no occasionally won't alienate them. (See *Planning, personal; Planning: priorities.*)

Stress reduction at work

Helpful techniques in your professional life

Stress is always a factor in your work, but you can minimize it with the following tips:

• *Maintain realistic expectations of your relationships on the job.* At various times in your nursing career, you may have conflicts with nursing administrators or colleagues. Remember, no person is perfect, including you. Accept other people's faults—and be kind to yourself, too.

• *Set realistic job goals.* Don't try to accomplish more than you humanly can. Pushing yourself beyond your limits will create unnecessary stress.

• *Ask for help from management.* If your job stresses are extreme and can't be reduced, you may need management's assistance.

• *Continue your education.* To keep up-to-date with the latest nursing developments, enroll in some continuing education courses that meet your needs, read professional nursing journals regularly, or get involved in a professional association. You'll gain new knowledge that you can apply to your nursing practice. And you may be relieved to discover that other nurses have the same problems and concerns you have.

• *Learn to say "no."* If you can't oblige your supervisor or a colleague who asks you to work overtime or change your days off, say no politely, and don't feel guilty about it. You're entitled to a personal as well as a professional life.

• *Look for new challenges.* If you're bored with your job, try to make it more challenging. Ask yourself how you can change it to better meet your patient's needs. Try to set new goals for yourself. If possible, assume new responsibilities.

• *Cultivate a supportive friendship or join a support group.* Discuss your concerns with understanding, supportive friends who will listen and keep the conversation confidential. This simple act can relieve much of your stress. And your friends may even suggest new ways to cope with a particularly stressful situation. Or join a nurses' support group. Most are led by a mental health specialist, a psychologist, or a psychiatrist, who guides the group in its discussions of job-related concerns.

• *Establish a "decompression routine."* Get involved in some activity right after your shift ends. This will help you forget about the job and relax before you get home. Try chatting with a friend over a cup of coffee before leaving work, or try walking home if possible. Experiment to discover what works for you.

• *Take a vacation or leave of absence.* Like anyone else, you have a limit to the amount of stress you can tolerate. Don't feel guilty about taking time off to regenerate your coping abilities.

• *Change your job.* If you've tried to deal with your job stresses constructively but have been unsuccessful, ask for a transfer to a new nursing unit, or request a shift change. Remember, prolonged excessive stress will take its toll on you as a nurse and affect the quality of your nursing care.

• *Value yourself.* You may forget that you need to care for yourself as much as for your patients. Stay alert to the warning signs of stress and burnout, and don't hesitate to do something about them. (See *Burnout; Burnout victims.*)

Stroke patients

Caring for them

Be aware of your patient's lack of proprioception when you care for him. Make sure his affected limbs are in a safe, secure position, especially when transporting him in a wheelchair or on a stretcher. When you help him walk, be sure his affected leg doesn't lag too far behind the other so that he won't trip.

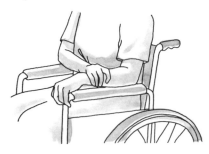

Remind him to check the positioning of his affected limbs before he moves—so he'll get into the habit of doing this when he's alone. This can spare him the embarrassment of accidentally hitting something with his arm or leg and might even save him from injury.

Strokes can rob their victims of any or all of the following sensations: pressure, touch, sharpness or dullness, heat or cold. Such sensory loss, coupled with the loss of proprioception, compounds the risk of injury for the stroke patient. You can ensure safety by keeping all potentially harmful objects away from his affected side. Be on the lookout for anything that might pose a danger to him—sources of extreme heat or cold, for example. And again, remind him of the importance of these precautions.

Stroke patients and fatigue

Helping your patients cope

Fatigue may cause a stroke patient's temper tantrums or other kinds of emotional outbursts. Fatigue can easily exacerbate a stroke patient's frustration at being unable to lift a fork to his mouth, for example, to the point where he'll push his dinner tray to the floor in anger.

To counterbalance the physically and emotionally draining experience of living with the aftereffects of a stroke, make every effort to bolster the patient's self-esteem. Praise his accomplishments, no matter how minor. For the stroke patient, pride can act like a surge of adrenaline, enabling him to surmount fatigue and push on to even greater accomplishments.

Be careful, though, not to ask too much of him. Establish goals that are realistic and short-term. Orchestrate his rehabilitation so that his progress involves a smooth, rising curve of small but consistent accomplishments, rather than erratic peaks and valleys.

Suicidal teenagers: postcrisis

Effective strategies

Clarifying what caused a teenager's suicidal feelings will allow him to focus on his main problem. Ask him what caused him to feel suicidal.

Use active listening skills to express your concern. Reflect his feelings. That will help him understand his feelings of hopelessness, helplessness, depression, fear, or ambivalence, and make them seem less overwhelming. (See *Listening to patients.*)

If you're not sure you understand his feelings, say so. Never say you

understand when you don't. If he says, "They said I was bad," ask who "they" are.

Reassure him that feelings are important and should be discussed. Encouraging discussion may also help improve his communication skills, making it easier to talk about alternative ways of coping with problems.

Explore options for dealing with problems. A hallmark of suicidal thinking is seeing "either/or" solutions—for example, "Either I pass this test or I kill myself." Your discussion may help him discover acceptable coping mechanisms.

It's better if the teenager thinks of these options himself. Finding his own solution will build his self-esteem as well as improve problem-solving skills. If you've ever had a similar problem and feel your solution might work here, offer it as a friend to a friend: "When I was in nursing school I was so afraid I'd flunk chemistry that I got a tutor. Do you think that would work for you?"

If the teenager comes up with a good solution, be sure to tell him so. But make sure you have some more. If the one solution fails, he may feel that suicide is the only option after all. If neither of you finds a solution, be honest about it. "You know, we haven't come up with a good solution yet. Let's get some help." If he sees that you're willing to ask for help, he'll understand that he can, too, and that seeking help is an acceptable coping mechanism in itself.

Minimize isolation, which is the suicidal teenager's worst enemy. Being alone or feeling that he's alone may convince him that suicide is an acceptable escape. So encourage him to talk to others about his feelings and to ask for (and accept) help.

Ask him whom he could talk with to make him feel better about himself. If he says "nobody," say, "I understand that you feel alone, but let's think again about people who care about you and want to help. What

S

about your parents, grandparents, neighbors, or teachers?"

Part of the teenager's problem may be that he can't make friends. He may say, "Can I get better by just staying home and reading books or watching TV?" Your answer should be a firm no—that being alone will only make his suicidal feelings stronger. Try to get him to discuss why socializing is so difficult. Ask him where he would find socializing most comfortable.

Finally, encourage him to seek professional counseling to prevent a recurrence. (See *Suicidal teenagers: prevention.*)

Suicidal teenagers: prevention

Implementing preventive actions

If you determine that a teenager's in immediate danger, your first concern is his safety. Stay with him until a person trained in crisis intervention arrives to help. Call for a stat psychiatric consultation and implement suicide precautions, following hospital policy. The usual precautions include:

• placing the patient in a room near the nurses' station (on the first floor, if possible)

• removing sharp and otherwise dangerous objects from the room

• inspecting the room for hidden dangerous objects (cracked windowpanes, protruding pieces of plastic or metal)

• monitoring him on a routine schedule (for example, every 15 to 30 minutes)

• observing him as he takes oral medications to ensure that he doesn't hide them in his cheek, then hoard them

• supervising his visitors if you suspect they're bringing him alcohol or drugs

• locking up his street clothes and keeping him in pajamas if you think he'll run away.

Be sure to document what you've done in the patient's care plan, and chart each time you checked on him. If he becomes more actively suicidal, arrange for continuous monitoring. Be especially watchful if he appears more energetic or less depressed; he may have made a firm decision to kill himself.

Suicidal teenagers: warning signs

Heeding them

The warning signs of an impending suicide attempt can be verbal or behavioral. To recognize them requires listening and observing. The most obvious verbal messages are such comments as "I'm just a burden to everyone," "I don't deserve to live," or "My parents will be sorry when I go to sleep and don't wake up again."

Behavioral clues may take more time to recognize. A teenager may daydream in front of a window, give away prized possessions, even tie a call bell cord around his neck for a "laugh." Or he may develop insomnia or anorexia, become withdrawn, or have trouble concentrating on what you're saying. While these behaviors may not always indicate an impending suicide attempt, they do warrant investigation, especially if they're markedly different from previous behaviors.

When you observe such clues, consider them a cry for help. Don't be afraid to explore the teenager's feelings, and don't be placated by a response that "everything is fine."

Consider asking about suicidal thoughts as part of your overall assessment—a step as basic as taking a pulse or temperature. If a teenager isn't suicidal, asking about suicide will not give him the idea to try it. But not asking may make a suicidal teenager feel even more hopeless and alone.

Suicide threats

When a patient threatens to jump from a window

Tell the patient you're going to stay with him, but you must let someone know where you are. Use the room phone to call the nurses' station or switchboard so that someone can notify the crisis intervention person. Identify yourself and report where you are. Say the patient needs someone to talk to right now, and you can't leave him. This statement should alert the staff that you need immediate help, yet should not further upset the patient.

Carefully move a little closer to the patient, watching for signs of increased agitation, such as his moving closer to the edge of the sill or his voice becoming loud. Don't rush toward him or he might jump.

Tell him you want to help. Remember, a person who has decided to commit suicide has reached a point where he can't see any other alternative to resolve his problems. Yet such a person is often as ambivalent toward death as he is toward life. So you must offer attractive alternatives and appeal to his desire to live.

For example, say something such as, "I want to help you; tell me what's bothering you." Involving the patient in relevant conversation will buy time, help calm him down, and bring a degree of normalcy to the situation.

Speak in a calm, steady voice. If you communicate anxiety to him, he'll sense that you've lost control of the situation (as he has) and can't help him. Try to make voice and eye contact; this will confirm your desire to help and divert his attention from the window. If anyone else is in the room, tell him to be quiet; if the radio or television set is on, turn it off, since excessive noise increases anxiety.

When you've established voice and eye contact and the patient appears calmer, say something such as, "Come down from the windowsill, and sit here so we can talk things over." By giving simple, direct commands, you relieve the patient of making decisions.

When a crisis intervention person arrives, introduce her to the patient. By showing respect for this person, you allow the patient to begin transferring some of his positive feelings for you to her.

What to do later

After the patient is safely down from the windowsill, arrange for a stat psychiatric consultation and transfer to a mental health unit. If a transfer isn't possible, place him in a room near the nurses' station, with a roommate. Review and implement the hospital's suicide precautions policy immediately. Then record your interventions in the patient's chart, and file an incident report if required.

Supervisors

Dealing with them effectively

Here are some strategies that'll help you get ahead when dealing with your supervisor.

• Be supportive. First, recognize your supervisor's goals and what she expects of you. By suggesting ways she can reach her goals, you'll become more valuable. And as you cooperate with her, she'll feel less need to directly monitor your activities. That increased autonomy means more power for you.

• Know when to back off from your own ideas and focus on what your supervisor thinks is important. For example, don't spend time revising a procedure manual if she thinks developing a new staffing plan is more urgent. When you help your supervisor look good, you're learning how to work the system—and that increases your power.

• Show your interest in learning. Many supervisors feel they have a

parentlike role: They want to pass on to others the knowledge they've gained from years of experience. So, for example, don't be afraid to ask your supervisor's advice on planning a better staff-development program or improving your assessment skills. She'll probably be glad you did. The more you show her she's an important resource, the more successful you'll be. Let her see that you can cope well during crises, do your work thoroughly and on time, and handle increased responsibility. A solid record of achievement helps increase your power.

• Network with recognized authorities at your hospital. (See *Networking*.) Volunteer to serve on committees, and meet with key people to learn more about their areas of expertise. The connections you develop will be useful to you—and your supervisors. (See *Career strategies*.)

Supplies

Helping nurses route them

If your unit frequently is staffed with nurses from a nursing pool who constantly ask where equipment and supplies are kept, try this: Make an alphabetical list of frequently used items and where they're stored. Post the list where all nurses can see it at the nurses' station.

Supply list	
Item	Location
Alcohol wipes	Medication room
Central I.V. line kit	Clean utility room
I.V. therapy equipment	Central supply room
Slippers, patient	Laundry closet
Tracheotomy tray	Crash cart

When new nurses come to the unit, show them the key supply areas: central supply room, clean and dirty utility rooms, medication room, and so on. Then when they need anything, they can just refer

to the posted list, go to the appropriate area, and get it themselves—without taking you away from your work.

Syncope

Immediate care and history taking

If you witness syncope, place the patient in a supine position, elevate his legs, and loosen any tight clothing. Ensure a patent airway and take vital signs. If you detect tachycardia, bradycardia, or an irregular pulse, have another nurse notify the doctor. Meanwhile, place the patient on a cardiac monitor to detect dysrhythmias. Give oxygen and insert an I.V. line for drug administration if dysrhythmias appear. Be prepared to begin cardiopulmonary resuscitation and to assist with cardioversion, defibrillation, or insertion of a temporary pacemaker, as needed.

If the patient reports an episode of syncope, collect information about the episode from the patient and his family. Did he feel weak, light-headed, nauseous, or sweaty just before he fainted? Did he get up quickly from a chair or from lying down? During the syncope, did he have muscle spasms or incontinence? How long was he unconscious? When he regained consciousness, was he alert or confused? Did he have a headache? Has he had syncope before? If so, how often did it occur? Next, take his vital signs and examine him for any injuries that may have occurred during a fall.

Syringe disposal

What to do with used syringes

Tell home care patients who use syringes to discard their used syringes in empty milk cartons. They can drop the syringes into the carton through the spout, then tape the carton shut before throwing it away.

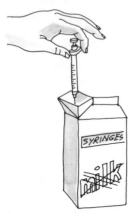

Disposing of syringes this way keeps children and others from hurting themselves with loose needles and may help conceal the fact that they're in the home.

Syringe filling

Technique for large ones

Filling a 50-ml syringe from several 10-ml vials is time-consuming and frustrating. To speed up the process, insert a needle without a syringe and another needle with a syringe into the vial. The syringe-

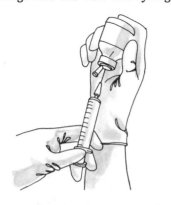

less needle will act as an air valve, allowing air into the vial so that the medication comes out faster.

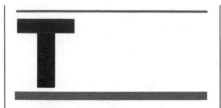

T tube: nursing measures

Guidelines

Avoid kinking of or tension on the T tube by securing it to the patient's gown with a pin or tape. Then:
• Place the drainage bag at abdominal level.
• Observe and record drainage amount, color, and any unusual conditions (for example, odor).
• After clamping the tube as ordered, check for and record such signs and symptoms as pain, nausea, vomiting, bloating, and chills.
• Monitor fluid, electrolyte, and acid-base status; report drainage amounts exceeding 500 ml in a 24-hour period.
• Return bile, as necessary, by replacing it orally or through a nasogastric tube (best given chilled in fruit juice).
• Protect the patient's skin from bile drainage. (See *T tube: wound care.*)

T tube: wound care

Preventing infection

Tell your patient to take care of his wound by doing the following:
• "Gather the necessary supplies: soap; a paper bag; five sterile 4" × 4" sponges; two sterile sponges soaked with povidone-iodine; one small, sterile povidone-iodine sponge and ointment packet; alcohol, sterile saline, and hydrogen peroxide solutions; a pair of sterile gloves; adhesive tape; a clean basin; a Velcro belt; and a sterile, disposable paper cloth.
• "Wash your hands thoroughly, using soap and water.
• "Remove the old dressing and discard it in the paper bag.

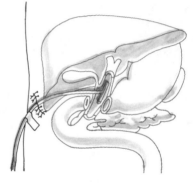

• "Wash your hands again.
• "Open the package containing the sterile paper cloth. Unfold the cloth to its full length, touching only its undersurface, and spread it onto a smooth, wide worktable.
• "Open a 4" × 4" sponge packet and carefully drop each one onto the sterile paper cloth surface—without touching them. Also, open the povidone-iodine sponge and ointment packet. Remove the tops from the bottles of alcohol, sterile saline solution, and hydrogen peroxide. Be careful to place the tops flat-side down on the worktable and away from the sterile cloth. Pour a little solution from each bottle into the basin—this will clean the lips of the bottles.
• "Put on the sterile gloves. Decide which hand will be your 'clean' hand and which one your 'sterile' hand.
• "Hold a 4" × 4" sponge in your sterile hand. Pick up the bottle of sterile saline solution with your clean hand, then thoroughly soak the sponge with saline solution. Wash around the wound site with the soaked sponge (still in your sterile hand). Wipe outward from the T tube wound in a spiral fashion to make a circle about 3" (7.5 cm) wide.
• "Repeat the procedure, using hydrogen peroxide solution.
• "Soak a 4" × 4" sponge in alcohol solution. Use it to wipe about a 6" (15 cm) length of tube, moving from the wound site toward the drainage bag. To prevent infection, never wipe the tube in the opposite direction.

S

• "Wipe the wound site a third time with the povidone-iodine sponges. Again, remember to clean outward from the wound in a spiral fashion.

• "Apply povidone-iodine ointment to the wound site by squeezing the packet with your clean hand, then letting the ointment drop onto the area. Use a sterile 4" × 4" sponge to spread the ointment with your sterile hand.

• "Again with your sterile hand, fluff open the remaining 4" × 4" sponge. Completely encircle the T tube at the wound site with the fluffed sponge. Tape this dressing securely to your abdomen. Also, tape a small segment of the T tube itself to your abdomen so you won't inadvertently pull on it. Pulling could enlarge the wound, increasing drainage and the risk of infection." (See also *Wound care dressings: taping.*)

TAC solution

Applying it to children

TAC (tetracaine, adrenaline, and cocaine) is used as a topical anesthetic before suturing. Here's how to apply it: Use a tuberculin syringe without the needle to slowly drip the solution into the laceration and onto the adjacent skin. (Usually, 4 to 5 ml are sufficient.)

A word of caution, though. Be sure to show the child that the needle's been removed and that you'll be using the syringe only to apply drops. Otherwise, he may fear he'll get a shot and not cooperate.

Keep TAC solution from mucous membranes. TAC will be absorbed systemically and cause adverse reactions.

Telephone advice: ED

Protecting yourself when you give it

First, devise a protocol for handling "routine" problems, such as diarrhea or sore throat (get the super-

vising doctor's approval first). That way, you'll be giving uniform advice at least some of the time and you'll have some legal protection if your advice is questioned.

Be meticulous about documentation. Besides the details you mentioned, also include the patient's name and a brief summary of any advice you give.

Refer unusual calls to the doctor, and document his involvement in the logbook.

Conclude all telephone conversations by advising the patient to seek medical treatment immediately if his condition doesn't improve or if any other signs or symptoms occur.

To be sure that your advice meets legal standards, write protocols incorporating the above measures, getting input from the emergency department doctors, hospital administrators, and the hospital lawyer.

Telephone guidelines

Dealing with a relative's rage

When a member of a patient's family calls angrily on the telephone to protest or demand, you can be caught in a particularly trying situation. Not only is the telephone by nature cold and impersonal, but it also fails to provide the nonverbal signals you need to complete the picture.

Here are some techniques for defusing the anger coming to you through the telephone.

• Always identify yourself by giving your name, position, and unit when answering the telephone. This puts you on a more personal footing with the caller.

• Avoid asking the caller to "hold"; waiting increases anger almost reflexively. If the caller requests information that will take time to get, tell him so. In the meantime, check back every couple of minutes to reassure him that he's not being neglected. If you have to call him back,

tell him why, and tell him when you plan to get back to him.

• When you hear anger in the caller's voice, acknowledge it. You can say, "I hear you're upset" or "I'd be upset, too, if that happened to me."

• Do not allow an angry caller to become abusive. Speak up at once. "I know you're upset, but yelling or becoming abusive won't help the situation. Let's talk in 15 minutes when we've both calmed down." (See also *Anger; Angry patients.*)

Telephone orders

Taking them prudently

To minimize your risks in taking any telephone orders, follow your hospital's policy to the letter. Document your actions and your conversations. Take these precautions:

• Write down the time, date, and doctor's name; describe the circumstances that prompted your call.

• Write down what you're going to tell the doctor, and read it to him.

• Write down his orders as he gives them to you.

• Read the orders back to him to be sure you've accurately recorded them.

• Record that you've read the orders back to him and that the doctor affirmed them as read.

If you accurately communicate the patient's symptoms, correctly record and follow appropriate orders, and question inappropriate orders, your risks will be minimal. If the patient later sues, the doctor alone will be charged for choosing to practice "telephone medicine." (See *Legal risks: doctors' orders.*)

Telephone technique

Giving bad news over the phone

When you must call a family with bad news about a patient, follow these practical guidelines.

T

Begin by identifying yourself and the hospital. Then give the reason for your call ("I'm calling about your wife . . ."). As you continue speaking to the family member, take care how you sound. A loud or high-pitched voice will signal alarm or anxiety, and that will increase the listener's anxiety. So keep your voice calm, lowering the pitch to accent certain points.

Avoid giving a lot of information all at once; give it in small doses. You might start with, "Your wife's condition has changed." Follow with a few details, then gradually progress to the worst. Don't overwhelm the listener with complex descriptions. In the midst of a crisis, he'll be too upset to comprehend blood pressure readings or names of medications.

Also of little comfort are vague and empty phrases such as "We're sure things will look up" or "We've done the appropriate things." Stick to simple facts: "Your wife developed some chest pain overnight. She's resting comfortably now and the pain is gone. As a precaution Dr. Gilbert wants her transferred to the coronary care unit, where she can be closely monitored."

If an emergency forces you to call a family member before you have all the details, be straightforward. Tell him that's all you know right now, but you'll convey the information as it's available.

Leave a brief moment for silence—to allow the news to sink in and the listener to express emotion. Be prepared for anything from crying to hysteria. This could, in fact, happen before you've finished giving the message. Just knowing someone's calling from the hospital may make the listener anticipate the worst. Also, his emotions may interfere with his ability to make decisions. He might say, "I'll be there in an hour or so; I can't get away right now." But by using a firm, direct approach—"We really need you here now"—you make the decision for him.

Giving reassurance

To alleviate some of his anxiety, reassure the listener by describing hopeful aspects of the patient's condition and concentrating on treatable symptoms. You might say, "Your wife has received pain medication and is resting comfortably." With that statement, you're letting him know that she's not suffering.

Other statements have calming effects, too. For instance, emphasize what the patient can do by saying "She can talk to us" or "She can breathe without assistance."

A worried family member may not hear or remember your entire message. For instance, to find out if he knows what unit his wife was taken to, ask "Do you know how to find the coronary care unit?" Show your concern by asking if he has any questions or by telling him, "I'll be waiting here to talk with you and answer your questions."

To ensure his safe arrival, encourage him to get a neighbor or friend to drive him to the hospital. If he must drive, tell him to be especially careful and to drive slowly; his state of mind could affect his judgment. Be sure to give him your name or the name of another nurse he can ask for when he arrives. Knowing that a specific "someone" is waiting will help him feel a little less anxious.

If the patient dies

What if the man's wife dies unexpectedly? Don't tell him this over the telephone. Instead, say, "My name is (blank), a nurse from (blank) Hospital. During the night your wife took a sudden turn for the worse. Could you come as soon as possible?"

Only under certain circumstances should the tragic news be given over the phone (for example, if relatives live out of town or can't get to the hospital). The doctor usually makes that call.

The message is brief and states:
• that this turn of events was unforeseen
• that the patient's medical condition was serious

• that appropriate medical care was available and was given
• that suffering was minimal
• that the patient did not die alone.

Saying that the patient "didn't survive" will soften the blow without hiding the message. If you say the patient "died" or "extinguished," you're more likely to shock the family or seem callous. Be sure to progress gradually to the bad news, leaving the worst for last, because the family member probably won't hear anything you say afterward. (See also *Communication: family; Death.*)

TENS

Attachment and regulation

If your patient is using transcutaneous electrical nerve stimulation (TENS) for chronic pain relief, help him apply, regulate, and care for the TENS unit properly.

Encourage him to rent a TENS unit for several months before buying one because pain relief may be transient. If you're assisting:
• Help him place the electrodes for optimal pain relief after applying conductive gel to them. Try placing electrodes directly over the painful

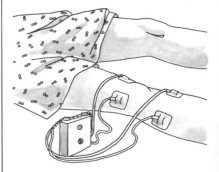

area, along the nerve pathways, or at points on the skin near the pain. Then secure them with adhesive tape.
• Turn on the unit and increase the wave amplitude (intensity) until the patient feels a tingling sensation.
• Set the amplitude, rate, and pulse width at prescribed settings; then

adjust these controls to fit the patient's comfort level.

• Monitor him for muscle twitching (indicating excessive stimulation).

• Remove the electrodes between uses or at least once a day if treatments are frequent. Wash the electrodes and the patient's skin with soap and water to remove gel, perspiration, and dead skin cells. Inspect his skin for redness and irritation. Let the skin dry thoroughly, then apply skin lotion. After putting fresh gel on the electrodes, reapply them in the same spots unless redness persists after skin care.

• Show the patient how to attach the TENS unit to his clothing for convenience.

Testicular self-examination

Teaching it

Monthly testicular self-examinations may help detect testicular cancer, which is the most common form of cancer in men between ages 15 and 35. Within the high-risk group, young white men have the highest incidence of testicular cancer; men with a history of undescended testes or a family history of testicular cancer are also at increased risk. All these patients should be taught to perform a testicular self-examination.

To teach it, first tell the patient that it's easy to learn and takes only a couple of minutes to do. The best time to perform the examination is during or after a hot bath or shower. That's because heat relaxes the scrotum and allows the testes to descend, making palpation easier.

While standing, the patient should place the index and middle fingers of both hands under one testicle and both thumbs on top of it. He should roll the testicle gently but firmly between his fingers and thumbs and

feel for any lumps or thickening. Then he should repeat the procedure with the other testicle.

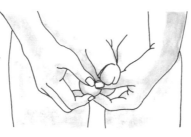

A normal testicle is egg-shaped, about 1½" (4 cm) long, and feels rubbery. The epididymis, behind the testicle, should feel soft, slightly tender, and tubelike. Most lumps or thickenings will develop on the sides and front of the testicle. Tell the patient to report any abnormalities to his doctor immediately.

Testifying: expert witness

When you're on the stand

When the opposing lawyer cross-examines you, don't forget: He's the enemy. He'll use any method to discredit your testimony. Further, no matter how much your lawyer has prepared, he can't predict questions completely. Also, if you're not careful, your answers can "feed" the opposing lawyer a whole new line of questioning. Keep these guidelines in mind:

• Answer only the question that's asked. Keep your answer short enough just to answer the question. If he asks "why" something happened, don't add "how."

• Bring notes, and refer to them. Even though you're an expert, you aren't expected to carry everything in your head.

• When you're sure of an answer, don't qualify it with "I think" or "perhaps." Be assertive. Look at the lawyer—don't look at the floor as if you have something to hide. If the

lawyer asks if you're paid to be a witness, don't act "guilty" when you say yes. It's an accepted practice.

• When using medical terminology, explain it for the jury.

• If the opposing lawyer quotes from material you're not familiar with or don't remember, ask to read it. Make sure he's quoted it accurately and in context. And give yourself plenty of time before answering.

• If he gets angry at you, don't show anger in return. Just remember you're a professional and act accordingly. Dress appropriately, too. Juries expect experts to act with dignity. (See *Witnessing, expert.*)

Testifying: preparation

What you need to know

Your best approach is to tell the truth—and to be prepared for the tactics lawyers use to try to weaken your credibility. Though they may use only one or two tactics, here are some they like to pick and choose from.

The plaintiff's lawyer may try to trick you by asking leading questions. Give yes-or-no answers whenever possible. And keep your answers to an absolute minimum. Don't stray from the main point.

Your recollection of events will be questioned, so always chart everything that might be important. What do you do if you haven't recorded a particular incident even though you remember it? Let your lawyer know before the trial. That will give him the chance, either before or after cross-examination, to let you explain why you remember the incident even though you didn't record it.

The plaintiff's lawyer will try to catch you in a contradiction. He will have carefully read the patient's chart and your signed pretrial deposition

T

before the case comes to court. You should, too. If you haven't, or you aren't sure of any answer when being questioned, don't hesitate to ask to see the chart to refresh your memory. The jury won't hold that against you. They have trouble remembering things, too. The same is true if you don't know something. Say you don't. The jury doesn't expect you to know everything.

Another common tactic is to weaken the nurse's testimony by trying to show she's biased in favor of the doctor or hospital. Not only is she employed by them, but she may also have social or business relations with, say, members of the doctor's family or with an executive of the hospital. You have nothing to fear in admitting social or business relations with people at your workplace. Jurors expect it. Just don't act evasive about it. And if the lawyer tries to give the impression that you're afraid of losing your job, simply state, "I took the oath, and I am here to tell the truth as I know it."

The lawyer will also attempt to uncover a bias you might have against the patient. If you ever have a difficult patient, make a note of it. Disagreeable patients are almost always the ones who sue.

Another common ploy is to try convincing the jury that at least one of your answers—or even a part of it—might have come straight from you lawyer's mouth. If the plaintiff's lawyer asks whether *your* lawyer went over questions that might be asked of you, say *yes*. But if he asks if your lawyer told you which *answers* to give, say, "I told him what I knew about the case and that I would answer any questions to the best of my recollection."

Besides avoiding defensiveness, make certain you don't use words you aren't familiar with. The plaintiff's lawyer might very well ask you what they mean.

Lawyers don't want to come across as being hard on you—in fact, they'll try to bait you; after all, the jury's on *your* side. But if you give lawyers the opportunity, they'll get tough with you.

If a plaintiff's lawyer is ever rude to you, don't be rude back. And don't lose your temper. That will just make the jurors think, "If she's like this here, what's she like in the hospital?" You'll then lose your credibility with them. And certainly don't disagree with the plaintiff's lawyer *just to disagree.* (See also *Witnessing, expert.*)

Tetanus prophylaxis

Guidelines

Proper wound care *always* includes appropriate tetanus prophylaxis. To determine the correct immunization for your patient, you must know:
• his wound classification (tetanus-prone or non-tetanus-prone)
• his history of tetanus immunization.

First, use the chart below to classify your patient's wound. Then, after determining his history of tetanus immunization, use the immunization schedule below to identify the prophylaxis he'll need now.

Features of tetanus-prone wounds include:
• wound age of greater than 6 hours
• stellate, avulsion, or abrasion configurations
• depth greater than 1 cm (3/8")
• missile, crush, burn, or frostbite injuries
• signs of infection
• devitalized tissue
• presence of contaminants (for example, dirt, feces, soil, saliva)
• denervated or ischemic tissue.

Tetanus-prone wounds
• If the patient is uncertain of his history of tetanus immunizations (number of doses), administer tetanus and diphtheria toxoids, adsorbed (for adult use), 0.5 ml (Td); and tetanus immune globulin (human), 250 units (TIG).
• If the patient has a history of 0 to 1 tetanus immunization, administer Td and TIG.

• If the patient has a history of 2 tetanus immunizations, administer Td. (Administer TIG only if 24 hours have elapsed since the wound was infected.)
• If the patient has a history of 3 or more tetanus immunizations, administer Td only if more than 5 years have elapsed since the last dose. Do not administer TIG.

Non-tetanus-prone wounds
• If the patient is uncertain of his history of tetanus immunizations, administer only Td.
• If the patient has a history of 0 to 1 tetanus immunization, administer only Td.
• If the patient has a history of 2 tetanus immunizations, administer only Td.
• If the patient has a history of 3 or more tetanus immunizations, administer Td only if more than 10 years have elapsed since the last dose.

When Td and TIG are given concurrently, separate syringes and separate sites should be used.

For children under age 7, diphtheria and tetanus toxoids and pertussis vaccine, adsorbed (DPT), is preferred to tetanus toxoid alone. If pertussis vaccine is contraindicated, administer Td.

Tetany

Nursing procedures

When you suspect that your patient has developed tetany after a thyroidectomy and you see positive Chvostek's and Trousseau's signs, notify his surgeon immediately. Then draw venous blood samples to check his calcium and phosphorus levels. Make sure you have previous blood values for comparison. (See *Chvostek's sign; Thyroidectomy; Trousseau's sign.*)

Obtain an order for 10 ml of a 10% solution of calcium gluconate. Administer the drug I.V. for 15 to 30 minutes. Because calcium gluconate's effects last only a few hours, you may need to repeat the infusion.

Or you can add 20 to 30 ml of the drug to 1 liter of dextrose 5% in water and infuse it over 12 to 24 hours.

If the patient is taking digitalis or if he has a history of cardiac problems, you should administer the calcium gluconate more slowly than indicated above. And you should continuously monitor his ECG because the combination of digitalis and calcium gluconate can cause life-threatening dysrhythmias.

Keep the bed's side rails up in case the patient has a seizure, and observe seizure precautions. (See *Seizures: precautions.*) If you can't prevent the seizures with calcium gluconate, the doctor may prescribe other drugs.

If the patient is anxious about his condition, stay with him and explain his treatment and medications. Continue to monitor his vital signs for changes, and check for symptoms of further calcium deficiency. To help the patient breathe more easily and to make him more comfortable, place him in high-Fowler's position. Keep his room quiet, draft-free, and dimly lit, and avoid sudden movements that may excite his nervous system.

If the patient is at risk for airway obstruction, make sure an oxygen source, suctioning equipment, and an emergency tracheotomy tray are ready in the patient's room.

What to do later
To make sure your patient is maintaining an adequate calcium level, monitor his serum calcium values, recheck for Chvostek's and Trousseau's signs, and note any complaints of paresthesia and cramping. Continue to assess his vital signs and respiratory status.

Thoracic outlet syndrome

Shoulder-girdle exercises

Instruct the patient to do 10 repetitions of each exercise twice a day.

She should increase the number of times she does each exercise as she gains strength in her shoulders and neck. Tell her:

"Stand with your arms at your sides, holding a 2-lb (0.9-kg) weight in each hand. (The weights can be sandbags or sand-filled bottles, jars, or sacks.) Shrug your shoulders forward and upward. Relax. Shrug your shoulders backward and upward. Relax. Shrug your shoulders upward. Relax, then repeat the exercise.

"Stand with your arms extended at shoulder level, holding a 2 lb weight in each hand. (Your palms should be facedown.) Raise your arms sideways and up over you head, keeping your elbows locked, until the backs of your hands meet. Relax, then repeat the exercise.

"As your strength improves and the above exercises become easier, increase the weights to 5 lb (2.3 kg) and, later, to 10 lb (4.5 kg).

"Stand facing a corner of a room, with one hand (palm forward) on each wall, elbows bent, and your hands at shoulder level. Contract your abdominal muscles. Slowly let your upper body lean forward, pressing your chest into the corner. Inhale as you lean forward. Then push out with your hands to return to your original position. Exhale as you push out. Relax, and repeat this exercise.

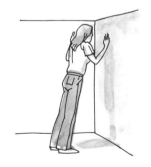

"Stand with your arms at your sides. Tilting your head to the left, try to touch your left ear to your left shoulder without raising the shoulder. Then try to touch your right ear to your right shoulder in the same way. Relax and repeat.

"Lie facedown on the floor with your hands clasped behind your back. Inhaling slowly, raise your head and chest from the floor as high as possible while pulling your shoulders back and your chin in. Hold this position for a count of three. Exhale and return to your original position. Relax, and repeat.

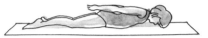

"Lie on your back with your arms at your sides. Place a rolled-up towel or small pillow under the upper part of your back between your shoulder blades. Inhaling slowly, raise your arms up, then back over your head. Exhale and return your arms to your sides. Relax, and repeat this exercise."

Thrombocytopenic patients

Bleeding precautions

Good communication among staff members is essential to proper care. You need to make the patient's condition known to all staff members involved in his care. Here's how:
• Write "Bleeding precautions" on his chart, patient care Kardex, and medication Kardex.
• Note on all requisition forms—in contrasting ink—that the patient is a potential bleeder.
• Request continuous updating of the patient's condition (including his latest platelet count and a description of any bleeding episodes) during end-of-shift reports.
• Place a sign above his bed or on the door to his room alerting staff members to take bleeding precautions.

To further ensure the safety and well-being of thrombocytopenic patients, bleeding precautions should be established as formal hospital policy. This will promote cooperation

T

among the various staff members—nurses, doctors, and laboratory technicians—involved in their care.

Thrombolytic therapy: bleeding

Guarding against the major complication

With thrombolytic therapy for acute myocardial infarction, the most common complications are bleeding, allergic reactions, serious reperfusion dysrhythmias, fever, and reocclusion.

Bleeding is the biggest risk. Avoid unnecessary I.V. or intra-arterial punctures and intramuscular or subcutaneous injections—especially during the first 24 hours of treatment. Limit your physical contact with the patient. Pad his side rails, and post a "Bleeding Precautions" sign.

Insert an arterial line before thrombolytic therapy is started so that you can draw blood later without risking a bleeding episode. Or, insert an 18-gauge heparin lock for withdrawing blood.

Another precaution to take before therapy: Double-check the patient's history for any recent invasive procedures or episodes of abnormal bleeding—contraindications to thrombolytic therapy.

If he does bleed from a puncture or an unavoidable injection, you may be able to control it simply by applying direct pressure. If bleeding persists, apply a gauze pad soaked in aminocaproic acid (Amicar) to induce clotting.

At the start of thrombolytic therapy, the patient's fibrinogen concentration and partial thromboplastin time (PTT) should be measured to establish baseline values, then reevaluated every 6 hours. If his fibrinogen concentration falls below 100 mg/dl, or his PTT is more than 2½ times the baseline value, the risk of bleeding increases.

Remember that the patient may bleed internally. To detect this, take his vital signs every 15 minutes until he's stable, then every hour. Watch for a drop in blood pressure, which may become apparent only over several readings, and a steadily increasing pulse rate. Observe for other signs and symptoms of internal bleeding—level of consciousness changes (such as confusion and disorientation), hematuria, hematemesis, hemoptysis, joint swelling, and flank or abdominal pain. Stools, urine, emesis, and nasogastric drainage should undergo guaiac testing. And, of course, urge the usual precautions for all patients at risk for bleeding: using a soft-bristled toothbrush, not straining during bowel movements, and so forth.

Get into the habit of monitoring for bleeding. After thrombolytic therapy, long-term anticoagulation therapy will probably begin. So watching for signs and symptoms of bleeding will remain high on your list of priorities. (See also *Anticoagulants.*)

Thrombolytic therapy: reperfusion

Signs and symptoms

Once your patient has been started on thrombolytic therapy, you should see indications that his heart muscle is being reperfused. His chest pain should stop abruptly. Also, elevated ST segments on his ECG should fall rapidly toward the isoelectric line. To observe for this sign, place your patient on a monitoring lead that would best show ST elevation, such as Lead II, modified chest Lead I, or modified chest Lead VI.

Another indication of reperfusion is resolution of an atrioventricular or idioventricular block.

When a thrombolytic agent dissolves a clot obstructing a coronary artery, the subsequent rapid reperfusion of the heart causes electrical instability. In about four out of five patients, this will produce dysrhythmias. About half of these patients develop an accelerated idioventricular rhythm that is usually transient and doesn't require treatment. These "reperfusion dysrhythmias" are another indication that adequate blood flow to the heart has been restored.

Watch for peak levels of the cardiac enzyme creatine phosphokinase (CPK) within 3 to 4 hours after treatment has begun. But don't confuse these peak CPK values brought on by successful thrombolytic therapy with increased CPK levels secondary to myocardial damage. In this case, increased values occur because CPK is washed out by the sudden influx of blood into the previously unperfused myocardium.

Thrombophlebitis, superficial

Diagnosis and treatment

Superficial thrombophlebitis differs from deep vein thrombosis in two important respects. First, superficial thrombophlebitis can be diagnosed easily from signs and symptoms. Look for the four "–ors" at the affected site—color, rubor, dolor, and tumor (heat, redness, pain, and

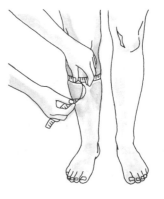

swelling, respectively); these are the cardinal signs and symptoms of inflammation. On palpation, the vein itself may feel like a firm, subcutaneous cord. Palpate gently—the vein may be tender. (See *Homans' sign.*)

Second, with prompt intervention, superficial thrombophlebitis should resolve with no further complications. One exception is thrombophlebitis of the greater saphenous system at the saphenofemoral junction, which could extend into the deep venous system. The saphenous vein may be divided as a preventive measure.

If an I.V. catheter appears to be causing the condition, remove it at once and find another insertion site. Then apply warm, moist soaks to the affected site. This will relieve the pain and reduce inflammation. (An analgesic or anti-inflammatory agent may be ordered for the same purpose.) Apply the soaks every 4 to 6 hours for 20 to 30 minutes, depending on the patient's activity level, until all signs and symptoms have been alleviated.

Also, to decrease swelling and enhance venous return, elevate the affected limb. If the condition has developed in his leg, keep the patient on bed rest; if his arm is affected, encourage him to use his other arm for activities.

To prevent superficial thrombophlebitis:
• Monitor I.V. sites closely for inflammation.
• Change I.V. tubing every 24 to 48 hours. Also, change the I.V. catheter site every 48 to 96 hours to prevent thrombus formation at an overused site.
• Avoid infusing irritating solutions through small veins.
• Follow instructions carefully when diluting I.V. medications.
• Observe for low-grade fever, indicating possible thrombophlebitis.
• Use restraints with caution to avoid a tourniquet effect on an arm or leg.
• When necessary, pad the side rails of the bed. (See *I.V. therapy: complications.*)

Thrombosis: activities

Preventing deep vein thrombosis

Encourage early ambulation in postoperative patients, explaining its importance in preventing deep vein thrombosis. And do the following:
• Perform passive range-of-motion exercises for bedridden patients. If the patient can do active range-of-motion exercises, teach him how. Also instruct him to dorsiflex his feet or move them in a walking motion against the footboard for 5 minutes every hour.

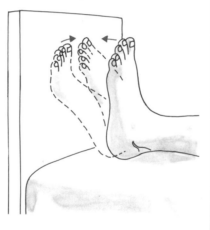

• Avoid elevating the patient's knees with pillows or by adjusting his bed because this can obstruct venous blood flow. If his knees must be elevated, raise the foot of the bed.
• Tell an ambulatory patient to avoid standing or sitting in one position for a long period. If he must do so, teach him to exercise his legs by repeatedly standing on his toes or shifting weight from one foot to another, or by alternately propping one leg, then the other, on a stool.
• Tell him to make sure his feet are flat on the floor when he sits on the side of the bed. This will avoid putting pressure on popliteal spaces.

Thrombosis: patient teaching

What to tell the deep-vein-thrombosis patient

Follow these guidelines:
• Put instructions for taking anticoagulants in writing. Tell your patient why he needs to take them. Warn him of possible adverse reactions and interactions with other drugs. Stress the importance of frequent follow-up examinations, and document your patient teaching in medical records. (See *Anticoagulants.*)
• Before discharge, teach him how to apply bandages or stockings correctly. Stress the importance of applying uniform pressure, not turning down the top of the bandage or stocking, and keeping the bandage or stocking wrinkle-free. Tell him to wear it until the doctor tells him otherwise. (See *Bandage, roller; Antiembolism stockings.*)
• Explain to him that elastic bandages and support stockings can be washed with mild soap and water but will shrink if dried in a clothes dryer. Tell him to replace bandages or stockings when they lose their elasticity. (He should have at least two pairs.)
• Encourage him to exercise regularly if possible. Recommend walking, jogging, bicycling, and swimming. Tell him to elevate his legs frequently.
• Warn him of the hazards of smoking and obesity: Nicotine constricts veins, decreasing venous blood flow. Extra pounds increase pressure on leg veins. Arrange consultation with a dietician if necessary.
• If the patient's female, tell her to discontinue use of oral contraceptives if diagnostic testing has confirmed thrombus formation.
• Advise the patient to avoid restrictive clothing. Such clothing reduces venous return, increasing pressure on leg veins.

T

• If the patient notices swelling, pain, tenderness, or sudden dilation of superficial veins in a leg or arm, urge him to notify his doctor immediately.

Thrombosis: prevention

Monitoring and precautions

Follow these steps to prevent your patient from getting deep vein thrombosis (DVT):

• Assess the patient's arms and legs regularly for swelling, asymmetry in size, inflammation, pain, deep muscle or generalized tenderness, cyanosis, and venous distention.
• Perform frequent checks of circulatory, motor, and neurologic function in arms and legs.
• Observe for low-grade fever, indicating possible thrombophlebitis.
• Maintain proper fluid balance. Both overhydration and dehydration can decrease venous return and cause venous stasis in legs. (Most patients need at least 3,000 ml of fluid every 24 hours.)
• Monitor the frequency of the patient's bowel movements. He may need stool softeners to avoid straining during bowel movements. Such straining can increase venous pressure in legs.
• Use limb restraints with caution to avoid a tourniquet effect.
• Pad the side rails of his bed, when necessary, to avoid leg trauma.
• Instruct him to perform deep-breathing exercises postoperatively to ventilate lungs and promote venous return.
• Observe him closely for signs and symptoms of pulmonary embolism (such as tachycardia, crackles, dyspnea, hemoptysis, hypotension, pleuritic chest pain, and cyanosis).
• If your patient smokes cigarettes, encourage him to quit.
• Leg compression is helpful in preventing DVT. Either antiembolism stockings or an intermittent pneumatic compression device can be used. The patient may also receive prophylactic heparin. (See *Antiembolism stockings; Pressure cuff.*)

Thyroid assessment

Guidelines

To inspect for enlarged thyroid tissue, stand in front of the patient and look closely at the lower half of his neck. Use cross light to help identify subtle neck movements and ascending masses.

Locate the thyroid and cricoid cartilages. Observe the area below the cricoid cartilage and to the sides of both cartilages. Assess these areas first when the patient's neck is in its normal anatomic position, then when it's slightly extended, and finally when the patient swallows. You should see the cartilages move when the patient swallows. Whether you'll be able to see the thyroid gland depends on its size and the patient's body build. Abnormal findings may include any unusual bulges of thyroid tissue.

Palpation
Normally, you can't palpate the thyroid gland itself. You should be able to palpate the isthmus if the patient has a thin neck. If he has a short, thick neck, the isthmus may be very close to the sternum and palpable only when he extends his neck.

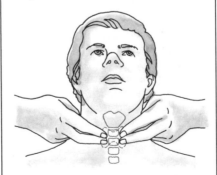

Palpate from both behind and in front of him. *From behind:* Ask him to sit while you stand behind him. Have him lower his chin to relax the neck muscles. Curve your index and middle fingers to the front so that your fingertips rest below the cricoid cartilage on the lower half of his neck, over his trachea. Palpate for the thyroid isthmus and the lobes' anterior surfaces.

Ask him to swallow as you palpate again. Because the thyroid gland is attached to the larynx and trachea, it will rise when he swallows. You should be able to feel the isthmus rising. Other structures, such as lymph nodes or any masses, won't rise.

Next, ask him to flex his neck slightly forward and to the right so that you can examine the right lobe. Use the fingers of your left hand to displace the thyroid cartilage to the right. With your right hand, palpate the area lateral to the cartilage. To palpate, place your thumb deep into and behind the sternocleidomastoid muscle and your index and middle fingers deep into and in front of it. Have him swallow as you palpate again. Reverse this procedure to examine the left lobe.

From in front: Stand in front of the seated patient and palpate below the cricoid cartilage for the thyroid isthmus with the pads of your index and middle fingers. Move your fingers laterally and to the back of the anterior borders of the sternocleidomastoid muscles to palpate each lobe.

Abnormal findings may include either a diffusely or locally enlarged thyroid gland. A diffusely enlarged gland usually doesn't have palpable nodules, whereas a locally enlarged gland may have one or more. A solitary nodule, which feels like a knot or protuberance, may be a cyst or a benign or malignant tumor. Document your findings.

Thyroid crisis

Actions to take

Thyroid crisis causes severe tachycardia, hypertension, hyperthermia, nausea, vomiting, diarrhea, confusion, and hyperexcitability. In caring for the patient with this disorder, you'll monitor his blood pressure, pulse rate, temperature, and any edema, and you'll try to keep him as calm as possible. Explain that his thyroid gland is overacting, causing his signs and symptoms. Assure him that he's going to get immediate treatment.

Check for dysphagia or respiratory distress, which could result from the enlarged thyroid gland. Administer oxygen and start an infusion of dextrose 5% in water or dextrose 5% in normal saline solution. Have another nurse set up for suctioning, and make sure emergency airway equipment, such as a tracheotomy tray, is available. Hook up the patient to a cardiac monitor, and watch his heart rate and rhythm closely. Stay alert for worsening signs and symptoms.

When the doctor arrives, he'll probably order propranolol to treat the patient's hypertension (and possible dysrhythmias) and to inhibit the conversion of thyroxine (T_4) to triiodothyronine (T_3). He'll also order specific antithyroid drugs (propylthiouracil, methimazole, iodine, or lithium) to minimize synthesis and secretion of these thyroid hormones.

Administer other drugs and treatments, as ordered. The doctor may also decide to insert a pulmonary artery catheter to monitor the patient's hemodynamic status.

What to do later
Continue to assess the patient's vital signs and condition. Maintain adequate fluid volume with I.V. infusions, checking his intake and output every hour. Observe for signs of hypoglycemia.

If the patient's thyroid crisis was precipitated by an infection, obtain urine, blood, and sputum specimens for testing. Broad-spectrum antibiotics can be prescribed until the results of culture and sensitivity testing are available.

Most patients who recover from thyroid crisis improve dramatically within 12 to 24 hours. During this period, some of the supportive therapy, such as corticosteroids, anti-

pyretics, and I.V. fluids, may be tapered off and withdrawn. This is a good time to implement patient teaching.

When the patient has completely recovered, his doctor will need to consider long-term management of his hyperthyroidism. His T_3 and T_4 levels should be measured periodically. Explain the importance of following his prescribed therapy and having his thyroid hormone levels measured as recommended.

Thyroidectomy

Managing respiratory distress after surgery

Respiratory distress may occur if your patient develops a hematoma postoperatlively, which puts pressure on his trachea.

Here's what to do when this emergency occurs: First, call for help. Remove the dressing to reduce pressure on the trachea. When another nurse arrives, ask her to get the surgeon. Don't leave the patient; his respiratory distress could worsen, leading to cardiac arrest.

Continue to check his vital signs. If he's hypotensive, speed up the drip rate of his I.V. fluids and *lower* the head of his bed as much as possible without compromising his respiratory status. (If he's not hypotensive, *elevate* the head of his bed to ease breathing and minimize swelling.) Begin administering oxygen.

Have another nurse set up for nasotracheal suctioning and get an emergency tracheotomy tray. Ask her to attach a preoperative checklist to the patient's chart and check off as much as possible. Be sure to locate the surgical clip remover. It should be at the patient's bedside.

While you're doing all this, constantly reassure the patient. Continue to monitor his respiratory status and vital signs, and be prepared to call the anesthesiologist or code team.

When the surgeon arrives, he'll also assess the degree of the pa-

tient's respiratory distress. He may decide to remove the surgical clips and evacuate the hematoma at the patient's bedside. But he'll probably have the patient transported directly to surgery for evacuation of the hematoma and repair of the bleeding vessel.

Tilt test

Assessing for hypovolemic shock

Tilt test results may help you assess a patient for volume depletion. With your patient supine, raise his legs above heart level. If his blood pressure rises significantly (indicating autotransfusion from his legs), consider the test positive—an indication of volume depletion. (See *Hypovolemic shock intervention.*)

Time management

Getting people to help

Co-workers, supervisors, doctors, families, and even patients can contribute to better organization and time management—if you'll only ask for their help.

Ask a co-worker, for example, to help you prepare several elderly patients for lunch. You can have the patients wash their hands while your co-worker sets up trays and raises the heads of their beds.

Are you running specimens to the lab, picking up late trays, and mopping up spills? Sometimes you won't have a choice, of course. But these responsibilities belong to nursing assistants, volunteers, and others, so let *them* manage these problems. Similarly, a little tact and common courtesy can smooth the way for emergency laboratory work, late diet changes, or help in finding missing supplies. Thank anyone who offers to help one of your less-able patients with lunch, freeing you to spend more time with other patients.

T

Don't let a doctor intimidate you by making unwarranted demands for immediate service.

Don't overlook anyone who can help you. Family members may be reluctant to help only because they're unsure of what to do. You'll need extra time to show a wife how to feed her husband, or give passive range-of-motion exercises. But it's a good long-term investment for you, the patient, and the family. Before explaining a procedure to family members, be sure they really want to help. Otherwise, they might think you're shirking your responsibility.

Be open with patients. They can sense when the unit's more chaotic than usual. And most will understand an occasional delay if you've established a trusting relationship and have shown them you care about their needs and feelings. You might say: "I've had some unexpected problems with another patient, Mr. Nelson. So I'd like to reschedule your dressing change for later this morning." Or if you know you'll be busy, you might tell a patient: "I need to help a doctor for the next half hour. Can I get you anything before I leave?" (See *Planning: priorities.*)

Toes

Removing incrustations

When even a vigorous soap-and-water scrub can't remove the incrustations from a patient's toes and nails, try a glycerin-and-lemon swab instead.

A single application will gently remove debris without causing discomfort or tissue damage.

Tourniquets

The best way to remove them

An experienced doctor or nurse can and should remove a tourniquet as soon as possible, since many are applied either too tightly or too loosely at emergency scenes. And, as you know, the longer a tourniquet is left in place, the greater the risk of tissue necrosis and limb loss.

The procedure recommended for safe tourniquet removal is:

1. Start an I.V. line and administer lactated Ringer's solution.

2. Elevate the extremity and apply a pneumatic cuff above the tourniquet. If a pneumatic cuff isn't available, use a blood pressure cuff.

3. Pump the cuff until systolic blood pressure is occluded.

4. Remove the tourniquet.

5. Deflate the cuff gradually, releasing pressure every 15 minutes or as necessary. When you're not releasing pressure, keep the cuff tubing clamped to maintain the desired pressure.

6. Monitor for a resumption of bleeding. Remember, even after you've stopped the bleeding, I.V. fluids can dislodge a clot and start the bleeding again.

Toxic shock syndrome

Patient-teaching guidelines

Diagnostic tests
• Explain to the patient that the disorder, most often affecting females, results from a toxin produced by *Staphylococcus aureus*. Tell her that diagnosis depends on several findings, including a fever exceeding 104° F. (40° C.); systolic blood pressure of less than 90 mm Hg; a desquamate rash; and at least three of the following: vomiting or diarrhea, myalgias or fivefold increase in creatine phosphokinase levels, hyperemia of mucous membranes, renal insufficiency, hepatitis, thrombocytopenia, or central nervous system disturbances.
• Inform the patient that examination of vaginal secretions can detect the causative organism and that a blood culture can detect *S. aureus* in the bloodstream.

Treatments
• Explain that drug therapy is specific to the causative organism. Stress the importance of completing the course of drug therapy to prevent recurrence.
• Teach the patient about the importance of volume replacement to maintain blood pressure. Stress the importance of liberal fluid intake—at least six to eight glasses of water daily.
• Educate the patient about risk factors, particularly cautioning against the use of hyperabsorbent tampons. Advise her to choose tampons made entirely of cotton.

TPN: administration

Beginning the infusion

To start total parenteral nutrition (TPN), remove the cap from the bottle, then remove the rubber diaphragm that's under the cap. Remove the protective cover from the I.V. tubing, and insert the spike into the larger hole in the rubber stopper. Be careful not to contaminate the spike with your hands.

Hang the bottle on an I.V. pole and use the gravity control clamp to prime the tubing with solution. Attach and prime the final filter, if the hospital where you work requires such a filter. Attach the tubing to the infusion pump. Then prime the pump chamber and pump tubing. Remove the tape from the tubing-catheter connection, and turn off the solution that's being infused.

Have the patient perform Valsalva's maneuver. Using a Kelly clamp to hold the catheter hub, quickly replace the old tubing with the new. The clamp will give you better leverage and will help prevent contaminating the hub with your fingers.

Adjust the infusion pump to the proper flow rate and volume. Open the gravity flow clamps and set the alarm. Most important, make sure you turn on the pump itself. Use a tape to secure the tubing to the catheter hub. Date the tubing. Secure the tubing-catheter connection to the dressing.

Check the flow rate every hour. To help you monitor the rate and check the pump's accuracy, apply a time tape, marked in hours, on the infusion bottle. Remember that pumps can malfunction, so keep monitoring both the system and the patient.

TPN: nursing considerations

What to look for

Before administering total parenteral nutrition (TPN), keep the solution refrigerated until needed; then warm to room temperature before infusion. Follow these steps:
• Administer the initial infusion gradually, until the patient can tolerate the concentrated glucose solution.
• Administer the solution at a steady rate. Don't increase the rate if administration falls behind schedule.
• Use sterile technique when changing the tubing or dressings.
• When changing the tubing, have the patient bear down or perform Valsalva's maneuver to prevent air embolism.
• Monitor serum and urine glucose levels. (See *Glucose monitoring.*)
• Assess for signs and symptoms of complications.
• Avoid using the TPN catheter for other procedures.
• To discontinue TPN, decrease the glucose solution gradually to prevent hypoglycemia. If TPN is stopped abruptly, administer dextrose 10% solution peripherally.

Tracheal deviation

Detecting slight deviation

Although gross tracheal deviation will be visible, detection of slight deviation requires palpation and perhaps even an X-ray. Try palpation first.

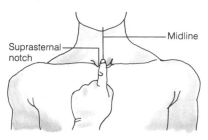

With the tip of your index finger, locate the patient's trachea by palpating between the sternocleidomastoid muscles. Then compare the trachea's position to an imaginary line drawn vertically through the suprasternal notch. Any deviation from this line is usually considered abnormal.

Tracheostomy: complications

Cuff pressure problems

To ensure that your patient's cuff (endotracheal or tracheostomy) pressure is within safe limits (lower than 18 mm Hg), measure the minimal occlusive volume (MOV), at least once a shift, if ordered, using the following procedure.

1. Gather the following equipment: stethoscope, three-way stopcock, 10-cc syringe partially filled with air, mercury manometer, and suction equipment.

2. Suction the endotracheal tube. (See *Endotracheal tubes: suctioning.*) Then suction the patient's oropharynx to remove secretions that have accumulated above the cuff.

3. Connect the ports of the three-way stopcock to the manometer tubing, the syringe, and the pilot balloon of the cuff. Close the port to the pilot balloon so that air can't escape from the cuff.

4. Instill air from the syringe into the manometer tubing until the pressure reading reaches 10 mm Hg. (Later, when you open the stopcock to the cuff and the manometer, this air will prevent a sudden deflation of the cuff.)

5. With the stethoscope, auscultate the patient's trachea. A smooth, hollow sound indicates a sealed airway; a loud, gurgling sound indicates an air leak.

6. If you detect an air leak, reinflate the cuff until you no longer hear an air leak on inspiration. (Airways are larger on inspiration than on expiration. So if you stop reinflating the cuff when you no longer hear a leak on expiration, a leak may still occur on inspiration.)

Certain patients—those receiving a high inspiratory pressure or positive end-expiratory pressure (PEEP), for instance—need an extremely high cuff pressure to seal the airway. If such a patient can tolerate the leak (if his arterial blood gas values stay normal), keep the cuff pressure within an acceptable limit. Otherwise, seal the airway.

If the tube is too small, you may be unable to seal the airway without overinflating the cuff. Report this to the doctor because the tube may need to be replaced with a larger one. When you no longer hear an air leak, go to the next step.

7. Turn off the stopcock to the manometer.

8. Continue to auscultate the trachea while you slowly deflate the cuff. (If deflating the cuff makes the patient cough, wait until he stops before going on.)

9. Turn off the stopcock to the syringe.

Endotracheal cuff pressure measurement

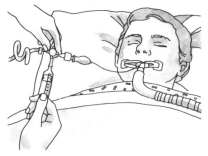

T

10. Record the manometer reading on expiration; this is the cuff pressure at MOV. (The mercury level will fluctuate as the patient inhales and exhales. The reading on inspiration reflects the effect of PEEP ventilation on the airways; the reading on expiration reflects the effect of cuff pressure on the tracheal wall.)

11. Turn off the stopcock to the pilot balloon, then disconnect the stopcock.

12. At least once a week, deflate the cuff completely, then reinflate it to MOV. Record the amount of air needed for reinflation. A gradual increase in the total amount needed to reach MOV may indicate tracheal malacia (an abnormal softening of the tracheal tissue). But maintaining cuff pressure at the lowest possible level and inflating it just to MOV will keep cuff-related complications to a minimum.

Tracheostomy: considerations

Concluding tracheostomy care

When you're finishing up, do the following:
• Change the tracheostomy ties if they're soiled, loose, or tight. (See *Tracheostomy: fastening.*)
• Replace the humidification device.
• Give oral care, as needed, because the oral cavity can become dry and malodorous or develop sores from encrusted secretions.
• Make sure the patient is comfortable and that he can easily reach the call light and other communication aids.
• Observe soiled dressings and any suctioned secretions for the amount, color, consistency, and odor of discharge.
• Properly clean or dispose of all equipment, supplies, solutions, and trash, according to hospital policy.

• Replenish any supplies used from the extra tracheostomy care set, and make sure all necessary supplies are readily available at the bedside.
• Repeat this procedure at least once every 8 hours or as needed. Change the dressing as often as necessary, whether or not you also perform the entire cleaning procedure, because a dressing wet with exudate or secretions predisposes the patient to skin excoriation, breakdown, and infection.

Tracheostomy: dislodged tube

Taking swift action

What if a patient's tracheostomy tube becomes dislodged? Call for help as you place the patient supine, hyperextend his neck, and assure him that you're going to help him.

If his chest isn't moving, listen for breath sounds or feel for air movement at the stoma. If there's no sign of air movement, or he's just gurgling around the stoma, you'll have to reestablish his airway. Adjust the bedside light so that it shines directly on the stoma. Look for stray sutures. (Some surgeons place these sutures at the top and bottom of the incision, so you can pull them up and out to open the stoma in an emergency.) If the patient doesn't have stray sutures, use a sterile Kelly clamp, which should always be kept at the bedside of a tracheostomy patient. Place the closed clamp into the center of the incision, then open it, spreading the incision. Hold the clamp in place.

If the clamp doesn't provide an adequate airway, you'll have to replace the tracheostomy tube. By now, at least one other nurse should have arrived to help. Tell her to unwrap the spare tracheostomy tube (also kept at the patient's bedside), to put the obturator in the outer cannula, and to hand you the assembled tube.

Ask this nurse to monitor the patient's vital signs and get the suction

equipment ready. Then, trying not to touch the end of the new tube, insert it into the incision. Remove the clamp. Hold onto the tube as you remove the obturator. You should hear a rush of air and see the patient's breathing become less labored. Anchor the tube with tracheostomy ties.

If the patient's breathing doesn't improve, the tube may be in the interstitial space. Remove it (keeping the incision open with the Kelly clamp) and reinsert it. If you can't get the tube inserted or you can no longer detect a pulse, call a code.

When the patient is breathing more easily, attach the humidified oxygen source to the new tracheostomy tube and determine whether he needs supplemental oxygen. Continue to monitor vital signs, color, and level of consciousness. Elevate the head of the bed unless this is contraindicated by his vital signs. Assure the patient that he's out of danger, and give him paper and pen so he can communicate his feelings.

After the new tube is in place, make sure an X-ray is taken to confirm that it's positioned correctly. Notify the surgeon. Then document what happened and what actions you took.

Be alert for increased bloody secretions and slight bleeding from the stoma because reinserting the tube was traumatic. Profuse bleeding, especially bright red blood, indicates vascular damage; call the surgeon immediately.

Because the tube wasn't inserted under controlled conditions, the patient's at high risk for infection, so plan to observe the stoma for at least a week after the insertion for induration, redness, and purulent drainage.

Replace the Kelly clamp and spare tracheostomy tube (one size smaller than the original one) at the patient's bedside. Check the suctioning apparatus. If any emergency equipment was *not* at the bedside, stock it, and find out why it wasn't there. Then find out what caused the tracheostomy tube to become dislodged.

Tracheostomy: double-cannula tube

Good cleaning method

After putting on gloves and setting up the equipment, proceed as follows:
• With your left hand, disconnect the ventilator or humidification device. Then, with the same hand, unlock the tracheostomy tube's inner cannula. Next, with your left hand, remove the inner cannula.

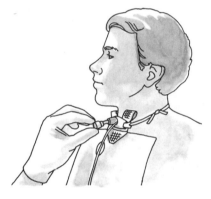

• Place the inner cannula in a container of hydrogen peroxide, and allow it to soak to remove encrustations.
• For the ventilator patient, use your left hand to remove the lid from the container with the spare inner cannula. Pick up the cannula with your right hand, and insert it into the outer cannula of the patient's tracheostomy tube. Use your left hand to reconnect the patient to the ventilator.
• Put a sterile glove on your left hand, and clean the skin, stoma, and tracheostomy tube flanges with normal saline solution–soaked gauze sponges and cotton-tipped applicators, as described for the single cannula. (See *Tracheostomy: single-cannula tube.*)
• Pick up the inner cannula with your right hand from the container

of hydrogen peroxide. Scrub the cannula with the sterile nylon brush. If the brush doesn't slide easily into the cannula, use a sterile pipe cleaner.

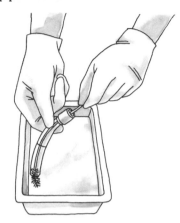

• Immerse the cannula in a container of sterile normal saline solution, and agitate it for about 10 seconds to rinse it thoroughly and provide a thin film of solution to lubricate it for replacement.
• Hold the cannula up to the light and inspect it for cleanliness. If encrustations are still present, repeat the cleaning process. If not, grasp the clean cannula and tap it gently against the inside edge of the sterile container to remove excess liquid and to prevent possible aspiration by the patient. Use three sterile pipe cleaners twisted together to dry the inside of the cannula. Don't dry its outer surface because a thin film of moisture acts as a lubricant during insertion.
• If the patient is not on a ventilator, gently reinsert the inner cannula (after cleaning it in a container of hydrogen peroxide) into the patient's tracheostomy tube. Lock it in place and then pull on it gently to ensure secure positioning. For patients on a ventilator, place the newly cleaned inner cannula in the sterile storage container (which now becomes the spare).
• Apply a new sterile tracheostomy dressing. If you're not using a commercially prepared dressing, avoid using cotton-filled gauze or a trimmed gauze sponge because as-

piration of lint and fibers can cause a tracheal abscess. Instead, open a sterile 4″ × 4″ gauze pad to its full length. With the folded edge facing downward, find the center of this edge; then fold each side straight up from this point to create a U-shaped pad. Slip this pad under the flanges of the tracheostomy tube so that the pad's flaps encircle and cushion the tube.
• Remove and discard your gloves. Replace and tighten the lid on the container with the spare inner cannula, if applicable. (See *Tracheostomy: considerations.*)

Tracheostomy: equipment

Setting up the equipment

Wash your hands and assemble all equipment and supplies in the patient's room. Then, do the following:
• Check the expiration date on each sterile package and inspect for tears.
• Open the waterproof trash bag and place it adjacent to your working area so you don't reach across the sterile field or the patient's stoma when disposing of soiled articles.
• Form a cuff by turning down the top of the trash bag, making a wide opening. This helps prevent contamination of instruments or gloves caused by touching the bag's edge.
• Wash your hands thoroughly.
• Establish a sterile field near the patient's bed (usually on the overbed table), and place equipment and supplies on it.

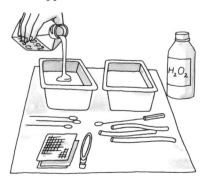

T

• For cleansing, pour sterile normal saline solution, hydrogen peroxide, or a mixture of equal parts of both solutions into one of the sterile containers; then pour sterile normal saline solution into a second container for rinsing. For double-cannula care, you may use the third basin to hold your gauze sponges and pads saturated with cleansing solution.

• Prepare new tracheostomy ties from twill tape, if indicated.

• If using a spare sterile inner cannula, unscrew the cap from the top of the sterile container, but do not remove it.

Tracheostomy: fastening

Securing a cannula properly

The usual method is to knot a string to each flange on the cannula, then knot both strings together behind the patient's neck. But the knot behind the patient's neck can cause skin breakdown. Or the knots on the flanges can pull the cannula to one side when the patient moves his neck, causing tissue damage, coughing, and ventilation leaks.

To avoid such problems, use a single string that's long enough to go behind the patient's neck twice. Here's how to attach the string:

First, slip one end through the front side of the flange opening.

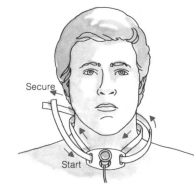

Secure

Start

Then, pass the string behind the patient's neck and through the back side of the opposite flange opening.

Next, pass the string behind the patient's neck again, and tie the two ends together. Knot the ends on the side of the patient's neck, and make sure the string isn't too tight over the carotid arteries.

Besides being easy to apply, the single long string is easy to remove. Simply untie the knot or cut through the string, then slip the string back through the flange openings.

Obtain the long string from a tracheostomy kit manufacturer or by using extra-wide, sterile umbilical tape.

Tracheostomy: occluded tube

What to do immediately

Signs and symptoms of tracheostomy tube occlusion include paleness, diaphoresis, and a whistling sound each time the patient inhales. His respirations will be labored, rapid, and shallow. And you'll feel minimal airflow at the stoma. Here's what to do if your patient's tracheostomy tube becomes occluded:

Call for help. Have the patient sit upright. Remove the tube's inner cannula and have him try to cough up the plug. This may be difficult if he's had his glottis removed; he won't be able to perform Valsalva's maneuver or cough with an effective force.

If this doesn't work, quickly attach a humidified oxygen source to his tracheostomy tube and assemble a tracheal suction setup. Prepare a syringe of 2 ml of sterile normal saline solution (without preservatives). Remove the oxygen source, quickly instill the saline solution, then vigorously suction. Apply suction for no longer than 10 seconds at a time, and replace the oxygen source between each suctioning attempt. (See *Tracheostomy: suctioning.*)

If the mucus plug still hasn't come out, call for the anesthesiologist, then cut the ties and gently remove the entire tube. Don't worry about the stoma closing; it's been permanently sutured open.

If the plug doesn't come out with the tube, use a flashlight to examine inside the tracheal stoma. If you see that the mucus plug is near the stoma, carefully try to remove it using a pair of sterile hemostats. Don't blindly grasp at it; you could push it down the trachea or damage the tracheal mucosa.

Repeat the procedure of instilling saline solution and applying suction. If these actions fail to remove the plug, replace the oxygen source and wait for the anesthesiologist.

Remember to remain calm and to continually reassure the patient throughout this ordeal. Don't leave him alone until the plug has been removed.

After the doctor has removed it, reassess the patient. Is he breathing without difficulty? Are his breath sounds clear? Are his vital signs stable? Does he require medication for anxiety? Is an analysis of arterial blood gases indicated?

Tracheostomy: patient preparation

Steps to take before cleaning the cannula

Here's what to do:

• Assess the patient's condition.

• Explain the procedure to him, even if he's unresponsive. Provide privacy.

• Unless contraindicated, place him in semi-Fowler's position to decrease abdominal pressure on the diaphragm, thereby promoting lung expansion.

• Disconnect any humidification or ventilation device.

• Using sterile technique, suction the entire length of his tracheostomy tube to clear the airway of any secretions that may hinder oxygenation. Follow appropriate suctioning procedures. (See *Tracheostomy: suctioning.*)

• Reconnect the patient to the humidifier or ventilator, if necessary.

• Remove and discard his tracheostomy dressing.

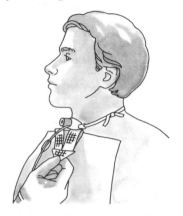

• Put a sterile glove on your dominant hand. Now you are ready to clean the cannula. (See *Tracheostomy: double-cannula tube; Tracheostomy: single-cannula tube.*)

Tracheostomy: single-cannula tube

Tips for proper cleaning

Follow these steps:

• With your gloved hand, wet a sterile 4″ × 4″ gauze sponge with the cleaning solution. Squeeze excess liquid from the sponge to prevent accidental aspiration. Then, wipe the patient's neck under the tracheostomy tube flanges and twill tapes.

• Saturate a second gauze sponge and wipe the patient's neck until the skin surrounding the tracheostomy is clean. Use additional sponges or cotton-tipped applicators to clean the stoma site and the tube's flanges. Wipe only once with each sponge and then discard it to prevent contamination of a clean area with a soiled sponge.

• If incrustations resist removal, clean with a sterile cotton-tipped applicator saturated in hydrogen peroxide (but pressed to remove excess liquid). Use each applicator only once and wipe gently, especially if the surrounding skin is excoriated.

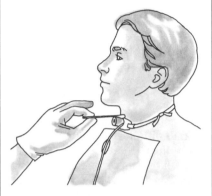

• Rinse any debris and hydrogen peroxide from the patient's skin with one or more sterile 4″ × 4″ gauze sponges dampened in sterile normal saline solution. Dry the area thoroughly with additional sterile gauze sponges. Remove and discard your glove. (See *Tracheostomy: considerations.*)

Tracheostomy: Stomahesive

Using it to reduce rubbing

If a patient with a tracheostomy tube complains that its faceplate rubs uncomfortably against his

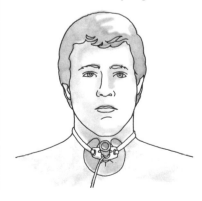

skin, try this: Cut a piece of Stomahesive in the shape of a "C." Apply it to the patient's skin around the stoma. (If you cut small slits along the inside edge of the Stomahesive, it will lie smoothly on the skin.) Besides cushioning the skin, the Stomahesive also acts as a barrier against secretions.

Tracheostomy: suctioning

Current procedure

Here's what to do:

1. Collect your equipment and wash your hands before starting. You'll need a suction kit containing a sterile suction catheter (usually a #12 or #14 French), a sterile cup for saline solution, a sterile glove, sterile normal saline solution, a plastic bag for used supplies, and tissues.

At the patient's bedside, you'll need an oxygen source, suction apparatus, connecting tubing, and a collection bottle.

2. Tell the patient what you're going to do. Listen to his breath sounds to determine whether he needs suctioning and to establish a baseline assessment. Also check heart rate and rhythm and assess his color.

3. Now prepare your equipment. Be sure the connecting tubing is within easy reach and that you'll have enough tubing to maneuver comfortably once the catheter is attached. If you're not sure, add extension tubing. Attach the tubing to the collection bottle.

With your equipment ready, open the suction kit.

4. Carefully spread open the sterile field, maintaining sterile technique. Place the glove on your dominant hand. (Hospital policy may require you to wear gloves on both hands.)

T

5. Set up the cup for the sterile saline solution, which is used to rinse and lubricate the catheter and to test its patency.

6. Using your ungloved hand, pour the sterile saline solution into the cup. Then, being careful to maintain sterility, remove the catheter from its plastic wrapper.

7. To lessen the risk of contamination, wrap the catheter around the fingers of your gloved hand. Then, insert it into the connecting tubing, which you hold in your ungloved hand. Turn on the suction with your ungloved hand.

8. Occlude the lumen of the catheter by pinching it between your fingers. Place the thumb of your ungloved hand over the suction port to apply suction, then look at the gauge on the suction apparatus. It should read between 80 and 120 mm Hg. Adjust the suction pressure accordingly, but be sure to release and reapply suction between test adjustments.

9. Lubricate the catheter and check its patency: Apply suction and draw up the sterile saline solution through the catheter and connecting tubing until you see it in the collection bottle.

10. Before suctioning, ask the patient to take a few deep breaths, and tell him that when you insert the catheter he'll probably cough. Loosen the tracheostomy collar to allow access to the tracheostomy.

11. As you gently insert the catheter, tell the patient to take a deep breath. Don't apply suction while inserting the catheter.

12. If the catheter meets resistance a short distance into the tube, it has probably met the curve of the tube. Continue to advance the catheter until it meets resistance again, which should be the carina. The patient will probably cough. When he does, withdraw the catheter about ½″ (1 cm), then apply suction.

While applying suction, gently rotate the catheter and withdraw it from the airway. Don't jab the cath-

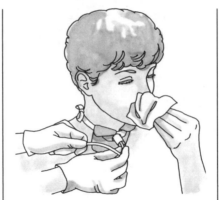

eter up and down, and don't apply suction for more than 10 seconds. The entire procedure—from insertion to withdrawal—should take no more than 15 seconds.

13. If the cuff of the tracheostomy tube has been deflated, the patient may be able to cough secretions up into his mouth as well as through the tube. So be sure to give him some tissues in case he needs to expectorate during suctioning.

If he can't expectorate the secretions, rinse the catheter and suction his mouth after you've finished suctioning his trachea. After suctioning his mouth, don't suction the trachea again because the catheter will now be contaminated. If you must suction the trachea again, use a fresh sterile catheter.

14. When you've finished suctioning, rinse the catheter and connecting tubing, then disconnect the catheter from the connecting tubing. Wrap the catheter around your gloved fingers.

15. Pull off the glove so that the catheter is inside it. Discard the catheter and glove in the plastic bag.

16. Make sure the patient is comfortable and breathing easily. Tell him to take a few deep breaths and give him supplemental oxygen, if necessary. Assess his color, breath sounds, and heart rate and rhythm, and compare your findings to the baseline assessments.

Discard any other used supplies in the plastic bag. Tie the bag and dispose of it in the contaminated trash, according to hospital procedure. Then wash your hands. Re-

stock any supplies that are needed at the patient's bedside.

Chart your findings, including the patient's vital signs and breath sounds before and after the procedure, and the color, consistency, and amount of secretions. Finally, document how the patient tolerated the procedure, whether he had any adverse reactions, and what steps you took to manage them.

Traction patients

Nursing tips

The doctor may order traction for a patient to treat a fracture or dislocation, to decrease muscle spasms, or to immobilize an injury before surgery.

Skin traction is used to treat fractures in small children or to reduce pain in adults by temporarily immobilizing their injuries.

Skeletal traction is used to treat long-bone fractures and cervical spine fractures.

Both types of traction work by exerting a pulling force on a body part. For skin traction, the doctor connects the weight system to a moleskin bandage and elastic; for skeletal traction, he connects it to a pin or wire. (You may be asked to apply some forms of skin traction.)

The following traction care tips will help you care for patients with skin or skeletal traction:

• Check for wrinkles in the moleskin; they may cause skin blisters.

• Monitor a patient with skin traction for itching, burning, or pain, possibly indicating an allergic reaction.

• Relieve pressure against bony prominences by placing sheepskin under them.

• Check for circulatory and neurologic impairment from an elastic bandage that's too tight or from splint pressure on the popliteal area.

• Maintain ropes and pulleys in straight alignment, with weights hanging free.

T

• For a patient in a pelvic sling, watch for signs and symptoms of abdominal organ injury. These include inadequate output, hematuria, rectal bleeding, abdominal pain, spasm, rigidity, distention, and shock from internal bleeding.

Transhepatic biliary catheter irrigation

Helpful pointers

Before irrigating the catheter, check the doctor's orders to confirm the amount of bacteriostatic saline solution you should use (usually between 5 and 20 ml). Also, make sure you know how often you should perform the procedure (at least once, preferably twice, a day in most institutions). Then gather the necessary equipment: the three-way stopcock, a small sterile cap, a padded tongue depressor, adhesive tape, two sterile syringes and one needle, and bacteriostatic saline solution. Use one syringe and needle to draw up the saline solution, then proceed as follows:

1. Using aseptic technique, attach the stopcock to the catheter tubing. Then connect the other end of the stopcock to the drainage bag tubing. Turn the stopcock so that it's opened to the patient and drainage bag, and closed to the external port. (Cover this port with the sterile cap.) Place the padded tongue depressor under the stopcock and secure it to the tubing with adhesive tape.

2. Remove the cap on the external port and insert the empty syringe. Then turn the stopcock so that it's opened to the patient, but closed to the drainage bag. Now aspirate a few milliliters of bile to rule out sediment, tissue, or a clot in the catheter. Discard the aspirate.

3. Warn the patient that he may feel some discomfort during the actual irrigation. The procedure may

irritate the liver bed and bile ducts, especially if cholangitis or edema has developed.

Irrigation

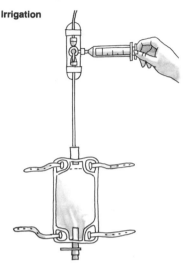

4. Insert the syringe that contains saline into the external port and gently instill the saline solution. If you feel resistance, don't force the instillation. Instead, stop the procedure and notify the doctor. The catheter may be occluded.

5. After you've instilled the irrigant, return the stopcock to its original position (opened to the patient and drainage bag). Remove the

Drainage

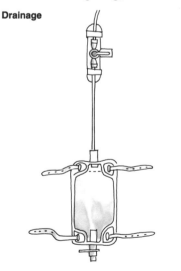

syringe, and cover the external port with the cap to preserve sterility and prevent contamination. Ob-

serve the patient carefully for adverse reactions. If he develops abdominal cramping or pain, you may have instilled too much irrigant. Notify the doctor; he'll probably want to reduce the amount of irrigant. If the pain grows increasingly severe and is accompanied by signs and symptoms of an acute abdominal disorder, such as peritonitis, notify the doctor immediately. The patient will probably need emergency cholangiography to evaluate the catheter's position and to rule out intra-abdominal bleeding or small-bowel perforation.

Transhepatic biliary catheter management

Preventing problems

The doctor may insert a transhepatic biliary catheter—an internal bile drain—as a palliative therapy when nonresectable liver, pancreatic, or biliary duct cancer obstructs a bile flow. This measure may also relieve signs and symptoms of biliary ostruction and hepatic dysfunction secondary to obstructive jaundice or biliary sepsis. Although not a cure, the procedure permits a normal life-style.

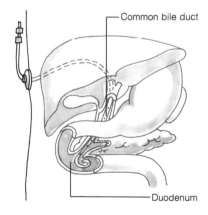
Common bile duct / Duodenum

The doctor will insert the catheter fluoroscopically through the abdominal wall, liver, and common bile duct, passing through or by the obstruction to the duodenum. Holes in the catheter allow bile to drain into the duodenum, preventing it from accumulating in the liver.

Before the procedure, explain to the patient that catheter insertion may take several hours and cause pain. Because the catheter will puncture the liver, the patient should have laboratory studies the day before to rule out bleeding disorders. If needed, also administer fresh frozen plasma, as ordered. Withhold food and fluids the day of the procedure. The doctor will order pain medication and possibly antibiotics.

After catheter insertion, monitor vital signs frequently for indications of hemorrhage and sepsis. An external drainage bag, attached for several days, allows ductal edema to subside. Observe drainage for quantity, color, odor, and consistency. Report excessively bloody drainage immediately—this may indicate catheter dislodgment in a hepatic blood vessel. If drainage exceeds 1,500 ml in 24 hours, suspect retrograde duodenal content flow, an intestinal obstruction, or both.

Irrigate the catheter with a syringe containing 5 to 20 ml of bacteriostatic saline solution, as ordered. A three-way stopcock, with the drainage bag attached, makes irrigation easier. (See *Transhepatic biliary catheter irrigation.*) When edema subsides, and if the patient shows no complications, remove the drainage bag and cap the catheter, as ordered, to allow bile to drain into the duodenum. With the bag removed, irrigation takes place through the external port. Don't force the irrigant against resistance, and don't aspirate it. If the patient develops cramping or pain, notify the doctor.

Keep the insertion site clean and dry. Report any bile leakage around the catheter.

Assess the patient for signs of adequate catheter function—for example, resolving jaundice and normal urine and stool color.

Before discharge, teach the patient and his family how to irrigate and care for the catheter. Also teach the patient which signs and symptoms of malfunctions or complications to report. Consider home health care referrals, if needed.

Transplant, corneal

Monitoring and aftercare

After the patient recovers from anesthesia, assess for and immediately report sudden, sharp, or excessive pain; bloody, purulent, or clear viscous drainage; or fever. Instill corticosteroid eyedrops or topical antibiotics, as ordered, to prevent inflammation and graft rejection.

Instruct the patient to lie on his back or on his unaffected side, with the bed flat or slightly elevated, as ordered. Also have him avoid rapid head movements, hard coughing or sneezing, bending over, and other activities that could increase intraocular pressure; likewise, he shouldn't squint or rub his eyes.

Clouded cornea removed

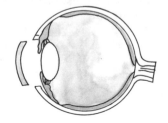

Replaced by clear cornea

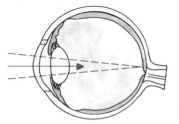

Home care instructions
• Teach the patient and his family to recognize the signs and symptoms of graft rejection (inflammation, cloudiness, drainage, and pain at the graft site). Instruct them to notify the doctor immediately if any of these signs and symptoms occur. Emphasize that rejection can occur many years after surgery; stress the need for assessing the graft *daily* for the rest of the patient's life. Also remind the patient to keep regular appointments with his doctor.
• Tell the patient to avoid activities that increase intraocular pressure, including extreme exertion; sudden, jerky movements; lifting or pushing heavy objects; or straining during defecation.
• Explain that photophobia, a common side effect, gradually decreases as healing progresses. Suggest wearing dark glasses in bright light.
• Teach the patient how to correctly instill prescribed eyedrops. (See *Eyedrops: patient teaching.*)
• Remind the patient to wear an eye shield when sleeping. (See *Cataract surgery.*)

Transsphenoidal surgery

Postop positioning

The transsphenoidal approach is used to excise pituitary adenomas and for performing a hypophysectomy to control bone pain in metastatic cancer.

When a patient returns from such surgery, elevate the head of his bed 30 to 45 degrees. This will minimize leakage of cerebrospinal fluid, reduce pressure on the surgical site, and facilitate venous drainage, thus decreasing the risk of edema.

Travel advice

Keeping travelers healthy

You can help keep your patient's trip free of medical—and medication—hassles. Tell him to:
• check vaccination requirements for every country he plans to visit.

T

• see his doctor for a pretravel evaluation, especially if he has a chronic illness, such as heart disease or diabetes.

• take along enough medication to last the entire trip. Just to be safe, he should ask his doctor to write a prescription for all his drugs, using generic names; trade names may vary among countries. If the patient's taking narcotics or sedatives, his doctor should write a letter documenting his need for them. Such drugs are sometimes difficult to bring into other countries.

• avoid packing his medication in luggage he's planning to check—it may become lost. He should keep his medicines with him at all times.

• be careful about buying over-the-counter drugs in foreign countries. Because of different drug laws, some potent and potentially dangerous drugs are available without a prescription outside the United States.

• beware of "medicine lag" when crossing time zones. To time his medication doses, tell him to use a watch set to the original time zone. Keeping the same schedule is especially important for such medications as oral contraceptives and insulin.

Trendelenburg's test

Testing venous retrograde filling

First, mark the distended leg veins with a pen while the patient stands. Then have him lie on the examining table and elevate his legs for about a minute to drain the veins. Next, have him stand while you measure venous filling time. Competent valves take at least 30 seconds to fill. If the veins fill in less than 30 seconds, have the patient lie on the table again and raise his legs for 1 minute. Then apply a tourniquet around his upper thigh. Next, have him stand. If his leg veins fill in less than 30 seconds, suspect incompetent perforating and deep-vein

valves (functioning valves block retrograde flow).

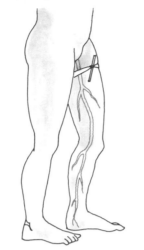

Now remove the tourniquet. If the veins again fill in less than 30 seconds, suspect incompetent superficial vein valves that allow backward blood flow.

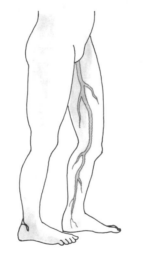

To pinpoint incompetent valve location, repeat this procedure by applying the tourniquet just above the knee and around the upper calf.

Triage, ED

Classification strategies

When a patient enters the emergency department (ED), his condition should be evaluated by the triage nurse, who will assign him to one of four classifications based on the urgency of his condition:

Class I (immediate). This category includes patients with life- or limb-threatening conditions that must be treated within minutes. Examples include acute cardiac or respiratory distress or arrest, severe multiple trauma, massive bleeding, major burns, and very abnormal vital signs.

Class II (urgent). These patients have potentially life-threatening conditions that require medical intervention within 30 minutes. The patient's condition is serious, but his vital signs don't require Class I attention. Examples include acute abdominal pain, open fractures, and bleeding lacerations.

Class III (semiurgent). Patients with potentially serious but not life-threatening conditions that require treatment with 2 hours are placed in this classification. Examples include nonacute abdominal pain, thrombophlebitis, cellulitis, minor burns, eye infection, and migraine headaches.

Class IV (nonurgent). These are patients whose conditions don't require priority attention. Examples are uncomplicated flu syndrome, rashes, minor toothaches, medication refills, suture removal, and nonexacerbated chronic conditions.

Develop a list of specific guidelines based on a patient's complaints, initial vital signs, and other signs and symptoms. When the triage nurse completes her assessment, she can compare it with the guidelines to determine under which classification the patient belongs. If a patient's problem is not represented on the list of guidelines, the triage nurse must use her judgment to determine the patient's classification. If in doubt, she should place a patient into a more urgent category. A patient assigned to Class II or Class III is continually observed by the nursing staff and can be moved from one classification to another if his condition changes.

Once a patient has been evaluated by the triage nurse, his chart

T

is flagged with a priority number within his classification and placed in the doctor's "to be seen" box. When a Class I patient has been assessed, the nurse gives the doctor a verbal report as well. A doctor must see all patients by order of class. For easy identification, color code each classification.

Trousseau's sign

Observing for hypocalcemia

Test for this sign by inflating a blood pressure cuff to a level above systolic pressure. Maintain this pressure for at least 2 minutes while observing the patient's hand for a carpal spasm. Then deflate the cuff. A spasm lasting 5 to 10 seconds after cuff deflation is a positive response. (An instantly disappearing spasm may be normal.)

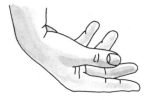

The most reliable sign of latent tetany, Trousseau's sign should be tested serially. (See *Chvostek's sign; Tetany*.)

U

Ulcers, arterial leg

Patient-teaching tips

Patients with poor circulation in their legs and feet may develop leg ulcers. To prevent this, teach your patient these rules.
• "Keep your legs and feet clean, soft, and dry. Wash daily and dry

thoroughly by patting with a soft towel, especially between the toes. Apply lanolin or a similar mild cream to keep your skin from cracking. And wear clean wool or cotton socks or stockings.
• "Inspect your legs and feet every day, because you may develop breaks in the skin that you can't feel. If breaks develop, keep the area clean, and contact your doctor if signs of infection appear.

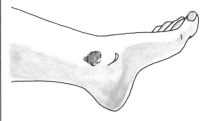

• "Avoid injury to your legs and feet. Wear shoes that aren't too loose or too tight. Put lamb's wool between your toes to prevent rubbing. Don't walk barefoot. Have a podiatrist cut your toenails.
• "Avoid temperature extremes. Keep your feet and legs warm at all times by wearing cotton or wool socks. Never put a hot object (for example, a hot water bottle) on your feet or legs. Test bathwater with your hand (not your foot) before getting into the bath. Avoid exposing your legs and feet to the sun, and don't swim in cold water.
• "Avoid over-the-counter foot preparations unless the doctor okays them. This is important because many foot plasters, corn removers, disinfectants, ointments, and the like are strong enough to injure your feet.
• "Avoid clothing that restricts your circulation. Don't wear girdles, garters, or socks that have tight elastic bands, and be sure your shoes have sufficient toe room.
• "Avoid smoking. This narrows blood vessels, further restricting the blood supply to your skin.
• "Notify your doctor if you get a wound on your leg or foot. Cover the wound with a plain, sterile gauze pad. Do not put ointments, such as hydrocortisone cream, on it."

Ulcers, decubitus

Managing aural lesions

If a bedridden patient develops a decubitus ulcer on her ear, you're in for a big challenge—trying to keep pressure off her ear so that it can heal while she's lying in bed.

To meet this challenge, use the following procedure: Make a pillow from foam rubber cut in the shape of a "C," and cover it with a pillowcase. (Fold and tape the case so that

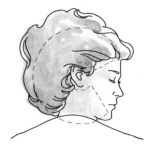

it doesn't cover the cut-out section.) The patient can lay her head on the pillow with her ear in the cut-out section so that no pressure is placed on the ulcer. Also, keep the ulcer clean, dry, and infection-free to speed healing.

Umbilical cord

Intervening quickly for prolapse

This is one of the most common—and most frightening—birth complications you'll ever witness. If it's not corrected within 5 minutes, expect fetal hypoxia, central nervous system damage, and possibly death. Fortunately, your quick assessment and intervention can help both mother and fetus survive this traumatic birth event.

A prolapsed cord is an umbilical cord that's displaced below the fetus' presenting part. It's common in women whose amniotic membranes rupture early in labor, carrying the long, loose cord below the unengaged presenting part in a sudden gush of fluid. The cord may slip through the mother's cervix into her vagina. But the most serious damage is done when the fetus compresses the cord, interrupting the blood flow from the placenta.

Watch for these signs and symptoms of a prolapsed cord:
• The mother feels the cord "slither" down after the membranes rupture.
• The umbilical cord is visible or palpable in the birth canal.
• Fetal activity is violent.
• Fetal bradycardia occurs with variable deceleration during contractions.

Your first priority is to relieve the pressure on the cord until the doctor can perform an emergency cesarean section (or, for a patient with a fully dilated cervix, a forceps delivery). Here's how to proceed:
• Place your patient in the knee-chest position to shift fetal weight off the cord.
• Using two gloved fingers, push the fetus' presenting part off the cord. Don't push the cord back into the uterus—this may traumatize the cord and stop blood flow to the fetus. You may also cause an intra-uterine infection.
• Notify the doctor and continue to relieve the pressure while the operating room's being prepared.
• Ask another nurse to give supplemental oxygen, to start a large-gauge I.V., to send blood for typing and crossmatching, and to insert a nasogastric tube, as ordered.
• Accompany the patient to the operating room, keeping pressure off the cord and watching for signs of maternal and fetal distress.

Unna's boot

Basic procedure for application

First, remove the Unna's boot bandage from its package. Then:
• Start wrapping from the inner ankle, making figure-eight turns around the ankle and foot. (Ask the

patient to flex his ankle so the bandage will fit properly without chafing.) Make overlapping turns as you move up the leg.

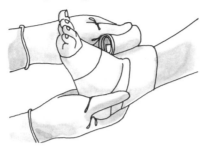

• Cut the bandage, or fold it in pleats, to keep it flat (remember, the bandage is nonelastic) as you apply it.
• Continue wrapping up to 1″ to 2″ (3 to 5 cm) below the knee. (The boot will be two or three layers thick.) Decrease the pressure gradually as you go up the leg.

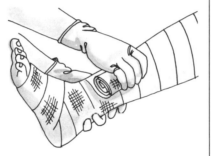

• Cover the boot with tube gauze or a 6″ (15-cm) wide Ace bandage to prevent soiling and provide additional support. (See *Bandage, roller.*)

Unsafe practices

Blowing the whistle

First, write a clear, precise description of the unsafe practice. It should answer these questions:
• What, exactly, is the dangerous practice?
• Who, exactly, is endangered and how?
• How, specifically, would your blowing the whistle be protective?

Make sure you can state in concrete, specific terms what's wrong and why.

Be accurate and credible. Your goal is to stop dangerous, unethical, or illegal behavior. Since this may entail discipline against the person responsible, you must have accurate, detailed, reliable information to back you up.

Document everything pertinent, seek verification from others, and stick to the facts.

After you've assessed the situation, assess your motives. Your testimony may be automatically dismissed or discounted if you have self-serving motives. Ask yourself:
• Is my reputation above reproach?
• What are my motives?
• What codes, rules, regulations, and laws support blowing the whistle in this case?

Try to find out if any hospital, local, and state regulations or licensing statutes have been violated.

Don't try to be a solitary whistle-blower. If you have to "go out on a limb," advisors are your guide ropes; friends, your safety net. Don't make your commitment a matter of record until you've recruited at least one trustworthy confidant and advisor. You need someone who's:
• stable, but willing to take a risk
• open-minded, but decisive
• caring, but clearheaded
• close enough to the situation to understand it, but far enough from it to be objective.

A nurse from another unit, a social worker, or a doctor may come closer to meeting these qualifications than a colleague on your unit.

Go through hospital channels. You want to get effective action at the lowest possible level. This usually means starting with your supervisor. (If the supervisor's the person you're reporting, go to *her* supervisor.) If necessary, go beyond the organization to regulatory agencies, law-enforcement bodies, licensing bureaus, and professional organizations.

Give your name. If you don't, those who review your charges may

U

have trouble evaluating their accuracy and won't know how to get more information. They're likely to suspect the motives of an anonymous tipster, too. Some won't consider a complaint seriously if the person bringing the charges isn't willing to stand behind them.

Once you blow the whistle, you're obliged to see the problem through.

Supervisors who want to cover up the situation may assure you that they'll "take care of the problem." You can show your persistence by following up your report to a supervisor with one of these comments or questions:

• "When may I expect a result?"
• "Let's look at your calendar . . . I'll check back with you Monday morning."
• "I could take this matter to the director. But I'd like to think we can solve the problem at this level."
• "I want you to understand that I think this is a very serious and dangerous problem. I must continue to press for action until it's stopped."

Ureteral stent

Essentials of management

Here's how to care for your patient who has a ureteral stent:

• If an indwelling (Foley) catheter is used with the stent, tape it to the patient's thigh and note on the chart that it's a ureteral stent catheter.
• Care for the tube site (which will be placed inside the ureter via cys-

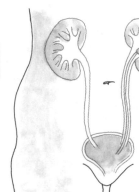

toscope, nephrostomy tube, or surgery and either taped to a ureteral catheter or connected to a drainage bag at the nephrostomy tube site).
• Watch for bleeding and signs of infection.
• Watch for signs of stent dislodgment, such as colicky pain and decreased urine output.
• Measure and record intake and output.
• Irrigate the ureteral stent slowly, never using more than 5 ml of warm saline solution, as ordered.

Urethral culture

Collecting one from a male patient

Instruct the patient not to void for an hour before the specimen collection to prevent eliminating any urethral secretions.

Provide privacy for him. Position him supine on an examination table, and expose his penis. Have him grasp and raise his penis to allow visualization of the urethra.

Wash your hands and put on sterile gloves. Then insert a thin, sterile urogenital alginate swab no more than ¾" (2 cm) into his urethra. Rotate the swab, and leave it in place for 10 to 30 seconds to absorb organisms.

Remove the swab, allow it to dry, and then send it to the laboratory. Assist the patient from the examination table and allow him to dress.

Urinary tract infections

Teaching your female patient

Tell your patient she can reduce discomfort during sexual activity by using a hormone cream or a water-soluble lubricant to relieve vaginal dryness, by taking pain medication before sexual activity, by using relaxation techniques (such as a hot

shower) before sexual activity, and by placing a pillow beneath her hips during intercourse to minimize urethral irritation.

Review with your patient the causes of urinary tract infection. Remind her to urinate before and after intercourse to flush the lower urinary tract, and advise her to drink two glasses of water right after intercourse to promote urination.

Urge her to avoid bubble baths, perfumed soaps, feminine hygiene sprays, and other irritants.

Urine glucose tests

Limitations

Urine glucose tests aren't always accurate because they measure blood glucose levels indirectly. A pregnant woman with a low renal threshold may have a positive urine test, even though her blood glucose level is low or normal. In contrast, an elderly patient with a high renal threshold could have a negative urine test despite an abnormally high blood glucose level. For accurate readings, patients like these must test their blood glucose levels as well as urine ketone levels.

Storage tips

Exposure to heat, light, and moisture can affect the reagent strips' accuracy. For reliable testing, encourage your patient to follow these storage guidelines:

• After removing a strip, close the bottle cap tightly.
• Store bottles in a dry, dark location—not in the refrigerator or bathroom.
• Discard strips that are darkened or discolored; also discard a bottle and its contents if the expiration date on the label has passed.
• After opening a new bottle, write the current date on the label. Dispose of the bottle and its remaining contents as the manufacturer directs or no later than 4 months from the date you've written. (See also *Urine self-testing.*)

U

Urine self-testing

Teaching your diabetic patient

Before discussing urine testing, ask your patient if he monitors his glucose levels with blood tests. If so, you'll have to review only urine ketone testing with him to reinforce your teaching.

Explain that even a small amount of glucose in the urine is abnormal and usually signals high blood glucose levels. Urine ketones, which are also abnormal, indicate that his cells are metabolizing fats because glucose is unavailable to them. So, if his test results are positive for either glucose or ketones, he must adjust his diet, medication, or exercise, as directed.

Review the procedure for obtaining a second-voided urine specimen.

Make sure he's familiar with the type of reagent strip or tablet he'll be using at home. Remind him, if he's a Type I diabetic patient, that he needs a product that measures up to 5% glucose; the Chemstrip uGK is one example. If he's a Type II diabetic patient, he can use a test such as Keto-Diastix, which measures only up to 2% glucose. Both these products also test for ketones. Products that measure only urine glucose include the Clinitest reagent tablet (which measures as high as 5% glucose, depending on the test method used), Tes-Tape, and Chemstrip uG. Acetate strips detect ketones only.

Urge the patient to check labels and package inserts before buying any product because manufacturers' recommendations may change.

If he's using a reagent strip, explain that the reagent blocks change color according to the composition of his urine. Point out the color key on the bottle's label. If he's using Tes-Tape strips, which have no reagent blocks, explain that the strips themselves change color.

Instruct him to remove one strip at a time—and only when he's ready to use it. If he accidentally touches

a reagent block, he should discard the strip and use a fresh one.

Advise him to use a watch with a second hand to time the test for the period the manufacturer specifies.

Instruct him to compare the reagent blocks to the color key under a bright light. If he's color-blind, teach a family member to help him with this part of the test. Or try a different reagent product; it may produce color changes in shades he can see. Another alternative: a blood glucose monitor that provides a digital reading.

Show your patient how to keep a record of all his test results. (See *Glucose monitoring; Urine glucose tests.*)

Urine specimen: catheters

Aspirating one properly

To aspirate a urine specimen from an indwelling (Foley) catheter, clamp the drainage tube just below where it's attached to the catheter for no more than 15 minutes. Or you can coil the tubing on the bed to avoid clamping. When urine has accumulated, clean the distal end of the catheter with alcohol or povidone-iodine. Then insert the sy-

Aspirating from drainage lumen

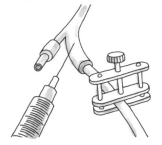

ringe needle into the catheter just above where it's attached to the drainage tube. This needle placement prevents accidental puncture of the lumen leading to the balloon holding the catheter in place in the bladder. Aspirating the water in this lumen can cause the catheter to fall

out of the bladder. After collecting the specimen, remove clamp.

Urine can also be aspirated from an indwelling catheter that has a

Aspirating from sampling port

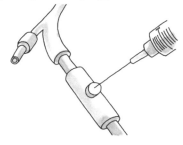

built-in sampling port. Follow the above instructions, but insert the needle into the sampling port.

Urine specimen: children

Effective collection method

Getting a child to void or drink at a certain time usually requires a little ingenuity. As an incentive, use a kitchen timer.

For example, if a child must give a second-voided specimen in 20 minutes or drink fluids every hour, set the timer accordingly. While it's ticking away, the child will mentally prepare himself for the task at hand. When the timer goes off, the child will know that he's "on" and usually perform with great enthusiasm.

Urine specimen: collection

When your patient has difficulty voiding

Here's a way to obtain a urine specimen when your patient can't start and stop voiding easily.

After cleaning the patient's genital area, spread a disposable pad under the commode and remove its collection container. Then seat him on the commode, and squat behind it.

U

Hold the collection container under the commode to catch the urine when he begins to void. Then lower

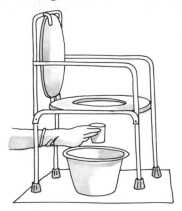

the container and hold a specimen cup under the commode to catch the midstream specimen. (Placing the container on the pad under the commode and holding the specimen cup above it works just as well.)

Urine specimen: elderly women

Collection techniques

Collecting a urine specimen from elderly women patients may be difficult when they have difficulty controlling urination. And if you can't get an order for an indwelling (Foley) or straight catheter, it can be even more difficult. So try using a pediatric urine collection bag. Tape the bag over the patient's perineum. It holds about 50 to 60 ml of urine—sufficient for most tests.

Urine specimen: incontinent patients

Recommended collection method

To get a clean-catch urine specimen from an incontinent man, first clean his penis with povidone-iodine and apply an external collection device

(such as a Texas catheter). Then cut a slit in the plastic lid of a sterile specimen cup. Insert the drainage end of the catheter through the cap and into the cup.

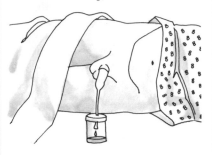

This way, you'll get the specimen without increasing the risk of a urinary tract infection.

Urine specimen: infants

Getting a sample

If you need to get a urine specimen from an infant or toddler, apply a pediatric urine collection bag. If you were to put a diaper over the bag, you'd risk squeezing the bag and causing the baby discomfort as well as having urine leak out. A safer, more comfortable alternative is this: Make a large, X-shaped slash in the diaper at the front of the crotch,

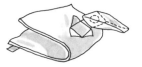

place the collection bag and diaper on the baby, and gently pull the bag out through the X-shaped opening.

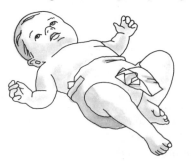

This way, there's no pressure on the bag, and you can readily see when the baby has voided.

Urine testing

Performing the three-glass test

Perform this test if your male patient complains of urinary frequency and urgency, dysuria, flank or lower back pain, or other signs of urethritis, and if his urine specimen is cloudy.

Ask him to void into three conical glasses labeled with numbers 1, 2, and 3. First-voided urine goes into glass 1; midstream urine goes into glass 2; and the remainder goes into glass 3. Tell him not to interrupt the stream of urine when shifting glasses, if possible.

Now observe each glass for pus and mucus shreds. Also note urine color and odor. Glass 1 will contain matter from the anterior urethra; glass 2 will contain bladder contents; and glass 3 will contain sediment from the prostate and seminal vesicles.

Urologic procedures

Improving care

Here's some advice on how to improve common urologic procedures:

1. Don't take a random urine specimen from a urinary drainage bag. As urine collects in a drainage bag, its pH changes from acidic to alkaline, and other components disintegrate. Instead, take the specimen directly from the drainage tube. (See *Urine specimen: catheters.*)

After collecting the specimen, withdraw the needle and unclamp the tube. When collecting 24-hour specimens from patients with indwelling (Foley) catheters, keep the bag on ice. If a preservative is ordered, empty the drainage bag into the container with the preservative at least every 2 hours.

2. Prepare the patient for changes in urine color during drug therapy. Some antimicrobials change the color of urine. For example, nitrofurantoin macrocrystals cause a brownish discoloration; drugs that contain phenazopyridine cause a reddish orange discoloration. If discoloration is expected and doesn't occur, it may indicate that the appropriate urine pH isn't being maintained or that the patient isn't taking his medication.

3. Encourage liberal fluid intake (2 to 3 liters/day) during antimicrobial therapy.

4. Explain that catheterization won't affect sexual functioning afterward.

5. Perform catheter care twice a day for patients who have an indwelling urethral catheter or an external collection device.

Clean the meatus with warm soap and water at least twice a day. External, condomlike collection devices provide a warm, moist environment—ideal for bacterial growth. To retard growth and prevent skin irritation, remove the device twice a day and leave it off for at least 15 minutes. Wash the penis and allow it to dry thoroughly. Before reapplying the device, sprinkle powder (preferably one with a cornstarch base) lightly around the penile shaft to prevent moisture buildup and to ease application of the device.

6. Don't allow an indwelling urethral catheter to hang freely. Excessive pressure on the urinary sphincter can cause damage, resulting in urinary incontinence after the catheter is removed. To prevent this, anchor the catheter securely. For women, anchor it to the thigh with enough slack for freedom of movement. For men, anchor it to the abdomen, especially in long-term use. This avoids pressure on

the penoscrotal junction that can lead to urethrocutaneous fistulas.

7. Do encourage liberal fluid intake (2 to 3 liters/day) while an indwelling catheter is in place and after it's removed.

8. Don't hang the urinary collection bag above the level of your patient's bladder.

9. Don't let a patient who's had urologic surgery be discharged without thorough instructions about resuming normal activities. Instruct him not to strain or lift heavy objects until his doctor permits. If he's had a flank incision, for example, he should avoid lifting heavy objects for at least a year.

Urologic surgery

When it involves pediatric patients

If a child has had urologic surgery, he may be ordered to stay on his back and not to touch his surgical site or catheter. How can you help the child comply without completely restraining him? Make a bed cradle with disposable bed pads, traction rope, and a large cardboard box that has one open side.

With the open side of the box facing down, cut a rectangular opening—large enough to fit over the child's waist—on one side. (The opposite side of the box can be cut away later to accommodate the child's legs, if necessary.) Then cut a small hole in the top of the box so you can see the dressing and catheter.

On the bottom of the other two sides, punch two holes 14″ (35 cm) apart. Thread the traction rope through the holes, and tie the ropes to the bed frame to keep the box securely in place. Then make a small notch near the bottom of one side of the box to extend the catheter tubing so that it won't become compressed.

Finally, cover the box with the disposable bed pads and ask the child's parents to help you draw pictures of his favorite things on it. You can also tie a rattle or small toy to the box within arm's reach of the patient.

Your bed cradle (which can be used with ankle restraints, if necessary) will restrain the child while still allowing him some mobility. It will help provide needed sensory stimulation, too.

Uterus, postpartum

Massaging it

If vaginal bleeding is heavier than it should be for your postpartum patient, stimulate uterine contractions by massaging her uterus. Simply place one hand just above her symphysis pubis, to support the bottom of her uterus, and cup your other hand around the fundus. Use a gentle but firm circular motion to massage the fundus.

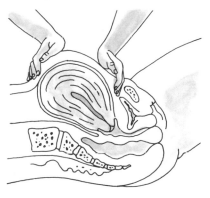

The uterus should respond quickly; stop massaging when it becomes apple-shaped and hard as wood. Be careful not to overdo the massage—this encourages muscle fatigue that can cause uterine relaxation and hemorrhage. And it's uncomfortable for the patient.

Reassess her uterus every 15 minutes for the first hour after it's contracted. If it starts to feel soft and boggy, like a very ripe tomato, begin massaging again.

U

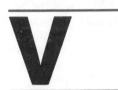

Valsalva's maneuver

When it causes decreased cardiac output

Just imagine you find a postop patient with a history of myocardial infarction (MI) seated on a commode and is barely responsive. He may have experienced decreased cardiac output from accidentally performing Valsalva's maneuver. He could be headed for cardiac arrest.

If the patient is still straining, tell him to stop and to remain still. Keep him in a position of rest—that is, with his head and arms on his knees and his feet spread shoulder-width apart. Also, encourage him to breathe in through his nose and out through his mouth. This will help increase pulmonary function and decrease intrapleural pressure and pressure on baroreceptors.

Remember, though, that these activities will now increase preload, causing more work for the heart. So continue to monitor his pulse, respiratory rate, color, and level of consciousness. Also check for evidence of bleeding.

Get help by switching on the emergency light, by having the patient's roommate summon another nurse, or by yelling for help. If it doesn't arrive quickly and you feel the patient's condition is worsening, lower him to the floor. Have the roommate call the operator and report a code, using the bedside telephone. Don't leave the patient.

When help and equipment arrive, move the patient to his bed and place him in a supine position. If his vital signs are satisfactory, elevate the head of his bed. Begin administering oxygen, and attach him to a cardiac monitor. Start an infusion of dextrose 5% in water at a keep-vein-open rate. You'll find it much easier to start an I.V. now than later if he does go into cardiac arrest.

What to do later

Monitor the patient for signs and symptoms of a new MI; remember, inadequate cardiac output will decrease oxygen supply to the myocardium. (See *MI: emergency intervention.*)

Tell him that from now on he should avoid bearing down while moving his bowels and urinating, as well as when coughing, turning, and moving up to a sitting position in bed. When doing these activities, he should not hold his breath but rather should breathe slowly in through his nose and out through his mouth. Practice this breathing pattern with him (it will have the added benefit of helping him relax).

Then review his bowel and bladder hygiene program. See that he's getting sufficient fluids, and consider increasing the fiber in his diet and getting an order for a stool softener or laxative.

Varicose veins

Doing a manual compression test

To assess venous valve competence, palpate the patient's dilated leg vein with the fingertips of one

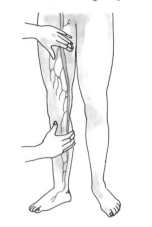

hand. Firmly compress the vein with the other hand at a point at least 8″ (20 cm) higher. Feel for an impulse transmitted to your lower hand. With competent saphenous valves, you won't detect any impulse. A palpable impulse indicates incompetent valves in a vein segment between your hands.

Venipuncture: blood specimen

Using a vacuum tube

Assemble the following supplies: a soft, flat tourniquet; a folded washcloth; an alcohol sponge; a vacuum specimen tube; a vacuum specimen tube holder; a sterile 2″ × 2″ gauze pad; a needle; gloves; and an adhesive bandage.

Connect the vacuum specimen tube holder to the needle. Then place the tube in the holder.

Tie the tourniquet 3″ to 5″ (8 to 12.5 cm) above the antecubital fossa. (If the specimen requires more than 25 ml of blood, tie the tourniquet 6″ to 8″ [15 to 20 cm] above the antecubital fossa.) Tell the patient to open and close his hand several times to engorge the veins. Have a patient with long fingernails hold the folded washcloth.

As the veins distend, instruct the patient to extend his arm with the palm facing up. To maintain venous distention, have him make a fist.

After putting on the gloves, palpate an antecubital vein, using your index finger. This will help you estimate blood volume in the vein. If you have difficulty palpating a vein, flick your finger at the area once or twice. This will cause blood to enlarge the vein. A well-distended vein should feel elastic when you depress it with your fingertip.

Clean the venipuncture site with the alcohol sponge. Start at the center and clean outward in a circular motion. Let the alcohol dry completely to prevent stinging when the needle pierces the skin.

Grasp the vacuum specimen tube holder with your dominant hand, placing your thumb on the tube. Insert the needle quickly and firmly into the vein at a 35- to 45-degree angle. As the needle enters the skin, lower the holder so that you pierce only the anterior vein wall. You should be able to feel when the needle enters the thick vein wall.

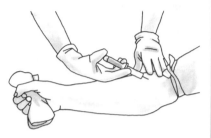

Push the vacuum specimen tube quickly and smoothly into the holder so that the tube can fill with blood. If you've punctured the anterior and posterior walls of the vein, you won't see blood return or you'll see blood only momentarily. When this happens, slowly and gently retract the needle until blood appears in the tube.

If you'll be obtaining several tubes of blood, release the tourniquet while the first or second one is filling. Leaving the tourniquet on too long may cause a hematoma. If you need only one or two tubes, release the tourniquet and have the patient open his hand when you're done drawing blood. Press the sterile 2″ × 2″ gauze pad over the site and remove the needle. Have the patient lift his arm and hold the pad in place for 1 to 3 minutes. Then, to prevent blood leakage, place the adhesive bandage over the venipuncture site.

Venous access device: blood specimen

Effective procedure

First, collect your supplies: a 3-ml syringe of normal saline solution, a 5-ml syringe of normal saline solution, a 5-ml syringe of heparin solution (100 units/ml), 6″ extension tubing with clamp, a ¾″ 90-degree-angle Huber point needle, two specimen tubes, a Vacutainer Luer adapter, alcohol sponges, povidone-iodine sponges, sterile gloves, and a sterile 2″ × 2″ gauze pad. Then, label one of the specimen tubes "discard."

Begin by connecting the 90-degree-angle Huber point needle to the proximal end of the extension tubing and connecting the 3-ml syringe of normal saline solution to the distal end. Open the clamp, prime the tubing with normal saline solution, and close it. Next, remove the syringe and replace it with the adapter.

Now, put on the sterile gloves. Then prep the patient's skin, using the alcohol sponges and povidone-iodine sponges. Following the manufacturer's directions, insert the Huber point needle into the venous access disk. Insert the adapter needle into the specimen tube labeled "discard," and open the clamp. If the specimen tube doesn't fill with blood, have the patient take a deep breath, cough, raise his arms, or change position. When the tube does fill, remove and discard it. Then, fill the other specimen tube.

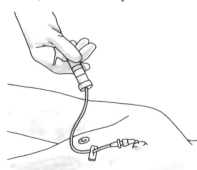

After you've collected the specimen, flush the line with 5 ml of normal saline solution and 5 ml of heparin solution. Then place the sterile 2″ × 2″ gauze pad over the needle, and remove the needle from the venous access disk.

Venous access device: bolus injections

Proper procedure

For I.V. bolus injections you'll need a sterile field, a pair of sterile gloves, three povidone-iodine sponges, and sterile extension tubing with a Luer-Lok and a stopcock.

Gather these additional supplies:
• a sterile 22-gauge, 1½″ Huber point needle (You must use a 22-gauge Huber point needle with an Infuse-a-Port; other needles will damage the entry septum.)
• two sterile 6-ml syringes of normal saline solution
• two sterile 6-ml syringes of heparin solution (100 units/ml)
• a sterile syringe containing the prescribed drug
• alcohol sponges
• a small bandage.

Inserting the needle
After putting on sterile gloves, palpate the Infuse-a-Port to find the entry septum. Then, using a povidone-iodine sponge, clean the injection site. Start at the center of the septum and wipe outward in a circular motion until you've cleaned an area at least 6″ (15 cm) in diameter. Repeat this procedure twice, using a new povidone-iodine sponge each time.

Attach a 6-ml syringe of heparin solution to the stopcock at the end of the extension tubing. Then connect the Huber point needle to the Luer-Lok at the other end and prime the tubing.

Insert the Huber point needle into the center, pushing until the needle stops. Then aspirate a small amount

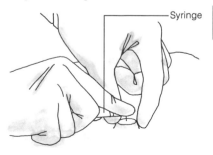

Syringe

V

of blood to make sure the needle is properly positioned.

Injecting

During the injection, hold the needle firmly in place. Twisting or tilting it may cut the septum, causing extravasation. Follow these steps:

• Using firm, steady pressure, flush the Infuse-a-Port with 6 ml of heparin solution at a rate of less than 5 ml/minute. If swelling occurs or the patient complains of pain or a burning sensation as you're injecting the heparin solution, you'll know the needle is improperly positioned. Withdraw it from the injection port and insert another sterile needle.

• Disconnect the syringe and discard it.

• Attach the syringe containing the prescribed drug. Slowly inject the drug.

• When finished, carefully disconnect the syringe to prevent any of the drug from dripping on the patient's skin.

• Attach the second 6-ml syringe of saline solution, and flush the injection port and catheter.

• Disconnect the syringe and discard it.

• Attach the second 6-ml syringe of heparin solution, and inject all 6 ml to prevent occlusion at the catheter tip.

• Withdraw the needle, being careful not to twist or tilt it.

• Observe the injection site for signs of extravasation. If the patient complains of pain or an abnormal sensation at the site, notify the doctor.

• Use alcohol sponges to remove the povidone-iodine from the area. Apply a small bandage if necessary.

Venous access device: continuous infusions

Start-up method

For a continuous infusion, prepare the injection site and insert the 90-degree-angle Huber point needle. Follow the steps for giving a bolus

injection, then proceed as follows. (See *Venous access device: bolus injections*.) You'll need these supplies:

• a sterile 6-ml syringe of normal saline solution

• a sterile 6-ml syringe of heparin solution (100 units/ml)

• a 22-gauge, 1″ 90-degree-angle Huber point needle

• a sterile 3″ × 3″ gauze pad

• tincture of benzoin

• ½″ Steri-Strips

• tape

• 5.6″ × 10″ (14 x 25 cm) Op-Site dressing

• I.V. tubing connected to an infusion pump.

Then proceed as follows:

• Roll up the sterile 3″ × 3″ gauze pad and place it under the needle hub and Luer-Lok to support the needle.

• Apply the tincture of benzoin to the skin on both sides of the gauze pad to help secure the Steri-Strips.

• Secure the needle and tubing by applying the Steri-Strips across the needle hub, using a chevron taping technique.

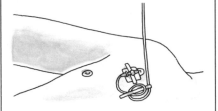

• Apply the Op-Site dressing.

• Attach the stopcock to the I.V. line from the infusion pump. Tape all connections to prevent any accidental disconnections.

• Begin the continuous infusion at the prescribed rate.

Change the I.V. line every 24 hours. The extension tubing and needle can remain in place for as long as 7 days, unless a problem develops. Change the dressing every 3 to 5 days, depending on the therapy and the condition of the site.

When the infusion is complete, disconnect the I.V. line and attach a 6-ml syringe of saline solution to the stopcock. Inject the saline so-

lution and disconnect the syringe. Then attach a 6-ml syringe of heparin solution to the stopcock and flush the Infuse-a-Port. Withdraw the needle without twisting or tilting it. Then remove the povidone-iodine and tincture of benzoin with an alcohol sponge, and apply a small bandage if necessary.

Venous access device: problems

Troubleshooting tips for clots and occlusions

If you have trouble withdrawing blood from a venous access device, the catheter tip may be resting against the vessel wall. Try changing the patient's position. Or ask him to bear down (Valsalva's maneuver) while you try to jog the catheter tip loose by alternating saline solution flushes with aspiration attempts.

Fibrin sheath formation

Over time, some catheters develop a fibrin sheath. Aspiration sucks the sheath into the tip, temporarily occluding it. If fluoroscopy confirms sheath formation, continue to use the device to infuse fluids, but obtain blood specimens from another site. The doctor probably won't replace the device because sheath formation tends to recur in susceptible patients.

Clotting problems

If permitted by hospital policy, you can easily solve some clotting problems by heparinizing the catheter and leaving it alone for about 45 minutes. Or, if the needle's occluded with tiny fibrin particles, a needle change may solve the problem. If these simple measures don't work, however, the doctor may try to alternately aspirate and irrigate the catheter. Always use a large-volume syringe for this procedure. A small syringe may exert too much pressure and rupture the catheter.

If the aspiration and irrigation method fails, administer a fibrinolytic agent (streptokinase or urokinase), as ordered, using a tuberculin syringe. Attempt to aspirate the clot after 10 minutes. Repeat the procedure at 5-minute intervals, as necessary.

Venous hum

Detecting it

To detect a venous hum, have your patient sit upright and then place the bell of the stethoscope over his right supraclavicular area. Gently lift his chin and turn his head toward the left, which increases the loudness of the hum. If you still can't

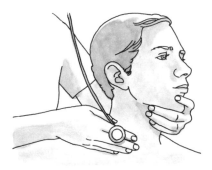

hear the hum, press his jugular vein with your thumb. The hum will disappear with pressure but will suddenly return, temporarily louder than before, when you release your thumb—a result of the turbulence created by pressure changes.

Ventilators: complications

What to watch for

Various complications may result from mechanical ventilation—for example, hyperventilation, hypoventilation, tracheal injury, pneumothorax, and impeded venous return.

Hyperventilation simply means the patient is being ventilated too fast or with too much air. Hypoventilation may result from too little air, an occluded airway or tubing, disconnected tubing, or a deflated endotracheal tube cuff or tracheostomy cuff. Tracheal injury is associated with excessive or prolonged cuff inflation. Air entering the lungs under pressure during positive-pressure ventilation may cause pneumothorax or impede venous return.

Ventilators: home care

Patient and family teaching before discharge

Teach the ventilator-dependent patient and his family the following procedures.

Airway assessment
Show the family members how to assess the patient's respiratory rate and recognize variations in breathing patterns, including shortness of breath and apnea. Then teach them how to describe the quality and amount of secretions.

Bagging technique
• Identify appropriate equipment.
• Connect the Ambu bag to the oxygen.
• Connect the Ambu bag to the patient's tracheostomy tube.
• Use the Ambu bag to give oxygen at a rate that's comfortable for the patient.

Sterile suctioning
• Explain the need for sterile technique.
• Wash your hands.
• Gather the appropriate equipment (catheter, gloves, Ambu bag, and a sterile packet of normal saline solution). (See *Tracheostomy: suctioning.*)

Cleaning the inner cannula of the tracheostomy tube
• Review aseptic technique and again wash your hands.
• Gather the necessary supplies: gloves, a mixture of one-half hydrogen peroxide and one-half normal saline or another appropriate solution, brush, pipe cleaners, sponges, tracheostomy tapes, and a 4" × 4" dressing. An extra tracheostomy set will already be at the bedside.
• Unwrap the equipment and disconnect the ventilator from the patient. Then put on gloves.
• Remove the inner cannula.
• Submerge the inner cannula in the mixture of hydrogen peroxide and normal saline solution. Be sure to assess the patient's respiratory status continuously while cleaning the inner cannula.
• Clean the inner cannula with the brush.
• Feed the pipe cleaner through the inner cannula.
• Shake excess fluid off the inner cannula.
• Reinsert it and lock it in place.
• Reconnect the ventilator to the patient.
• Remove the 4" × 4" dressing around the tracheostomy.
• Clean peristomal skin with the mixture of hydrogen peroxide and normal saline solution or another solution, as ordered.
• Record peristomal skin condition.
• Place a new 4" × 4" dressing around the tracheostomy.
• Change tracheostomy tapes only if another person is available to help. This can be the patient if he's able to assist.
• Explain the danger of the outer cannula coming out. Describe what to do if it does: Immediately replace it with a sterile tracheostomy tube and tie it securely; notify the doctor, and assess the patient's respiratory status. (See *Tracheostomy: dislodged tube.*)

Troubleshooting ventilator problems
• Teach family members how long the patient can tolerate being off the ventilator. Tell family members if this isn't enough time to troubleshoot ventilator problems, they should call the respiratory therapist, doctor, or ambulance service immediately.
• Teach family members how to identify the possible causes of re-

V

spiratory distress or why the ventilator alarm went off. Explain how to deal with these problems:

Obstructed tracheostomy tube

1. Preoxygenate the patient using an Ambu bag.

2. Irrigate with normal saline solution if necessary.

3. Suction the patient.

4. Connect the patient to the ventilator and assess respiratory status.

5. If the patient is still in distress, dial the emergency phone number to arrange transportation to the nearest health care facility.

Water in tubing

Here's what to do:

1. Disconnect the tubing from the ventilator.

2. Empty the water from the tubing.

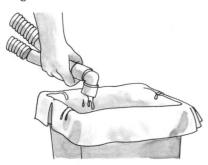

Improper cuff pressure

Follow these guidelines:

1. Inflate the cuff with the appropriate amount of pressure. (Explain the importance of cuff inflation.)

2. During the patient's next visit to his doctor and respiratory therapist, they should report problems that arose and what they did to solve them.

Ventilators: patient care

Keeping your patient comfortable

One of your nursing responsibilities is keeping your intubated patient on a ventilator as comfortable as possible. The endotracheal tube, which must be taped in place or secured with another device, can cause skin irritation. You'll have to remove (and change) the tape periodically to clean the skin and to shave a male patient. Moving the tube to the opposite side of the mouth will also help prevent tissue breakdown. (See *Endotracheal tubes: discomfort.*)

Be careful not to dislodge the tube when you're retaping it or giving mouth care. Having another nurse hold the tube in position while you're moving and retaping it is a good idea. Remember to check the number on the side of the tube to make sure it hasn't changed since the last time you checked it.

In most hospitals, a chest X-ray is taken routinely to confirm that an endotracheal tube is in the correct position. If that's the procedure in your hospital, try to plan your tube care so that it's done right before a scheduled chest X-ray. And remember that if an endotracheal tube does become dislodged, you can use an oral airway and the chin-lift maneuver to help keep the patient's airway open. Notify the doctor immediately. You may have to ventilate the patient with a manual resuscitation bag until he can be reintubated.

Because an intubated patient can have nothing by mouth, he may require total parenteral nutrition or liquid feedings through a nasogastric or gastrostomy tube. Monitor his fluid status closely. To prevent pressure sores and to ensure optimal ventilation, turn him every 1 to 2 hours. If he can tolerate sitting in a chair for a short while, it'll help prevent pressure sores and also boost his spirits.

Violent patients

Effective strategies

Most hospitals provide protocols for dealing with violent patients. Make sure you're familiar with them and with protocols for physical and chemical restraints. Here's some practical advice:

• Call for help at the first sign or threat of violence. Often the mere presence of other medical personnel can defuse it.

• When help arrives, isolate the patient as much as possible. Evacuate visitors and other patients to avoid potential hostage taking. And, if possible, move chairs and other objects out of the area.

• Watch the patient's hands. Most of us naturally tend to look into a person's face or eyes. But they can't hurt you. The patient's hands can. If he's getting ready to strike you or reach for a weapon, you'll know only by watching his hands.

• If the patient's armed with a gun, knife, or other weapon, call the police to handle the situation. But remain alert and watch for seemingly harmless objects that can be used against you. A lit cigarette flipped into your face can distract you for a split second—long enough for an attack. And if the patient has kept his hand clenched for a while, he may be holding ground pepper or cigarette ashes to throw in your eyes. Even a pen can be dangerous.

Finally, remove your necktie, scarf, and stethoscope, placing them out of the patient's reach so they can't be used against you.

• Before approaching the patient, appoint a team leader, preferably the staff person who's been dealing with him for the longest time. That leader should then assign each staff member a specific area of responsibility, such as a certain limb to control during the actual restraint effort. Remember to control the patient's head, as well as his arms and legs, to prevent him from injuring himself and to reduce the risk of his butting or biting you.

• The team leader should be the only person who talks to the patient; that way, he won't feel threatened or confused by a lot of voices. The rest of the staff should spread out evenly around the patient so that they won't trip over each other when it's time to move in. Then, when the leader moves in, everyone else should move in together.

• No one should relinquish control of the patient until he's been restrained. Restraining him in a face-down position will reduce his leverage for breaking free and make medicating him easier.

• After the patient is restrained, a security guard should be called in to search him for weapons or other objects that could endanger himself or others. Be sure to document and store all confiscated items in a safe place.

• Use extreme caution when approaching the patient, even if he's securely restrained. He still may be able to grab or scratch you if you come close. Or he may be able to twist his upper body to butt you with his head or to bite you.

• Last but not least: Protect yourself legally. Within 24 hours, obtain a doctor's written order for the restraints. While a patient's restrained, observe him closely. Check that restraints are secure but don't restrict his circulation or breathing. (See *Legal risks: restraints.*)

As with all unusual situations involving patients, document the incident carefully, explaining why you had to use restraints and which alternative methods you tried.

Vision loss

When it occurs suddenly

Sudden vision loss can signal central retinal artery occlusion or acute closed-angle glaucoma—ocular emergencies that require immediate intervention. If your patient reports sudden vision loss, immediately notify an ophthalmologist for an emergency examination, and perform these interventions, as ordered:

For suspected central retinal artery occlusion, perform light massage over the patient's closed eyelid.

Increase his carbon dioxide level, as ordered, by administering a set flow of oxygen and carbon dioxide through a Venturi mask. Or have him rebreathe in a paper bag to retain exhaled carbon dioxide. These steps will dilate the artery and, possibly, restore blood flow to the retina.

Central retinal artery occlusion

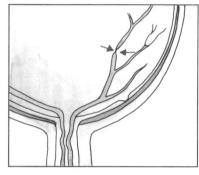

For suspected acute closed-angle glaucoma, help the doctor measure intraocular pressure with a tonometer, as ordered. (You can also estimate intraocular pressure without a tonometer by placing your fingers over the patient's closed eyelid. A rock-hard eyeball usually indicates increased intraocular pressure.) Expect to administer timolol drops and I.V. acetazolamide to help decrease intraocular pressure.

Visitors

Asking them to leave

When should you ask your patient's visitors to leave? These questions and answers can help you decide:

• *Are they interfering with the patient's rest?* If so, they'll have to leave. You might direct them to a waiting area and tell them you'll let them know when the patient's awake.

• *Is the patient undergoing an intimate or invasive procedure?* If the patient wants privacy, ask the visitors to step out into the hallway for a few minutes.

If the doctor is performing a medical procedure, he may want the vis-

itors out of the room. But if the patient prefers company—and the doctor agrees—let him choose one person to remain with him. Show this person where to stand, and advise him how he can best support the patient.

• *Are the visitors interfering with the patient's care?* If visitors are keeping you from getting your job done either because they're in the way or they're disrupting successful communication with your patient, ask them to step out until you're finished with the patient.

• *Are the visitors ill?* Tell any visitor who's obviously ill and whose presence isn't critical that he might help the patient more by staying home until he's well.

• *Do the visitors hover?* If so, chances are that's their style of coping. This trait, in fact, may comfort the patient. So don't banish the visitors because you find their behavior offensive.

• *Are the visitors disturbing the patient's roommate?* If he complains that they're loud or disruptive, ask the visitors to be quieter. If that doesn't work and the patient can't meet them in a waiting area, the visitors will have to go.

Using diplomacy

If they feel you're being fair and have the patient's best interests at heart, few visitors will argue about leaving. Be sure to stress how it will benefit the patient. Before they go, give them a report on his condition and, if possible, tell them when they can return.

Visual aids: patient teaching

Using them to help your patients

V

Here's a way to use photographs when teaching your patient about his illness or treatment.

Make an album for patients undergoing total hip replacement surgery. Write a simple explanation for each part of the patient's preoperative and postoperative care. With the help of the hospital photographer, take pictures of traction equipment and other materials the patient will use, the way the patient will be moved, and so on. Put all the explanations and photos together in the album. Now give the album to each patient who will undergo this procedure so that he can read about it and understand what to expect.

This album will answer your patient's questions and alleviate his fears. (See also *Patient-teaching timesavers.*)

Visual aids: transparencies

Using X-ray film

Is the cost of audiovisual aids hampering your in-service style? If so, use X-ray film (with the coating removed) instead of costly overhead transparencies.

The film's light-blue color and sturdy composition make it a perfect substitute for a transparency. You can use permanent or washable felt-tip markers on it. And if you can get the X-ray film to fit into your copying machine, you can copy more detailed pictures and graphs right onto it.

Visually impaired patients

Helping them

To help the patient feel safe and comfortable, orient him to his hospital environment. Let him feel the length, width, and height of his hospital bed. Using the bed as a focal point, guide him along the walls so he can locate the bedside table, window, bathroom, closet door, and hall door. Then return him to the bedside. Next, let him feel his way into the hallway; help him find specific areas he may

need, such as the nurses' station or patients' lounge. This hands-on orientation will help him develop a mental image of his room and the surrounding environment.

Carefully inspect his room and remove any obstacles. Make sure the lighting is appropriate: bright for patients with dimming vision, subdued for those with photophobia. Always keep the furniture and the contents of his bedside table in the same place. He'll become accustomed to their locations and expect them to always be there. Place the side rails in the low position, but instruct him to ask for assistance if he wants to get out of bed.

Sounds are especially important to a visually impaired patient. Learning to identify certain sounds—the noise of traffic, for instance—helps him protect himself against hazards. In the hospital, certain sounds can help orient him to the time of day. Identify the sounds he might hear, such as: "That rumbling noise is the laundry cart. It usually arrives about 9 a.m." Or, "Dinner is served at 6 p.m. You'll hear the rattling of the trays."

Explain other hospital routines in detail, such as the times for medications, personal care, and visiting hours.

Schedule a time to discuss his feelings about his vision problem. Explore any alterations in his self-image. If he feels that he needs to change his life-style, support and encourage this effort.

In cases of sudden, total blindness, as in optic neuritis, use crisis intervention techniques. The patient's high stress level will prevent him from accurately interpreting what he hears. So give clear, simple directions. Empathize with him to gain his trust. Discuss his past coping behaviors and use them to help him adjust to his blindness.

Note the patient's visual impairment on the Kardex. All staff members should identify themselves when they enter the room; they should also tell him when they're leaving. You may want to put a sign in the room

to inform other hospital personnel of his visual impairment. (See *Blind patients.*)

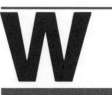

Walkers: carryalls

Making a carryall

A strap-on bicycle basket makes an inexpensive carryall for a patient using a walker. Strap the basket to the outside of the walker so that it doesn't interfere with the patient's mobility. It'll be large enough to

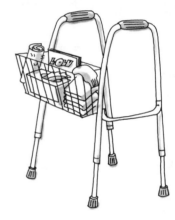

carry magazines, bath articles, clothing, and so on. And these lightweight baskets are available in various sizes and colors.

Walkers: patient teaching

Do's and don'ts for patients

Here are some guidelines to follow when your patient needs a walker.
Do:
• Give the patient a walker that is the correct height. When standing upright, he should be able to grasp the bars with his arms slightly bent at the elbows.

• Make sure he uses the handles on the *sides* of the walker.
• Tell him to look ahead when he's walking.

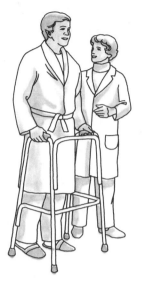

• Remind him to keep his feet flat on the floor, about 2′ to 3′ apart, for a wider base of support. And make sure he stands between the back legs of the walker for maximum stability.

Don't:
• Give the patient a walker that's too low for him. If he has to stoop over the walker, straighten his arms to grasp the bars, or tip the walker toward himself, he's using the wrong size.
• Let him grasp the front bar of the walker. He won't be able to lift it to step forward.
• Let him step up against the front bar. This position offers little stability, and he's likely to fall.
• Let him look down.
• Stand in his way—watch your feet if you're near the walker. (See also *Walkers: carryalls.*)

Walking

Motivating your patient

If verbal prodding won't get your patients walking after surgery, hang a bulletin board at the nurses' sta-tion, with the heading "You've come a long way." Post pictures on the board of patients walking with I.V. poles, drainage bags, and various encumbrances. Then attach a sheet of paper and a pencil so that pa-tients can sign their names on their first postop walk to the nurses' sta-tion. The sheet provides a goal for patients to work toward and shows the world (or at least the staff and other patients) that they've gone the course.

Another suggestion: Use positive reinforcement. Set up a juice and ice cart in the hall. When the pa-tients want a drink, they can walk to the cart and help themselves.

Wheelchair patients

Helping them maneuver better

For wheelchair-bound patients, so-cialization has its price: long hours of sitting uncomfortably in one po-sition. To help these patients, put them in reclining chairs that have wheels, and wheel them wherever they want to go. If they get tired or uncomfortable, they can just change the position of their chairs—for example, they can move from a sitting position to a lying position and back to a sitting po-sition again.

Wheelchairs

Repositioning a patient

Use a towel to reposition a patient in a wheelchair. Fold it in half lengthwise and place it on the chair's seat so that it extends slightly over the front and back edges. When the patient slides for-ward, stand behind the wheelchair, lock the wheels, and pull the back edge of the towel. He will be pulled back on the seat and you won't strain your back.

If too much of the towel hangs out in back and it drags on the floor,

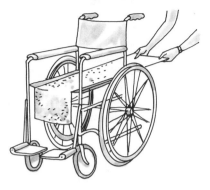

bring the end up and over the back-rest, placing it behind the patient's shoulders. (See also *Wheelchair transfers.*)

Wheelchair transfers

Transferring patients safely

A simple procedure—transferring a patient to a wheelchair—can have disastrous results. The patient could fall, or you could injure your back. Here's a guide to safe transfers.

Do:
• Place the wheelchair alongside the bed so that the patient can get into it with a 90-degree pivot. If she has an affected side, put the chair on that side so she can raise herself on her unaffected leg and pivot on that foot back into the wheelchair.

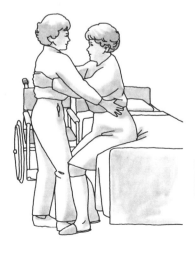

W

• Put the footrests up and lock the brakes.
• Tell the patient to hold onto you between your shoulders and your waist.
• Spread your feet to give yourself a wide base of support. Place one foot forward so that your leg presses against the patient's affected leg. Then, on a count of three, rock back (one), forward (two), and back (three), pulling him up on three.
• Protect your back by using your legs to help you lift. If the patient loses his balance or becomes too heavy, lower him back to bed simply by bending your knees.
• Hold the patient at the waist to provide support—or use a transfer belt.

Don't:
• Angle the wheelchair away from the bed.
• Leave the wheelchair's footrests down.
• Let the patient grasp your neck. You could be seriously injured if he slips and all of his weight is hanging from your neck.
• Bend too far at the waist; you may strain your lower back.
• Grab onto your patient's clothing. If it rips, you won't be able to provide much support. (See also *Wheelchairs.*)

Winged-tip needle: blood specimen

The best technique

Gather these supplies: a soft, flat tourniquet; a folded washcloth; an alcohol prep pad; a syringe; a winged-tip needle set; a vacuum specimen tube; a sterile 2″ × 2″ gauze pad; gloves; and an adhesive bandage. Attach the syringe to the proximal end of the winged-tip needle set.

Prepare the arm for insertion of the needle. (See *I.V. therapy: insertion.*)

Then, hold the wings of the needle set with the thumb and forefinger of your dominant hand; tuck your other fingers under your hand. Because of the long tubing, you can lay the attached syringe on the bed next to the patient while you're inserting the needle. Insert the needle at a 10- to 45-degree angle, depending on the position of the vein. As soon as the needle enters the vein, blood will rush into the tubing. When you have a good blood return, stop advancing the needle.

Keep holding the skin taut and let go of the needle. Gently aspirate blood into the syringe with your dominant hand.

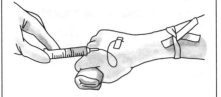

When you've collected the required amount of blood, lay the syringe on a flat surface near the patient. Release the tourniquet. Then press a sterile 2″ × 2″ gauze pad over the venipuncture site. Remove the needle quickly and smoothly. Have the patient lift his arm and hold the pad in place for 1 to 2 minutes. Then place the adhesive bandage over the site.

Insert the winged-tip needle into the specimen tube; the negative pressure in the tube will make it fill with blood.

Withholding information

When it's appropriate

Suppose a doctor decides to withhold information from your patient and you believe he has no therapeutic basis for his decision. You know the patient has a legal right to be told about his condition, but you don't want to interfere with the doctor-patient relationship. Here's what to do:

1. Discuss the situation with the doctor. Ask him why he withheld information. If you disagree with him, tell him you intend to discuss the matter with your supervisor.

2. Inform your supervisor, in writing, that you disagree with the doctor's decision. Give her the facts about the patient's condition and explain your feelings. She'll either handle the matter from that point or tell you why she thinks the doctor is right. If you still feel you're right, tell her you intend to take the matter to someone else in the nursing chain of command.

3. Then submit a written explanation to her supervisor regarding your disagreement with the doctor and what steps you've taken so far. This supervisor will tell you whether or not she intends to pursue the matter. If she isn't going to pursue it, tell her you will on your own.

4. Submit your disagreement, in writing, to your institution's committee on multidisciplinary practice. The committee should issue a ruling on the matter. (See *Confidentiality; Doctors' orders.*)

Witnessing, expert

Preparation guidelines

If you're hired to work as a nurse expert witness, you'll review the voluminous medical records and depositions of witnesses for the plaintiff and the defense. Start with the medical records.

Read the patient's chart carefully to be sure it's complete. Check the chronologic order to detect any missing pages, and verify that the necessary laboratory slips, flow charts, and graphs are included. Always take notes as you read and flag critical areas for later review.

Then cross-check sections. For example, how do the doctor's progress notes compare with the nurses' notes? Were the doctor's orders properly documented and carried out? Were the consents signed and witnessed? Do the laboratory data support the treatment ordered? Don't overlook graphs. Did the nurse take vital signs as ordered? Did the nurse use proper judgment if vital signs needed to be taken more often? Did the nurse administer drugs that the patient was allergic to? Although some attorneys are knowledgeable about certain medical and nursing issues, they're still lay people. Never assume that they've noted basic facts in the medical record.

Next, check for tampered records, an unfortunate (and all-too-common) practice. Watch for data that could have been inserted after the fact. You should know which hospital records are filled out in duplicate or triplicate; ask the attorney to subpoena all copies if you suspect that they were altered after being separated.

Once you know the facts, review current literature to help determine the standard of care. Compare the care the plaintiff received to the care the plaintiff would have received from a reasonably prudent nurse—not by the best nurse you've ever known. Ask yourself: What would I have done in this situation? Does the care meet the standards of the health community? If not, precisely how does it deviate?

After inspecting the medical records, examine the deposition of witnesses involved in the case and other expert witnesses. (See also *Testifying: Expert witness.*)

Wound assessment

Postoperative care

Do you sometimes have trouble remembering the basics of postoperative wound assessment? If so, you may find this memory-jogging technique helpful:

S—Seepage from the wound (Is the seepage serous or purulent? What's the color, amount, odor, and consistency?)

C—Color of the incision area (Is it bruised, inflamed, or necrotic?)

A—Approximation of wound edges (Are they sutured, intact, swollen, or dehisced?)

R—Reaction of the patient (Is he in pain? Does he feel pressure or general malaise?)

Next time you need to determine whether a patient's incision is healing properly, just think SCAR.

Wound care: pressure sores

Choosing the right dressing and applying it properly

Follow these guidelines to determine which dressing is best to use on your patient's pressure sore:

Transparent dressing
Use a transparent dressing if your patient's pressure sore is in Stage I (red skin; relieving pressure and massaging the skin won't return it to its normal color) or Stage II (blistered, peeling, or cracked skin).

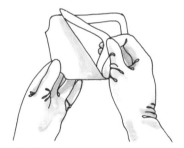

Application
When you use a transparent dressing, follow the manufacturer's instructions for applying it properly. Here are some general guidelines you should keep in mind:
• Use a dressing that's large enough to cover a 2″ margin of healthy, dry skin around the wound.
• Clip—don't shave—excessive hair at the site.
• Don't use creams, oils, or detergents because they'll interfere with adhesion.
• To prevent skin shearing, gently lay the dressing on the skin. Don't

stretch it before applying it. Press firmly on the edges to make sure it adheres properly.
• If necessary, tape the dressing edges to prevent them from rolling.
• Before applying the dressing to the sacrum, spread the gluteal fold. Then center the dressing and gently lay it on the skin. Press down firmly from the center toward the edges of the dressing. (Follow this same procedure to apply a hydrocolloid dressing to the sacrum.)
Removal
Grasp the edge of the dressing, anchoring the skin as you do so, and slowly pull it back. (Make sure you pull it in the direction in which the hair is growing.) If you have trouble doing this, try any of these tips:
• Use a cotton swab and mineral oil to soften the adhesive and ease the dressing off the skin.
• Attach a piece of tape to one corner of the dressing. Then slowly pull the tape back across the dressing.
• Lift a corner of the dressing and gently stretch it straight out, away from the wound. This "pops" the dressing, releasing the adhesion and minimizing skin trauma. Then slowly pull the dressing back over itself.

Hydrocolloid dressing
Use a hydrocolloid dressing if your patient's pressure sore is in *Stage III* (broken skin; a full thickness of skin is lost and subcutaneous tissue may be damaged; you may see serous or bloody drainage).

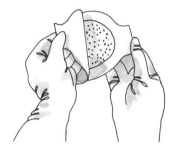

Application
Make sure you follow the manufacturer's directions. And remember these points:
• Clip excessive hair at the dressing site.

• Choose a dressing that will cover at least 1″ of healthy, dry skin around the wound. An oval-shaped dressing, such as Tegasorb, works well in the sacral area.

• Use hydrocolloid granules, powder, or paste to fill wounds that have a lot of exudate. Fill the wound to just below skin level to leave room for expansion. Granules and powder are easier to apply if the wound is level.

• If the dressing doesn't have an adhesive border, frame its edges with tape or strips of transparent dressing to prevent the edges from rolling and to extend wearing time.

Removal

Press down on the skin and loosen the corner of the dressing. Continue to loosen the edge, moving toward the center of the dressing. Carefully lift the dressing from the wound. To remove any remaining gel, irrigate the area with normal saline solution, according to hospital protocol.

One last point about hydrocolloid dressings: They're impermeable to odor, so when you remove the dressing, you may think the yellow, malodorous gel that has formed in the wound bed is purulent drainage. After irrigating the wound, assess its appearance to rule out this possibility.

If your patient's pressure sore is in *Stage IV* (deep, craterlike ulcer forms; full thickness of skin and subcutaneous tissues is destroyed; fascia, a connective tissue, bone, or muscle beneath the ulcer are exposed and may be damaged), both dressings are contraindicated.

Wound care dressings: changes

Procedure for minimizing infection

Follow these steps when changing dressings:

1. Put on nonsterile gloves. To remove the tape, apply gentle tension to the skin with one hand, then pull the tape toward the wound with your other hand. Place the soiled tape in a plastic bag. Gently remove the soiled dressings one at a time and put them in the plastic bag. Never pull on a dressing—this may disturb sutures or newly formed tissue. If you have trouble removing a dressing, moisten the area with sterile water or normal saline solution. Remove your gloves and place them in the plastic bag, too. Then wash your hands.

2. After putting on *sterile* gloves, inspect your patient's wound for any discharge or redness. Then, fold a 4″ × 4″ gauze pad into quarters and grasp it with forceps. Make sure the folded edge faces outward.

3. Dip the folded gauze into sterile water.

4. Starting at the top of the incision, gently wipe from top to bottom in one motion. Then, discard the gauze pad, putting it in the plastic bag. To avoid contamination, be careful not to touch the bag with the forceps.

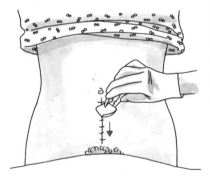

Repeat this procedure, wiping in the same direction each time—be sure you always move from the least contaminated area to the most contaminated area. Using a clean gauze pad with each wiping motion, repeat the procedure until you've cleaned the entire wound.

5. Pat the area dry with a clean 4″ × 4″ gauze pad.

6. If the wound is infected, apply an ointment. Remove the cap from the ointment tube with your nondominant hand. (This hand is no longer sterile.) With the same hand, squeeze a small amount of ointment onto a 4″ × 4″ gauze pad. Doing so will ensure sterility.

Squeeze ointment over the entire wound from top to bottom. Be sure to use only your dominant hand to apply the sterile dressings, because your nondominant hand is no longer sterile.

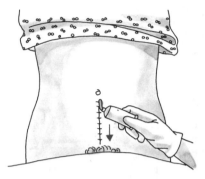

To prevent the primary dressing from sticking to the wound, place a nonadhesive dressing over the wound. Be sure the wound is completely covered—use two nonadhesive dressings if necessary.

7. A primary dressing will help absorb drainage from the wound surface. Remove a 4″ × 4″ gauze pad from its open wrapper and place it over the nonadhesive dressing.

8. To apply the secondary dressing, which will act as a drainage reservoir if necessary, place a Surgipad over the gauze pads. (If necessary, apply a second Surgipad to cover the entire wound.)

Remove your gloves and discard them in the plastic bag.

9. Tape the dressing in place and dispose of the plastic bag according to your hospital's infection-control standards. (See *Infection control; Wound assessment; Wound cleaning: problem solving*).

Wound care dressings: taping

Recommended methods

Teaching a patient or his family how to dress and redress wounds on hairy areas of the body can be a problem: The tape sticks to and pulls the patient's hair when it's removed. Shaving the area helps, but the tape still tends to catch some hair. Pink hairdressing tape solves the problem by keeping dressings as secure as regular tape while lifting off easily.

Wound cleaning: power spray

Proper use

Before you can spray the wound, prepare the patient, the wound itself, and the equipment. Here's how:

Make the patient comfortable and explain what you're going to do. Power-spray cleaning is usually painless—but not always. Administer analgesics, as ordered, 30 to 45 minutes before starting.

Remove the old dressing. Note the amount of drainage, as well as its color, type, consistency, and odor. Note the skin condition around the wound and any wound trauma. Discard the dressing. If indicated, gently examine the wound for sinus tracts. Document any active bleeding, hematoma, edema, erythema, or tenderness around the wound. (See *Wound assessment.*) Don't use the power spray on a wound that's actively bleeding, because it could aggravate bleeding or force bacteria into the circulation.

Using aseptic technique, arrange the following equipment on a sterile field: sterile gloves and masks, bed protector, two sterile basins, sterile 4″ × 4″ gauze pads, bulb syringe and a bottle for the cleaning solution, sterile atomizer with nozzle, the Devilbiss spray pump, the prescribed solution, plastic bag for soiled dressings, sterile towel, tape, sterile gauze for redressing the wound, and suction equipment.

Wear a mask and perform the procedure away from other patients, because the force of the spray could loosen bacteria, making them air-

borne. (See *Infection control.*) Give the patient a mask if indicated. Assemble the suction equipment and keep it ready; you may have to suction gently if the solution stays in the wound or doesn't flow out of the body cavity. (Never leave cleaning solution in a body cavity.) When power-spray cleaning a patient with a tracheostomy, inflate the cuff, cover the stoma with a sterile 4″ × 4″ gauze pad, and keep the patient upright.

Here's how to set up and use the power-spray equipment:

1. Put a sterile glove on your hand, and pick up the bottle. Use your ungloved hand to fill the bottle with the prescribed solution, and turn the machine on. (Don't use more than 20 lb of pressure.) Put a sterile glove on your other hand, and screw the glass rod onto the top of the bottle to form a tight seal.

2. Attach the nozzle to the top of the bottle.

3. Using a sterile 4″ × 4″ gauze pad, attach the tubing from the spray pump to the connector on the top of the power-spray bottle.

4. Keep the top 4″ to 6″ (10 to 15 cm), or as ordered, away from the wound while spraying. Spray the wound from all angles. Don't spray exposed nerve endings (which may cause pain), and don't spray around exposed large vessels (which may cause hemorrhage). Use sterile basins to collect the drainage.

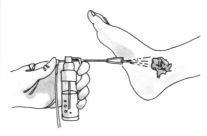

5. Repeat if necessary. Remove excess moisture.

6. After applying a new dressing, record the procedure and the wound's condition before and after the procedure. Clean the equipment and have it sterilized. (See *Wound care dressings: changes.*)

Wound cleaning: preparation

Steps needed before suturing

When a patient with an open wound comes into the hospital, your first priority is to control the bleeding. Do this by applying pressure to the wound, applying a cold pack, or elevating the injured part. Cover the wound with a sterile gauze pad to prevent contamination.

When you inspect and clean the wound, do so gently to avoid destroying delicate tissue cells. Shave the surrounding area as little as possible, if at all, because shaving increases desquamation of the epithelium. It also increases the risk of contamination. Thoroughly evaluate the wound. Then, using sterile technique, clean the skin around the wound with povidone-iodine surgical scrub soap for 5 to 10 minutes. Flush the skin with sterile water or sterile saline solution.

If cleaning and irrigating the wound will cause the patient discomfort, the wound will need to be anesthetized first. Ask the patient if he's ever had a reaction to an anesthetic. If he hasn't, prepare the anesthetic. For wounds on the leg, forearm, upper arm, back, chest, or scalp that are bleeding copiously, prepare 1% lidocaine (Xylocaine) with epinephrine in a 5- to 10-ml syringe with a needle no larger than 27G (preferably a 30G). For wounds in the same areas that are not bleeding copiously, as well as for wounds on fingers, toes, ears, the penis, the nose, and for all wounds on elderly patients, prepare only lidocaine. Don't prepare more than 20 ml of lidocaine for adults (2 to 3 ml usually suffice). Don't prepare more than 3 mg/kg of lidocaine for children. (See also *TAC solution.*)

After the doctor anesthetizes the area, watch the patient for signs and symptoms of an allergic reaction. If adverse reactions develop, admin-

W

ister high-flow oxygen immediately. Have 10 mg of diazepam (Valium) ready for immediate intravenous administration if the patient convulses.

After the area's prepared and the anesthetic has taken effect, use a Toomey or control syringe with a 18G needle to irrigate the wound. Follow the Kirz rule: Irrigate with 50 ml of normal sterile saline solution per inch of wound per hours of age of wound. This rule applies to most open wounds. Use more irrigant when flushing dirty, older wounds; less when flushing small, clean wounds. When flushing small wounds, use a 5-ml syringe with a 22G needle to create an irrigating jet stream.

After you've cleaned and irrigated the wound, carefully inspect it for clots or foreign bodies, such as dirt, pieces of wood, hair, grass, and so forth. If you find clots or foreign bodies, remove them and re-irrigate as described. The wound will then be ready for suturing. (See also *Infection control; Wound irrigation.*)

Wound cleaning: problem solving

Tips for cleaning wounds in inaccessible spots

Washing can effectively reduce bacteria in the infected wound, especially when you use large quantities of liquid. But how do you avoid messes or spills when the wound is in a hard-to-reach location?
• *Arm and lower leg wounds.* These may be soaked in a large vessel of *warm* irrigating fluid: water, normal saline solution, or an appropriate antiseptic. An agitator can help dislodge bacteria and loosen debris.

If possible, rinse the wound several times and carefully dispose of the infected liquid. Reserve the utensils you used for that particular

patient only, and store them after soaking them in disinfectant and letting them air dry. (See also *Soaks: arms and legs; Soaks: home care.*)
• *Trunk or high leg wounds.* A recently developed device uses Stomahesive and a plastic irrigating chamber applied over the wound. You run the warm irrigating liquid through an infusion set and collect it in a drainage bag.

A syringe irrigation at the time of dressing is another alternative. Where possible, direct the flow at right angles to the wound, and allow the fluid to drain by gravity. This requires careful positioning of the patient, either in bed or on a chair. (See *Wound irrigation.*)

If irrigation isn't possible, sponge cleaning will be necessary. Wipe away exudate before using antiseptic or saline solution to clean the wound (taking care not to push loose debris into the wound). Use sharp scissors to snip off loose dead material—never pull it off.

Wound dehiscence

Emergency intervention

You're caring for a patient who has had an appendectomy and is receiving tube feedings. You note that his nasogastric tube is clamped and his abdomen is distended. He tells you that his incision felt wet after he vomited. You remove the dressing and see open wound edges with loops of bowels protruding.

Summon help, and tell the patient to remain still. Ask the nurse who responds to bring supplies for sterile saline dressings. Place the dressings over the wound.

Call the patient's doctor immediately and ask for an order to resume suctioning on the nasogastric tube to relieve abdominal distension and vomiting. Also ask for an order for I.V. fluids, because the patient probably wasn't receiving them with his tube feedings. Start

an I.V. line if the patient doesn't already have one.

Because the patient is awake and realizes something has happened, tell him that his wound has opened. Explain that you've notified his doctor, who will be there soon. Reassure him that you've covered the wound to keep it clean. Continue to monitor his vital signs.

What to do later

When the patient returns to the unit after surgery, monitor him carefully for new signs of infection—for example, increased heart rate, elevated white blood cell count, and fluctuating blood glucose levels. Teach him how to prevent straining his incision by splinting it with a pillow when he coughs and calling for help when he wants to get out of bed. Tell him *not* to strain when reaching for things—and make sure the call bell and other items he needs are close at hand.

Wound drainage

Using a Penrose drain

To collect wound drainage from a Penrose drain, place an ostomy appliance over the drain, taking care not to irritate the suture line. The drainage will accumulate in the appliance, away from the patient's skin.

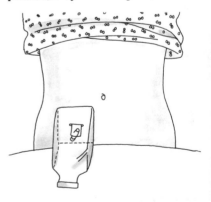

This will not only prevent skin breakdown and decrease the number of dressing changes, but it will also allow you to evaluate the color, consistency, and amount of drainage in the appliance.

Wound irrigation

Using small vials for small wounds

When a patient has a small fistula or wound that needs to be irrigated frequently, don't use a big 1,000-ml bottle of normal saline solution. It just clutters the patient's bedside table, and the unused solution will have to be discarded later.

Use 5-ml vials of the solution instead. They can be stored easily, and a couple of vials are usually sufficient for each irrigation. (See also *Wound cleaning: problem solving.*)

Wound packing

An easy and effective method

To pack deep, large wounds after irrigations or dressing changes, use a roll of sterile stretch gauze instead of 4" × 4" gauze pads. Wearing gloves, hold the roll in one hand and a sterile hemostat in the other, releasing the

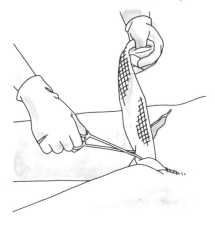

dressing gradually and packing it in the wound. Since the stretch gauze is fluffier and smoother than 4" × 4" gauze pads, it packs better. And be-

cause it's all one piece, the gauze can be removed easier and faster—a feature patients appreciate.

Writing

Getting your work published

If you want your colleagues and supervisors to recognize your abilities in a particular area, consider writing an article from your expert point of view. If you've never written an article before, you'll appreciate these seven tips.

1. *Write only what you know about.* Reading a few references at the library won't give you the expertise to write about a particular topic. Instead, base your article on firsthand knowledge. And to help make your points clear, use concrete examples from real life.

2. *Familiarize yourself with each professional magazine's philosophy, audience, and style.* Before submitting your manuscript, request a copy of the journal's author guidelines. When you submit your manuscript, include a cover letter and your resume.

3. *Give yourself enough time to write.* Formulating ideas, researching information, completing rough drafts, and writing a final version of your article can take months. You won't find a shortcut; it takes hard work.

4. *Get help from others when possible.* Set up brainstorming sessions with two or three coauthors to spark your creativity. Depending on your topic, you may want to collaborate with doctors, dietitians, social workers, or other professionals.

5. *Recognize the importance of timing.* When a new product or procedure is developed, writing an article about it could turn into a scoop for you and the journal you submit it to. Make sure you're writing about a truly new topic by checking if it's been covered in other journals.

6. *Make writing enjoyable—not a chore.* Keep each writing session short enough to avoid frustration.

7. *Be patient.* After submitting an article, you may have to wait 3 to 6 months to find out whether it's been accepted for publication. If it is accepted, the journal's editors may want you to revise it or may work with you on revising it. If it isn't accepted, don't despair. You can submit it to another journal. Just make sure you submit the same article to only one journal at a time.

X-rays

Radiation precautions

When patients can't be transferred to the radiology department for testing because of their unstable conditions, you may have to assist with portable X-rays in their rooms or with angiography or fluoroscopy in the ICU or the operating room. What's your risk?

With portable X-rays, you're vulnerable to inadvertent exposure because of "leaks" from faulty equipment and radiation "scatter" (deflection of the X-rays that aren't absorbed by the patient).

Fluoroscopy can be especially hazardous to health care personnel. Although fluoroscopy emits lower radiation than standard X-rays, extended testing periods can cause a greater cumulative exposure.

To avoid unnecessary exposure, follow these guidelines when assisting with diagnostic X-rays:
• Wear a lead apron if you must remain in the same room with patients receiving portable X-rays, fluoroscopy, or angiography. Stand behind a protective lead shield or barrier, if available.

X
Y
Z

• If you must restrain patients receiving portable X-rays, stand to the side, away from direct X-ray beams.

• When assisting with fluoroscopy, remind the technician or doctor to turn off the fluoroscope except when a view is actually needed. For example, if the doctor's inserting a Swan-Ganz catheter, the fluoroscope should be on only to check the catheter's position, not while it's being inserted.

• If you frequently restrain or accompany patients getting diagnostic X-rays, wear a film badge to monitor cumulative exposure. (See *Radiation monitoring.*)

• If you're pregnant or think you might be, wear a 0.5 mm–thick lead apron that wraps completely around your body. (See *Pregnant nurse: radiation hazards.*)

Yeast infection

Nursing interventions

Most often, candidiasis infects the nails, skin, or mucous membranes, especially the oropharynx, vagina, esophagus, and GI tract. Rarely, the *Candida* fungi enter the circulation and invade the kidneys, lungs, endocardium, brain, or other structures, causing serious infections.

With patients using nystatin solution for oral infections, advise swishing it around the mouth for several minutes before swallowing. Swab nystatin on the oral mucosa of an infant with thrush. Provide a nonirritating mouthwash to loosen tenacious secretions and a soft toothbrush to avoid irritation. Relieve mouth discomfort with a topical anesthetic, such as lidocaine, at least 1 hour before meals. (It may suppress the gag reflex and cause aspiration.)

Provide a soft-food diet for patients with severe dysphagia. Tell them to chew food thoroughly, and make sure they don't choke.

Use cornstarch or dry padding in the intertriginous areas of obese patients to prevent irritation.

Assess patients with candidiasis for underlying systemic causes, such as diabetes mellitus. If a patient is receiving amphotericin B for systemic candidiasis, he may have severe chills, fever, anorexia, nausea, and vomiting. Premedicate with aspirin, antihistamines, or antiemetics to help reduce adverse reactions.

Frequently check vital signs of patients with systemic infections. Provide appropriate supportive care. In patients with renal involvement, carefully monitor intake and output, and urine blood and protein levels.

Check high-risk patients daily (especially those receiving antibiotics) for patchy areas, irritation, sore throat, bleeding of mouth or gums, or other signs of superinfection. Check for vaginal discharge; record color and amount.

Encourage women in their third trimester of pregnancy to be examined for vaginal candidiasis to protect their infants from infection at birth.

Yellow jacket sting

Nursing guidelines

Since a yellow jacket retains its stinger, you won't be able to remove it. Instead, follow these steps:

• Clean the site and apply ice.

• Watch the patient carefully for signs of anaphylaxis; keep emergency resuscitation equipment on hand.

• If anaphylaxis develops, administer oxygen, epinephrine, and other drugs, as ordered. (See *Anaphylaxis: emergency care; Anaphylaxis: emergency kit.*)

Zipper injuries

Managing them

Zipper injuries are common and painful. A zipper injury occurs when the skin of the patient's penis gets caught in his trousers' zipper—and stays caught.

Obviously, this is an injury that's both extremely painful *and* embarrassing. Your first priority is to lessen your patient's anxiety: Tell him exactly what the doctor's going to do to help him.

The doctor will begin treatment immediately by applying a topical anesthetic, such as lidocaine (Xylocaine 2% jelly). (Depending on the patient's age, cooperativeness, and degree of pain, the doctor may also ask you to give him a sedative.) When the anesthetic has taken effect, the doctor will hold the zipper firmly and ease it down, a notch or two at a time, while gently disentangling the patient's skin. (This is *never* a surgical procedure; cutting the skin free of the zipper would increase the tissue trauma and could result in deformity or erectile dysfunction.)

Before the patient is discharged from the emergency department, expect to apply an antiseptic ointment and a sterile dressing. Then give him (or his parents, if the patient's a child) these instructions for home care:

• Apply cold compresses for 12 hours to reduce swelling and pain.

• If the patient is an adult, he should wear scrotal support temporarily to relieve discomfort and to protect delicate tissues.

Z-track injections

Essential steps

If you're administering iron dextran complex (Imferon), you must use the Z-track method. It involves pulling the skin so that the needle track is sealed off after the injection. Doing this minimizes subcutaneous irritation and discoloration.

Attach a needle to the syringe, and draw up the prescribed medication. Then, draw 0.2 to 0.5 cc of air (depending on hospital policy) into the syringe. Remove this needle, and attach a second needle to prevent leakage into subcutaneous tissue as the needle is inserted. Then follow these steps:

• Place the patient in the lateral position, exposing the opposite gluteal muscle to be used as the injection site. Or place him in the prone position.

• Cleanse an area on the upper outer quadrant of the patient's buttock with a sterile alcohol sponge.

• Displace the skin laterally by pulling it about ½″ (1 cm) away from the injection site.

• Insert the needle into the muscle at a 90-degree angle.

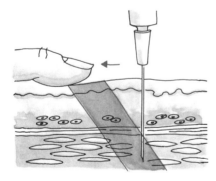

• Aspirate for blood return; if none appears, inject the drug slowly, followed by the air. (Injecting air after the drug helps clear the needle and prevents tracking of the medication through subcutaneous tissues as the needle is withdrawn.)

• Wait 10 seconds before withdrawing the needle to ensure dispersion of the medication.

• Withdraw the needle slowly. Then release the displaced skin and subcutaneous tissue to seal the needle track.

• Encourage the patient to walk or move in bed to facilitate absorption of the drug from the injection site.

Never inject more than 5 ml into a single site, using the Z-track method. Don't massage the injection site, because this might force the drug into subcutaneous tissue. Alternate gluteal sites for repeat injections. If the patient is on bed rest, encourage active range-of-motion exercises or perform passive range-of-motion exercises to facilitate absorption from the injection site.

X
Y
Z

Acknowledgments

The editors gratefully acknowledge the kind cooperation of the following publishers and authors.

"CPR: aftercare" was excerpted from *The Cardiac Patient: A Comprehensive Approach* by Richard Sanderson, MD, FACS, FACC, and Chestine L. Kurth, RN, MSN, CCRN, published by W.B. Saunders Co., © 1983. Reprinted by permission of W.B. Saunders Co.

"Feeding tube: diarrhea" was excerpted from *Nutrition Handbook for Nursing Practice* by Susan G. Dudek, RD, BS, published by J.B. Lippincott Co., © 1987. Reprinted by permission of J.B. Lippincott Co. and Susan G. Dudek, RD, BS.

"Instructions" was excerpted from *Effective Communication in Nursing: Theory and Practice* by Joseph F. Ceccio and Cathy M. Ceccio, published by John Wiley & Sons, copyright © 1982. Reprinted by permission of John Wiley & Sons.

"I.V. therapy: infection control" was excerpted from *Critical Care Procedures and Protocols: A Nursing Process Approach* by Carol B. Persons, RN, MSN, EdD, published by J.B. Lippincott Co., © 1986. Reprinted by permission of J.B. Lippincott Co. and Carol B. Persons, RN, MSN, EdD.

"Leadership strategies" was excerpted from *The Persuasive Manager* by Thomas L. Quick, published by Chilton Book Company, © 1982. Reprinted by permission of Chilton Book Company.

"Medication, topical" was excerpted from *The Nurse's Atlas of Dermatology* by Marilyn B. Lanning, RN, BSN, Theodore Rosen, MD, and Marcia J. Hill, RN, MSN, published by Scott Foresman & Co., © 1983. Reprinted by permission of Little, Brown, & Co.

"Pain detection" was excerpted from *Pain: Nursing Approach to Assessment and Analysis* by Noreen T. Meinhart, RN, MS, and Margo McCaffery, RN, MS, FAAN, published by Appleton & Lange, formerly Appleton-Century-Crofts, © 1983. Reprinted by permission of Appleton & Lange.

"Pain, postoperative" was reproduced by permission from Lewis, Sharon Mantik, and Collier, Idolia Cox: *Medical-Surgical Nursing: Assessment and Management of Clinical Problems*, ed. 2, New York, 1987, McGraw Hill Book Co.; copyrighted by the C.V. Mosby Co., St. Louis, MO.

"Panic attacks" was reprinted from *Emergency Medicine: A Comprehensive Review* by T.C. Kravis and C.G. Warner, pp 538-539, with permission of Aspen Publishers, Inc., © 1983.

"Prostatectomy: complications" was excerpted from *Care of Patients with Urologic Problems* by Edwina A. McConnell, RN, PhD, and Mary F. Zimmerman, RN, BS, published by J.B. Lippincott Co., © 1983 . Reprinted by permission of J.B. Lippincott Co. and Edwina A. McConnell, RN, PhD.

"Radiation reactions" was excerpted from *Care of the Client Receiving External Radiation Therapy* by Joyce Yasko, RN, PhD, published by Appleton & Lange, formerly Appleton-Century-Crofts, © 1982. Reprinted by permission of Appleton & Lange.

"Visually impaired patients" was excerpted from *Guide to Neurological and Neurosurgical Nursing* by Mariah Snyder, RN, PhD, published by John Wiley & Sons, © 1983. Reprinted by permission of John Wiley & Sons.

"Wound cleaning: preparation" was excerpted from *Assessment and Intervention in Emergency Nursing*, 2nd ed., by Nedell E. Lanros, RN, published by Appleton & Lange, formerly Appleton-Century-Crofts, © 1983. Reprinted by permission of Appleton & Lange.

The editors gratefully acknowledge the following sources for portions of this book.

The information in "AIDS: self protection" is derived from guidelines recommended by the American Hospital Association and the Centers for Disease Control.

The information in "Anger" is based on information that appeared in *Executive Fitness Newsletter*.

The information in "Antineoplastic drugs: handling" is adapted from guidelines published by the National Study Commission on Cytotoxic Exposure.

The information in "Appraisals: records" is adapted from *Writing on the Job: A Guide for Nurse Managers* by Kathleen Garver Mastrian, RN, MSN, and Eric Birdsall, PhD.

The information in "Catheterization: patient teaching" is adapted from *SCI Nursing*.

The information in "Conflicts" is derived from *Anger: The Misunderstood Emotion* by Carol Travis.

The information in "Criticizing others" first appeared in *Nursing Business News*.

Portions of "Death: child" were recommendations given by the organization Compassionate Friends.

The information in "Hickman catheter: patient teaching" was originally adapted with permission from *Home Parenteral Nutrition Therapy for the Adult Client*, Geriatric Pharmacy Systems.

The information in "Infection control" originally appeared in guidelines from the American Hospital Association and the Centers for Disease Control.

The information in "Interviewing techniques" first appeared in *Successful Woman* magazine.

The information in "I.V. therapy: blood specimen" first appeared in *The New England Journal of Medicine*.

The information in "Job change: relocation" was adapted from *Strategic Career Planning and Development for Nurses* by Russell and Phillip Swansburg.

The information in "Job change: resignation" first appeared in *Communication Briefings*.

The information in "Osteoporosis" came from the National Institutes of Health.

The information in "Planning, personal" was adapted from *Getting Noticed: A Manager's Success Kit* by Dennis J. Kravetz.

The information in "Public speaking: visual aids" first appeared in *Communication Briefings*.

The information in "Staff management: communication" first appeared in an article by Arlene Yerys in *Management Review*.

The information in "Staff management: hiring" first appeared in *Folio* magazine.

The information in "Staff management: supervision" is adapted from *Supervisory Management*.

The information in "Travel advice" first appeared in *U.S. Pharmacist*.

Index

10 Principles of infection control

Use precautions with all blood and body fluids. To minimize the risk of contracting or spreading an infection, consider all blood and body fluids as potentially infectious. (See *AIDS: self-protection.*) Pregnant nurses should follow these precautions meticulously. Hospital policies vary as to whether pregnant nurses should care for patients with certain infectious diseases or not. (See *Pregnant nurse: infection risks.*) With *all* patients, use the following precautions.

1. Wash your hands.
Wash them before and after contact with patients, even if you wear gloves. Wash your hands *immediately* if you come in contact with blood or body fluids. Review these basic hand-washing techniques:
• Remove all rings, except a plain wedding band, if you're wearing one. Then, wet your hands under warm, running water.
• Apply the proper amount of soap or antiseptic cleaning agent. Work up a lather by vigorously rubbing your hands together, fingers intertwined. Doing so

Lathering

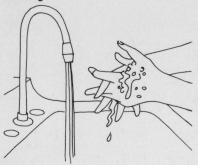

creates friction, which loosens dirt and organisms. If necessary, use a scrub brush. Scrub for at least 15 seconds over every part of your hands, including between your fingers, knuckles, and over your wrists.
• Now, you're ready to rinse your hands. Place them under warm, running water.

Point your fingertips downward to prevent bacteria from running onto your forearms and becoming a possible

Rinsing

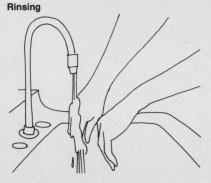

source of infection. Make sure you don't touch the sides of the sink. If you do, wash your hands again.
• Now, dry your hands with a paper towel. Discard the paper towel. If your sink doesn't have foot or knee controls for the water, turn off the faucets with the paper towel before discarding it.

2. Wear gloves.
Wear them when you anticipate contact with blood, body fluids, tissues, or contaminated equipment. Change gloves between patients. Wear gloves when

Putting on gloves

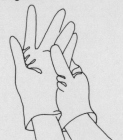

handling blood specimens or emptying fluid-filled containers. (See *Chest drainage bottles.*) Wear gloves on both hands when suctioning a patient. (See *Tracheostomy: suctioning.*) Wear gloves to bathe a patient if you have a cut or dermatitis on your hands. Wear gloves to examine mucous membranes, such as the mouth or rectum, and to examine

any skin area that is not intact. In some hospitals nurses wear gloves to perform venipuncture, arterial puncture, or any

Arterial puncture

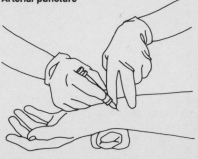

procedure involving I.V. lines. Gloves are also being worn to perform CPR in the hospital. Gloves are meant to be used once and should not be disinfected for reuse, except for rubber gloves.

3. Wear a gown.
Wear one when your clothes are likely to be soiled during patient care and when emptying fluid-filled containers.

Emptying chest tube bottle

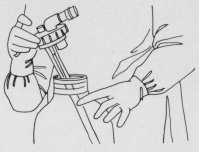

Examples of procedures that would require you to wear a gown include nasopharyngeal suctioning, cleaning a large amount of feces, and assisting with invasive procedures. Gowns are also worn to perform CPR. When laundering your soiled uniforms at home, wash them separately from the rest of the family's clothing, using hot water, detergent, and bleach.
    To put on a gown, follow these steps:
• Unfold the gown with the opening facing you.
• Then, slip your arms through the gown's sleeves. Make sure the gown opening is in the back.